ESSENTIALS OF
MENTAL HEALTH
NURSING

PRAISE FOR THE BOOK

'This is a valuable addition to the literature on mental health nursing which will surely become an essential part of teaching for undergraduate students.'

Laurence Baldwin, Senior Lecturer in Mental Health Nursing, Coventry University

'A contemporary mental health nursing textbook with a range of approaches and underpinning theory and practice guides'

Jude Ibe, Principal Lecturer and Programme Leader Family Care & Mental Health, The University of Greenwich

'*Essentials of Mental Health Nursing* provides a comprehensive commentary on the nature of contemporary mental health nursing. It draws on expertise from a range of contributors, including highly skilled practitioners, researchers and service users. Its focus is on enhancement of knowledge and understanding as well as enabling its readers to deliver reflective and recovery focused, evidence-based care.'

Tracey Cassidy, Senior Lecturer and Programme Lead for Mental Health, University of Plymouth

'An interesting and engaging text that challenges nurses to think critically, creatively, therapeutically and autonomously.'

Vickie Glass, Senior Lecturer in Mental Health Nursing, University of Suffolk

'A contemporary, informative, innovative book (and resources) which provides readers with information, opportunities to critically appraise evidence, and activities from which to develop a range of skills and approaches which should lead to the delivery of compassionate, recovery focussed evidence-based care.'

Amanda McGrandles, Lecturer in Mental Health, University of West of Scotland

ESSENTIALS OF
MENTAL HEALTH
NURSING

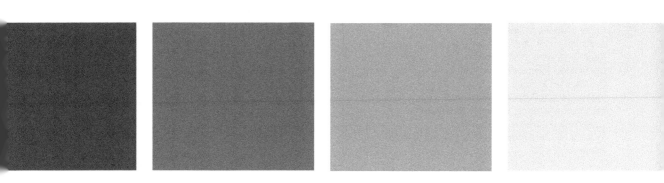

EDITED BY
KAREN M. WRIGHT AND MICK McKEOWN

ADVISORY EDITORS:
IAN HULATT, JONATHAN GADSBY, KEVIN MOORE,
MARIE O'NEILL, STEVEN TRENOWETH AND SUE BARKER

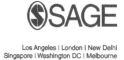

Los Angeles | London | New Delhi
Singapore | Washington DC | Melbourne

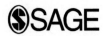

Los Angeles | London | New Delhi
Singapore | Washington DC | Melbourne

SAGE Publications Ltd
1 Oliver's Yard
55 City Road
London EC1Y 1SP

SAGE Publications Inc.
2455 Teller Road
Thousand Oaks, California 91320

SAGE Publications India Pvt Ltd
B 1/I 1 Mohan Cooperative Industrial Area
Mathura Road
New Delhi 110 044

SAGE Publications Asia-Pacific Pte Ltd
3 Church Street
#10-04 Samsung Hub
Singapore 049483

Editor: Becky Taylor
Development editor: Christofere Fila
Editorial assistant: Jade Grogan
Assistant editor, digital: Chloe Statuam
Production editor: Katie Forsythe
Copyeditor: Sharon Cawood
Proofreader: Philippa May
Indexer: Adam Pozner
Marketing manager: Tamara Navaratnam
Cover design: Wendy Scott
Typeset by: C&M Digitals (P) Ltd, Chennai, India
Printed in the UK

Library of Congress Control Number: 2017944170

British Library Cataloguing in Publication data

A catalogue record for this book is available from the British Library

ISBN 978-1-4129-6197-4
ISBN 978-1-4129-6198-1 (pbk)
ISBN 978-1-5264-4716-6 (pbk & Interactive eBook)

At SAGE we take sustainability seriously. Most of our products are printed in the UK using FSC papers and boards. When we print overseas we ensure sustainable papers are used as measured by the PREPS grading system. We undertake an annual audit to monitor our sustainability.

To our partners, Phil and Lynda, whose love and tolerance
have made this endeavour possible, and our wonderful children,
John, Caraline and Rachael for being our inspiration.

CONTENTS

GUIDE TO YOUR BOOK

We are the student panel for this book and we are all currently mental health students. We've road tested the features in this book and the additional exercises online at **https://study.sagepub.com/essentialmentalhealth** to make sure they work for you – wherever you are in your journey to becoming a mental health nurse. We hope you enjoy the book and the online resources, and that it helps you succeed in your degree and your future career. **Good luck!**

AMY, ANITA, EDWARD, AOIBHIN, APRIL, DANIEL AND KASMINDAR

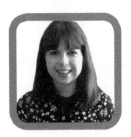

'Throughout the book, the **voices** give direct access and valuable insight into true experiences from mental health service users.They provided me with practical ideas and techniques communicated in a user-friendly way.' **Amy**

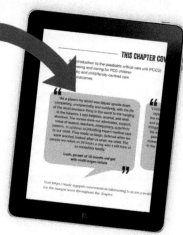

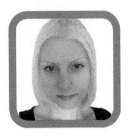

'**Knowledge links** in each chapter show where topics are related in other chapters. This helps to reinforce our knowledge.' **Anita**

SEE ALSO CHAPTER 5

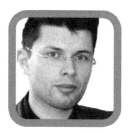

The **critical thinking stop points** in the book helped me to assess my own knowledge and expand on it, before I needed to implement it in practice. For additional exercises check out the multiple-choice questions for each chapter at **https://study.sagepub.com/essentialmentalhealth** to help you further test your knowledge.' **Edward**

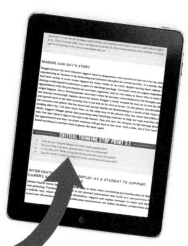

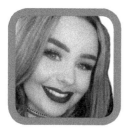

'The **critical debates** are an excellent feature of the book which introduce various view points on a particular issue and help stretch and challenge the reader. It makes you think and question what would be the best solution for a situation and it prepares you for going into the ward and possible debates among staff for a patient's care.'
Aoibhin

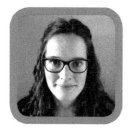

'The **case studies** show real world examples of how the content of the chapter applies to practice. I really enjoyed those, they are a chance to see what is being taught in relation to your future role and presented in a very accessible way.' **April**

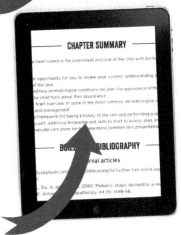

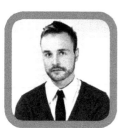

'The **chapter summary** at the end allows you to reflect back on the chapter and tests whether you have learned what you should have given the information presented.'
Daniel

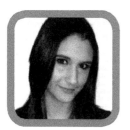

'I personally found the inclusion of **websites, video links, books and journal articles** at the end of chapters particularly useful. It provides a starting point to where to research and revise further.' **Kasmindar**

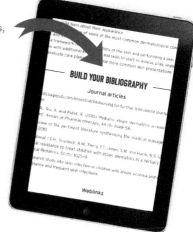

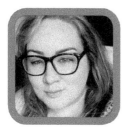

'The **What's the Evidence** feature gives a good starting point for essays – it highlights the many contentious areas in mental health nursing and it's also helpful for references.' **Bethany**

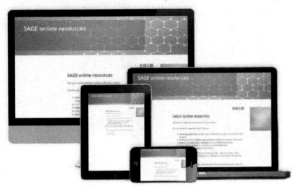

Don't forget – you can find great online resources at **https://study.sagepub.com/essentialmentalhealth** for more help with your learning, whether you are revising, doing assignments or preparing for placement. We've found these really helpful when you want a break from reading and to reinforce your learning in a different way – from reading a case study to taking a quiz. The icons throughout the book will remind you where there is a resource available on the website.

Answer available: When you see this icon, you'll be able to find an answer or guidance to an activity online so you can be sure you are on the right track.

Further reading and useful websites, including selected free journal articles, can be found online whenever you see this icon. These will help you when writing assignments or if you are interested in exploring a topic further.

Preparing for placement can be nerve racking. The extra case studies online will help you to think through real-life scenarios and be prepared.

Revise - Multiple choice questions and extra exercises: each chapter has a set of MCQs and exercises online to help you test and reinforce your knowledge online.

NOTES ON THE EDITORS AND CONTRIBUTORS

EDITORS

Karen M. Wright is Professor of Nursing and the Head of School of Nursing at the University of Central Lancashire. Previously, Karen was Nurse Consultant for Personality Disorder within a high secure hospital. She has subsequently developed acclaimed curriculum, research and practice initiatives in this field and also in the care and support of individuals with eating disorder. Her research into how the police assess mentally distressed people in public places and custody areas established the Public Psychiatric Emergency Assessment Tool, adopted by the College of Policing and cited in Department of Health policies including Closing the Gap and the Crisis Concordat.

Mick McKeown is Professor of Democratic Mental Health, School of Nursing at the University of Central Lancashire and trade union activist with Unison. He supports service user and carer involvement at the university and union strategising on nursing. He has taken a lead in making the case for union organising to extend to alliance formation with service users/survivors.

The editors have donated fees and royalties to the Abaseen Foundation UK which supports sustainable health and education initiatives in north western Pakistan.

ADVISORY EDITORS

The following advisory editors helped work to ensure this book contained accurate and equal coverage of all fields of nursing in a variety of settings:

Jonathan Gadsby, Steven Trenoweth, Sue Barker, Kevin Moore, Marie O'Neill and Ian Hulatt.

CONTRIBUTORS

Anthony Ackroyd is a mental health nurse, non-medical prescriber and Specialist Clinical Lead for the Wellbeing Health Improvement Service (WHISe), part of Navigo CiC.

Kevin Acott was Senior Lecturer at Middlesex University, London at the time of writing.

Alan Armstrong is Senior Lecturer in Adult Nursing at Teesside University.

Laura Baker is a writer who specialises in mental health care and a visiting lecturer at University of Worcester, where she is a member of the service user group Impact.

Sue Barker is a Lecturer in Mental Health, Learning Disabilities and Psychosocial Care at the University of Cardiff. She is a registered mental health nurse and chartered psychologist.

Megan Beadle At the time of writing the chapter, Megan was a final year mental health nursing student and is now a community mental health nurse working with older people with complex functional mental health needs.

Richard Bentall is Professor of Clinical Psychology at the University of Sheffield.

Nick Bohannon is Senior Lecturer in Mental Health at the University of Central Lancashire.

Jess Bradley is Trans Officer, National Union of Students.

Jayne Breeze is Senior Lecturer in Mental Health at Sheffield Hallam University.

Mick Burns is Head of Mental Health (Interim)/Co-Commissioner PD Offender Pathway (North), NHS England North of England Specialised Commissioning Team.

Maddie Burton is Senior Lecturer in Child and Adolescent Mental Health at the University of Worcester.

Don Bryant is a service user representative at Mersey Care NHS Foundation Trust.

John Butler was Senior Lecturer (retired) in Mental Health at the University of Central Lancashire. He led the MSc in pre-registration Mental Health Nursing.

Jane Cahill is a Senior Research Fellow at the School of Healthcare, University of Leeds.

Ian Callaghan is the Recovery and Secure Care Manager at the national mental health charity Rethink Mental Illness.

Lynda Carey is Associate Head of Nurse Education, Faculty of Health and Social Care, Edge Hill University.

Jenelle Clarke is a Research Fellow at the University of Nottingham's Business School.

Simon Clarke is a clinical psychologist and works as a Senior Lecturer in the Department of Psychology at Nottingham Trent University.

Michael Coffey is Associate Professor of Public Health, Policy and Social Sciences at Swansea University.

Rachel Cohen is Senior Research Associate, Centre for Academic Mental Health, University of Bristol & project manager on the National Evaluation study of the Offender Personality Disorder Pathway for women Offenders (W-NEON).

Alison Commissiong is a nurse consultant with Lancashire Care NHS Foundation Trust.

Carol Cooper is Senior Lecturer in mental health at Sheffield Hallam University.

Rhiannon Corcoran is Professor of Psychology and Public Mental Health at the University of Liverpool.

Christine Crossman is a registered mental health nurse working in Lancashire Care NHS Foundation Trust.

Jennie Day is Director of Studies of the Master of Public Health programme at the University of Liverpool, a researcher and a pharmacist.

Stephanie de la Haye is an independent user consultant, educator and researcher in mental health.

Tommy Dickinson is Senior Lecturer in Mental Health at King's College London and Talbott Visiting Professor of Nursing, School of Nursing, the University of Virginia, USA.

Duncan Double is a consultant psychiatrist, Norfolk and Suffolk NHS Foundation Trust and honorary Senior Lecturer, Norwich Medical School at the University of East Anglia.

Joy Duxbury is Professor of Mental Health Nursing at the University of Central Lancashire.

Bethan Edwards is a research occupational therapist at Cwm Taf University Health Board and a PhD student at Cardiff University.

Chris Essen is an involvement facilitator for Comensus at the University of Central Lancashire.

Simon Fletcher is a research associate in interprofessional education at the Centre for Health and Social Care Research, Kingston and St George's University.

Joe Forster previously worked in NHS secure mental health care and is now self-employed in the participatory design field.

Amanda Francis is a carer.

Jonathan Gadsby is a mental health nurse and a founder member of the Critical Mental Health Nurses' Network. His research interests are voice-hearing and the politics of health. He is a Research Fellow for Learning Disability and Mental Health Nursing at Birmingham City University.

Emily Griffin was a student nurse at the time of writing.

Simon Hall is a Senior Lecturer at the University of West of England.

Ben Hannigan is Professor of Mental Health Nursing, School of Healthcare Sciences at Cardiff University.

Susan Henry is a Peer Support coordinator at the Hackney Centre for Mental Health, East London NHS Foundation Trust.

Ian Hulatt is a consultant Editor of *Mental Health Practice*.

Karen James is a researcher at the Centre for Health and Social Care Research, Kingston and St George's University.

Annie Jeffrey is a mother and Open Dialogue advocate.

Claudette Kaviya was a third-year mental health nursing student at the time of writing.

Michael Kelly is Director of Programmes for Mental Health at Middlesex University.

Sumaiyaa Khoda is Mental Health Clinical Lead, Student Wellbeing Services, at the University of Central Lancashire.

Angela Kydd is Associate Professor, Edinburgh Napier University.

Sarah Loughran (a student at the time of contributing to this book) is a Registered Mental Health Nurse working as a staff nurse in the NHS.

Rachel Lyon is a registered nurse (mental health), Greater Manchester Mental Health NHS Foundation Trust.

Ged McCann works for NHS England commissioning specialist secure mental health services.

Robert G. MacDonald RIBA is an architect and Mersey Care NHS Foundation Trust Design Champion expert by experience.

Karen Machin works freelance in mental health and writes from the perspective of lived experience.

Doug MacInnes is Professor of Mental Health, Faculty of Health and Wellbeing, Canterbury Christ Church University.

Nick Manning is Professor of Sociology at King's College London.

Rosie Mansfield is a researcher at the University of Manchester, exploring mental health and well-being in schools.

Alan Meudell is Chair of Trustees at Caerphilly Borough Mind, and is a service user researcher and activist.

Natalie Miles is a CBT therapist and counsellor, accredited with BABCP and BACP.

Suzanne Monks is a Lecturer in Adult Nursing, specialising in end-of-life care, at Sheffield Hallam University.

Nicki Moone is a Senior Lecturer practitioner in Berkshire Healthcare NHS Foundation Trust and the University of West London.

Kevin Moore is Lecturer in Nursing, Academic Lead, Continuing Professional Development Provision, and an associate member of the Institute of Nursing Research in the School of Nursing at Ulster University.

Amrita Mullan is a community mental health nurse, Sheffield Health & Social Care NHS Foundation Trust.

Karen Newbigging is Senior Lecturer in Health Policy and Management, Health Services Management Centre, at the University of Birmingham.

Samantha O' Brien is a qualified teacher and also works with a number of organisations and universities.

Marie O'Neill is Lecturer in Nursing, School of Nursing at the Ulster University.

David Pilgrim is Professor of Health and Social Policy at the University of Liverpool and co-author of the award-winning book: *A Sociology of Mental Health and Illness.*

Steven Pryjmachuk is Professor of Mental Health Nursing Education at the University of Manchester.

David Pulsford is a retired Senior Lecturer in Mental Health Nursing previously at the University of Central Lancashire.

Julian Raffay is Specialist Chaplain (Research, Education and Development) at Mersey Care NHS Foundation Trust.

Mandy Reed is Senior Lecturer in Mental Health Nursing at the University of the West of England

Scott Reeves is Professor in Interprofessional Research at the Centre for Health and Social Care Research, Kingston University and St George's University of London. He is also Editor-in-Chief, *Journal of Interprofessional Care.*

Julie Ridley is Reader in Applied Social Sciences, School of Social Work, Care and Community at the University of Central Lancashire and an experienced social researcher.

June Sadd is an independent survivor consultant, educator and researcher.

Isaac Samuels is a trustee for a national HIV/Aids charity and advises different organisations on how to engage people from LGBT and other seldom-heard communities.

Bob Sapey is retired social worker academic and co-editor of the recent book: *Madness, Distress and the Politics of Disablement.*

Amy Scholes is a clinical psychology student at the University of Manchester.

Alan Simpson is Professor of Collaborative Mental Health Nursing at the Centre for Mental Health Research, School of Health Sciences, City University London.

Julie Skilbeck is Senior Lecturer in adult nursing and research theme lead for cancer and life-limiting illness at Sheffield Hallam University.

Helen Spandler is Reader in Mental Health in the School of Social Work, Care and Community at the University of Central Lancashire.

Donna Taylor Learning Disability Commissioning Case Manager at Heywood, Middleton and Rochdale Clinical Commissioning Group.

Julia Terry is Associate Professor in Nursing at the College of Human and Health Sciences, Swansea University.

Mike Thomas is Vice-Chancellor and Professor of Organizational Leadership at the University of Central Lancashire.

Tim Thornton is Professor of Philosophy and Mental Health, Faculty of Health and Wellbeing at the University of Central Lancashire and senior editor of *Philosophy, Psychiatry & Psychology*.

Adam Traill is a mental health nurse and therapist who works with children and young people (CAMHS services).

Sarah Traill is the Academic Team Leader for Mental Health at the University of Central Lancashire. She is a mental health nurse and cognitive behavioural therapist.

Steve Trenoweth is a Senior Lecturer in Mental Health Nursing at Bournemouth University.

James Turner is Principal Lecturer Mental Health Nursing and Professional Lead End of Life and Supportive care at Sheffield Hallam University Centre for Health & Social Care Research.

Lauren Walker is a Mental Health Research Assistant, University of Manchester.

Emma Watson is a peer researcher and peer support development lead in Nottinghamshire Healthcare NHS Foundation Trust.

Harvey Wells is Senior Lecturer in Medical Education, Barts and The London School of Medicine and Dentistry, Queen Mary, University of London.

Jacquie White is Associate Dean Education, Faculty of Health Sciences, at the University of Hull.

Sophie Williams is a staff nurse working within mental health services for older people in Cardiff and Vale UHB. At the time of writing she was a student nurse at Cardiff University.

Eleanor Wilson is Senior Research Fellow in the Nottingham Centre for the Advancement of Research in supportive, palliative and end of life care.

Gary Winship is Associate Professor at the School of Education, and Senior Fellow at the Institute of Mental Health at the University of Nottingham.

ACKNOWLEDGEMENTS

VOICES

The editors and SAGE would like to thank all the students, service users, families, carers and practitioners who contributed their stories to the book. The book is much richer for your contribution.

REVIEWERS

We would also like to thank all the students, lecturers and practitioners and service users who helped review this book's content, design, and online resources to ensure it is as useful as possible. These include the following:

Student Reviewers

Special thanks to our student review panel: Amy Penny, Anita Juzevski, April Langton, Edward Charles Parker, Daniel Peay and Bethany Slater at Bournemouth University; Kashmindar Badsha at UCLAN and Aoibhin Lennon at Ulster University.

Thanks also to the students from the University of Dundee, Abertay, and Birmingham City University who took part in focus groups on the book's content and suitability for study, making sure the book meets students' needs.

Academic Reviewers

Shelley Allen, University of Salford

Susan Barker, Cardiff University

Diane Carpenter, University of Southampton

Fiona Carver, Edinburgh Napier University

Tracey Cassidy, University of Plymouth

Angelina Chadwick, University of Salford

David Coyle, Bangor University

Audrey Cund, University of the West of Scotland

Tommy Dickinson, King's College London

Keith Ford, Fatima College of Health Sciences

Iris Gault, Kingston University

Linda Goddard, London Southbank University

Scott Henderson, University of Abertay

Val Howatson, Glasgow Caledonian University

Ada Hui, University of Nottingham

Yvonne Middlewick, University of Southampton

David Price, Middlesex University

Marc Roberts, independent researcher and lecturer

Rebecca Rylance, University of Salford

Gary Souter, Sheffield Hallam University

Julie Teatheredge, Anglia Ruskin University

Steve Trenoweth, Bournemouth University

Andrew Walsh, Birmingham City University

Karen M. Wright, University of Central Lancashire

Service Users and Practitioners

Special thanks to all the service users and practitioners who reviewed the content of this book throughout its writing, many of whom contributed their voices to the chapters.

PUBLISHER'S ACKNOWLEDGEMENTS

The authors and publisher are grateful to the following parties for permission to reproduce their material:

Table 2.4 Instructional architectures in higher education, Clark, R.C. (2008) Building expertise: Cognitive methods for training and performance improvement, 3rd edition. San Francisco, CA: Pfeiffer. Reproduced with permission.

Figure 4.1 Arnstein's ladder of citizen participation, Arnstein, S.R. (1969) A ladder of citizen participation. Journal of the American Planning Association, 35(4), 216–224. Adapted with permission.

Excerpt from the NHS constitution for England 2013, Department of Health (DH) (2013a) The NHS Constitution: the NHS belongs to us all. London: DH © Crown copyright.

Figure 4.2 Whole-person approach, Hafal (2012) A recovery approach to mental illness: A guide for students developed by people with a serious mental illness and their carers. Neath: Hafal. Reproduced with kind permission.

Page 69, Hearing Voices Network, (2016) Sheffield Hearing Voices Group. Available at: www.hearing-voices.org/groups/sheffield/ (accessed 20.9.17). Reproduced with kind permission.

Excerpt from Brown, M. (2015) The best effing lonely: social media and #mentalhealth. The New Mental Health. Available at: http://thenewmentalhealth.org/?p=136 (accessed 03.08.17). Reproduced with kind permission.

Table 6.1 Culture, race and ethnicity, Fernando, S.J.M. (2010) Mental Health, Race and Culture, 3rd edition. Basingstoke: Palgrave. Reproduced with permission.

Figure 6.2 Spiral of oppression, Trivedi, P. (2002) Racism, social exclusion and mental health: a black service user's perspective.' In K. Bhui (ed). Racism and Mental Health: Prejudice and Suffering. London: Jessica Kingsley. Reproduced with permission.

Excerpt from Fulford, K.W.M. (1999) Analytic philosophy, brain science and the concept of disorder. In S. Bloch, P. Chodoff & S.A. Green (eds) Psychiatric ethics, 3rd edition. Oxford: Oxford University Press. pp. 161–192. Reproduced with permission.

Excerpt from Jay, C. (2013) What is spiritual care? In C. Cook (ed.) Spirituality, theology and mental health: Multidisciplinary perspectives. Norwich: SCM Press. © Christopher C. H. Cook, SCM Press 2013. Reproduced with permission of Hymns Ancient & Modern Ltd.

Figure 17.2 Duai Axis Model of Mental Health, Keyes, C.L. (2007) Promoting and protecting mental health as flourishing: a complementary strategy for improving national mental health. American Psychologist, 62(2), 95. American Psychological Association, adapted with permission.

Table 30.1 Core standards of Enabling Environments, Royal College of Psychiatrists (2016b). Reproduced with kind permission.

Table 30.2 A meta-recovery framework, Winship, G. (2016) A meta-recovery framework: positioning the 'New Recovery' movement and other recovery approaches. Journal of Psychiatric and Mental Health Nursing, 23, 66–73. Reproduced with permission under the terms of the Creative Commons Attribution License.

Page 482, Joint Commissioning Panel for Mental Health (JCPMH), 2013, Royal College of Psychiatrists. Reproduced with kind permission.

Page 510, UK National Statistics – Total SSRI, SNRI Annual Prescription & Increase Data England 1998–2011. Copyright © 2016, Re-used with the permission of NHS Digital. All rights reserved.

Figure 36.1 relationship-centered care, Nolan, M., Davies, S., Brown, J., et al. (2004) Beyond person-centred care: a new vision for gerontological nursing. *Journal of Clinical Nursing*, 13, 45–53. Reproduced with permission.

INTRODUCTION

MICK McKEOWN, KAREN WRIGHT AND JONATHAN GADSBY

Nurses make up the majority of the workforce in mental health services and are usually associated with the organisation and delivery of that relatively indeterminable endeavour, *mental health care*: a therapeutic use of self, at once elusive of definitive description yet essential for positive outcomes (Altschul, 1971; Barker, 1989; Freshwater, 2002; Hewitt & Coffey, 2005; Morse et al., 1990; O'Brien, 2001; Paley, 2001; Peplau, 1952). Any attempt to account for different forms of mental health care, let alone advocate for the value of one approach over another, must first address critical questions regarding what mental health care is, or is not, and, specifically, concentrate on nursing practice. Hence, we question in what ways it might imaginatively or potentially be given license for development and refinement, or even whether proposed interventions are required or requested on the part of recipients of care or their families.

In many respects, these are as much political and societal questions as matters of practice alone. Hence, we wish this book to assist mental health nurses to possess the necessary critical and political acumen to be able to reflect and deliberate on the complexities of both the nursing role and the societal context within which it is practised. It has never been more essential for nurses and other disciplines to understand the range of critical ideas brought to bear on their practice, and to have some sense of where these ideas come from (Reynolds et al., 2009).

Mental health nursing has much to be proud of with respect to providing timely, consensual, cooperative and compassionate care that is very much appreciated by service users, and delivered despite the challenges of the operating environment. Caring mental health nurses have also faced up to the challenges of forging supportive and therapeutic alliances within the constraints of compelled and coercive services. Conversely, mental health nursing and other psy-disciplines stand accused of presiding over systems of abuse, neglect and injustice, too readily accommodating themselves to an oppressively dominant bio-psychiatry. Historical approaches to care and treatment now viewed as oppressive were previously considered from within a '*cruel to be kind*' frame, and certain contemporary practices appear to remain in this category, calling attention to issues of power and conflict in relationships between service users and nurses (Jacob et al., 2016; Melia, 1987).

Such concerns have arguably been complicated by nursing's historical professionalisation journey. This mission to garner esteem, respect and higher wages, and to escape the identity of the asylum attendant has, to some extent, denied nurses opportunities for occupational self-determination beyond the limiting confines of a psychiatric orbit. Furthermore, this leads us to neglect some of the experience-focused aspects of our work in favour of questionable forms of objectivity. Thus, we have conceptual confusions of nomenclature, with many professional trailblazers, even in the humanist tradition, preferring the somewhat ugly and oxymoronic title: *psychiatric and mental health nursing*.

The standpoint we adopt in framing this text, and in the selection of a plurality of contributing authors, reflects our openness to criticism of nursing and mental health care. Alongside this, however, we maintain passionate enthusiasm for work that can transcend this critique and make a genuinely positive difference to the lives of distressed individuals, their families and the communities in which they live.

COMPLIMENTS, CONTROVERSIES AND CRITIQUE

Arguably, through their history, mental health services have been consistent in few respects other than being controversial and provoking criticism. Answers to relevant critical questions usher in considerations of the role of the state and institutions of welfare amidst a prevailing neo-liberal polity and matters of freedom, compulsion and coercion in the organisation of mental health care services and associated legislation.[1] In the extreme, certain critics would urge us to dismantle or radically redesign mental health services and professional roles as we know them (Burstow, 2014). Others align us to psychotherapeutic and counselling models where we focus in on the finer details of the one-to-one relationship, and thus direct us away from the context in which we operate. Despite this, and alternately, mental health nursing can legitimately lay claim to a set of values, virtues and characteristics that speak of the powerful role that healing, supportive, salutogenic and loving human relationships must play in the care of people in profound mental distress and the minimisation or prevention of such distress in the first place.

Nurses are often singled out for praise and appreciation when individuals speak of positive experiences of services, and a lack of time with nurses and other practitioners is often cited as a reason for dissatisfaction (Mind, 2011). There is almost a dichotomy between the 'angel' on the one hand, where the nurse is held in high moral esteem and, on the other hand, 'nurse Ratched', identified with uncritically dolling out medication and restrictive practices. Pivotal to the administration of health care systems, nurses operate on the frontline of eking out limited and stretched resources. So much so, that, to borrow from Tolkien (1954, p.32), nurses' own sense of value can mirror the degradation of care, becoming attenuated 'like butter scraped over too much bread'.

The fact that the very idea of mental health nursing can be a slippery concept, difficult to define (Barker & Buchanan-Barker, 2011; Chambers, 2006), is, for some, its main weakness but for others it is a strength. Such matters of definition can play into questioning the very legitimacy of the mental health nursing role and whether it is distinct enough from other, perhaps more focused, disciplines or, indeed, whether nursing is necessary in any mental health professional taxonomy. Compatibilities have been highlighted between conceptualisations of mental health nursing favouring 'art or science' (Norman & Ryrie, 2013; Peplau, 1988); though, arguably, tensions have not been satisfactorily resolved (see Repper, 2000). We might even contend that our collective professional fumbling around such terms is indicative of much deeper problems, which the conceptually elusive notion of 'mental health' fudges (Pilgrim, 2005).

We agree with Phil Barker's (2008) emphasis on *caring* as the central feature of nursing's role in responding to mental distress and the conception of nursing work as *craft*. That said, it is also palpably the case that we can't assume that being 'caring' is unproblematic and, indeed, it may not be enough just to be caring. Within such a frame, mental health nursing involves a diverse set of human responses, acting to:

---

[1] It is worth noting that different international jurisdictions have their own mental health law. Indeed, the UK has different mental health law for: England and Wales (Mental Health Act 1983, revised 2007); Scotland (Mental Health Care & Treatment Act 2003); and Northern Ireland (Mental Health Order 1986). See the Appendix for further information.

- be supportively present with people at times of crisis and distress
- aid such individuals and their social networks to cope with problems of living
- properly listen to narratives of distress and coping in ways that assist people to find meaning in their experiences
- ultimately, reclaim a valued sense of self and social role that, for some, is referred to as recovery.

This notion of mental health nursing is essentially communicative, democratic and relational, chiming in with appreciation for the ideals of therapeutic alliance (McAndrew et al., 2014). Ideally, these caring, supportive and therapeutic relations are transacted consensually and cooperatively with willing service users. Similarly, we favour a framing of such relations and the need for them in primarily social, rather than primarily biological, terms (Beresford et al., 2010; Wallcraft & Hopper, 2015).

Notwithstanding the opportunity to define mental health nursing in such wholesome terms, the reality for many people who find themselves in mental health crisis is to face a service response that is legally compelled, coercive, quite often violent, and hugely dominated by biological understandings and physical or pharmacological interventions (Read, 2005). These services exist primarily to contain people designated as mentally ill, and the nursing role within them has become increasingly subordinate to psychiatric knowledge and power and commensurate with social control (Bracken & Thomas, 2001; Gastaldo & Holmes, 1999; Pilgrim, 2016; Thomas, 2016). Relations with service users are increasingly fraught with conflict, proximally and emotionally distant, and authoritarian rather than democratic (Csipke et al., 2016; Rose et al., 2015). In the extreme, practices within such services are traumatic or reinvent the trauma that often lies behind people's mental distress or crisis, such that they may be better referred to as 'trauma-organised systems' (Bloom & Farragher, 2010; Sweeney et al., 2016). Even within apparently 'softer' recovery-orientated circumstances, where service user autonomy and involvement are fostered and supported by nurses, the controlling nature of the psychiatric gaze, whereby services exert a social control function, may never be far away (Cooke & Kothari, 2002; Harper & Speed, 2012; O'Donnell, & Shaw, 2016). This is apparent where services have become a conduit for the scrutiny of the Department of Work and Pensions (Friedli & Stearn, 2015). For these and other reasons, many individuals have quite negative experiences of nursing care and might prefer to avoid the reach of services altogether (Mental Health Recovery Study Working Group, 2009).

CRITICALLY INFORMED CARE

To meet the challenges posed by the various criticisms of mental health care, it is essential that mental health nurses have the capacity and resources to constructively engage with this critique. Marc Roberts (2016) makes a persuasive case for nurse education to prioritise critical thinking and reflection skills, especially challenging tendencies to assume that aspects of knowledge or practice are settled or 'self-evident'. We concur, and also maintain that such learning is best achieved via democratic pedagogies that promote critical self-awareness and an equally critical disposition to the context of practice (Freire, 1971; McKeown et al., 2015). Paulo Freire's critical pedagogy relies on dialogue and cooperative and supportive relationships that are at one and the same time democratic and radical. Mutual learning pivots on a process of *conscientisation*, a political awakening amongst participants underpinned by understanding, hope and love (Apple, 2014; Giroux, 2007; Glass, 2001; Roberts, 2000). According to Freire (1998: 59), such approaches to learning are implicitly concerned with criticality and, ultimately, empowerment: 'respect for the autonomy and dignity of every person is an ethical imperative and not a favour that we may or may not concede to each other'. For learning to actually be emancipatory, it must raise the consciousness of and promote resistance to forms of oppression: 'Learners together, in the act of analysing a dehumanising reality, denounce it while announcing its transformation in the name of ... liberation' (Freire, 1971: 4).

Both Freire and Campbell (1984) refer to love as a central theme, an emotion which can often be shied away from under the guise of professionalism. For Freire (1971), education and, for that matter, political organising are acts of love. Beyond this, educators have a responsibility to create an environment where loving others is easier. Indeed, a space where a person feels loved, nurtured and cared for is what Gesler (1996: 96) refers to as a place of healing or a therapeutic landscape: 'physical and built environments, social conditions and human perceptions combine to produce an atmosphere which is conducive to healing'.

Further, Stickley and Freshwater (2002: 253) propose that we 'foster a therapeutic alliance that is founded within love' in order to realise its healing potential. Campbell, in his 1984 text, *Moderated love: A theology of professional care*, suggests that nurses should indeed love people under their care within the concept of companionship, personal involvement and giving. This transcends skill or technique to create authentic and restorative interpersonal connections resonating with Yalom's (1980: 5) premise that 'it is the relationship that heals'. We suggest that the virtues that enable such care include humility, humanity and honesty. In the current health care context, where building self-defined resilience and recovery is high on the agenda, we argue that these 'softer' qualities which enable a person to 'be themselves' are fundamental to both the nurse's personal strength and the service user's sense of being 'cared for'.

The value of socially and politically aware learning is not confined to early career nurses and students, but must involve all of the nursing workforce, ideally in conjunction with other critically minded interdisciplinary colleagues and service user groupings (McKeown et al., 2017). Various strands of critical thinking exist to support such endeavours and these can be associated with collegiate and activist networks. Such networks formed by professional groupings have included: the *Critical Psychiatry Network; Politics, Psychology, Resistance; Psychologists against Austerity*; and, importantly, the relatively new *Critical Mental Health Nurses Network*. To some extent, complementing these groups or offering interesting openings for forging alliances, but necessarily also presenting a more radical or even oppositional perspective, are service user/survivor-led sites of activism such as *Recovery in the Bin* (see Thomas, 2016), *Mad Studies* (LeFrançois et al., 2013) and new variations on *anti-psychiatry* (see Burstow, 2016; Virden, 2016).

CRITICALITY FOR CHANGE

Organised service users, refusers and survivors of mental health care have variously aligned with critical perspectives on psychiatry, and nurses do not escape this critique (Crossley, 2006; LeFrançois et al., 2016). That said, many nurses have contributed to critical analyses of mental health care and forged practical and political alliances with service users and survivors, with a view to either making care the best it can possibly be under constrained circumstances or working towards transforming those circumstances (McKeown et al., 2014). It is our contention that continuous nurse education, pre- and post-qualifying, ought to be reflexively engaged with such critical ideas so that mental health nurses are always able to exhibit informed critical thinking when faced with the complexities of contemporary services and the society within which these are situated. To these ends, we intend that this text offers readers an opportunity to access a range of critical perspectives and bring their own critical faculties to bear on identified key issues for mental health care and the content of the various chapters. In doing so, we hope that this will involve challenging taken-for-granted assumptions or professional positions taken up with regard to contemporary practices and orthodoxies.

It is not our intention to necessarily promote particular policy priorities, however progressive they may appear on the surface, as these often date quite quickly. Nor do we intend to single out specific conceptual frameworks or critical accounts as ideal. Rather, the goal is to support reflexively critical nurses, who are able to function humanely, with kindness, compassion and respect within currently constituted psychiatric services at the same time as being able to imagine, and work for, *alternative* visions for more humane, democratic, less coercive approaches to care. At the very least, the desired critical disposition might extend to consideration of the appropriate *limits* of biological psychiatry and the *legitimacy* of compulsion and coercion. Equally, we need to bring our criticality to the critical perspectives on offer. In this way, critical accounts may become progressively more mature, nuanced and sophisticated and furnish greater insights into the nature of mental distress and relevant services, so that the latter can be incrementally improved or, indeed, transformed. In this sense, it is our belief that mental health nurses need to understand the political and economic landscape we are working in and how to effect change.

A critical standpoint does not mean we desire to do away with mental health care – in these neo-liberal times, we actually need *more* services rather than *fewer*, and much better funding of them. We do, however, need to organise mental health care services and the work of mental health nurses in much better ways than those which attract the legitimate criticism of service users and other commentators. The *psychopolitics* of Peter Sedgwick (1982, 2015) and the recently emergent *Mad Studies* (LeFrançois et al., 2013) are promising sources to nourish the sorts of alliances required to plausibly critique contemporary services, contemplate alternatives and prefiguratively work together to bring them into being. *Mad Studies*, in particular, is notable for privileging survivor knowledge at the core of its critique (Russo & Beresford, 2015), whilst this and Sedgwickian psychopolitics (Spandler et al., 2016) move beyond simple *anti-psychiatry* to further the case for the movement alliances necessary for envisaged changes to both services and society (McKeown et al., 2014).

We have structured the book into sections dealing with:

1. Contextual matters – the backdrop against which mental health nurses must practise.
2. Key concepts and debates surrounding mental health, care and treatment – competing ideas and contextualising theory.
3. Skills necessary for mental health care and therapeutic approaches.
4. Transition to practice – the knowledge required to support the change of role from learner to registrant.

The authors of each chapter have been encouraged to apply critical and up-to-date ideas and research to their subject matter. The included chapters reflect some of the diversity of mental health nursing practice and theory. As such, there is not necessarily consistent agreement across critical points, and nor, in our view, should there be – these are quite rightly debated and contested, and we encourage you, the reader, to engage in the debate. Similarly, authors have been free to use their favoured language and terminology. As such, this represents the diversity of language and terms that people are likely to come across within the real-world policy and practice context, rather than suggesting an editorial endorsement of all terms or limiting expression. Where appropriate throughout the text, language is contested from the aforementioned critical standpoints. On these points and others, readers are encouraged to consider and develop their own views and affinities, and every chapter includes points of critical reflection relating to key debates in the field that are designed to support such contemplation.

It is worth distinguishing between a critical standpoint and mere criticism, favouring the former over the latter. It is easy to criticise, and, to some extent, psychiatry and mental health services can be a straw man to be readily knocked down by easy criticism. Equally, it can be just as easy to offend or upset people, including colleagues and service users, who do not agree with or recognise themselves in the critique. This is not our goal. Rather, we hope to encourage a critical disposition that is reasoned, respectful, well informed, enlightening and *always* concerned with forging solutions for change rather than stopping at criticism alone.

We are also conscious that a critical disposition can potentially render individuals vulnerable to isolation or vexation amongst colleagues. Again, this is not our intention, though we do accept that critical ideas can be provocative and energising. Perhaps of more concern is the dissonance that is likely for critically minded practitioners who work within services that are not always in tune with a more progressive world view. We do not have any easy answers for this, other than to note it may be such discomfort that niggles all of us to strive for better forms of care and outcomes. Moreover, the relational approaches to care and political solidarity that we advocate ought to afford some protection against alienation and upset in one's job role.

CONCLUSION

These are interesting and challenging times for mental health nurses and service users. The future of mental health care services, as we know them, is uncertain, as is the future of mental health nursing and associated education. We may be living through a period of consolidation of the power of bio-psychiatry to subjugate service users and subordinate disciplines alike, or we are on the threshold of significant transformation towards progressive alternatives within a plurality of provision. We hope that this book furnishes mental health nurses, particularly students embarking on their career, with useful information and critical tools for making sense of their work and how to make the most of it, creating benefit for service users and rewarding and fulfilling experiences for themselves.

REFERENCES

Altschul, A.T. (1971) Relationships between patients and nurses in psychiatric wards. *International Journal of Nursing Studies, 8*(3), 179–187.

Apple, M. (2014) *Official knowledge: Democratic education in a conservative age*. Abingdon: Routledge.

Barker, P. (1989) Reflections on the philosophy of caring in mental health. *International Journal of Nursing Studies, 26*(2), 131–141.

Barker, P. (ed.) (2008) *Psychiatric and mental health nursing: The craft of caring*, 2nd edition. Boca Raton, FL: CRC Press.

Barker, P. & Buchanan-Barker, P. (2011) Myth of mental health nursing and the challenge of recovery. *International Journal of Mental Health Nursing, 20*, 337–344.

Beresford, P., Nettle, M. & Perring, R. (2010) *Towards a social model of madness and distress: Exploring what service users say*. York: Joseph Rowntree Foundation.

Bloom, S. & Farragher, B. (2010) *Destroying sanctuary: The crisis in human service delivery systems*. New York: Oxford University Press.

Bracken, P. & Thomas, P. (2001) Postpsychiatry: a new direction for mental health. *British Medical Journal, 322*(7288), 724.

Burstow, B. (2014) The withering away of psychiatry: an attrition model for antipsychiatry. In B. Burstow, B.A. LeFrançois & S.L. Diamond (eds) *Psychiatry disrupted: theorizing resistance and crafting the revolution*. Montreal, QC: McGill/Queen's University Press. pp. 34–51.

Burstow, B. (ed.) (2016) *Psychiatry interrogated: An institutional ethnography anthology*. New York: *Springer*.

Campbell, A.V. (1984) *Moderated love: A theology of professional care*. London: SPCK.

Chambers, M. (2006) The case for mental health nurses. In J. Cutcliffe & M.F. Ward (eds) *Key debates in psychiatric/mental health nursing*. London: Churchill Livingstone. pp. 33–45.

Cooke, B. & Kothari, U. (2002) *Participation: The new tyranny?* London: Zed Books.

Crossley, N. (2006) *Contesting psychiatry*. London and New York: Routledge.

Csipke, E., Williams, P., Rose, D., et al. (2016) Following the Francis report: investigating patient experience of mental health inpatient care. *The British Journal of Psychiatry, 209*(1), 35–39.

Freire, P. (1971) *Pedagogy of the oppressed*. Harmondsworth: Penguin.

Freire, P. (1998) *Pedagogy of freedom: Ethics, democracy and civic courage*. Lanham, MD: Rowman & Littlefield.

Freshwater, D. (2002) The therapeutic use of self in nursing. In D. Freshwater (ed.) *Therapeutic nursing: Improving patient care through self-awareness and reflection*. London: Sage. pp. 1–15.

Friedli, L. & Stearn, R. (2015) Positive affect as coercive strategy: conditionality, activation and the role of psychology in UK government workfare programmes. *Medical Humanities, 41*(1), 40–7.

Gastaldo, D. & Holmes, D. (1999) Foucault and nursing: a history of the present. *Nursing Inquiry, 6*(4), 231–240.

Gesler, W. (1996) Lourdes: healing in a place of pilgrimage. *Health and Place, 2*, 95–105.

Giroux, H. (2007) Introduction: democracy, education and the politics of critical pedagogy. In P. McLaren & J. Kincheloe (eds) *Critical pedagogy: Where are we now?* New York: Peter Lang. pp. 1–8.

Glass, R. (2001) On Paulo Freire's philosophy of praxis and the foundations of liberation education. *Educational Researcher, 30*(2), 15–25.

Harper, D. & Speed, E. (2012) Uncovering recovery: the resistible rise of recovery and resilience. *Studies in Social Justice, 6*(1), 9.

Hewitt, J. & Coffey, M. (2005) Therapeutic working relationships with people with schizophrenia: literature review. *Journal of Advanced Nursing, 52*, 561–570.

Jacob, J., Peron, A. & Holmes, D. (2016) Introduction: unmasking the psychiatric apparatus. In D. Holmes, J. Jacob & A. Peron (eds) *Power and the psychiatric apparatus: Repression, transformation and assistance*. London: Routledge. pp. 1–22.

LeFrançois, B., Beresford, P. & Russo, J. (2016) Editorial: destination mad studies. *Intersectionalities: A Global Journal of Social Work Analysis, Research, Polity, and Practice, 5*(3), 1–10.

LeFrançois, B., Menzies, R. & Reaume, G. (eds) (2013) *Mad matters: A critical reader in Canadian mad studies*. Toronto: Canadian Scholars Press.

McAndrew, S., Chambers, M., Nolan, F., et al. (2014) Measuring the evidence: reviewing the literature of the measurement of therapeutic engagement in acute mental health inpatient wards. *International Journal of Mental Health Nursing, 23*(3), 212–220.

McKeown, M., Carey, L. Rhodes, C., et al. (2015) Democratic learning for democratic practice: co-operation and deliberation. In G. Brewer & R. Hogarth (eds) *Creative education, teaching and learning: Creativity, engagement and the student experience*. Basingstoke: Palgrave Macmillan.

McKeown, M., Cresswell, M. and Spandler, H. (2014) Deeply engaged relationships: alliances between mental health workers and psychiatric survivors in the UK. In B. Burstow, B.A. Lefrançois and S.L. Diamond (eds) *Psychiatry disrupted: Theorizing resistance and crafting the revolution*. Montreal, QC: McGill/Queen's University Press.

McKeown, M., Jones, F. & Spandler, H. (2017) Conscientization and transformation in the workplace: new forms of democracy for mental health services. In A. Melling & R. Pilkington (eds) *Paulo Freire and transformative education: Changing lives and transforming communities*. Basingstoke: Palgrave Macmillan.

Melia, K. (1987) Everyday ethics for nurses: balance of power. *Nursing Times, 83*(25), 42.

Mental Health Recovery Study Working Group (2009) *Mental health 'recovery': Users and refusers*. Toronto: Wellesley Institute.

Mind (2011) *Listening to experience: An independent inquiry into crisis and acute mental health care*. London: Mind.

Morse, J., Solberg, S., Neander, W., et al. (1990) Concepts of caring and caring as a concept. *Advances in Nursing Science*, 13, 1–14.

Norman, I. & Ryrie, I. (2013) *The art and science of mental health nursing: Principles and practice*, 3rd edition. Maidenhead: Open University Press/McGraw-Hill Education.

O'Brien, A.J. (2001) The therapeutic relationship: historical development and contemporary significance. *Journal of Psychiatric and Mental Health Nursing*, 8, 129–138.

O'Donnell, A. & Shaw, M. (2016) Resilience and resistance on the road to recovery in mental health. *Concept*, 7(3), 1–18.

Paley, J. (2001) An archaeology of caring knowledge. *Journal of Advanced Nursing*, 36(2), 88–198.

Peplau, H. (1952) *Theory of interpersonal relations in nursing*. New York: Putnam.

Peplau, H. (1988) The art and science of nursing: similarities, differences, and relations. *Nursing Science Quarterly*, 1(1), 8–15.

Pilgrim, D. (2005) *Key concepts in mental health*. London: Sage.

Pilgrim, D. (2016) Psychiatric coercion: some sociological perspectives. In A. Molodynski, J. Rugkasa & T. Burns (eds) *Coercion in community mental health care: International perspectives*. Oxford: Oxford University Press.

Read, J. (2005) The bio-bio-bio model of madness. *The Psychologist*, 18(10), 596–597.

Repper, J. (2000) Adjusting the focus of mental health nursing: incorporating service users' experiences of recovery. *Journal of Mental Health*, 9(6), 575–587.

Reynolds, J., Muston, R., Heller, T., et al. (2009) *Mental health still matters*. Houndmills: Palgrave/Open University Press.

Roberts, M. (2016) Critical thinking and reflection in contemporary mental health care: a Foucauldian perspective. *Nurse Education Today*, 45, 48–50.

Roberts, P. (2000) *Education, literacy, and humanization: Exploring the work of Paulo Freire*. Santa Barbara, CA: Greenwood Publishing Group.

Rose, D., Evans, J., Laker, C., et al. (2015) Life in acute mental health settings: experiences and perceptions of service users and nurses. *Epidemiology and Psychiatric Sciences*, 24, 90–96.

Russo, J. & Beresford, P. (2015) Between exclusion and colonisation: seeking a place for mad people's knowledge in academia. *Disability and Society*, 30, 153–157.

Sedgwick, P. (1982) *Psychopolitics*. London: Pluto.

Sedgwick, P. (2015) *Psychopolitics*, new edition. London: Unkant.

Spandler, H., Moth, R., McKeown, M., et al. (2016) Editorial: psychopolitics in the twenty first century. *Critical & Radical Social Work*, 4, 307–312.

Stickley, T. & Freshwater, D. (2002) The art of loving and the therapeutic relationship. *Nursing Inquiry*, 9(4), 250–256.

Sweeney, A., Clement, S., Filson, B., et al. (2016) Trauma-informed mental healthcare in the UK: what is it and how can we further its development? *Mental Health Review Journal*, 21(3), 174–192.

Thomas, P. (2016) Psycho politics, neoliberal governmentality and austerity. *Self & Society*, 44(4), 382–393.

Tolkien, J.R.R. (1954) *The Lord of the Rings*. London: Allen & Unwin.

Virden, P. (2016) Garth Daniel's struggle against vindictive psychiatry. *Asylum: the Magazine for Democratic Psychiatry*, 23(4), 18–24.

Wallcraft, J. & Hopper, K. (2015) The capabilities approach and the social model of mental health. In H. Spandler, J. Anderson & B. Sapey (eds) *Distress or disability? Mental health and the politics of disablement*. Bristol: Policy Press. pp. 83–97.

Yalom, I. (1980) *Existential psychotherapy*. New York: Basic Books.

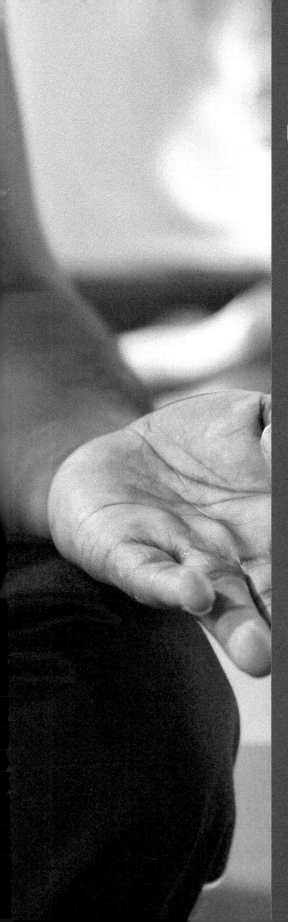

PART A   CONTEXT OF MENTAL HEALTH

THE CONTEXT AND NATURE OF MENTAL HEALTH CARE IN THE 21ST CENTURY

MICK McKEOWN, KAREN M. WRIGHT AND JONATHAN GADSBY

THIS CHAPTER COVERS

- The context in which mental health nursing takes place
- The importance of social and political factors in framing this context
- The legitimacy of mental health nursing and mental health services
- The role of the mental health nurse in engaging in critical thinking and action for change.

"

Mental health services are in a state of crisis. Despite government rhetoric to the contrary, services have been decimated. People in distress have had to travel hundreds of miles for a bed on an acute ward. More and more children are being diagnosed with mental health problems and CAMHS are struggling to cope. IAPT therapy is being delivered, not so much to help people in distress but as a cheap, short-term behaviour modification process to get people into the right frame of mind for work at the cost of longer-term, more useful and efficacious psychotherapies.

I belong to a mental health organisation called reVision. We are of the belief that mental distress is predominantly caused by social factors and we are critical of the unscientific and reductionist medical model. It is telling that the rate of suicide and of self-harm and the number of prescriptions of antidepressants have all increased dramatically in these times of austerity. The potential for the mentally distressed to recover is hindered significantly by the way people on benefits are portrayed in the media as lazy scroungers who claim benefits fraudulently.

(Continued)

Visit **https://study.sagepub.com/essentialmentalhealth** to access a wealth of online resources for this chapter – watch out for the margin icons throughout the chapter. If you are using the interactive ebook, simply click on the margin icon to go straight to the resource.

I facilitate groups at a local mental health resource centre. The effect of Work Capability and Personal Independence Payment assessments have been devastating. Levels of ill health have spiralled, service users have disclosed suicidal thoughts and attempts to end their lives, incidents of self-harm are on the rise and many have had medication increases. Letter phobia is rife amongst welfare recipients – an aptly named response of pure fear and trepidation at the sight of a letter from the DWP.

I was involved in a campaign we called SOS (Save Our Sanity) to keep the running of the mental health resource centre I volunteer at in the hands of the local authority and prevent it being tendered out to private companies. The success of this campaign I believe was due to the fact it was fought as an alliance: service users, academics, the Social Work Action network, reVision, Unite, Unison and Liverpool Against the Cuts. Although campaigning can be stressful, especially for those with mental distress, it can also bring rewards. Many service users blossomed during the campaign. We played to our strengths. I did the media stuff, talking to local papers and radio. A colleague with computer skills enabled the different organisations who were campaigning to keep connected and others lobbied council meetings. We were fortunate to be successful in our protest but just doing something, not being passive as service users so frequently are, but fighting for a Centre we felt strongly was integral to our recovery journey was empowering.

The staff at the Centre were as supportive as they could be without any actual involvement that could have resulted in their dismissal. I know that many were impressed at the power of our campaign and the alliances we had formed. It says a great deal about the service provided by the Centre that it supported service users who felt confident to use their voices, were angry enough to act, and loved their Centre enough to fight for it.

I still remember with pride the public meeting we held. The almost tangible feeling of solidarity in the room. It was well attended and funded by a TUC donation. We used this money to pay for service users from two other successful campaigns against cuts to services in Salford and Cambridgeshire to attend our public meeting. Our message was loud and clear – that campaigns can and do succeed. Activism, although stressful, tiring and frustrating really can be good for your mental health.

While services are based on a medical model of mental health with questionable basis in scientific fact and while we live in a neoliberal society that is toxic, cruel and unfeeling and sees service users as defective commodities and demonises and dehumanises them, the rate of mental distress will not decrease. Tory rhetoric and promises of more money for mental health will not stop the continuing increase in mental distress that is, as Wilkinson and Pickett demonstrate so convincingly in *The Spirit Level*, predominantly the result of living in an unequal society.

Patricia Stoll, service user

Right now, working as a mental health nurse in a community mental health team the effects of neoliberalism and austerity can be felt close up. Care has become a technical enterprise without political colour. It must be actioned, administrated and documented: real human feeling occurs, but can be superseded by the desire to be seen to be doing the right thing, both for those that govern the service that employs and the profession that gives status. Resources are few: these can be whittled away in discussions about 'appropriateness' for a particular service, form filling, reporting, writing letters, sending work elsewhere. The plethora of numbers, outcomes and data management that proliferated after Tony Blair's New Labour administration is a substantial burden. These tasks must be completed around real patient contact, which grows more difficult to establish. Patient discharge is a triumph. Patients must engage: they must utilise and respond to what is offered. The good patient is grateful, shows up, takes medication (if she is on any) and if not introjects whatever psychotherapeutic discipline is offered, changing his behaviour in the process. Time is rushed, accelerating, impacting upon the quality of thinking and the shape of subsequent work. I learn to accept how things are, to do my best within limitations, to stick to the Code, to offer as much real relating, help and availability as I can. I work extra hours but develop a healthy life to sustain the level of anxiety I inevitably must accumulate. I aim to be ethical. I am aware that every minute is another few pounds of the public purse spent and that someone, somewhere, be it patient or finance officer, is counting on me.

Peter Bull, mental health nurse

INTRODUCTION

Mental health nurses comprise the majority of the workforce in mental health care services. They are acknowledged as having a very demanding job and are appreciated by service users for providing skilled and compassionate support, which, for many, results in positive outcomes and an amelioration of mental distress. At its best, the role is intensely relational and humane, drawing heavily on interpersonal resources and communication skills and informed by progressive **values** concerning health, wellbeing and society (Dziopa & Ahern, 2009; O'Brien, 2001). To be able to practise such skills well to the benefit of individuals is a most rewarding role, and such job fulfilment pivots on the shared humanity of nurses and service users. Indeed, one of the biggest contemporary complaints from service users is when they feel they are denied sufficient time to talk or simply be with nursing staff.

Mental health nursing has always been as much concerned with the prevention of mental distress as responding to it once it is present in people's lives (Calloway, 2007). Modern mental health services, however, are often overwhelmingly reactive, and contemporary circumstances across society and mental health services appear increasingly inimical to good mental health. Hence, mental health nursing presently operates in a highly challenging **environment**. This is framed by, amongst other things, adverse socio-economic conditions that diminish people's mental health and the capacity of services to deal with the consequent distress. Neo-liberal austerity politics have resulted in cuts to the extensiveness and quality of mental health services, which have always struggled to assert a fair claim on funding and esteem compared with general health care services. Moreover, a number of spectacular service failings have ushered in a degree of public disquiet with the quality of care and perceived levels of compassion amongst the workforce, such that nursing faces profound criticisms of its very legitimacy. This legitimacy crisis is compounded by a sharp critique of biological psychiatry (Read, 2005; Sidley, 2015) and mental health nursing's supposed subordination to this (Abbott, 2014). Increasingly coercive systems of care, the public perception of dangerousness and all-pervading legislation further complicate matters of nursing identity and experience, alienating service users and the nursing workforce alike and undermining efforts to forge therapeutic alliances.

We contend that the question of what is the context for critical reflection on mental health care depends on the consideration of a territory comprising conceptual framings and influencing factors that are contentious and contested. Ultimately, this requires an appreciation of the prevailing social, political and economic conditions, the political nature of the very notions of health and mental health, and some sort of politically inspired solutions for extant problems. Despite previous calls for mental health nurses to demonstrate critical political understanding and action (e.g. Hart, 2004; Hopton, 1997; Leiba, 2001), a generally poor recognition of this politicised backdrop is why so much writing about mental health fails, in our view, to satisfy. We concern ourselves within this chapter with making sense of this difficult context in which mental health nursing finds itself, offering optimistic suggestions for escaping these circumstances; and avoiding any self-defeating spiral of pessimism and despair whilst simultaneously facing up to salient critique.

Interestingly, much of the better informed, progressive critique of mental health care has emerged from two important sources. First, an increasingly confident radical **service user** and **survivor** movement is asserting user-defined and articulated knowledge and action. Second, critical practitioners and researchers from amongst the psy-workforce are also finding their voice, raising the potential for radical alliances seeking transformational change and alternative forms of care.

HELPFUL FOR
ASSIGNMENTS!

CASE STUDY:
ROBERTA

QUO VADIS MENTAL HEALTH NURSES?

Arguably, the future of mental health nursing as a distinct occupational group is open to some doubt. At the very least, a consensus over professional regulatory identification of relevant competencies and the most appropriate education of practitioners is somewhat in flux (Hemingway et al., 2016; McKeown & White, 2015). Nevertheless, the need for mental health care, whilst disputed by some critics, is unlikely to diminish, and we would not have bothered producing this book if we didn't feel that mental health nursing had an important and valuable role to play in shaping the future.

A recent politics of austerity has raised the stakes for users of mental health services, exacerbating levels of mental distress at the same time as diminishing welfare entitlements and demonising recipients of benefits (McKeown et al., 2013; Orton, 2015; Thomas, 2016). Consequently, the confluence of neo-liberal political ascendancy and a recent rise in right-wing populism has led to calls for more assertive expressions of nursing resistance to this hegemony (Goodman & Grant, 2017). Arguably, for mental health nurses to take up this challenge they need a clearer and stronger sense of who they are, and who they could be.

Interested interlocutors with mental health nursing are frequently presented with a dichotomous choice for understanding matters of role, function and identity:

1. Mental health nursing is a legitimate branch of nursing, and like other forms this is subordinate to medicine (read psychiatry). Debates concerning context are thus of a piece with professional politics. Such professional concerns focus on: government funding, a battle to continue to get mental health accepted as 'an illness like any other', and the concomitant needs of a discipline engaged in the attempt to produce increasingly rigorous research to furnish an evidence base for practice. OR	2. Potentially a fundamentally different context – a context in which the main questions are about power in society, inequalities, discrimination, ethnic supremacy and capitalism, human/civil rights issues, and consideration of alternative models of provision. From this perspective, science and medicine are seen as a sham or depoliticised smokescreen for powerful elites, or even a means by which people can be made responsible for their own oppression. At its logical conclusion, this view must also contemplate the idea that mental health services could NEVER be of benefit to those deemed in need of it – in other words, that reform of services is impossible.

Of course, most people wholly subscribe to neither set of views but say and do things that reflect a range of competing assumptions. That these assumptions have a tendency to map on to political philosophies and philosophies of identity make it clear that resolving them is, at the very least, likely to pose huge challenges. Plausible and persuasive arguments can exist on either side, and meaningful and compassionate views are spread across what must be seen as a (mostly) legitimate diversity ('mostly' because some values may be founded on ignorance, and, by definition, lack legitimacy). Either side can resort to throwing 'evidence' down on the table like trump cards, thus avoiding a more respectful, deliberative engagement with each other's views. Nevertheless, just such dialogue may be the only means for arriving at an agreeable solution to these points of contention. Of course, agreeing to disagree may be a palatable outcome, as long as the debate moves us towards a more plural range of alternative services beyond simple bio-psychiatry.

THE POLITICAL ECONOMY OF MENTAL HEALTH

Since the great banking crisis of 2007, UK public services have been starved of resources and the poorest in society have paid a disproportionate price in a huge redistribution of wealth towards those already most affluent (Krugman, 2012; Kushner & Kushner, 2013; Piketty, 2014). Mental distress and other health and social problems are most evident when such income **inequality** is most stark (Wilkinson & Pickett, 2009). This politics of austerity has adversely affected the nation's mental health, so much so that contemporary times may best be referred to as a new age of **anxiety** (Orton, 2015; Stossel, 2014). Coinciding with the period of recession and subsequent austerity policies, previously falling suicide rates have substantially risen since 2007, alongside huge increases in prescriptions for antidepressants (Barr & Taylor-Robinson, 2016; Davies, 2017). Amidst this adverse economic and emotional climate, services are cut, reconfigured or privatised and uncertainties and discontinuities are consolidated, so that service users and staff struggle to establish meaningful, supportive relationships and the quality of care is put at risk (Bauman, 2000).

In parallel, the **stigma** that mentally distressed individuals face has mutated to reflect a wider demonisation of the poor, and their legitimate entitlement to welfare is cynically questioned by right-wing zealots wishing to recreate previously left-behind distinctions of deservingness (Patrick, 2016; Tyler, 2013). Mental health services have become swept up in this, with psychological therapists located in job centres and failures to comply with treatment subject to benefit sanctions – processes that have been termed psycho-compulsion (Friedli & Stearn, 2015; Thomas, 2016). Moreover, the same period has seen ever increasing levels of compulsory admission to inpatient units and **community treatment orders** under the Mental Health Act in England and Wales (Care Quality Commission, 2016).

Such developments may come as no surprise to critics who view mental health services as playing a significant role in social control within a society increasingly obsessed with containing risk (Beck, 1992; Rose, 1990). From this perspective, mental health nursing is one of a number of *psy*-professions who labour under the aegis of an over-arching *psy-complex*, the prime function of which relates to governance rather than care and support, regardless of the supposed motivations of individuals (Ingleby, 1985). One important consequence is risk aversion and the proliferation of technologies of risk assessment and management. Nurses can find themselves caught up in ever expanding paperwork and administrative tasks, taking them further away from the interface with patients. Ironically, prioritising paperwork over care work may render services more, rather than less, risky, and the written record may become compiled of available fictions instead of authentic observations (Coffey et al., 2016; McKeown et al., 2017).

A SHARED INTEREST IN TACKLING CRITICAL CHALLENGES?

One possible outcome of consciousness raising around critical perspectives is the reinforcement of division and conflict between practitioners and service users. Alternately, and a position we align with, is that reflection on cogent critique of mental health care holds emancipatory potential for both staff and service users, and that this goal may be best achieved in constructive alliance.

Arguably, the mental health system can be damaging for both admitted service users and the staff who work in it. Overly simplistic demarcations of identity are unhelpful, as the mental health workforce is not immune to mental health difficulties and staff can be service users themselves. The traumatising and re-traumatising effects of mental health services for service users have been well documented. This is so much the case that critical commentators have referred to psychiatric services as 'trauma-organised systems' (Bloom & Farragher, 2010; Sweeney et al., 2016) resulting in 'iatrogenesis' (Breggin, 1991). This is most obviously connected to experiences of **compulsion** and **coercion**, including such fairly routine practices as physical restraint, seclusion and forced medication (Frueh et al., 2005). Other coercions also occur which may not be so immediately obvious, such as commonplace interactions that more subtly reinforce powerlessness by restricting liberties or pushing compliance with professional treatment priorities (Bloom & Farragher, 2010). There has been longstanding disquiet regarding the over-use of medication with seriously harmful consequences, based on quite equivocal evidence (Moncrieff, 2013; Whitaker, 2010).

All of this is especially problematic when we recognise that trauma, particularly distressing childhood experience, is the most plausible factor implicated in the cause of mental health problems (Varese et al., 2012). Moreover, individuals' distress can be compounded by unsympathetic, pathologising responses from services interpreting reactions to abuse as symptomatic of mental **illness**, notably the diagnosis of borderline **personality** disorder (Asylum, 2004). Furthermore, appropriate or helpful forms of care that are sensitive to abuse experiences are rarely routinely available (Read et al., 2016; Sweeney et al., 2016). Mental health nurses need to take seriously this important work around the links between abuse and all kinds of mental health problems, including **psychosis**. Together with the profound questions raised by critical thinkers such as David Smail (e.g. 2005), we may conclude that diagnoses themselves cause a shift of attention away from personal abuse and systemic oppressions that may almost be thought of as colluding with that abuse – regardless of other questions about the validity of diagnoses.

The mental health care workforce may face numerous **alienation** hazards implicated in high rates of sickness/absence, stress and mental distress (Health and Safety Executive, 2016; Rössler, 2012). Notably, these are associated with: lack of control over how care work is organised; stress and uncertainty stemming from working in under-funded or poorly managed services; associated worries regarding outcomes for service users; and fear of, or actual experience of, violence. A dissonance between aspirations for a wholesome, caring professional identity and the actualities of conflictual relationships with service users can result in particularly pernicious alienation from one's ideal sense of self or species-being (McKeown & Spandler, 2006). Staff can also experience vicarious trauma in caring for traumatised people – described variously as compassion fatigue or secondary trauma, with empathic practitioners perhaps most vulnerable (Figley, 1995; Sabin-Farrell & Turpin, 2003). Whistleblowing staff, who call attention to organisational wrongdoing or inadequate care, are unfortunately as likely to be victimised by colleagues and employers as celebrated for their courage (Jackson et al., 2014).

Research has shown that mental health nurses and other staff are at the very least ambivalent about compulsion and coercion, and many would prefer not to engage in physical restraint (Perkins et al., 2012). It is also the case that nurses have historically objected to policies likely to exacerbate compulsion and coercion (Hannigan & Cutcliffe, 2002). Despite this, the fact that these interventions that many service users object to or view as harmful are legitimated within the mental health system suggests that all of us mental health care workers are complicit in such harms. Workers may bear responsibility for quite serious consequences without necessarily having sufficient authority to alter systemic practices or overarching power relations (McKeown & Foley, 2015). The overwhelming majority of mental health nurses did not begin with the intention to be part of an abusive or oppressive system, and not all service users are at all times against all compulsion and coercion (Katsakou et al., 2012). For example, Dina Poursanidou (2013) has recalled times when she was able to abscond from a coercive ward environment that she intensely disliked and found to be depressingly therapeutically limited, but with hindsight acknowledged her vulnerability, suggesting staff ought to have more competently confined her to the ward.

One of the unfortunate consequences of compulsory and coercive services is that staff aspirations to build therapeutic alliances are complicated and compromised. Inpatient settings especially can be typified by conflictual relationships that, in turn, are a major source of workplace stress for staff and compound service users' distress (Rössler, 2012; Unison, 2014). Because of the complexities of these aspects of care provision, such conflictual relationships require sophisticated understanding, beyond simplistic 'us and them', oppositional framings – even though this is how they often might feel to protagonists. Unanticipated and regrettable cycles of **aggression** and hostility with resulting reciprocal traumatisation can occur and re-occur, establishing many units as distinctly uneasy or untherapeutic environments. Such cycles of aggression or violence feed off feelings of fear or powerlessness, escalate suspicions and mistrust, and lead to further coercive responses, exacerbating situations, spoiling relationships or leading to further aggression. Taken together, this provides misplaced justification for coercive practices, legitimating an ongoing deployment that avoids attention placed on their role in potentiating rather than minimising fear and violence (McKeown et al., 2017). **Advocates** for alternative approaches, such as trauma-informed care models, argue for more considered reflection on the intricacies of service users and staff relations to better understand and thus avoid the potential for mutual mistrust, violence and oppression (Bloom, 2013; Sweeney et al., 2016).

What should be done?

We suggest that there are at least two elements that should be present in any attempt to respond to the difficulties outlined above. First, mental health nurses and any others wishing to improve the lives of mental health service users need to work in ways that make the philosophical tensions, political context and contested nature of the field clear. Moreover, they should always assertively raise awareness of the range and significance and credibility of the contest, and all of what the currently most accepted practices assume and conceal. It is probable that, in doing so, nurses will have to renegotiate their relationships with other professionals and their knowledge bases, towards much more genuinely holistic approaches and flatter hierarchies. This process is also an opportunity to reassess our relationships with survivor groups and their knowledge, promoting equality. Mental health nurses therefore need to open spaces characterised by dialogue and democracy. We feel that this is very much with the grain of some of our best instincts historically, but we continue to view it as a challenging or even revolutionary practice requiring great thoughtfulness and skill.

Second, while creating and upholding such spaces, we must continue to focus on service user experience. It would be very possible for such a space to appear to be wonderfully inclusive of many perspectives but in effect merely pass on conceptual confusion to service users. Yet it should be remembered that, despite current attempts at certainty and objective expertise, this is already the result of mental health services. The need for more explicit skills might focus nurses towards ideas such as 'Evidence-based practice vs **value-based practice**' (Morgan et al., 2015), **Open Dialogue** (Seikkula & Arnkil, 2014), Trialogue (Amering, 2016) and perhaps hitherto unexplored ways of conducting our work.

Any constructive alliance requires a progressive politics of mental health, a view on what needs to change, including options for alternative forms that services might take, and a process for achieving the desired change. Various critical thinkers from within practitioner ranks have articulated elements of this and organised into critical/radical networks. Notably, a grouping of radical nurses led by Jonathan Gadsby have formed the *Critical Mental Health Nurses Network* to facilitate the discussion of critical ideas and develop thinking about solutions to key problems. One strand of this activity is influencing mental health nursing education, whilst another seeks to engage public sector trade unions in critical debate and alliances with service user and survivor activist groups.

In an earlier wave of criticality, Pat Bracken and Phil Thomas (2001), prominent members of the Critical Psychiatry Network, coined the term *post-psychiatry* to refer to more humane practices that are alternatives to simplistic bio-psychiatry and inspired by critical social, ethical and philosophical theoretical ideas. Thomas (2014) rightly emphasises the context in which people live and under which care is provided as the most important consideration for those interested in progressive change and better outcomes. Ultimately, he settles on narrative ways of making sense of mental distress, and thus helping through various means of constructive talking, as a more fruitful alternative to the unproductive search for biological causes and remedies.

This chimes in with service user calls for humane, person-centred approaches to extreme mental distress. In addition, it is increasingly recognised that not all human experiences eligible to be considered as psychiatric symptoms are unique to supposed categories of mental illness and ought to be left alone, especially in the absence of distress or where this can be minimised by non-medical or **peer support**. It is such reasoning that lies behind the successes of movements like the Hearing Voices Network (Escher & Romme, 2012) and clinical approaches that are formulation-based and less invasive (Johnstone & Dallos, 2014).

FIND OUT
MORE

ELEANOR
LONGDEN'S
TED TALK

The desirability of making sense of madness and unintelligibility is marvellously depicted in Eleanor Longden's TED talk (www.ted.com/talks/eleanor_longden_the_voices_in_my_head), which narrates her personal, triumphal, transcendence of massively distressing experiences despite, rather than because of, standard psychiatric treatment. However, although the often unexplored possibilities for supporting such recoveries should be a priority for mental health nurses, we feel that we must also remain a **profession** able to be with people for whom many simple notions of **recovery** would involve a denial of the complexities and ongoing distress of their experience, and perhaps even a **denial** of their financial and social impoverishment.

One way to resolve the various crises facing mental health care and mental health nursing is to consider avowedly political solutions, but to do so in an inclusive, participatory, deliberative spirit that has most chance of engaging with interested parties to the debate. Psychosocially inclined mental health nurses and others have recognised the virtues of dialogue and democracy as both therapeutic and political tools (see Winship, 2003, 2013). A provocative template for a democratic politics of mental health is provided in the work of Peter Sedgwick, scholar, activist, service user and psychologist. Sedgwick's (1982/2015) seminal text, *Psycho Politics*, offers a prescient critique of the shortcomings of both psychiatry and **anti-psychiatry** before turning to a relational prescription for change rooted in the potential power of alliances between social movements comprising radical service users and staff. Arguably, before the labour movement, and by inference, mental health nurses and their trade unions can fruitfully enter such alliances, they must appreciate and embrace an alternative politics of mental health, or at the very least begin to consider taken-for-granted understandings in more politicised terms (McKeown et al., 2014). The call for a new politics of mental health and constructive movement alliances resonates strongly with aspects of the **Mad Studies** vision for change (Beresford, 2016).

HOPE FOR A BETTER FUTURE

Arguably, we already have numerous fitting ideas for better, more humane mental health care. Similarly, we have methods and communicative tools to help us realise these. We may not immediately be able to provoke large-scale transformative change but, following Sedgwick's call for prefiguration, we may be able to create smaller-scale, situated alternatives (Cresswell & Spandler, 2016; Moth & McKeown, 2016). Such openings can be sought in the interstitial spaces of public services, in the places where neo-liberal power does not absolutely reach (Clarke, 2007). This may involve working the contradictions of policies that serve consumerism but to some extent create openings for democracy, dialogue and empowered voice. In this way, service user movement-led alternatives have emerged from time to time in history, having the appearance of mini working utopias (Crossley, 1999) and recent movement activism has presented a blueprint for wide-ranging alternatives grounded in survivor knowledge (Russo & Sweeney, 2016).

We started this chapter by highlighting the substantial challenges that frame the context within which mental health nurses must practise. We suggested that mental health care and nursing are beset with crises of legitimacy, assailed from various quarters with pointed and justified criticism. The prevailing, iniquitous, unjust social relations that typify **neo-liberalism** are not just stifling for mental health care, they also underpin the major problems facing the world: rampant poverty and inequality, climate change, perpetual war and the rise of populist right-wing authoritarian politics. Rather than view all of this as grounds for fatalistic pessimism, we can contemplate, and work for, alternatives.

A reconfigured, critically informed mental health care system and the actions required to achieve it would emphasise positive human relationships. Similarly, agreeing with Sedgwick, the cooperative, relational task of transforming psychiatry could model broader transformations across society as a whole, towards achieving more just distribution of economic resources and fairer social relations. To be in a legitimacy crisis is not the same as saying everything is bad. The endemic nature of mental distress suggests we do not need to do away with mental health care; rather, we need more of it and to do it much better. Ideally, skilled, empathic, critically minded mental health nurses will remain central to such services and play a key role in their creation.

CHAPTER SUMMARY

This chapter has covered:

- The discussion of different aspects of the context of mental health care
- A consideration of various critiques of established services, including the potential for services to do harm as well as good
- Contemplation of the implications for mental health nursing as a distinct practice discipline
- The possibilities for imagining and working towards more progressive models of care.

BUILD YOUR BIBLIOGRAPHY

Books

- Sedgwick, P. (2015) *Psycho Politics*. London: Unkant. The reissued classic by Peter Sedgwick with a very good new introduction by Spandler, Dellar and Kemp that makes the case for continued relevance of Sedgwick's critique.

- Kushner, B. & Kushner, S. (2013) *Who needs the cuts? Myths of the economic crisis.* London: Hesperus. Not directly about mental health, but a very accessible analysis of the problems with the economics of austerity – how the poorest are paying for a crisis they didn't cause.
- Tummey, R. & Turner, T. (eds) (2008) *Critical issues in mental health.* Basingstoke: Palgrave Macmillan. This edited collection showcases many of the critical ideas and authors drawn upon in our introduction to this book. In their preface, Tummey and Turner correctly emphasise vigilance over complacency.

SAGE journal articles

FURTHER
READING:
JOURNAL
ARTICLES

Go to https://study.sagepub.com/essentialmentalhealth for further free online journal articles related to this chapter. If you are using the interactive ebook, simply click on the book icon in the margin to go straight to the resource.

- Clarke, J. (2010) Public management or managing the public? The Frank Stacey Memorial Lecture 2009, presented at the Public Administration Committee Conference, University of Glamorgan, 8 September 2009. *Public Policy and Administration, 25*(4), 416–433.
- Maslin-Prothero, S. & Masterson, A. (2002) Power, politics, and nursing in the United Kingdom. *Policy, Politics, & Nursing Practice, 3*(2), 108–117.
- Springer, S. (2014) Neoliberalism in denial. *Dialogues in Human Geography, 4*(2), 154–160.

Weblinks

FURTHER
READING:
WEBLINKS

Go to https://study.sagepub.com/essentialmentalhealth for further weblinks related to this chapter. If you are using the interactive ebook, simply click on the book icon in the margin to go straight to the resource.

A number of websites provide further information regarding the context of mental health care and the potential for change:

- Critical Mental Health Nurses website: https://criticalmhnursing.org
- Gary Sidley's Tales from the Madhouse blog: www.talesfromthemadhouse.com/blog – this series of blogs is a useful introduction to critical ideas written by a progressive author who has worked as both a mental health nurse and a clinical psychologist.
- Recovery in the Bin: https://recoveryinthebin.org; www.facebook.com/search/top/?q=recovery%20in%20the%20bin – this is a user- and survivor-led group with website and Facebook pages; has critical debates and humorous observations on the uses and misuses of the recovery concept under neoliberalism.

ACE YOUR ASSESSMENT

ONLINE
QUIZZES &
ACTIVITY
ANSWERS

Revise what you have learned by visiting https://study.sagepub.com/essentialmentalhealth. If you are using the interactive ebook, simply click on the tick icon to go straight to the resource.

- Test yourself with multiple-choice and short-answer questions and flashcards.

REFERENCES

Abbott, A. (2014) *The system of professions: An essay on the division of expert labor.* Chicago: University of Chicago Press.

Amering, M. (2016) Trialogue: an exercise in communication between users, carers, and professional mental health workers beyond role stereotypes. In W. Gaebel, W. Rössler & N. Sartorius (eds) *The stigma of mental illness: End of the story?* New York: Springer. pp. 581–590.

Asylum (2004) Women at the margins: special issue on women and borderline personality disorder. *Asylum: The Magazine for Democratic Psychiatry, 4*(3).

Barr, B. & Taylor-Robinson, D. (2016) Recessions are harmful to health. *British Medical Journal,* 354, i4631.

Bauman, Z. (2000) *Liquid modernity.* Cambridge: Polity Press.

Beck, U. (1992) *Risk society.* London: Sage.

Beresford, P. (2016) From psycho-politics to mad studies: learning from the legacy of Peter Sedgwick. *Critical and Radical Social Work, 4*(3), 343–355.

Bloom, S. (2013) *Creating Sanctuary: Toward the Evolution of Sane Societies.* New York, NY: Routledge.

Bloom, S. & Farragher, B. (2010) *Destroying sanctuary: The crisis in human service delivery systems.* New York: Oxford University Press.

Bracken, P. & Thomas, P. (2001) Postpsychiatry: a new direction for mental health. *British Medical Journal, 322*(7288), 724.

Breggin, P. (1991) *Toxic psychiatry: Why therapy, empathy and love must replace the drugs, electroshock, and biochemical theories of the 'new psychiatry'.* New York: St. Martin's Press.

Calloway, S. (2007) Mental health promotion: is nursing dropping the ball? *Journal of professional Nursing, 23*(2), 105–109.

Care Quality Commission (2016) *Monitoring the Mental Health Act Report 2015/16.* Newcastle upon Tyne: CQC. Available at: www.cqc.org.uk/content/monitoring-mental-health-act-report (accessed 04.05.17).

Clarke, J. (2007) Citizen-consumers and public service reform: at the limits of neo-liberalism? *Policy Futures in Education, 5,* 239–248.

Coffey, M., Cohen, R., Faulkner, A., et al. (2016) Ordinary risks and accepted fictions: how contrasting and competing priorities work in risk assessment and mental health care planning. *Health Expectations, 20*(3), 471–483.

Cresswell, M. & Spandler, H. (2016) Solidarities and tensions in mental health politics: mad studies and psychopolitics. *Critical and Radical Social Work, 4*(3), 357–373.

Crossley, N. (1999) Working utopias and social movements: an investigation using case study materials from radical mental health movements in Britain. *Sociology, 33*(4), 809–830.

Davies, J. (2017) Introduction. In J. Davies (ed.) *The sedated society: The causes and harms of our psychiatric drug epidemic.* New York: Springer. pp. 1–22.

Dziopa, F. & Ahern, K. (2009) What makes a quality therapeutic relationship in psychiatric/mental health nursing? A review of the research literature. *Internet Journal of Advanced Nursing Practice, 10*(1), 1–19.

Escher, S. & Romme, M. (2012) The hearing voices movement. In *Hallucinations.* New York: Springer. pp. 385–393.

Figley, C. (1995) Compassion fatigue: towards a new understanding of the costs of caring. In B.H. Stamm (ed.) *Secondary traumatic stress: Self care issues for clinicians, researchers, and educators.* Baltimore, MD: The Sidran Press. pp. 3–27.

Friedli, L. & Stearn, R. (2015) Positive affect as coercive strategy: conditionality, activation and the role of psychology in UK government workfare programmes. *Medical Humanities* 41(1): 40–7.

Frueh, B., Knapp, R., Cusack, K., et al. (2005) Special section on seclusion and restraint: patients' reports of traumatic or harmful experiences within the psychiatric setting. *Psychiatric Services*, 56(9), 1123–1133.

Goodman, B. & Grant, A. (2017) The case of the Trump regime: the need for resistance in international nurse education. *Nurse Education Today*, 52, 53–56.

Hannigan, B. & Cutcliffe, J. (2002) Challenging contemporary mental health policy: time to assuage the coercion? *Journal of Advanced Nursing*, 37(5), 477–484.

Hart, C. (2004) *Nurses and politics: The impact of power and practice.* Basingstoke: Palgrave Macmillan.

Health and Safety Executive (2016) *Work Related Stress, Anxiety and Depression Statistics in Great Britain 2016.* London: HSE.

Hemingway, S., Clifton, A. & Edward, K.L. (2016) The future of mental health nursing education in the United Kingdom: reflections on the Australian and New Zealand experience. *Journal of Psychiatric and Mental Health Nursing*, 23(5), 331–337.

Hopton, J. (1997) Towards a critical theory of mental health nursing. *Journal of Advanced Nursing*, 25(3), 492–500.

Ingleby, D. (1985) Professionals as socialisers: the 'psy-complex'. In A. Scull & S. Spitzer (eds) *Research in law, deviance and social control.* New York: Jai Press. pp. 79–109.

Jackson, D., Hickman, L., Hutchinson, M., et al. (2014) Whistleblowing: an integrative literature review of data-based studies involving nurses. *Contemporary Nurse*, 48(2), 240–252.

Johnstone, L. & Dallos, R. (2014) *Formulation in psychology and psychotherapy: Making sense of people's problems*, 2nd edition. Hove: Routledge.

Katsakou, C., Rose, D., Amos, H., et al. (2012) Psychiatric patients' views on why their involuntary hospitalisation was right or wrong: a qualitative study. *Social Psychiatry and Psychiatric Epidemiology*, 47(7), 1169–1179.

Krugman, P. (2012) *End this depression now.* New York: W.W. Norton & Co.

Kushner, B. & Kushner, S. (2013) *Who needs the cuts? Myths of the economic crisis.* London: Hesperus.

Leiba, T. (2001) An introduction to the history of mental health nursing. In S. Forster (ed.) *The role of the mental health nurse.* Cheltenham: Nelson Thornes. pp. 1–12.

McKeown, M. & Foley, P. (2015) Reducing physical restraint: an employment relations perspective. *Journal of Mental Health Nursing*, 35(1), 12–15.

McKeown, M. & Spandler, H. (2006) *Alienation and redemption: the potential for alliances with mental health service users.* Published conference proceedings: Alternative Futures & Popular Protest. 11th International Social Movements Conference, 19–21 April. Manchester: Manchester Metropolitan University.

McKeown, M. & White, J. (2015) The future of mental health nursing: are we barking up the wrong tree? *Journal of Psychiatric and Mental Health Nursing*, 22, 724–730.

McKeown, M., Cresswell, M. & Spandler, H. (2014) Deeply engaged relationships: alliances between mental health workers and psychiatric survivors in the UK. In B. Burstow, B.A. LeFrançois and S.L. Diamond (eds) *Psychiatry disrupted: Theorizing resistance and crafting the revolution.* Montreal, QC: McGill/Queen's University Press.

McKeown, M., Jones, F. & Spandler, H. (2013) Challenging austerity policies: democratic alliances between survivor groups and trade unions. *Mental Health Nursing*, 33(6), 26–29.

McKeown, M., Wright, K. & Mercer, D. (2017) Care planning: a neoliberal three card trick. *Journal of Psychiatric and Mental Health Nursing*, 24, 451–460.

Moncrieff, J. (2013) *The bitterest pills: The troubling story of antipsychotic drugs.* Basingstoke: Palgrave Macmillan.

Morgan, A., Felton, A., Fulford, B., et al. (2015) *Values and ethics in mental health: An exploration for practice.* Basingstoke: Palgrave Macmillan.

Moth, R. & McKeown, M. (2016) Realising Sedgwick's vision: theorising strategies of resistance to neoliberal mental health and welfare policy. *Critical and Radical Social Work*, 4(3), 375–390.

O'Brien, A.J. (2001) The therapeutic relationship: historical development and contemporary significance. *Journal of Psychiatric and Mental Health Nursing*, 8, 129–138.

Orton, M. (2015) *Something's not right: insecurity and an anxious nation.* London: Compass. Available at: www.compassonline.org.uk/wp-content/uploads/2015/01/Compass-Somethings-Not-Right.pdf (accessed 01.08.17).

Patrick, R. (2016) Living with and responding to the 'scrounger' narrative in the UK: exploring everyday strategies of acceptance, resistance and deflection. *Journal of Poverty and Social Justice*, 24(3), 245–259.

Perkins, E., Prosser, H., Riley, D., et al. (2012) Physical restraint in a therapeutic setting: a necessary evil? *International Journal of Law and Psychiatry*, 35(1), 43–49.

Piketty, T. (2014) *Capital in the 21st century.* Cambridge, MA: Belknap Press.

Poursanidou, D. (2013) Being against compulsion in mental health care and upholding service users' right to free decision making: any questions? Available at: www.asylumonline.net/being-against-compulsion-in-mental-health-care-and-upholding-service-users-right-to-free-decision-making-any-questions (accessed 23.05.13).

Read, J. (2005) The bio-bio-bio model of madness. *The Psychologist*, 18(10), 596–597.

Read, J., Sampson, M. & Critchley, C. (2016) Are mental health services getting better at responding to abuse, assault and neglect? *Acta Psychiatrica Scandinavica*, 134, 287–294.

Rose, N. (1990) *Governing the soul: The shaping of the private self.* London: Routledge.

Rössler, W. (2012) Stress, burnout, and job dissatisfaction in mental health workers. *European Archives of Psychiatry and Clinical Neuroscience*, 262(2), 65–69.

Russo, J. & Sweeney, A. (2016) *Searching for a rose garden: Challenging psychiatry, fostering mad studies.* Wyastone Leys: PCCS Books.

Sabin-Farrell, R. & Turpin, G. (2003) Vicarious traumatization: implications for the mental health of health workers? *Clinical Psychology Review*, 23, 449–480.

Sedgwick, P. (1982) *Psycho Politics.* London: Pluto.

Sedgwick, P. (2015) *Psychopolitics.* London: Unkant.

Seikkula, J. & Arnkil, T. (2014) *Open dialogues and anticipations: Respecting otherness in the present moment.* Tampere, FL: National Institute for Health and Welfare.

Sidley, G.L. (2015) *Tales from the Madhouse: An insider critique of psychiatric services.* Monmouth: PCCS Books.

Smail, D. (2005) *Power, interest and psychology: Elements of a social materialist understanding of distress.* Ross-on-Wye: PCCS Books.

Stossel, S. (2014) *My age of anxiety.* London: Windmill Books.

Sweeney, A., Clement, S., Filson, B. & Kennedy, A. (2016) Trauma-informed mental healthcare in the UK: what is it and how can we further its development? *Mental Health Review Journal*, 21(3), 174–192.

Thomas, P. (2014) *Psychiatry in context: Experience, meaning and communities.* Wyastone Leys: PCCS Books.

Thomas, P. (2016) Psycho politics, neoliberal governmentality and austerity. *Self & Society*, 44(4), 382–393.

Tyler, I. (2013) *Revolting subjects: Social abjection and resistance in neoliberal Britain*. London: Zed Books.

Unison (2014) *Stress at work: A guide for Unison safety reps*. London: Unison. Available at: www.unison. org.uk/content/uploads/2014/10/On-line-Catalogue227032.pdf (accessed 22.05.17).

Varese, F., Smeets, F., Drukker, M., et al. (2012) Childhood adversities increase the risk of psychosis: a meta-analysis of patient-control, prospective- and cross-sectional cohort studies. *Schizophrenia Bulletin, 38*(4), 661–671.

Whitaker, R. (2010) *Mad in America: Bad science, bad medicine, and the enduring mistreatment of the mentally ill*. Cambridge, MA: Basic Books.

Wilkinson, R.G. & Pickett, K. (2009) *The spirit level: Why more equal societies almost always do better*. London: Allen Lane.

Winship, G. (2003) The democratic origins of the term 'group analysis': Karl Mannheim's 'third way' for psychoanalysis and social science. *Group Analysis, 36*(1), 37–51.

Winship, G. (2013) A genealogy of therapeutic community ideas: the influence of the Frankfurt School with a particular focus on Herbert Marcuse and Eric Fromm. *Therapeutic Communities: The International Journal of Therapeutic Communities, 34*(2/3), 60–70.

E-RESOURCES

Eleanor Longden TED Talk – The Voices in My Head: www.ted.com/talks/eleanor_longden_the_ voices_in_my_head

OVERVIEW OF MENTAL HEALTH NURSE EDUCATION AND TRAINING

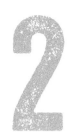

STEVEN PRYJMACHUK

THIS CHAPTER COVERS

- The knowledge, skills and attitudes required of registered mental health nurses
- The regulatory framework surrounding nurse education and training
- The personal obligations you have if you are to be successful in your studies
- The teaching and learning methods used in mental health nurse education and the evidence for their effectiveness.

> " As both an educator and a researcher in mental health nursing, I strongly believe that mental health nursing should be a *graduate* profession because, as you will discover throughout this book, the issues surrounding mental health and mental ill health in today's society are complex and subject to a variety of cultural, political, social and philosophical influences.
>
> **Steve, mental health nurse** "

Visit **https://study.sagepub.com/essentialmentalhealth** to access a wealth of online resources for this chapter - watch out for the margin icons throughout the chapter. If you are using the interactive ebook, simply click on the margin icon to go straight to the resource.

Amy and Grace from Common Room (www.commonroom.uk.com), a young people's consultancy group, offer some excellent advice for budding mental health nurses below, advice which neatly reflects the content of this chapter:

> We can't proclaim what all service users think makes a good mental health nurse, but here are four things we think might help along the way:
>
> - **Treat us as individuals.** You will probably find you need a different set of skills to work with each service user.
> - **Be honest with us.** If you are not sure about something, remember that it is fine to not have all the answers straightaway, providing you work with us to find a solution or enhance your understanding. Remember that while you must learn how and when to trust an individual service user, it is also important for the service user to trust you, and honesty is a big part of this.
> - **Be patient** (even when we are being hard work!) You would not be studying mental health nursing if you weren't wanting to be approachable and kind. But sometimes you need a bit of extra patience. We know it can be very difficult being nice all the time in such a stressful occupation, but it can make such a difference.
> - **Don't beat yourself up.** Sometimes you may be scared of saying or doing the wrong thing, or you might be worried that your actions may aggravate a situation or upset a service user. What we really appreciate is you trying, being responsive and learning as you go. Nobody gets it right all the time; the best mental health nurses are those who try their hardest to learn from their mistakes.
>
> **Amy and Grace, service users**

From the quotations above, it is clear that mental health nurses require a degree of intelligence if they are to comprehend – perhaps even reconcile – the sometimes disparate views of how someone might become mentally unwell and how someone might find the strength and resources to recover from mental ill health. If mental health nurses are to provide the best possible care, they will need to be able to: analyse information for its credibility and validity; search for, and interpret, evidence of the best ways to help and support **service users** and their families; challenge poor, outdated or restrictive practices; and work with other professionals and with service users and their families as 'co-producers' of care. Mental health nurses also require a degree of self-awareness and appropriate attitudes and **values** if they are to provide care that is ethical, compassionate and service user-centred.

In this chapter, I will explain how your mental health nursing course is designed so as to ensure that those entering the **profession** have the right personal qualities and the necessary knowledge and skills to become caring and effective mental health nurses.

INTRODUCTION

You are probably reading this book because you are doing a mental health nursing course (or you are seriously thinking about doing one). It is highly likely that that course is delivered by a university or some other higher education (HE) institution. Hopefully, you will be successful in your studies and, at the end of three-or-however-many years, you will come out with two qualifications (or 'awards'): a licence to practise as a mental health nurse; and an academic award, most likely a degree titled something like 'BSc Hons Mental Health Nursing'.

However, have you ever stopped to think about why you need a licence to practise or why you are studying in a *university* rather than on the job or in a local college? Surely, joining one of the 'caring' professions only requires an ability to care?

This chapter will try to answer these questions and, in the process, hopefully help you understand the rationale behind why you get tested so much, why you have to essentially do unpaid work while also attending university, why your lecturers harp on about 'critical analysis', '**reflective practice**' and 'the evidence base', and why becoming a registered nurse will constrain how you behave publicly and socially.

THE REGISTERED MENTAL HEALTH NURSE

Before moving on, it is worth dissecting three components in the title allocated to your chosen profession: *Registered nurse, mental health*.

Registered

Registration is intrinsically connected to the regulation of the professions. 'Profession' is a somewhat complex and controversial concept that has kept sociologists busy for decades (see, for example, Freidson, 1970; Macdonald, 1995), but, briefly, a profession can be seen as something more than a mere occupation or job.

All of the UK health care professions are regulated by law, via a statutory council. The *Nursing and Midwifery Order (2001)* established nursing's statutory council, the *Nursing and Midwifery Council* (or 'NMC'). Each statutory council controls a 'register' of those licensed to practise in their respective professions. Moreover, each sets the standards for entry to their respective profession: each council determines the criteria individuals need to meet in order to become registered. The following are characteristics of a profession:

* ownership of a specific body of knowledge
* a prolonged period of training, ideally in a university setting
* a high degree of autonomy
* some sort of service is provided for the benefit of the public
* explicit organisation: professional associations, committees, etc.
* monopolistic control over a specific area of practice, including rights to restrict entry into the profession.

Nurse

Mental health nursing is a sub-specialty (or 'field') of nursing, along with adult, children's and learning disability nursing. This seemingly benign statement has the potential to be controversial, however, in that some see nurses as a homogenous group and thus question the need for specialisation at a pre-registration level. However, our history is different to that of general nurses, emerging from the asylum attendants of the late 19th and early 20th centuries. 'Psychiatric' nursing developed alongside the medical specialty of psychiatry, with the forerunner of the Royal College of Psychiatrists providing the first qualifications for asylum attendants (or 'mental nurses' as they would later be called). Indeed, for a long time, nursing would not accept mental nurses as 'proper' nurses (Nolan, 1993), a position that still resonates in some quarters today.

CRITICAL DEBATE 2.1

To specialise or not?

The UK is one of a small number of countries that produces specialist nurses at first registration. Most other countries produce *generalist* practitioners at first registration, with mental health being a post-registration/postgraduate specialty. If this applied in the UK, there would only be one type of nurse at registration (a generic nurse) and becoming a mental health nurse would require a further period of education and training.

What do you think are the advantages and disadvantages of the UK's current set-up? Do you think we should consider having something like the recently introduced *Think Ahead* system for mental health social work (see https://thinkahead.org) where specialty is retained at first registration but you have to be a *graduate* (of any subject) to enter the profession?

Mental health

Some people still refer to qualified (registered) mental health nurses as 'RMNs', an abbreviation for 'registered mental nurse', the profession's title when it was first established in the early 20th century. Currently (2017), the NMC register has just three parts – *nurse, midwife* and *specialist public health nurse* – so mental health nurses are not legally distinct from other nurses being simply 'registered nurses' (RNs) like their adult nursing counterparts. Our current official title is *registered nurse, mental health*, though, colloquially, (registered) mental health nurse is more frequent.

The issue here, however, is not whether we are nurses or not (we touched on that earlier) but whether we are *mental health* nurses. As you will discover elsewhere in this book, mental health and mental illness, though related, are distinct concepts. Being a mental health nurse implies that our primary purpose is protecting and promoting the mental *health* of the population. Yet much of what we currently do is care for those with mental *illness*, so why are we not called 'mental illness nurses' or, indeed, 'psychiatric nurses'?

Whatever we call ourselves, the context is changing. Ageing populations coupled with austerity measures have made governments increasingly worried about the costs of sustaining hospital- and illness-focused care both in physical and mental health. NHS England's *Five Year Forward View for Mental Health* (Mental Health Taskforce, 2016) makes the salient point that half of all mental health problems are established by the age of 14 (rising to three quarters by the age of 24) and that most of the £34 billion spent on mental health care each year is spent on *treatment*. If the focus shifted to promotion, prevention and early intervention – i.e. to mental *health* and away from mental *illness* – then not only would many families escape the misery and trauma associated with mental illness, governments could also escape having to pump more and more money into institutional systems that do not always help people and which often stigmatise them.

So, while 'mental health nurse' might not accurately reflect the nature of our work currently, my prediction is that it will be a much more accurate description of what we will be doing in the future. Or, maybe, there will be both mental health nurses and mental illness nurses in the future?

BECOMING A REGISTERED MENTAL HEALTH NURSE

So now you know the statutory and regulatory underpinnings of the registered mental health nurse, what is actually required to become one? The NMC has two sets of standards that impact on nurse education: *Standards for Pre-Registration Nursing Education* (NMC, 2010) and *Standards to Support Learning and Assessment in Practice* (NMC, 2008). There is no point being too specific about these standards because they will probably be obsolete by the time you are reading this, as both sets are currently under review. A few aspects are worth mentioning, however, because they are highly likely to continue in any new standards.

First, in line with a core criterion defining a profession (see the bullet points on p. 19), the NMC insists on an extended period of training: currently, this is a specified number of hours (4,600) which must be completed in no less than three years and split 50–50 between theory and practice. Second, following a long campaign to professionalise nursing, the standards have brought nursing into line with other health care professions by specifying that the minimum level at which registered nurse education and training must be set is *degree* level; prior to 2010, it was HE diploma level.

Bringing nursing into universities, however, created additional demands because it is the universities, not regulatory bodies like the NMC, who set the standards for awards (degrees, diplomas, etc.). Thus, to become a registered mental health nurse you not only need to meet the NMC's demands for registration but also the demands of the university awarding the degree. Do not worry about this, however. Since a university can only deliver a nursing degree with NMC approval, graduates from UK pre-registration nursing degrees automatically qualify for entry onto the NMC register – so long as the university is also able to sign off a candidate's 'good health and character', a point we will return to shortly.

KNOWLEDGE, SKILLS AND ATTITUDES

The standards set by the NMC and the university awarding a mental health nursing degree reflect three essential qualities: (a) intellectual capacity; (b) psychomotor skills; and (c) appropriate values and attitudes. In other words, mental health nurses need the **right knowledge**, the **right skills** and the **right attitudes**. All three aspects are necessary: if an individual is weak in *any* area, chances are they will not be allowed to progress on their course or onto the register.

These aspects also underpin current educational practice in that they reflect an influential educational model called 'Bloom's taxonomy' (Anderson & Krathwohl, 2001; Bloom, 1956). Bloom's taxonomy divides learning into three domains: **cognitive**, **psychomotor** and **affective**. These translate roughly as *knowledge*, *skills* and *attitudes* and are useful in helping educators determine what students should learn in a specific module or course. In particular, they are helpful in establishing and grouping **intended learning outcomes** (ILOs), the things a student might expect to learn as a result of a particular block of learning. Table 2.1 gives some examples of ILOs for a hypothetical degree module and outlines how these map onto Bloom's domains. You should be able to find the ILOs for your module or course by checking its handbook or by asking your lecturers.

ILOs help both student and educator understand what a particular block of learning is all about: they determine the module's content, the ways in which that content is delivered or accessed, and the assessments used. For example, an educator could check whether intended learning outcome P1 (and also A1 and A2) has been achieved through a simulated mental health assessment that uses role play or has actors playing service users.

Much of the remainder of this chapter will be spent exploring these three learning domains in more detail because they determine what it is you will learn during your time as a student mental health nurse and because they are critical to you achieving NMC registration.

Table 2.1 Learning outcomes for MHN105: assessment in mental health nursing

Domain	Focus	Intended learning outcomes *At the end of the module, students will be able to:*
Cognitive *Thinking*	knowledge and understanding; intellectual skills	C1. explain the biological, psychological, social and cultural factors underpinning the concepts of 'mental health' and 'mental illness'
		C2. compare and contrast different mental health assessment frameworks, outlining the strengths and weaknesses of each
		C3. argue for the benefits of involving service users in assessments as co-producers of care
Psychomotor *Doing*	practical skills; intellectual skills; transferable skills	P1. conduct a comprehensive, service user centred mental health assessment
		P2. agree with the service user a summary of the main issues emerging from the assessment
		P3. keep accurate, comprehensive notes of any assessment they conduct
Affective *Feeling*	transferable skills; personal qualities; values and attitudes	A1. introduce themselves to service users and their significant others in a professional and caring manner, fully explaining the process behind the assessment
		A2. converse openly with a service user and any significant others during the assessment, demonstrating compassion, empathy, warmth, genuineness and self-awareness
		A3. identify any safeguarding issues that emerge from an assessment, knowing when to discuss these with senior colleagues

KNOWLEDGE ACQUISITION: WHAT YOU NEED TO KNOW

The cognitive domain (or 'knowledge') is concerned with what you need to know to become a registered mental health nurse. In the past, topics to be covered would simply appear as a list in a 'syllabus of training'. However, learning-to-the-syllabus tends to lead to 'surface' rather than 'deep' learning. **Surface learning** is characterised by the uncritical learning of 'facts' (usually through rote), a passive acceptance that there is usually a 'right' way of doing things and a detachment of theory from practice. This is fine if you want passive nurses who act ritualistically or merely on the orders of others (doctors, for example) rather than autonomous practitioners who are able to make robust clinical decisions in the face of complexity. **Deep learning**, however, is about understanding information and challenging it, thinking for yourself and establishing links between theory and practice.

Running alongside the debate on the professionalisation of nursing in the late 20th century was the emergence of **evidence-based practice** (see, for example, Sackett et al., 1996), an approach to health care which necessarily requires practitioners to be information-savvy, critical thinkers who are able to forge strong theory–practice links if they are to enhance care through effective clinical decision making. Modern nurse education thus requires deep, rather than surface, learning.

Academic levels

Another influence of Bloom's taxonomy on education was the establishment of hierarchies of learning within its domains. In the cognitive domain, mere knowledge sits at the bottom of the hierarchy, with higher-order cognitive and intellectual skills at the top (see Table 2.2).

Table 2.2 Bloom's taxonomy and academic levels

Bloom's Taxonomy (Cognitive)		Academic Level		Typical descriptors for this level	Awards at this level
		EW&NI	Scotland		
Creating synthesis	Postgraduate	Level 8	Level 12	synthesis; originality	doctorates
Evaluating		Level 7	Level 11	synthesis	master's degree; PG diploma; PG certificate
Analysing		Level 6 Year 3 of 3	Level 10 Year 4 of 4	critical evaluation	bachelor's degree with honours
			Level 9 Year 3 of 4	critical analysis; critical evaluation	ordinary bachelor's degree
Applying	Undergraduate	Level 5 Year 2 of 3	Level 8 Year 2 of 4	critical analysis; application to practice	diploma of HE; foundation degree
Understanding (comprehension)		Level 4 Year 1 of 3	Level 7 Year 1 of 4	understanding; application to practice; describing	certificate of HE
Remembering (knowledge)		Pre-university			

Notes: EW&NI = England, Wales and Northern Ireland; PG = postgraduate

The hierarchy in the cognitive domain has been instrumental in determining what is expected of university students as they progress through their studies. These **academic levels** not only reflect incremental learning but also help students and educators determine the expectations at each stage (year) of their studies. Thus, early on in your studies, you may only be expected to demonstrate knowledge and understanding of the concepts and theories you encounter (which you do through *describing*, in your own words); as you progress, you will increasingly be expected to demonstrate **critical ability** and, at the point of graduation, perhaps even **synthesis** and **evaluative** skills (at postgraduate level, you will almost certainly be expected to demonstrate these skills).

Academic levels guide the development of university courses and play a role in determining what we should test in examinations and assessments.

Examples of assessment tasks at various undergraduate levels

The descriptors typical of each level are highlighted:

- **Describe** in your own words the main biopsychosocial determinants of mental health (Level 4; Scottish Level 7).
- In helping people with low **mood**, **analyse critically** a current intervention that mental health nurses might be involved in (Level 5; Scottish Level 8).
- **Critically evaluate** the barriers and facilitators to setting up an evidence-based school mental health service for children and young people (Level 6; Scottish Levels 9 and 10).

Credit and units of learning

A degree course is typically made up of modules (or units) of learning and associated with each module will be a number of **credits**. How credits are calculated depends on your university's regulations but, typically, one credit equals 10 hours of learning or 'student effort' (importantly, credit is related to *learning*, not teaching). Thus, a 20-credit, Level 5 module requires 200 hours of student effort and will be pitched at a level appropriate for second-year undergraduates.

Credits build up into recognisable awards. For example, the standard English and Welsh Bachelors-with-Honours degree results from a cumulative total of 360 credits over three years (Year 1: 120 Level 4 credits + Year 2: 120 Level 5 credits + Year 3: 120 Level 6 credits). Credits may be transferable across universities via a process known as **accreditation of prior (experiential) learning** or 'AP(E)L'.

CRITICAL THINKING STOP POINT 2.1

The hours you do

The wily among you will have spotted an anomaly: for a degree, you need 360 credits in total or 3,600 hours of student effort. The NMC demand 4,600 hours for registration.

Does this mean a nursing course is more demanding than other university courses? Does this have any implications if you share accommodation, make friends and socialise with non-nursing students?

SKILLS ACQUISITION: WHAT YOU SHOULD BE ABLE TO DO

At this point, you probably realise that two sets of skills are required to be a mental health nurse: **intellectual skills** and **practical skills**. These also reflect the NMC's 50–50 theory–practice split.

Intellectual skills: critical thinking

Intellectual skills are the skills required to ensure that learning becomes more than simply remembering. The most important intellectual skill is **critical thinking** but it is also perhaps the most challenging.

Scholars often talk of *theories*, *hypotheses*, *models*, *concepts* or *ideas* rather than facts. If a scholar puts forward a theory, hypothesis, model, etc., it is likely that other scholars will *criticise* that view and put forward alternatives. This may be because the opposing scholar views the world in a different way to the proposing scholar or because she or he has found holes in the proposing scholar's theory that cannot be explained. Typically, there is amicable, healthy debate over these disagreements, the primary platforms for such debate being the scholarly journals and conferences. The debate tends to be 'won' by the side that has the most convincing portfolio of evidence *at a given point in time*. The italicised part of this statement is important: as time passes and as more research is undertaken, 'losers' in a debate sometimes become the victors.

A relevant example here is the concept of *schizophrenia*: critical exploration of the concept over time has led to differing views on its causes. As Table 2.3 shows, there are currently a number of competing views on **schizophrenia**, so how do you reconcile these? In terms of critical thinking, the answer is that you do not have to. Instead, you need to ensure that you are aware of the **evidence** for each view before you make any judgements about the one (if any) you are most convinced by. To get the evidence, you must **read widely**, which is why your lecturers ask you to look at lots of journal articles and books when putting essays and assignments together.

One good analogy for critical thinking is to think of a court case. We can, for example, put 'biological schizophrenia' into the dock. 'Defence' and 'prosecution' scholars provide evidence (ideally from research) to persuade you to side with them. When you have heard or read the evidence, you can then make an *informed* decision. Your decision can be one of three options: side with the prosecution (disagree with biological schizophrenia), side with the defence (agree), or sit on the fence because neither

Table 2.3 Theories of the aetiology of schizophrenia over time

Era	Theories (proponents)	Notes
Pre-industrialisation	Demonic possession	Still a common perspective in some cultures, e.g. in developing nations
1880s	Dementia praecox (Emil Kraeplin)	Schizophrenia was seen as an early form of dementia; biological origin
1910s	'Split mind' (Eugen Bleuler)	The term 'schizophrenia' is introduced to reflect the view that it is a thinking disorder not a dementia; biological origin still suspected
1940s–1960s	Psychodynamic theories (Sigmund Freud, Carl Jung)	Schizophrenia is caused by unresolved childhood conflicts; more popular in the USA than the UK
1940s–1970s	Schizophrenogenic mothers (Theodore Lidz)	Psychosocial theory whereby cold, distant parents (particularly mothers) were blamed for causing schizophrenia
1950s–present	Chemical imbalance	Schizophrenia is caused by a brain chemical imbalance; the discovery of antipsychotics (which supposedly correct the imbalance) reinforced this neurobiological view
1960s–1970s	Critical anti-psychiatry (Ronnie Laing, David Cooper)	Diverse criticisms of bio-psychiatry that pointed to certain alternative understandings and treatment options, such as Kingsley Hall and Philadelphia Houses
1970s–2000s	Stress vulnerability/'stress bucket' model (Joseph Zubin, Bonnie Spring)	Biopsychosocial view whereby everyone has an innate (genetic?) vulnerability towards developing mental illness; those with high vulnerability need little stress to be tipped into schizophrenia and vice versa
1980s–present	Humanistic views (Maurius Romme, Sandra Escher)	People with so-called schizophrenia experience the world differently; hearing voices is not a symptom of illness but a reaction to trauma or simply an aspect of some people's lived experience
1990s–present	Scientific anti-psychiatry (Richard Bentall, Mary Boyle, David Harper, Peter Kinderman, Dave Pilgrim)	A group of mostly psychologists who argue that there is no scientific evidence that schizophrenia is a disease
2000s–present	Big neuroscience	The advent of powerful brain-imaging techniques has led to a resurgence of interest in a biological view of schizophrenia

argument was strong enough to sway you. As long as you can demonstrate an appraisal of the available evidence (through reading and referencing), any one of these decisions is fine.

Practical skills

As well as intellectual skills, there are some specific practical skills that are necessary in mental health nursing. These include simple psychomotor skills associated with specific clinical procedures, such as giving depot injections, manual handling and handwashing, as well as first aid and emergency procedures like stemming blood flow from wounds and cardio-pulmonary resuscitation (CPR). As with driving and riding a bike, these skills require little intellectual input and are best learned through repetition, ideally in real or simulated practice settings.

Some practical skills, however, require greater intellectual input. These skills require the critical appraisal of specific theories and concepts and – as you will shortly discover – perhaps even a critical appraisal of yourself. They include communication and interpersonal skills, assessment skills, team-working skills, self-awareness skills and self-management skills. These higher-level practical skills are crucial for effective and compassionate mental health nursing and you will find reference to them throughout this book.

Practice assessment

As you know, your course is notionally 50% theory and 50% practice, although this divide is somewhat arbitrary because theory and practice are interdependent (see Table 2.2). Having a notional 50–50 split does, however, mean that practice as well as theory needs to be assessed.

Practice assessment tends to focus on the practical skills outlined above (whether they are simple psychomotor skills or those with a greater intellectual element) and it will often be based on a series of practice learning outcomes that you will be expected to achieve. Some examples can be found below.

Examples of practice outcomes

- PO1: The student is able to introduce her- or himself to service users and their families in a professional and approachable manner.
- PO2: The student is able to administer depot injections safely, with courtesy and compassion.
- PO3: The student is sensitive to the cultural, religious and/or spiritual needs of service users.
- PO4: Within legal and ethical bounds, the student is able to respond compassionately and sensitively to enquiries from service users' relatives and friends about their loved ones' progress and care.

CASE STUDY: DEALING WITH A DIFFICULT MENTOR

Although practice outcomes are technically a subset of ILOs, they differ subtly from the more general module or course outcomes. First, while module outcomes can be met in a variety of ways (via lectures and seminars, directed study, group work, tests, etc.), practice outcomes can only be met in practice. Second, the person assessing practice outcomes needs to be rooted in practice and she or he is normally a registered nurse from the same field of practice (the NMC call this 'due regard') who has also undertaken a course in how to assess students in practice. These assessors even have their own name: **mentors**. Finally, practice outcomes are usually 'threshold' outcomes in that students are not graded numerically but judged merely on a pass/fail basis as to whether they meet a standard or not (in some sense, they are more **competencies** than outcomes).

> The relationship with your mentor is crucial to your success in practice. A mentor can make or break a placement. Most mentors are great: they will hold you back when you're over-confident and encourage you when you lack confidence. Good mentors will help you identify your strengths and the areas in which you need to develop, and they will encourage you to reflect on your practice, perhaps by sharing some of their experiences as a student.
>
> Of course there are some poor mentors. It's important that if you feel placement is not going well or you have a 'clash of personality' with a mentor that you discuss this with someone like a practice education facilitator, the unit manager or your personal tutor or module lecturer.
>
> **Peter, third-year mental health nursing student**

ATTITUDES AND VALUES: PERSONAL QUALITIES

The third domain important for NMC registration concerns the personal qualities – the attitudes, values and beliefs – of the people entering, and pursuing a career in, nursing. Indeed, 'values-based recruitment' has been an essential element of all NHS recruitment since the Francis Report (2013). These personal qualities also matter because the NMC requires a statement of good health and *good character* from the university before a student can first enter the register, and continuing good health and character are a requirement for remaining on the register at periodic revalidation. This latter point is particularly important because, once on the register, your behaviour is expected to be fitting to that of a nurse, or, as the Code states, is such that you 'uphold the reputation of your profession at all times' (NMC, 2015: 15). Even something as seemingly trivial as posting a picture on social media of you 'worse for wear' can threaten the reputation of mental health nursing; making racist, sexist, ageist or homophobic comments certainly will, and is likely to lead to disciplinary action from your employer, the NMC or indeed both.

Compassionate care

Think about what might determine 'good character' and you have a list of the values that are essential for nursing: trust, honesty, a caring nature, compassion, empathy, and so on. Recent scandals – the serious care failings at the Mid Staffordshire Trust during 2007–2009 (Francis, 2013), the mistreatment of people with learning disabilities at Winterbourne View in 2011 (Department of Health, 2012) and, more recently, the failure to investigate unexpected deaths at Southern Health Trust (Mazars, 2015) – have meant that the attitudes and values of nursing staff have been under intense scrutiny. Some used these failings to argue against graduate nursing (the 'too posh to wash' argument; see Rolfe, 2014), while others welcomed an opportunity for nursing to reaffirm its core principles. England's Chief Nursing Office, for example, reinforced *care, compassion* and *commitment*, along with *courage, competence* and *communication* in her '6Cs' initiative (Department of Health/NHS Commissioning Board, 2012).

Common factors and the therapeutic alliance

Another core reason as to why the attitudes and values of those working in mental health matter, arises from research into 'common factors' in therapy. These are the factors which consistently appear in analyses of successful outcomes in therapy. Contrast them with therapy-specific factors such as the theoretical perspective (psychodynamic, humanistic, cognitive-behavioural, etc.) or treatment modality (face to face, online, telephone, etc.). Common factors include things such as the **therapeutic alliance**, the **warmth** of the therapist, a feeling of **partnership**, therapist **self-awareness** and **self-reflection**, and the use of **feedback**. Importantly, these are also the sorts of things that the service user voice at the beginning of this chapter alluded to. As much as 70% of the effect in therapy may be down to common factors compared to as little as 15% for specific factors (Imel & Wampold, 2008). In other words, the 'active ingredient' in any therapy may be dependent on the therapist's – *your* – personal qualities more than anything else.

Attitudes towards learning

Since nursing is now firmly embedded in the university sector, another important personal quality is a student's attitude towards learning and her or his expectations of university-level study. If you are straight out of school or college, the educational approaches we use may be very different to what you are used to. We expect you to be an *independent* learner who takes responsibility for your own learning. While we create **environments** and use techniques to help you think and act independently, you need to show **initiative**, **motivation** and a certain degree of **self-discipline** and **resilience** if you are to succeed in your studies. This is especially important given that nursing degrees, in combining work and study, demand 1000 hours (around a day a week) more learning than most other degrees.

REFLECTION POINT 2.1

Linking theory and practice

In a practice-based discipline like mental health nursing, learning can be seen as a cyclical process whereby both theory and practice develop through two complementary processes (see Figure 2.1). I have called the theory-to-practice link **testing** simply because ideas or theories are tested out in practice. There is, however, also a practice-to-theory link which I have termed **refining** because theories might be refined as a result of the student *reflecting* on practice.

Being able to reflect on your experiences, actions or practice (and write about them) is a skill that can enhance your learning dramatically: because the process is cyclical, it can both change your way of thinking (theory) and the way in which you practise.

Reflection is not merely describing or passively observing something that has happened. It is a skill that is closely related to **critical thinking**; indeed, reflection is perhaps nothing more than a *critical appraisal of yourself and your actions*.

Writing reflectively

Being able to write reflectively is one of the easiest ways of demonstrating an ability to reflect. You will have to write reflections throughout your career: as assessments of formal learning, for personal and professional development, to remain on the register at periodic revalidation and to enhance clinical practice. Reflective writing sometimes permeates whole modules, or even entire courses of study, via **reflective diaries** (sometimes called reflective journals or logs). Reflective diaries are a key component of **professional portfolios**.

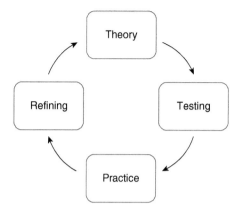

Figure 2.1 A learning cycle for the acquisition of knowledge

Source: Pryjmachuk, 1996

The **critical incident technique** (see, for example, Smith & Russell, 1991) is useful for helping students both identify events that are good for reflection and as a reflection framework. A critical incident is an event or situation, positive or negative, that is incredibly important – *critical* – in defining who you are. Obvious critical incidents include the death of a loved one or the birth of your first child, but events such as your first day on placement, failing an assessment or receiving a thank you card from relatives can all be critical to your development as a mental health nurse.

Students sometimes find it useful to use a reflective model to help them write reflections, the most well-known being *Gibbs' Reflective Cycle* (Gibbs, 1988), the *Model of Structured Reflection* (Johns, 2013) and the *What? Model* (Driscoll & Teh, 2001).

CRITICAL THINKING STOP POINT 2.2

Reflection and feedback

Receiving feedback, whether verbally or in writing, is an ideal opportunity for reflection. If some specific feedback has made you upset (or, indeed, happy), try to work out what it is about the feedback that has made you feel that particular way and whether there is anything from your analysis (your reflections) that can help you grow and achieve in the future. For example, if you have just received a low mark or a ward manager has taken issue with your behaviour, ask yourself whether you are upset simply because you have been (rightly) criticised or because you do not agree with the feedback and want to challenge it.

A particular form of reflective practice common in mental health is **clinical supervision** (see, for example, Butterworth et al., 2007; Cassedy, 2010). Clinical supervision has its roots in counselling and psychotherapy, and is an approach whereby a practitioner meets regularly with a supervisor to discuss and reflect on their caseload or clinical practices. There is more on clinical supervision in Chapter 42 of this book.

FACILITATING AND ENHANCING LEARNING: THE STAFF-STUDENT PARTNERSHIP

Education is essentially the process of facilitating and enhancing learning. Primary and secondary education – education aimed at *children* – is often 'didactic': a one-way process where the teacher imparts information to a hopefully willing recipient. Higher education necessarily focuses on *adults* and the process tends to be two-way, reflecting a staff–student partnership philosophy that most universities have. Though some didactic methods are used in higher education (the lecture being the obvious example), most universities employ a variety of teaching and learning methods. In this final section, we will explore the principal teaching and learning methods employed in (mental health) nurse education and consider the staff and student factors that underpin successful learning.

Student factors in successful learning

Earlier, when talking about attitudes, I mentioned that success in your studies requires initiative, motivation, self-discipline and resilience. Being reflective is also likely to enhance your learning. While these are prerequisites to successful learning, there are other factors that may influence how you learn. In particular, acknowledging any personal learning (or learning style) preferences you have might also help you succeed. You may be reflective enough to already know what works for you but, if not, there are some tools out there that can help identify your learning preferences: the *Learning Styles Questionnaire* (Honey & Mumford, 1986) and the *VARK* questionnaire (Fleming & Mills, 1992), for example, are easy enough to find on the Internet.

Educator factors in successful learning: alignment and evidence-based teaching

There are two key ways in which educators can help you succeed in your studies. The first is to ensure that what you learn is relevant to what you need to do as a future mental health nurse; the second is to ensure that the teaching and learning methods employed are appropriate and effective.

Constructive alignment (Biggs & Tang, 2011) is an approach that ensures that what you learn will be relevant to mental health nursing. In this approach, educators directly *align* any teaching and learning activities (assignments, projects, seminars, etc.) to the ILOs. Rather than passively receive information, students *construct* meaning from these activities which helps them not only achieve the ILOs but also engage in deeper learning.

The best lecturers always explain at the beginning of a session or activity what it is all about and why it is relevant to me as a future mental health nurse. They encourage us to think for ourselves, ask questions without us feeling stupid and give us feedback on how we are doing.

Aleah, mental health nursing student

Table 2.4 Instructional architectures in higher education

Architecture	Examples	Notes
Receptive *Little student–teacher interaction; passive learning experiences*	*Traditional* Attending a lecture Reading a textbook *Technology enhanced* Watching a video Lecture capture	Likely to lead to surface learning Good for briefings; poor for skills development
Directive *Generally short sessions with immediate feedback*	*Traditional* Seminars and tutorials *In vitro* (lab-based) practice learning; clinical skills laboratories *Technology enhanced* Simulated skills training xMOOCs	Good for teaching novices or procedural skills An xMOOC is a type of MOOC or *Massive Open Online Course*. xMOOCs are short online courses based on traditional university courses that are open to anyone but with limited teacher–student interaction
Guided discovery *Problem-focused learning where teachers are essentially coaches*	*Traditional* Enquiry-based learning (problem-based learning, case studies) *In vivo* (real-life) practice learning Collaborative learning Game-based learning Role play *Technology enhanced* Simulated learning Digital games (gamification)	In *collaborative learning*, students work together on a task assigned by a teacher but without the interdependence of cooperative learning (see below) *Simulated learning* can involve either virtual patients (no specialist equipment is needed; its simplest form is *role play*) or specialist equipment, e.g. interactive resuscitation mannequins
Exploratory *Learning where there is a high degree of learner control*	*Traditional* Projects Cooperative learning *Technology enhanced* Internet courses with significant learner control, e.g. cMOOCs	In *cooperative learning*, students are required to work *interdependently* to complete a task assigned by a teacher – the opposite of *competitive* learning A cMOOC is a MOOC where groups of students *construct* (hence the 'c') knowledge without a formal instructor

Source: Clark, 2008

Regarding teaching and learning methods, Clark (2008) argues that there are four broad types of what she calls 'instructional architecture'. These are the design frameworks in which various teaching and learning methods sit (see Table 2.4).

It is likely that you will be exposed to almost all of the methods within these architectures during your course, but how effective are they?

CRITICAL DEBATE 2.2

Evidence-based teaching and learning?

- Despite a significant amount of literature arguing that learning is most effective when 'meshed' with **specific learning styles** ('mind-maps' for visual learners, audio-recordings for auditory learners, etc.), a comprehensive literature review (Pashler et al., 2008) found no evidence for meshing.
- **Passive learning** approaches like the lecture are not especially effective (which begs the question why we continue to use them); **active learning** (guided discovery and exploratory) methods, on the other hand, are (Freeman et al., 2014).
- **Cooperative learning** can promote the acquisition of higher-order intellectual and interpersonal skills; the evidence for **collaborative learning** is not as robust but there is some evidence of positive effects; **problem- and other enquiry-based styles of learning** elicit positive results for cognitive, developmental and affective outcomes but mixed results for knowledge acquisition (Davidson & Major, 2014).
- **Simulated learning** has some evidence of effectiveness but it is not necessarily superior to other methods (Cook et al., 2013); **virtual patients** are cheap compared to other simulation methods and can be helpful in developing clinical reasoning skills (Cook & Triola, 2009).
- The evidence for **game-based learning** and **gamification** is mixed: Domínguez et al. (2013) found that gamified experiences can result in higher motivation and better scores in practical assignments but weaker performance in written assignments and lower participation in class activities.

CONCLUSION

Hopefully, at the end of this chapter, you are fully aware that a combination of knowledge, skills and attitudes are required for entry onto the NMC register. You should be aware of the contributions that you personally and your lecturers need to make in order for you to achieve in your studies. You should also now know why your lecturers emphasise critical analysis and thinking skills, reflective practice and the evidence base, and why you need to keep tabs on how you behave – professionally, publicly and socially – in your journey to become a compassionate, service user-centred, effective mental health nurse.

CHAPTER SUMMARY

This chapter has covered:

- The range of knowledge and skills possessed by registered mental health nurses
- The necessity of developing critical thinking skills
- The importance of reflective practice
- The importance of linking evidence, theory and practice
- Different models and approaches for effective learning.

BUILD YOUR BIBLIOGRAPHY

Books/book chapters

- Aveyard, H., Sharp, P. & Woolliams, M. (2015) *A beginner's guide to critical thinking and writing in health and social care*, 2nd edition. Milton Keynes: Open University Press. A useful text on understanding critical thinking and writing.
- Johns, C. (2013) *Becoming a reflective practitioner*, 4th edition. Oxford: Wiley-Blackwell. A good text for health care practitioners from the originator of Johns' Model of Reflection.
- Knowles, M.S., Holton, E.F. III & Swans, R.A. (2015) *The adult learner: The definitive classic in adult education and human resource development*. Abingdon: Routledge. A classic text on adult learning (or 'andragogy' as it is known).

SAGE journal articles

Go to https://study.sagepub.com/essentialmentalhealth for further free online journal articles related to this chapter. If you are using the interactive ebook, simply click on the book icon in the margin to go straight to the resource.

FURTHER READING: JOURNAL ARTICLES

- Goldfinch, J. & Hughes, M. (2007) Skills, learning styles and success of first-year undergraduates. *Active Learning in Higher Education*, 8(3), 259–273. A Scottish study identifying traits of successful first-year university students.
- Hansson, L., Jormfeld, H., Svedberg, P. & Svensson, B. (2013) Mental health professionals' attitudes towards people with mental illness: do they differ from attitudes held by people with mental illness? *International Journal of Social Psychiatry*, 59(1), 48–54. A study identifying that many mental health staff hold negative attitudes and beliefs about people with mental health problems.
- Pashler, H., McDaniel, M., Rohrer, D. & Bjork, R. (2008) Learning styles: concepts and evidence. *Psychological Science in the Public Interest*, 9, 105–119. A literature review challenging the value of personal learning styles.

Weblinks

Go to https://study.sagepub.com/essentialmentalhealth for further weblinks related to this chapter. If you are using the interactive ebook, simply click on the book icon in the margin to go straight to the resource.

FURTHER READING: WEBLINKS

- LearnHigher's critical thinking and reflection resources: www.learnhigher.ac.uk/learning-at-university/critical-thinking-and-reflection
- Some great e-learning resources on reflection from NHS Scotland: www.flyingstart.scot.nhs.uk/learning-programmes/reflective-practice
- An online learning styles quiz based on Honey & Mumford's questionnaire: www.brainboxx.co.uk/A2_LEARNSTYLES/pages/roughandready.htm

GREAT FOR REVISION

ACE YOUR ASSESSMENT

Revise what you have learned by visiting https://study.sagepub.com/essentialmentalhealth. If you are using the interactive ebook, simply click on the tick icon to go straight to the resource.

- Test yourself with multiple-choice and short-answer questions and flashcards.

ONLINE QUIZZES & ACTIVITY ANSWERS

REFERENCES

Anderson, L.W. & Krathwohl, D.R. (eds) (2001) *A taxonomy for learning, teaching, and assessing: A revision of Bloom's taxonomy of educational objectives* (abridged edition). London: Longman.

Biggs, J. & Tang, C. (2011) *Teaching for quality learning at university: What the student does*, 4th edition. Maidenhead: McGraw-Hill.

Bloom, B.S. (ed.) (1956) *Taxonomy of educational objectives: The classification of educational goals. Handbook I: Cognitive domain*. London: Longman.

Butterworth, T., Bell, L., Jackson, C., et al. (2007) Wicked spell or magic bullet? A review of the clinical supervision literature 2001–2007. *Nurse Education Today*, 28(3), 264–272.

Cassedy, P. (2010) *First steps in clinical supervision: A guide for healthcare professionals*. Maidenhead: Open University Press.

Clark, R.C. (2008) *Building expertise: Cognitive methods for training and performance improvement*, 3rd edition. San Francisco, CA: Pfeiffer.

Cook, D.A. & Triola, M.M. (2009) Virtual patients: a critical literature review and proposed next steps. *Medical Education*, 43, 303–311.

Cook, D.A., Hamstra, S.J., Brydges, R., et al. (2013). Comparative effectiveness of instructional design features in simulation-based education: systematic review and meta-analysis. *Medical Teacher*, 35(1), e867–e898.

Davidson, N. & Major, C.H. (2014) Boundary crossings: cooperative learning, collaborative learning, and problem-based learning. *Journal on Excellence in College Teaching*, 25(3&4), 7–55.

Department of Health (DH) (2012) *Transforming care: A national response to Winterbourne View Hospital*. London: DH. Available at: www.gov.uk/government/uploads/system/uploads/attachment_data/file/213215/final-report.pdf (accessed 06.05.16).

Department of Health/NHS Commissioning Board (2012) *Compassion in practice: Nursing, midwifery and care staff – our vision and strategy*. London: DH. Available at: www.england.nhs.uk/wp-content/uploads/2012/12/compassion-in-practice.pdf (accessed 13.05.16).

Domínguez, A., Saenz-de-Navarrete, J., de-Marcos, L., et al. (2013) Gamifying learning experiences: practical implications and outcomes. *Computers & Education*, 63, 380–392.

Driscoll, J. & Teh, B. (2001) The potential of reflective practice to develop individual orthopaedic nurse practitioners and their practice. *Journal of Orthopaedic Nursing*, 5, 95–103.

Fleming, N.D. & Mills, C. (1992) Not another inventory, rather a catalyst for reflection. *To Improve the Academy*, 11, 137.

Francis, R. (Chair) (2013) *Report of the Mid Staffordshire NHS Foundation Trust public inquiry: Executive summary*. London: The Stationery Office. Available at: www.gov.uk/government/uploads/system/uploads/attachment_data/file/279124/0947.pdf (accessed 06.05.16).

Freeman, S., Eddy, S.L., McDonough, M., et al. (2014) Active learning increases student performance in science, engineering, and mathematics. *PNAS*, 111(23), 8410–8415.

Freidson, E. (1970) *Profession of medicine: A study of the sociology of applied knowledge*. New York: Dodd Mead & Co.

Gibbs, G. (1988) *Learning by doing: A guide to teaching and learning methods*. Oxford: Oxford Polytechnic.

Honey, P. & Mumford, A. (1986) *The manual of learning styles*. Maidenhead: Peter Honey Publications.

Imel, Z.E. & Wampold, B.C. (2008) The importance of treatment and the science of common factors in psychotherapy. In S.D. Brown & R.W. Lent (eds) *Handbook of counseling psychology*, 4th edition. Hoboken, NJ: John Wiley & Sons.

Johns, C. (2013) *Becoming a reflective practitioner*, 4th edition. Chichester: Wiley.

Macdonald, K.M. (1995) *The sociology of the professions.* London: Sage.

Mazars (2015) *Independent review of deaths of people with a learning disability or mental health problem in contact with Southern Health NHS Foundation Trust, April 2011 to March 2015.* London: NHS England. Available at: www.england.nhs.uk/south/wp-content/uploads/sites/6/2015/12/mazars-rep.pdf (accessed 06.05.16).

Mental Health Taskforce (2016) *The five year forward view for mental health.* London: NHS England. Available at: www.england.nhs.uk/wp-content/uploads/2016/02/Mental-Health-Taskforce-FYFV-final.pdf (accessed 06.05.16).

Nolan, P. (1993) *A history of mental health nursing.* London: Chapman & Hall.

Nursing and Midwifery Council (NMC) (2008) *Standards to support learning and assessment in practice.* London: NMC.

Nursing and Midwifery Council (NMC) (2010) *Standards for pre-registration nursing education.* London: NMC.

Nursing and Midwifery Council (NMC) (2015) *The Code: Professional standards of practice and behaviour for nurses and midwives.* London: NMC.

Nursing and Midwifery Order (2001) *Statutory Instrument 2002: No. 253.* London: HMSO.

Pashler, H., McDaniel, M., Rohrer, D. et al. (2008) Learning styles: concepts and evidence. *Psychological Science in the Public Interest, 9,* 105–119.

Pryjmachuk, S. (1996) A nursing perspective on the interrelationships between theory, research and practice. *Journal of Advanced Nursing, 23*(4), 679–684.

Rolfe, G. (2014) Editorial: educating the good for nothing student. *Journal of Clinical Nursing, 23,* 1459–1460.

Sackett, D.L., Rosenburg, W.M., Gray, J.A., et al. (1996) Evidence-based medicine: what it is and it isn't. *British Medical Journal, 312,* 71–72.

Smith, A. & Russell, J. (1991) Using critical learning incidents in nurse education. *Nurse Education Today, 11*(4), 284–291.

WORKING WITH OTHER PROFESSIONALS

3

SCOTT REEVES AND SIMON FLETCHER

THIS CHAPTER COVERS

- The key concepts and principles which have foregrounded interprofessional teamwork
- The factors responsible for the emergence of interprofessional teamwork and its establishment as a globally relevant aspect of health and social care
- The successes and tensions embedded in interprofessional teamwork, and how nuanced dynamics influence the production and restriction of team-based activity
- The elaboration of a key conceptual framework for interprofessional teamwork
- Proposals for the future direction of interprofessional teamwork.

I have come to realise, over time, that (i) I don't know everything and (ii) I can't do everything that the service user in my care needs. When I was first qualified in the 1980s nurses were certainly seen as part of the 'team', but there was a very clear hierarchy where some members of the team were viewed as more important and more powerful. Additionally, other team members were seen as less important, were paid less, and their opinion was rarely sought; in those days they were called the 'auxiliary nurses' who, by their very title, were ascribed a marginal role. Moving from surgical nursing to mental health nursing created an immediate transition, to a sense of equality between workers and joint responsibility for care, perhaps, in part, due to the lack of uniforms worn.

However, it wasn't only about status, power and hierarchy: the knowledge and skills of other professionals such as occupational therapists, social workers and pharmacists were clearly different to mine. I realised that I could learn from them, not to be like them – their role is different to mine – but how we could each contribute different approaches and interventions to the plan of care. Without the sense of hierarchy, joint working feels easier; I felt more able to ask for opinion and less fearful of criticism for 'not knowing'. Take yesterday, for example, I saw the dietician, the psychologist, the psychiatrist, the nurse, the 'meal coordinator' and the art therapist all working together to assist a woman with anorexia to accept care and treatment and to help her to understand how she can contribute herself to her plan of care.

Michael, mental health nurse

Two service user experiences (Michelle and Julie) can be heard later on in this chapter. Their stories illustrate the benefit of interprofessional teamwork (Michelle) and how the absence of teamwork adversty affect a service user (Julie).

INTRODUCTION

In this chapter, we look at how we work with other professionals, and how we might do that positively and collaboratively. There has been growing academic and clinical attention given to interprofessional **collaboration** in health and social care over the last three decades. 'Teamwork' has developed in tandem with this, moving from a corporate buzzword into a central aspect of practice. Strategically established interprofessional agendas not only encourage teamwork, but actively facilitate and constructively critique it, enabling the notion to evolve alongside the changing imperatives of health and social care. The recognisable need for successful **interprofessional teamwork** has warranted a universal understanding of intention, objective and outcome, however there remains a lack of distinction, both terminological and practical, when the idea is discussed and implementation is attempted. It is hoped here that we can situate teamwork within this, and then use the idea to explore the extent to which the significance of **interprofessional collaboration** can not only undermine any confusion, but also foreground a more widely applicable standard of practice.

In this chapter, we will attempt to chart the core concepts and principles of teamwork, the development of teamwork amongst health and social care professionals with a deconstruction of the interprofessional teamwork literature, as well as the professional, organisational and contextual issues which **affect** interactions when working together to provide care, including the successes and tensions of interprofessional working. It will also outline key concepts and theories which help to illuminate and understand the nature of teamwork, describing the growing evidence base for the effects of teamwork interventions across clinical contexts and exploring a framework which supports this. Finally, it will discuss a range of ideas in relation to developing the conceptual, empirical and theoretical understanding of interprofessional teamwork in health and social care settings, in a way which encourages a focused model for progression.

CONCEPTS AND PRINCIPLES OF TEAMWORK

Interprofessional teamwork in health and social care settings is guided by a selection of key aims (CAIPE, 2011; Carpenter & Dickinson, 2008; Freeman et al., 2010; Hammick et al., 2007; Oandasan & Reeves, 2005; WHO, 2010). These cover the following: the collective consolidation of professional skills and knowledge in the interests of mutual benefit and enhanced **service user** care; the sharing of information about the organisation of care to ensure patients' needs are well met; the continuity of care through ongoing interaction, discussion and communication, through which interprofessional teamwork aims to reach agreement about apportioning and ensuring responsibility for patient care; and a joint approach to work which ensures that health and care services are delivered in a coordinated and effective fashion (Hughes, 2007; Miers et al., 2002).

To achieve these aims, the literature (e.g. Barr, 1998, 2003, 2013; Barr & Low, 2011, 2013; Freeth et al., 2005; Howkins and Bray, 2008) suggests that interprofessional teamwork should follow a framework based on the following:

* a common purpose – individual practitioners need to agree on and share a common purpose or aim for their collaborative work
* role definition – effective interprofessional teamwork depends on each professional having a clear role in their group or team, and also a series of meaningful tasks that they undertake
* systemic relationships – there needs to be a mutual interdependence of different health and social care professionals in their collaborative work

- shared knowledge – as no single practitioner can meet the range of needs of their patients, there needs to be a reliance on the clinical and professional expertise of others to provide care
- regular interaction – professionals need to regularly interact with one another in both a synchronous and asynchronous manner to agree on how to provide care together
- varied communication – communication needs to be undertaken in a flexible manner using both formal and informal mechanisms such as team meetings and more casual conversations
- balanced hierarchy – there needs to be a balance of leadership and democracy. We know that the hierarchical division of labour between the health **professions** can undermine interprofessional relations. Therefore, effort needs to be made to ensure that these arrangements are offset by local arrangements that encourage a more horizontal or flattened approach to leadership in teams (see Chapter 41 for a more in-depth discussion of leadership).

Other important underlying elements which interprofessional teamwork rests on include an individual willingness – individual practitioners need to be willing to engage in teamwork and to support its aims and goals. Also needed are shared planning and decision making – where there is agreement, reached by negotiation, that professionals will adopt a shared approach to planning and decision making in their collaborative work. Further, organisational support is required to ensure that senior management invests in the resources required to nurture and promote interprofessional teamwork. This creates an understanding that **interprofessional education** is needed to provide opportunities for colleagues to collaboratively enhance their teamwork skills. Regular feedback is needed to create opportunities for practitioners to discuss joint approaches to overcoming any shortfalls identified, and to also share their successes.

Additionally, a shared philosophy is a requirement to encourage agreement and a shared agenda for collaborative working. Finally, respect, trust and humour between colleagues are seen as critical to good teamwork (see Case study 3.1). Indeed, trust and respect are in many ways cornerstones of good teamwork ensuring a mutually agreed approach. But humour is also vital, as we need to be able to stand back and laugh together (Barr et al., 2005; Freeth et al., 2005; Griffiths, 1998; Hewitt et al., 2015; Reeves et al., 2010; Thomson et al., 2015).

CASE STUDY 3.1

Griffiths (1998) explores the role and influence of humour within two community mental health teams (CMHTs). Both teams consisted of doctors, nurses, social workers and occupational therapists. Audio-taped recordings of team meetings were gathered over a 12-month period to develop an in-depth understanding of how each team used humour in their collaborative work.

Findings from the study revealed that humour in both teams was used as a way of 'letting off steam' (p. 892) in relation to the general stresses and strains of working together. Humour was also regarded as a mechanism that helped team members support one another in their difficult work with patients who had serious mental health problems. It was also seen as useful in helping to maintain a cooperative relationship between the team leader and the other team members.

Griffiths further found that humour could be employed by team members to question their team leader's approach to, or opinion on, issues related to the delivery of care. Specifically, the study revealed that team members used humorous comments to 'signal their unease about certain referrals' (p. 884) to their team leader, or question their leader's preferred course of action on a patient. Often, team members' use of humour resulted in a changed course of action by the team leader.

All of the above should combine to contribute to an interprofessional **environment** which functions well and naturally evolves. These factors foreground work by Henneman and colleagues (1995), who have argued that effective teamwork 'requires many types of sharing: shared knowledge, shared values, shared responsibility, shared outcomes and shared visions', and build on Kraus's (1980) comment that interprofessional teamwork 'is a cooperative venture based on shared power and authority. It is non-hierarchical in nature'. Indeed, interprofessional tension often manifests in the distortion, exploitation or abuse of power, therefore an early and enduring recognition that hierarchy is conditional, and that professional roles and their associated perceptions are interchangeable, goes some way towards facilitating a healthy interprofessional set-up.

Reeves et al. (2010) have developed a typology which builds on the ideas presented in the interprofessional literature, and this allows us to situate teamwork with a view to defining its contemporary

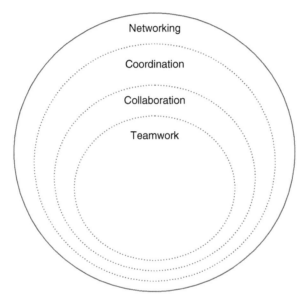

Figure 3.1 A typology of different forms of interprofessional practice

role both conceptually and clinically. The model provides a holistic analysis of the principles of interprofessional interaction, and by taking the ideas which have been collectively applied to interprofessional practice it becomes possible to see how these concepts would be enacted in a contemporary clinical setting. Figure 3.1 displays the typology, with teamwork at the centre of the model.

Interprofessional teamwork can be regarded here as the most focused activity (see Case study 3.2), requiring high levels of interdependence, integration and shared responsibility, whilst collaboration, coordination and networking represent interprofessional characteristics which are increasingly broad. We are able, in addition, to situate this typology within a clinical context by describing the interprofessional adaptation which takes place alongside a patient's trajectory of care. From hospital admission to **recovery** and rehabilitation, it is possible to follow this typology outwards. Assessing and responding to the needs of a patient who is acutely unwell requires high levels of interdependence and integration between health professions, in which teamwork, in a number of guises, is fundamental. As the patient moves through treatment and then recovery progresses, we see collaboration, coordination and finally networking emerging. Levels of urgency decrease, and discussions around **appropriate treatment** and prevention take place with a focus which encompasses wider possibility and more diverse scope for intervention. Interprofessional work is more predictable at these levels, and the collaborative imperatives are driven by long-term clinical targets. It is possible to glean from this that differing forms of work are not only important to the successful functioning of an interprofessional environment, but also needed to respond to change, as outlined throughout the operation of the typological model.

Remaining at the core, interprofessional teamwork, in its most essential state and then adapting towards the outer layers, interaction is a constant and foundational aspect of interprofessional practice.

CASE STUDY 3.2

Principles in action

Norman and Peck (1999) ran a number of workshops in which community mental health team (CMHT) members (nurses, occupational therapists, social workers, doctors) were asked to generate accounts of their own roles and identities as CMHT members. Data gathered from the workshops revealed a range of successes associated with working in a CMHT.

A number of areas were identified in which team members felt they were working well together, in an environment of focus and structure. These included:

- a strong commitment to teamwork
- a shared understanding of each other's roles and professional cultures
- regular contact between team members
- clear systems for referring clients between members and across different care agencies
- senior management support for teamwork.

CRITICAL THINKING STOP POINT 3.1

Consider the following:

- How do each of the key principles of interprofessional collaboration collectively facilitate successful teamwork?
- Can you think of an occasion where you have encountered similar collaborative interaction?
- Can you identify the motivating factors which cause teamwork to adapt as treatment moves from acute to chronic?

EMERGENCE OF INTERPROFESSIONAL TEAMWORK

CASE STUDY:
CRITICAL
INCIDENT
TECHNIQUE

There are a number of global developments which have shaped the emergence of interprofessional teamwork. Taking place over the last three decades, there have been landmark changes centring around six key areas: quality and safety; patient-centred care; chronic care; rising costs; education and training; and media coverage.

Improving *quality and safety* has provided principle justification for the implementation of effective interprofessional teamwork. The publication of the Institute of Medicine's (2000) report, *To Err is Human*, foregrounded a shift towards a public and professional recognition that the reduction of error and improvement of safety strategies should be formally prioritised. As a result, there have been a number of national quality improvement initiatives launched in an attempt to respond to a universal call for a rise in standards.

Patient-centred care represents the growing need to adapt intervention towards the needs of the patient, rather than focus specifically on the **illness**. Each individual is unique, and a fully functional treatment team will be able to provide tailored care based on reciprocal collaboration (Little et al., 2001). Whereas an approach which focuses on illness and treatment may not necessarily benefit from intervention in which there are extant hierarchies and conflicting outlooks, a collective recognition of the experience, characteristics and history of the patient serves to diminish some of these fault lines.

Chronic care signals another shift – as increasing life expectancy gives rise to more long-term illnesses, the need for calculated, prolonged therapeutic collaboration which responds to and evolves with the changing characteristics of the illnesses becomes greater. The complexity of an illness which develops over many years can be accommodated and, to a certain degree, controlled under a collaborative approach, as the adaptive qualities of teamwork and consistent evaluative communication are of particular **value**.

Rising costs can be partially reversed by a well-organised and externally supported collaborative framework. The growing impact which interprofessional teamwork has had on cost reduction has been recognised by various governments, subsequently placing collaboration in health care at the forefront of national agendas. Interprofessionalism is therefore both politically useful, as it is recognised in a way which goes beyond partisan division, and measurably influential, serving to safeguard its role as a fundamental aspect of practice.

Various approaches to *education and training* are now designed around interprofessional collaboration, although an identification that a more structured curriculum in health care education which directly explores interprofessional collaboration again reinforces how significantly collaborative interaction has developed over recent years (Barr et al., 2005; Zwarenstein et al., 2005; Reeves et al., 2013). There is now a range of learning activities aimed at engaging students and professionals in collaborative practice, as teamwork has become a subject of diverse reach and pedagogical prominence.

The heightened saturation of *media coverage* over recent years has been particularly influential in the growth and establishment of interprofessional collaboration. Increasing scrutiny and a necessary rise in standards, invoked by a heavily pluralised media marketplace, have both bolstered the uptake of interprofessional education and intervention and publicised the notion as a fundamental characteristic of contemporary health care. The way in which collaborative problems are now generally broadcast in some form encourages a transparency in health care intervention which is rendered less potent when interprofessional teamwork is in evidence.

Of course, there are other contributing factors which have led to the establishment of interprofessional teamwork, however the six mentioned above have combined to create the idea which is recognised today. Whilst teamwork is clearly a significant, even critical, aspect of a well-rounded modern health care approach, there are, as with any collaborative effort, sources of tension. In order to complete a more nuanced, critical introduction to teamwork practice, it is as important to problematise the notion in addition to its celebration. This takes place below, as we analyse both the successes and tensions of interprofessional team dynamics.

CRITICAL THINKING STOP POINT 3.2

Consider the following:

- What are the shifts which have been responsible for a move towards greater team-based intervention?
- Think about each of the six contributing factors mentioned above. How do the issues listed in Case study 3.2 fit with these areas and can you think of a specific example?

INTERPROFESSIONAL TEAMWORK DYNAMICS: SUCCESSES AND TENSIONS

As West (1996: 13) states: '[team reflexivity] involves the members of the team standing back and critically examining themselves, their processes and their performance to communicate about these issues and to make appropriate changes.' Whilst we have established that interprofessional success can be measured through the evolutionary and adaptable characteristics of teamwork, it should also be noted that collective reflexivity is central to this. The significance of self-criticism cannot be underestimated here, as we are able not only to highlight the advantages of collaborative communication, but also draw attention to the conflict which is resident when different professionals come together. Being reflexive and encouraging reflexive exchange directly address team conflict in a way which can nurture a rational, measured response to dispute. However, there remain a number of potential sources of fracture which can impede the successes which are described above and throughout.

There are, at the most basic level, temporal–spatial restrictions to consider when an interprofessional team is evaluated. For example, Handy (1999) found that placing colleagues on two different floors in a building can reduce interaction by 30%. In addition, heavy profession-specific workloads can limit time for interprofessional meetings and interactions, which in turn can undermine the quality of interprofessional teamwork. Collectively, difficulties related to time–space can result in the emergence of what Engeström and colleagues (1999) termed 'knotworking' – a state of affairs in which professionals' interactions are like threads of activity, which are temporarily tied, then untied, as they work. This type of working arrangement can be seen as a useful response to working interprofessionally over time and space (Oandasan et al., 2009; Seneviratne et al., 2009), providing a concentrated collaborative focus which is necessarily adaptable.

Miller et al. (2008) have explored the subject of emotion in nursing and its role in determining professional dynamics. They argue that greater emotional sophistication amongst nurses can lead to an authoritarian distortion when enacted under the auspices of professional hierarchy (see Case study 3.3). In addition to this is a form of isolationism motivated by what Miller and colleagues have described as a robust 'esprit de corps', serving to separate nurses from other medical staff by virtue of an emotional response to workplace tension which can only be professionally specific. Teamwork subsequently becomes difficult to accommodate, dependent as it is on emotional sensitivity, or even emotional compromise. There is almost a requirement for emotional neutrality when operating in a team, and the tendency to develop emotional **coping** strategies which emphasise professional distinction can potentially undermine this.

Responding to this in any durable sense will be challenging, as the professional individualism we refer to here is rooted in wider misconceptions about the professional context in which nurses operate. The reaction to this by nursing staff has demonstrated both pragmatism and nuance, as the mediated methods by which they communicate and interact with other professionals reflect the distorted perceptions which have shaped this working landscape. Miller et al. (2008) state that 'nurses calibrated relational attachments on the basis of perceived co-worker status. They strove to maintain "a smile on their face" when dealing with physicians, and displayed politeness rather than authority when supervising subordinates' (p. 334). The way in which they reinterpret, and to an extent avoid altogether, the hierarchies which have been reported in collaborative health care contexts, is a novel and effective way of overcoming the difficulties associated with professional isolation. Miller et al. (2008: 334) comment that as 'most health professionals have been socialized into **cultures** with strong uniprofessional foci, interprofessional relationships are often approached with some degree of **anxiety**'. This is, however, tempered by an ability to empathetically communicate with other professionals whilst simultaneously maintaining a strong sense of disciplinary identity.

The idea of exchange should also be considered, as arguably a great deal of interprofessional interaction takes place under the auspices of self-interest. As Hudson (1987) states, one needs to remember that the act of collaboration is not an altruistic one; it is important therefore to establish the parameters of mutual gain before collaboration is undertaken, in order to avoid a problematic, potentially divisive disparity in delivery. Of course, as with any collaboration, when there is mutual reliance on the fulfilment of promises there is a strong element of risk involved. Team dynamics are often highly unpredictable and an ultimate inability to account for each member makes some disagreement inevitable. Acknowledging this risk at the outset, just as the notion of exchange should be highlighted, will help to encourage a more comprehensive understanding of the nuances of collaborative teamwork, and allow for an early identification of role expectation and behavioural standards. There will obviously be tacit opposition and challenges to authority in team situations, evidenced by Beattie (1994: 115) who states, 'when individuals and groups come together ... there is representation of different and often competing interests [which] can generate tensions and conflicts'. Not only are these tensions and conflicts motivated by divergent interests, but they also potentially stem from a fear of failure and a fear of the unknown. When we join a team, we are often forced to adapt, and a subsequent collective recognition of risk can help to assuage some of the natural and, by extension, counterproductive concerns which are encountered here.

The notion of groupthink, as explored by Janis (1982), presents a further potential barrier to coherent team-working. The idea suggests that in high-pressure situations, where the consequences of error are particularly **acute**, there is a tendency amongst groups to merely agree with each other, rather than suggest an alternative. This in itself can have disastrous consequences, as an individually self-serving consensus can obscure or prevent an analysis of crisis which carries any genuine depth.

CASE STUDY 3.3

Hierarchy

Cott (1998) examined the meanings and structures of teamwork of nurses, doctors and therapists who worked in a hospital-based, long-term older adult care unit. Interviews with team members revealed the existence of two distinctive sub-groups within their interprofessional team:

- a sub-group consisting of doctors, therapists and social workers who occupied a high position in the team hierarchy
- a sub-group consisting of junior qualified and unqualified nursing staff who occupied lower positions in the hierarchy.

Cott's study also revealed that while team members in both sub-groups held favourable perceptions of teamwork, these views were largely dependent on their location in the team hierarchy. As Cott (1998: 849) states: 'Staff in different structural positions held different perceptions of meanings of teamwork because they were engaged in different kinds of teamwork.'

It was found that the sub-group consisting of doctors, therapists and social workers collaborated as equals in the team, discussing and agreeing aspects of patient care. When they needed to ask one of the nurses to undertake a task, they generally spoke to the senior nurses, who in turn would talk to one of their juniors or one of the unqualified staff. In addition, for the sub-group of doctors, social workers and therapists, teamwork was essentially viewed as vital for improving the quality of care they delivered to the patient. In contrast, the sub-group consisting of junior qualified and unqualified nursing staff viewed teamwork in less positive terms, as it involved being told what to do by their senior colleagues.

Cott goes on to conclude that teamwork for the doctors, therapists and social workers was regarded as a rewarding activity, as they occupied a high position in the team hierarchy and could influence the work of the junior nurses and the unqualified staff. Indeed, for the junior nurses and the qualified staff, who had little influence on patient care, teamwork was regarded in a different light.

Finally, and in some ways most significantly, one needs to be aware of the range of professional issues that exist, which can undermine interprofessional teamwork. The sheer diversity of medical and therapeutic professions, and their differing and, in some instances, starkly opposing processes of interaction and socialisation, make collaboration across such a network fraught with potential disruption (Leathard, 1994; Payne, 2000; Whitehead, 2001). Professional idiosyncrasy is not always conducive to collaborative engagement. As Daly (2004: 78) states:

Everyone in the NHS shares a common goal – the wellbeing and health of patients. However, this goal becomes a singular ideal within each discipline, based on the 'cure or care' aim of that discipline and the role of the professionals within it. It is this strong identity of professional groups that has led to rigid distinctions between them.

There remains a fine line between the retention of professional identity and a well-rounded collaborative experience. It should be the intention of interprofessional teamwork strategies to accommodate this and develop an appropriate, productive balance.

With these rigid professional distinctions comes the potential for power structures, and struggles, to emerge. We should acknowledge the complex politics involved in professionalisation and can use the work of Michel Foucault to enable this. Exploring the relationship between power and knowledge, Foucault has argued (1977, 1981) that perceptions of knowledge, or in this case the professional distinction which nurses display and reinforce, are wholly dependent on wider power structures. According to Foucault, knowledge is couched in social control, and it is possible to describe the complexity related to interprofessional politics described above and throughout as being embedded in this. It is also possible to assert the view that team-based collaboration is enacted as a means of responding to the problematic distinctions which professional politics create and maintain. By avoiding, or at least offsetting, the myriad power dynamics in the affirmation of a form of knowledge which has been distorted under a regime of wider social dominance, it becomes possible to regard collaborative efforts as both a product of and a reaction to broad-based systems of control. The issue of power imbalances was explored in some depth by Baker et al. (2011), who reported that interprofessional politics tended to either reinforce or attempt to restructure traditional power relationships between nursing and other professional groups.

There has been a call to develop a key framework which allows a critically conceptual and practically applicable solution to some of the challenges which are discussed above and the next section explores such intervention in more detail.

CRITICAL THINKING STOP POINT 3.3

Consider the following:

- What issues can lead to the creation of conflict in interprofessional teams?
- Why do these issues emerge in interprofessional contexts?
- What steps can be taken to remedy conflict in interprofessional teams?

A CONCEPTUAL FRAMEWORK FOR TEAMWORK

Reeves et al. (2010) have offered a useful framework for teamwork, which enables greater understanding of the factors which are necessary to both emphasise the efficacy of team collaboration and respond to the well-documented tensions that emerge in such environments. Reeves and colleagues have synthesised these factors into four main domains:

- Relational – factors which directly affect the relationships shared by professions such as professional power and socialisation.
- Processual – factors such as space and time which affect how the work of the team is carried out across different workplace situations.

- Organisational – factors that affect the local organisational environment in which the interprofessional team operates.
- Contextual – factors related to the broader social, political and economic landscape in which the team is located.

Although presented as separate, Reeves et al. acknowledge that there is some overlap here, offering further justification of a sociologically informed approach to an analysis of interprofessional teamwork. That this has not been widely explored within previous teamwork literature further supports an exploration which maps the intersections and dynamics of professional interaction and serves to suggest productive, catalytic intervention. Figure 3.2 provides a representation of the functioning of these teamwork factors.

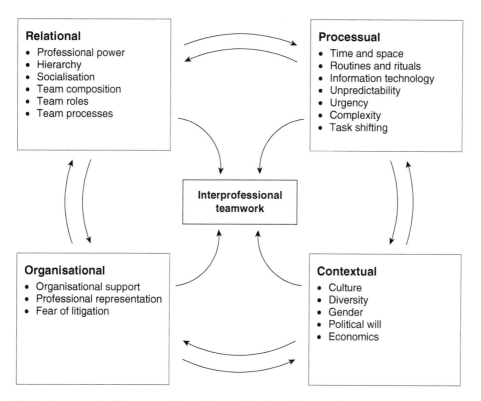

Figure 3.2 A conceptual framework for interprofessional teamwork

The interdependence displayed in Figure 3.2 should be situated within a wider recognition of the collective and individual interpretations of each factor, and how the additional points provide further explanation. For example, hierarchical differences between team members place them in different social and economic relations with one another, thereby undermining the quality of their relations. In addition, the roles which members adopt can either generate friction (if roles are unclear) or support team performance (if roles are negotiated and agreed between members). The processual factors presented indicate how the nature of elements such as time and space, routines and rituals and unpredictability can affect how interprofessional teamwork is actually undertaken. Limited time and too many demands can mean professionals have little opportunity to focus on strengthening their collaborative work. Organisational factors including support for resources are key to the effective functioning of interprofessional teams. The focus related to the contextual factors presented above adds width to the issues surrounding teamwork and moreover allows practitioners and service users alike to benefit from a systematic understanding of the myriad challenges associated with collaborative effort.

CRITICAL THINKING STOP POINT 3.4

Consider the following:

- How does the conceptual framework allow us to highlight the benefits of interprofessional teamwork?
- How does the conceptual framework allow us to respond to the tensions which can be generated by interprofessional teamwork?
- How well does the model represent your experiences of interprofessional teamwork?

TEAMWORK SUCCESSES AND FAILINGS: STORIES FROM THE BEDSIDE

The following vignettes are representations of the real-life experience of instances which benefitted from effective interprofessional teamwork (Michelle) or were affected by its absence (Julie) in two different clinical settings:

My nine year old son, Gary had been complaining of nausea and severe headaches so we made an appointment with our GP. She carried out a number of tests on him and asked us all sorts of questions about his diet and medical history. After pressing his stomach and asking if it hurt, Gary said yes, although as the pain wasn't significant this didn't seem to give us any definite diagnosis so we were all left unsure.

He was referred to a gastroenterology specialist, Dr Malik, at the local hospital who we met with the following week. We sat down in his office and he began to talk through the information which our GP had provided him with. By this time Gary had been feeling a lot worse and had been off school. He said that he had spoken with Dr Allen from our surgery on the phone last night and they were both in agreement that an ultrasound scan would be the way forward. I must have looked concerned as the doctor quickly emphasised that this was simply routine, saying that they just wanted to rule out anything nasty. We braced ourselves for what would no doubt be a protracted wait for an appointment, however Dr Malik quickly picked up his phone and started tapping in a number. He liaised with the person on the other end, appearing friendly, jovial and personable. After the conversation had ended he announced that he had managed to pull some strings and there was an opening this afternoon at 3 o'clock.

We were met by Dr Malik outside the ultrasound room on the fourth floor. As we entered he greeted the nurse and began another playful interaction with her. It was revealed that she had also been in contact with our GP, Dr Allen, that day and began to talk through the particulars of the conversation with Dr Malik. As the scan was taking place he called Dr Allen. He walked back into the room, surveyed the screen and nodded. He pointed to something in the top right-hand corner and uttered something indiscernible to the nurse who smiled in what seemed to be agreement and admiration. He announced that Gary had a bowel condition called *diverticulitis* and would need to stay in hospital overnight as a precaution. They put him on a course of antibiotics, however his symptoms remained and he was still in a great deal of pain. He was required to remain in hospital for a further three days during which time Dr Malik organised a consultation with the nurses who had seen Gary, a pharmacist and a nutritionist. Together they devised a more 'holistic' treatment plan, as they called it, and rather than just giving him pills they looked at the problem from a range of angles.

I was struck by the way that the staff who helped worked together to get to the bottom of my son's condition as quickly and efficiently as they could. Whilst the problem isn't that serious, the symptoms were worrying and it was a real relief to have been dealt with by staff who not only placed Gary's welfare at the forefront but also knew instinctively what steps needed to be taken to get round a tricky diagnosis.

Michelle, service user

I had been suffering with migraines for a number of weeks and decided to visit my GP. I made an appointment and saw the doctor who assessed me and my history and asked me to monitor the situation. I was rather frustrated by what I felt was a hurried dismissal. I had been a patient of his for nearly 20 years so this felt rather callous under the circumstances. I sought a second opinion at the same surgery. Whilst the original doctor, one who has treated myself and my family for many years was the practice manager, the doctor that I elected to gain a second opinion from was much younger and in his first post. Having been seen by him, after the migraines had continued and if anything, intensified, he suggested that I should be referred to a specialist at the local hospital. He said he would liaise with the nursing staff and arrange an appointment for me. I was pleased as it felt as though we were making progress, not to mention the fact that I was in some discomfort. I had a brief discussion with one of the senior nurses who reassured me that an appointment would be made soon.

Weeks went by without any indication of when I would be seen. I made another appointment for the GP, this time with my original doctor in a deliberate attempt to get things moving. As I was in the waiting room I saw the nurse who assured me that I would get a quick referral. She explained that she had been advised by one of her nursing colleagues to talk to a more senior GP before actioning the request, as the second doctor had not been in post long and was therefore under what they described as 'diagnostic scrutiny'.

I spoke to the doctor and explained the situation. He had no knowledge of the original intention for referral and on assessment agreed that I would need to see a specialist in the next few days. I was asked to wait for a short while after the consultation and was approached by a different nurse who gave me a date and time for my hospital appointment. I was both relieved and angry, not just at the lack of communication, but at the way in which my referral was delayed by nothing more than an assumption. There was a lot of manipulation here which could have been responsible for me not getting a referral at all. Whilst in hospital the scan revealed that I would require surgery to remove an awkwardly placed ganglion which if left, could have caused a blood clot.

Julie, service user

CRITICAL THINKING STOP POINT 3.5

Reflect on these narratives and try to identify the following:

- the advantages of communication between staff members
- the problems associated with role definition and hierarchy.

MODELS OF PROGRESSION

The complexities involved in working collaboratively and furthermore forming and sustaining teams are both numerous and challenging. There is, however, considerable potential in the organised, systematic and sensitive development of teamwork in health and social care. In order to bolster our understanding of the efficacy of collaborative teamwork and the influence of the practice itself, there are a number of possible ways forward. These cluster around developing, implementing and influencing a range of interprofessional interventions linked to:

- *Interprofessional education* – interventions that could aim at delivering formal collaborative learning activities such as simulated learning or team retreats, as well as informal learning activities.
- *Interprofessional practice* – interventions aiming at changing the nature of interprofessional meetings to ensure they have more opportunities for shared problem solving, the development of interprofessional checklists and pathways, and the use of information technology to support interprofessional activities that span time and space.
- *Interprofessional organisation* – interventions could produce organisation-wide guidelines and procedures that strengthen teamwork, as well as reconfiguring workplace space to foster more opportunities for interprofessional interaction and communication.
- *Interprofessional policy* – attempting to influence the production of regional and national health policies to ensure an explicit focus on interprofessional teamwork, and also similarly target professional regulatory bodies and accreditation agencies to lobby for the adoption of more team-based approaches in policy and regulation.

Combining aspects of each of these areas will help foster a collaborative climate which benefits from an interprofessional foundation. Attempting to form team-based strategy will be far easier if enacted within a climate which readily facilitates this, and by reinforcing a collaborative narrative from conceptual, practical, political and educational positions, it becomes possible to (i) influence perceptions surrounding teamwork and (ii) tailor intervention around collaboration instead of vice versa. Rather than focusing efforts on implementing single interventions, which can only generate limited results, there is a need to design, implement and evaluate multiple interventions consisting of education, practice and organisational activities. As such, any potential impact can be further-reaching and hopefully more sustainable.

CRITICAL THINKING STOP POINT 3.6

Consider the following:

- What can be done in order to maintain an effective approach to interprofessional teamwork?

- How effective will the suggestions stated above be when it comes to safeguarding the future of interprofessional teamwork?
- Think about what has facilitated your own interprofessional teamwork and how this can be applied to future interventions.

CRITICAL DEBATE 3.1

Give some thought to the different multi-professional teams you may have worked in. Call to mind two examples: (i) the team that exhibited the best team-working; (ii) the team that didn't really work as a team.

1. Make a list of the characteristics of each team that, in your view, help make the distinction between good and not-so-good team-working.
2. Consider your list in relation to the categories of 'relational', 'processual', 'organisational' and 'contextual', discussed in this chapter. How might these concepts help you to make sense of what makes a good team and how you might think about improving the team-working of your weaker team?
3. What relational nursing skills, in particular, might you transfer to the context of improving team-working?

CONCLUSION

Given what has been discussed above and throughout, if interprofessional teamwork is to establish itself in health and social care in a meaningful and sustainable way, it will be important to consider the following issues. First, it will be particularly important to focus on generating robust, clinically significant outcomes in relation to both team performance and patient care. An interprofessional operation which overlooks the experiences of the service user is, by definition, poorly functioning, and this must be made explicit to the team from the outset. Second, there is a real need for the generation of good quality qualitative data which seeks a full understanding of the changing nature of team dynamics in tandem with the shifting imperatives of health and social care. Talking with key stakeholders, in both treatment and recovery contexts, will encourage the generation of a fuller picture of the failures and successes of contemporary teamwork and, as such, processes of narrative development should not be overlooked. Third, the aim and scope of interprofessional teamwork research should be more far-reaching. Rather than focusing on single-site studies, work should take place which accommodates multi-institutional investigations, itself engendering greater collaborative possibility. Fourth, there is genuine value in an explicit economic measurement of both the cost and benefit of interprofessional teamwork intervention. Financial constraints are often responsible for the restriction of team-based strategies, however when the intervention itself is responsible for raising costs, specific analysis will also be required. Finally, the study of interprofessional teamwork will benefit greatly from the application of social science which accommodates and deconstructs the intricacies of team-working. Diversifying conceptual approaches, and encouraging methodological techniques which have seldom been seen in the study of team-based interaction, will potentially enable the consolidation of interprofessional teamwork as a fundamental aspect of health and social care, and also uncover new meaning in an area which is clearly rich in revelatory potential.

CHAPTER SUMMARY

This chapter has covered:

- The value of interprofessional teamwork within contemporary services
- The key concepts and principles which help make sense of interprofessional teamwork
- The factors responsible for the emergence of interprofessional teamwork and its establishment as a globally relevant aspect of health and social care
- The successes and tensions embedded in interprofessional teamwork, and how nuanced dynamics influence the production and restriction of team-based activity
- The elaboration of a key conceptual framework for interprofessional teamwork: relational, processual, organisational and contextual
- Proposals for the future direction of interprofessional teamwork.

BUILD YOUR BIBLIOGRAPHY

Books

- Day, J. (2013) *Interprofessional working: An essential guide for health and social care professionals.* London: Cengage Learning.
- Pollard, K., Thomas, J. & Miers, M. (2009) *Understanding interprofessional working in health and social care: Theory and practice.* Basingstoke: Palgrave Macmillan.
- Reeves, S., Lewin, S., Espin, S., et al. (2010) *Interprofessional teamwork for health and social care.* Oxford: Wiley-Blackwell.

Journal articles

- Hall, P. (2005) Interprofessional teamwork: professional cultures as barriers. *Journal of Interprofessional Care, 19*(s1), 188-196.
- Hewitt, G., Sims, S. & Harris, R. (2014). Using realist synthesis to understand the mechanisms of interprofessional teamwork in health and social care. *Journal of Interprofessional Care, 28*(6), 501-506.
- Thistlethwaite, J., Jackson, A. & Moran, M. (2013) Interprofessional collaborative practice: a deconstruction. *Journal of Interprofessional Care, 27*(1), 50-56.

Weblinks

Go to https://study.sagepub.com/essentialmentalhealth for further weblinks related to this chapter. If you are using the interactive ebook, simply click on the book icon in the margin to go straight to the resource.

FURTHER
READING:
WEBLINKS

- Canadian Interprofessional Health Collaborative: www.cihc.ca
- Centre for the Advancement of Interprofessional Education: www.caipe.org.uk
- European Interprofessional Practice and Education Network: www.eipen.eu

ACE YOUR ASSESSMENT

Revise what you have learned by visiting https://study.sagepub.com/essentialmentalhealth. If you are using the interactive ebook, simply click on the tick icon to go straight to the resource.

- Test yourself with multiple-choice and short-answer questions and flashcards.

ONLINE
QUIZZES &
ACTIVITY
ANSWERS

REFERENCES

Baker, L., Egan-Lee, E., Martimianakis, M.A. et al. (2011) Relationships of power: implications for interprofessional education. *Journal of Interprofessional Care, 25*, 98–104.

Barr, H. (1998) Competent to collaborate: towards a competency based model for interprofessional education. *Journal of Interprofessional Care, 12*(2), 181–187.

Barr, H. (2003) Ensuring quality in interprofessional education. *CAIPE Bulletin, 22*, 2–3.

Barr, H. (2013) Enigma variations: unravelling interprofessional education in time and place. *Journal of Interprofessional Care, 27*(S2), 9–13.

Barr, H. & Low, H. (2011) *Principles of interprofessional education*. Fareham: Centre for the Advancement of Interprofessional Education.

Barr, H. & Low, H. (2013) *Introducing interprofessional education*. London: CAIPE.

Barr, H., Koppel, I., Reeves, S., et al. (2005) *Effective interprofessional education: Argument, assumption and evidence*. Oxford: Blackwell.

Beattie, A. (1994) Healthy alliances or dangerous liaisons? The challenge of working together in health promotion. In A. Leathard (ed.) *Going interprofessional: Working together for health and welfare*. London: Routledge.

CAIPE (2011) *Principles of interprfessional education*. Fareham: CAIPE Centre for Advancement of Interprofessional Education.

Carpenter, J. & Dickinson, H. (2008) *Interprofessional education and training*. Bristol: Policy Press.

Cott, C. (1998) Structure and meaning in multidisciplinary teamwork. *Sociology of Health and Illness, 20*, 848–873.

Daly, G. (2004) Understanding the barriers to multiprofessional collaboration. *Nursing Times, 100*(9), 78–79.

Engeström, Y., Engeström, R. & Vahaaho, T. (1999) When the center does not hold: the importance of knotworking. In S. Chaklin, M. Hedegaard & U. Jensen (eds) *Activity theory and social practice*. Aarhus: Aarhus University Press.

Foucault, M. (1977) *Discipline and punish: The birth of the prison*. Paris: Gallimard.

Foucault, M. (1981) *The history of sexuality*. Paris: Gallimard.

Freeman, S., Wright, A. & Lindqvist, S. (2010) Facilitator training for educators involved in interprofessional learning. *Journal of Interprofessional Care, 24*(4), 375–385.

Freeth, D., Hammick, M., Reeves, S., et al. (eds) (2005) *Effective interprofessional education: Development, delivery and evaluation*. Oxford: Blackwell.

Griffiths, L. (1998) Humour as resistance to professional dominance in community mental health teams. *Sociology of Health and Illness, 20*, 874–895.

Hammick, M., Freeth, D., Koppel, I., et al. (2007) A best evidence systematic review of interprofessional education. *Medical Teacher, 29*, 735–751.

Handy, C. (1999) *Understanding organizations*, 4th edition. London: Penguin.

Henneman, E., Lee, J. & Cohen, J. (1995) Collaboration: a concept analysis. *Journal of Advanced Nursing, 21*, 103–109.

Hewitt, G., Sims, S., Greenwood, N., Jones, F., Ross, F. & Harris, R. (2015) Interprofessional teamwork in stroke care: is it visible or important to patients and carers? *Journal of Interprofessional Care, 29*(4), 331–339.

Howkins, E. & Bray, J. (2008) *Preparing for interprofessional teaching: Theory and practice.* Oxford: Radcliffe Publishing.

Hudson, B. (1987) Collaboration in social welfare: a framework for analysis. *Policy and Politics, 15*(3), 175–182.

Hughes, L. (2007) *Creating an interprofessional workforce: An education and training framework for health and social care.* London: CAIPE.

Institute of Medicine (2000) *To err is human: Building a safer health system.* Washington, DC: National Academies Press.

Janis, I. (1982) *Groupthink: A study of foreign policy decisions and fiascos,* 2nd edition. Boston, MA: Houghton Mifflin.

Kraus, W.A. (1980) *Collaboration in organizations: Alternatives to hierarchy.* New York: Human Sciences Press.

Leathard, A. (1994) *Going interprofessional: Working together for health and welfare.* London: Routledge.

Little, P., Everitt, H., Williamson, I., et al. (2001) Preferences of patients for patient centred approach to consultation in primary care: observational study. *British Medical Journal, 24*(322), 468–472.

Miers, M., Barrett, G., Clarke, B.A., et al. (2002) *Evaluating an interprofessional curriculum: Meeting the research challenge.* Bristol: FHSC/UWE.

Miller, K.-L., Reeves, S., Zwarenstein, M., et al. (2008) Nursing emotion work and interprofessional collaboration in general internal medicine wards: a qualitative study. *Journal of Advanced Nursing, 64*(4), 332–343.

Norman, I. & Peck, E. (1999) Working together in adult community mental health services: an interprofessional dialogue. *Journal of Mental Health, 8*, 217–230.

Oandasan, I. & Reeves, S. (2005) Key elements for interprofessional education part 1: the learner, the educator and the learning context. *Journal of Interprofessional Care, 19*, 21–38.

Oandasan, I., Gotlib, C.L., Lingard, L., et al. (2009) The impact of time and space on interprofessional teamwork in Canadian primary care settings: implications for healthcare reform. *Prim Health Care Res Dev, 10*(2), 151–162.

Payne, M. (2000) *Teamwork in multiprofessional care.* Basingstoke: Macmillan.

Reeves, S., Lewin, S., Espin, S., et al. (2010) *Interprofessional teamwork for health and social care.* Oxford: Wiley-Blackwell.

Reeves, S., Perrier, L., Goldman, J., et al. (2013) Interprofessional education: effects on professional practice and healthcare outcomes (update). *Cochrane Database of Systematic Reviews, 28*(3), CD002213.

Seneviratne, C., Mather, C. & Then, K. (2009) Understanding nursing on an acute stroke unit: perceptions of space, time and interprofessional practice. *Journal of Advanced Nursing, 65*(9), 1872–1881.

Thomson, K., Outram, S., Gilligan, C., et al. (2015) Interprofessional experiences of recent healthcare graduates: a social psychology perspective on the barriers to successful communication, teamwork and patient centred care. *Journal of Interprofessional Care, 29*, 634–640.

West, M. (1996) *Handbook of work group psychology.* Chichester: Wiley.

Whitehead, C. (2001) Collaborative practice. *Nursing Standard, 15*(20), 33–38.

World Health Organization (WHO) (2010) *Framework for action on interprofessional education and collaborative practice.* Geneva: WHO. Available at: www.who.int/hrh/resources/framework_action/en/index.html (accessed 02.08.17).

Zwarenstein, M., Reeves, S. & Perrier, L. (2005) Effectiveness of pre-licensure interprofessional education and post-licensure collaborative interventions. *Journal of Interprofessional Care, S1*, 148–165.

MEANINGFUL SERVICE USER INVOLVEMENT

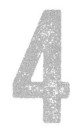

JULIA TERRY AND THE SWANSEA UNIVERSITY SERVICE USER AND CARER INVOLVEMENT GROUP FOR HEALTH PROGRAMMES

THIS CHAPTER COVERS

- What helps make service user involvement meaningful
- How mental health nurses and student nurses can facilitate meaningful service user involvement
- Different types of involvement.

> I am a survivor
> I am a survivor and I don't know how and I don't know why
> But I know I will feel even better when I have had a little cry
> The nurses appear, take my pulse and listen to my chest
> Then whisper to themselves 'all she needs is a good night's rest'
> So I'll just lay here and contemplate my life
> And imagine a world that's free from strife
> It will feel good again to feel the warm sun on my face
> I will be free once more to greet the human race
> So I'll gather my scars and my old sore bones and soldier on
> I will learn once more to fight another cold grey morn
> I will not just lie here and die
> I'll leave this ward with my head held high
> And if I can't run anymore who gives a jot?
> I have got my sanity and today that's worth such a lot
> I'll try to be patient
> I'll try to be brave
> Because I know that even I
> Will one day keep my appointment
> with that good survivor in the sky
>
> **Lucy, service user**

> During my career as a mental health nurse I have seen a mixed picture of people being involved in their care. I have seen many service users worried and uncomfortable in ward rounds and excluded from care planning in a system that can seem all powerful. I have also seen people starting to challenge, to ask more questions, to debate care with health workers which fills me with hope. I believe that people can be involved in their own care in both big and small ways, and that these are all achievements. I believe that nursing students need to have the opportunity to learn how people can be involved in their own care, in service development and in education programmes. This can be best achieved by listening, thinking and either taking action or encouraging service users to take action themselves.
>
> **Jenny, mental health nurse**

INTRODUCTION

This chapter explores the subject of meaningful **service user** involvement and relates to involvement activities in both individual care and treatment in mental health services, as well as involvement in the planning and delivery of those services. The term service user refers to people who use services in health or social care (Levin, 2004).

USEFUL FOR
ASSIGNMENTS!

CASE STUDY:
HARRY

The chapter starts with discussion about the term meaningful user involvement, and service users' expectations of involvement. This will be followed by a section on how involvement has changed and progressed over time, including a look at the advantages and disadvantages of being involved. **Stigma** and attitude change to mental health problems will briefly be explored, as these have relevance for meaningful involvement. This will be followed by a discussion about involvement in care planning, shared decision making and the benefits for all involved. The issue of representation will be examined, including related factors that **affect** both individuals and services. This will be followed by user involvement in service development, along with examples. User involvement in nurse education has become a focus across the UK, as all health professional programmes are required to demonstrate how service users are included in the teaching, planning and delivery of programmes – and this will briefly be explored. As there are many barriers to meaningful involvement, solutions to address these will be discussed at the end of the chapter, along with ideas on how professionals might listen to service users in different ways. Service user involvement is a two-way opportunity – for service users to voice their views and concerns and for professionals to listen to those concerns. The chapter will conclude with key messages for mental health nurses.

REFLECTION POINT 4.1

Take a few minutes to think what meaningful service user involvement means to you, and of good examples you have seen or been part of in practice:

- What helped to make the involvement meaningful?
- What did the service user say about their involvement?

THE LANGUAGE OF HEALTH CARE

Language defines and shapes our understanding and has been used to wield power. As such, it has been used to pathologise, dominate and discriminate against people who have lived experience (National Survivor User Network, 2014).

The terms used to refer to people who use mental health services have changed significantly over the past 30 years. Traditionally, the NHS has used the term 'patient' or 'client'. Such terms have received criticism from those who argue that it incorrectly positions people who use mental health services (particularly those with long-term conditions) as passive recipients of care (McLaughlin, 2009; Coldham, 2012). The political context of the 1980s and 1990s, with its emphasis on the growth of the market economy, saw a move towards the privatisation of mental health services. Within this discourse, health and social care was viewed as a product. It led to the view that patients or clients should be viewed as 'customers' or 'consumers' (Rush, 2004; McLaughlin, 2009). Mental health services became commodities to be bought and sold and the 'customer' or user of services was positioned as someone who was able to choose between the different public, private and voluntary sector services on offer. The terms 'customer' and 'consumer' have been widely critiqued for their emphasis on the notion of individual 'choice'. Choice is empowering if it genuinely enables a person to make decisions about their health and life. However, such choice may not be afforded to all service users as people may be disadvantaged by geographical differences in provision, service criteria and financial constraints, to name just a few.

Another key term is that of **carer**, which is widely used to refer to family members or friends who provide frequent support to someone experiencing mental distress. However, this term is also fiercely contested. Sayce et al. (2012) use the more inclusive term 'families, friends and carers' for three related reasons:

- Many people experiencing mental distress have objected to the term 'carer'. This is because key relationships, such as spouse, parent, child or friend, are ignored and the reciprocity and complexity of these relationships are reduced to a 'one-way street of care'.
- Some carers see their role as part of their family responsibility and do not readily identify with the label carer.
- There are diverse socio-cultural views on caring, and support within families and friendship circles differs between communities. For example, many community languages do not have a term for carer. (Sayce et al., 2012)

The term family also varies widely between communities and is not easily translatable. Furthermore, the categories of 'service user' and 'carer' are not necessarily distinct as carers can also be service users themselves (Coldham, 2012).

WHAT IS MEANINGFUL USER INVOLVEMENT?

Meaningful service user involvement indicates that there is active engagement and participation from individuals who use services at all levels of service provision. Service user involvement can take many forms and occurs in many different ways. Essentially, it is about making sure that the views of the people who use services have the opportunity to be heard, in order to make real, sustainable changes and improvements, both to their own care and to services generally.

As nurses, we need to ask ourselves if service users are really involved in situations, and question how truly empowered they actually are. Nurses can experience challenges with service user involvement and may not understand the best way forward. We may have to wrestle with what real levels of involvement are and consider whether people feel meaningfully involved. Nurses can feel that involvement is tokenistic, or be part of a system that some mental health service users feel is against them.

As there are many ways that service users can get involved in the development and delivery of services, it is good practice to assess the level of actual user participation. One of the available tools to assess user involvement is Arnstein's (1969) ladder of citizen participation (see Figure 4.1). Arnstein's ladder shows eight different types of participation, with minimal participatory activities at the bottom, moving up to increasing amounts of participation at the top. Whilst there is a sense that the participation or involvement of citizens is a desirable activity, there is a sense of power present, by 'those' who allow participation in the first place. Power and involvement will be explored later in the chapter. Suffice it to say that user involvement can be meaningful, with individuals experiencing a sense of partnership and influence. Conversely, user involvement may be minimal and tokenistic. This chapter will explore some of these differences, along with the issues that impact on the actual type of involvement people experience.

Meaningful service user involvement takes time and effort to develop, and needs constant monitoring and improvement to meet people's changing needs.

CRITICAL THINKING STOP POINT 4.1

What types of skills are essential for nurses to facilitate meaningful service user involvement?

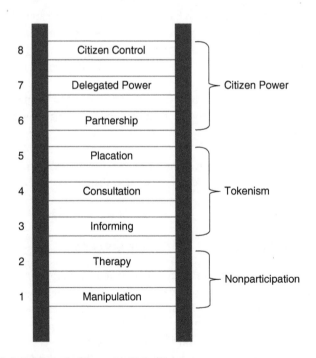

Figure 4.1 Arnstein's ladder of citizen participation

Source: Arnstein (1969) Taylor and Francis, adapted with permission

REFLECTION POINT 4.2

What do you think service user expectations are of service user involvement?

CASE STUDY 4.1

Ask a service user you are working with about their expectations in relation to their current care.

Service users' expectations of involvement

Service users' expectations of involvement may vary. Historically in health services, a culture of paternalism has existed. The notion that the doctor or nurse knows best has permeated both health service culture and mainstream society. Traditionally, service users were not accustomed to being asked their views, or given choices regarding their health care and treatment.

The NHS Constitution for England 2013 sets out patients' rights and states that patients have the right to be involved in discussions and decisions about their health and care. Equally, this extends to involvement in health service provision:

> You have the right to be involved, directly or through representatives, in the planning of healthcare services commissioned by NHS bodies, the development and consideration of proposals for changes in the way those services are provided, and in decisions to be made affecting the operation of those services. (DH, 2013: 9)

Similar policies exist in other parts of the UK. Scotland has the Patient Rights (Scotland) Act (Scottish Government, 2011), which aims to improve people's experience of using health services, and encourages increased involvement. Ireland has the European Charter of Patients' Rights 2002. Wales does not appear to have an actual charter, but NHS patients' rights in the NHS in Wales are available. Focusing on mental health, Wales is the only part of the UK that has unique mental health legislation that centres on the support that should be available for people with mental health problems. The Mental Health (Wales) Measure 2010 was passed by the then National Assembly for Wales and has the same legal status in Wales as other mental health acts.

Integrated care is about improving the service user experience and there being increased efficiency from health care services (Lawn, 2015). It is important that patient care is better coordinated and more continuous, and that the patient's perspective remains a central organising principle throughout (Shaw et al., 2011). Such integration can only be brought about by relevant models and methods that involve a shared vision to improve the care experience.

The National Institute for Health and Care Excellence (NICE, 2011) quality standard for service user experience in adult mental health outlines the level of service that people using NHS mental health services should expect to receive. This NICE standard seeks to **drive** quality improvement regarding the experience of people using adult NHS mental health services, with a focus on easy access to services. The 15 statements in the NICE quality standard are aspirational and include statements such as:

- Service users are actively involved in shared decision making and supported in self-management.
- People using mental health services feel confident that the views of service users are used to monitor and improve the performance of services. (NICE, 2011)

These types of statements certainly encourage an ethos of involvement and may result in raising users' expectations:

> Since I came into mental health nursing over 20 years ago I have seen a lot of change. It is fundamentally a good thing that people are more aware of their rights, and that service users can be involved in their care. My role in this is about promoting choice and working together with people to promote recovery. It is a journey that sometimes neither the service user nor me know where we will go, but if we walk the path together we will learn a lot along the way. Essentially user involvement is about lots of things especially trust on both sides and ensuring people have a choice.
>
> **Jill, mental health nurse**

CRITICAL THINKING STOP POINT 4.2

How would you have a conversation with a service user about their experience of being involved in their mental health care?

CASE STUDY 4.2

Since Cris arrived on the unit, he had spent a lot of time talking with Marie, the nurse responsible for coordinating his care. They had looked together at the leaflets about care planning and discussed Cris' expectation about being in hospital and thinking about the steps he wanted to take over the next few months. Cris said he was keen to be discharged home soon, but needed help with things to do with his accommodation and finances. He said he had got very stressed in the last few months which led to an increase in drinking alcohol. Cris told Marie that he had lost confidence in going out socially and become quite withdrawn.

Together, they looked at different options in the community that could be helpful. At Cris' request, Dave from the DrinkAware team visited Cris on the unit and made an appointment to meet up after Cris' discharge home. Marie asked Cris about the relationship with his community mental health nurse, who used to visit a long time ago. Cris said he didn't want to see anyone regularly, and had been discharged, but said he did want to join a local group that got him out of the house. Marie talked with Cris about a local mental health charity, and asked Cris if he would like to meet the charity's peer support worker who visited the ward each week.

Questions

- Did you think Cris was involved in his care?
- How could he have been more involved?

USER INVOLVEMENT: CHANGING TIMES

It has been suggested that if you want to know how good a restaurant is, you should ask the diners (according to Matt Muijen, former director of the Sainsbury Centre for Mental Health); hence the concept of asking service users how services might be improved (McGowan, 2010).

While we may consider user involvement in service improvement a new venture, in fact it has been around for a long time. One early example of mental health service users lobbying for improved care dates back to 1620 when people from the House of Bedlam petitioned the House of Lords, stating that they were being treated inhumanely by being forced to entertain the public in exchange for clothing and food, as well as being physically mistreated and shackled.

A wide range of legislation and policy has gradually developed the concept of user and carer participation in the provision and evaluation of services. This previously included the Care Standards Act 2000, the Health and Social Care Act 2001 and the Carers Recognition and Services Act 1995. However, much of this legislation has been superseded by the recent Health and Social Care Act. It remains to be seen how far service user and carer involvement will continue to be embraced by the current government. Participation has developed at different rates throughout the UK, with a range of national and international projects arising mainly from campaigning bodies and voluntary organisations.

Since the 1990s, there has been increased user involvement activity across the NHS, in think-tank report groups, government policy and local services (McGowan, 2010). The implication has been that since the NHS and Community Care Act 1990, the message from government has been to get service users involved wherever possible. The NHS and Community Care Act 1990 required local authorities to prepare care plans and to consult with groups that represented people who used services. However, there are many examples where user involvement has been considered purely tokenistic. For example, inviting one or two service users to meetings about service developments, where plans may be underway and service users have limited information, is unethical, and implies participation at a very low rung on Arnstein's ladder. Situations where people are consulted or informed does not equate to meaningful involvement. Instead, users should have a sense that their views matter and their input can impact on service changes.

Mental health service users have a unique **insight** into the very nature of mental **illness** and mental health care, putting them in a position of expertise. However, this expertise, although readily available, has been largely ignored and untapped by mental health professionals, & has not been valued by those in power to make a difference (Campbell, 1998). Perkins & Goddard (2004) argue that meaningful user involvement requires far more than getting a service user to add their signature to a **care plan** or to be part of a committee meeting. Meaningful involvement requires a major cultural change at strategic, operational and individual levels – strategically in relation to the planning and development of services; operationally in terms of service users evaluating their experience of services; and at an individual level, involvement means making choices and decisions about individual treatment and support (Perkins & Goddard, 2004).

A range of sectors, including the voluntary sector and charitable organisations, are more actively involving their users. For example, the Big Lottery Fund stipulates that beneficiaries should be involved at the beginning of the process of applying for grant funding. Regardless of the sector, whether health services, education, research or voluntary organisations, relevant principles concerning involvement are recognised. These include:

* being clear about the purpose of involvement and being open about boundaries
* service users choosing to be involved at a level that they feel is appropriate to them and their circumstances at the time
* appropriate supports to become involved and sustain, develop or withdraw (this includes payment and feedback)

- respect for people's contribution and time
- making involvement accessible by providing information and guidance in good time
- trying to recognise and overcome barriers to involvement.

It is acknowledged that whilst user involvement is generally thought to be a good thing, there will naturally be advantages and disadvantages (see Table 4.1). If those facilitating involvement as well as those users involved are aware of these, solutions are far more likely to be found. Frequently, individuals and organisations report that the biggest barriers to user involvement activities are money and time (Terry, 2013).

Table 4.1 Advantages and disadvantages relevant to user involvement

Advantages	Disadvantages
<ul><li>Empowering for individuals</li><li>Opportunity to learn skills and build confidence</li><li>New opportunities</li><li>Can monitor progress and provide feedback</li><li>Have the benefits of user insight re impacts and approaches</li></ul>	<ul><li>People may not wish to be involved</li><li>Expectations may be raised and lead to disappointment</li><li>May be conflict between users and others in terms of what is best</li><li>Time and commitment required to involve users</li></ul>

There are a range of terms used to refer to people who use mental health services, with perhaps service user being the most in use at the moment. You will also hear the word '**survivor**', which refers to people who have lived through mental health problems or the consequences of a life event. Another version of this term is 'psychiatric survivor'. This is more a rights-based term which implies that a battle has been won, that someone encountered mental health services and lived to tell the tale. Psychiatric survivors might say that some forms of mental health treatment are abusive, and campaign for reforms to end the powers of psychiatry. Psychiatric survivors are particularly concerned about issues that relate to compulsory detention and enforced treatments that are against people's will.

REFLECTION POINT 4.3

It is worth taking time to consider how an individual service user views themselves. Do they see themselves as someone who engages with or uses mental health services, or as someone who has survived the system?

In user involvement literature, reference is often made to the limited empowerment that is actually on offer in mental health services. Such limited empowerment devalues involvement, and users are frequently aware that professionals will always have a higher status and therefore hold more power than them (McKeown et al., 2014). The service user themselves is an expert with lived experience and may be far more knowledgeable than the mental health nurse about what it's like to live with a particular mental health problem.

Service user involvement rather unsettles the power and control dynamics in the very fabric of health and care services, particularly those sited in more traditional institutions (Carr, 2007). There is a clash of concepts and principles apparent between **citizenship** and consumerism, which often only comes to light when challenges are wrought by service users, their families or recovery-focused workers. Carr (2007) highlights that power is all-pervasive within mental health services, yet often overlooked in discussions about user involvement.

Social movements can be described as groups of people who actively resist dominant forms of power and seek social change (Toch, 1965). Such groups of people may share an oppressed identity, which would certainly ring true for mental health service users. The mental health service users' survivor movement can be described as being in opposition to 'expert' medical knowledge. In this sense, service user/survivor activism is a form of identity politics framed by people's relationship to mental health problems and contact with services (Rogers & Pilgrim, 2010). Some commentators have questioned whether institutional approaches to service user involvement go far enough to give authentic voice to these political aspirations, or might be organised in ways that limit true democratic involvement (Hodge, 2005). Cooke and Kothari (2002) go further to claim that government interest in involvement is a smokescreen for broader social control objectives.

McGowan (2010) notes that some users have been around services long enough to have a greater depth of knowledge than many staff. Indeed, it is suggested that mental health services are a major disappointment to many who come to work in them (Brandon, 1991). Whether through staff burnout or low morale, there is a sense that user involvement as a driver for change will challenge the status quo, where motivation may be lacking in NHS staff.

CRITICAL THINKING STOP POINT 4.3

Why are mental health survivors ideally placed to be meaningfully involved in user involvement activities, whether to do with their individual care or service development?

REFLECTION POINT 4.4

'User involvement ... remains in the gift of provider managers, in so far as they retain control over decision making and may expect users to address the organisation-set agendas and conform to their management practices' (Rogers & Pilgrim, 2010: 257). Do you think this is true, and if so why?

Getting involved in ward based activities is a creative way to learn about service users; don't be afraid to join in and potentially look silly! You often learn a lot about someone when they feel relaxed and they can witness your fun side. Also don't be afraid to be human. My fear of balloons bemuses a lot of patients, but it also makes me relatable in the sense that no one has it all together all of the time. Service users respect honesty.

Lisa, mental health nursing student

STIGMA AND ATTITUDE CHANGE

It is worth noting that although many positive changes have taken place regarding the status and treatment of people living with disabilities, traces of tradition still influence present-day practices (Wa Munyi, 2012). It has been reported that mental health service users do feel stigmatised. This includes feeling shunned by mental health professionals, particularly in relation to certain diagnoses, such as **personality disorder** and post-traumatic stress disorder (Mental Health Council of Australia, 2011).

Public attitudes to mental illness are changing for the better. It is hoped that as mental health problems become more acknowledged, there will be wider acceptance in communities of people experiencing mental distress. Rethink, along with other leading mental health charities, researched public attitudes to mental illness as part of the anti-stigma programme Time to Change. The aim of the research, commissioned by the Department of Health (Time to Change, 2013), was to monitor changes in public attitudes towards mental illness over time. It was reported that attitudes towards integrating people with mental illness into the community have generally improved since 1994. For example, agreement with the statement 'The best therapy for many people with mental illness is to be part of a normal community' increased from 76% in 1994 to 81% in 2012, and agreement with 'No-one has the right to exclude people with mental illness from their neighbourhood' increased from 76% in 1994 to 83%. This indicates that the views of the general public have improved towards people with mental health problems.

Health promotion programmes such as the Time to Change campaign suggest that we should help end mental health discrimination by raising awareness about the stigma of mental illness. This campaign proposes that by talking with and supporting people we help to reduce isolation. There is a suggestion in Time to Change that the effects of mental illness are as real as a broken arm or leg, which may be offensive to service users, who would suggest there is little comparison.

In relation to staff attitudes, a significant correlation was shown between those who reported optimistic views of their own personal **recovery** and those who perceived the professionals they saw as holding positive views about their recovery too (Mental Health Council of Australia, 2011). This indicates that the attitudes of others do impact on how people view their mental health.

On British television, the first programme about mental illness was screened in 1957, called *The Hurt Mind*, featuring people from Warlingham Park Hospital (Croydon), who spoke about their experiences of mental distress. There was much controversy about the powerful psychiatrists depicted in the series and their biased explanations of physical treatments of mental illness. However, such programmes may have exposed the general public, perhaps for the first time, to the experiences of people living with mental illness.

The idea of service users having a voice in the nature and delivery of their treatment or services provided was a concept that was not readily accepted initially by all professionals and managers. The attitude of many was 'we know best what is good for you'. Many also feared that people were going to shout and make unrealistic demands, and were concerned there would be unmanageable requests when the authorities were financially challenged.

From 1969, strategies and white papers for people with learning disabilities began to include the opinions of people who needed support services. The intention was that they have a say in their lives. Progress for people with physical disabilities and mental health problems developed many years later.

REFLECTION POINT 4.5

What have you witnessed regarding meaningful user involvement in mental health services? Thinking of some examples where you have seen progress, how was that achieved?

MEANINGFUL INVOLVEMENT IN CARE PLANNING

In health and social care, a care plan is a way of signposting care and agreeing service provision. There is little focus on this in the policy and practice literature regarding the skills involved (Lloyd, 2010), so it is imperative that time is spent developing the necessary knowledge in professional education programmes. It is important for mental health nurses to develop the skills of how to involve service users in care planning. This will ensure that nurses learn how service users can be meaningfully involved in developing and evaluating their care experiences.

There is an onus on health professionals to provide accessible and timely information to new and existing service users about ways in which they can be involved in discussions and decisions about the care they receive. For example, on admission to an **acute** admission unit service users (and their carers) need to be provided with information about the **environment**, day-to-day amenities and activities, as well as about services users' rights. Equipping and facilitating individuals (and their families) to be involved is the first step. Service users may be unwell and find it difficult to concentrate on a wealth of verbal information. The provision of written information in an accessible format, in the service user's language of choice, is vital:

As a student nurse I have found that working closely with service users and involving them in their own care planning has the best outcomes. Those who have a say in and control over steering the direction of their own care seem more confident to make beneficial changes with the added benefit of staff support to succeed. This creates truly holistic, balanced relationships based on mutual trust and respect. Bear in mind that we may have differing ideals to that of the service user but we are not planning care for ourselves; it is for them. We must be mindful of differing beliefs and respect this.

Lisa, student

Knowing what to expect from a hospital admission or a community team intervention will go some way to allay anxieties, and will also provide service users and their families with useful contact details and information. Service users who are detained in hospital under a section of the Mental Health Act (England & Wales 1983, revised 1997) need to have prompt information about their rights and access to an **advocate**. Advocacy services in mental health have developed significantly in the last 20 years, and seek to challenge the discrimination often experienced by mental health service users. Advocacy ensures that people are able to speak out and enables people to:

- express their views and concerns
- access information and services
- defend and promote their rights and responsibilities
- explore choices and options. (Mind, 2010: 3)

The provision of health care has been influenced by a number of models over time. In terms of those models and those most suited to user involvement, this is worth some exploration. The medical model, which has been dominant in psychiatry since its inception, is **disease**-focused and relies on diagnosis and treatment. The service user is expected to comply with such treatments and report on their progress. This makes user involvement unlikely, as the power differential between doctor and patient is rather skewed. However, models such as the biopsychosocial model or the holistic model open up far more opportunities for users to be fully involved in their care. Such models give more scope for users to discuss their strengths and aspirations, and create an environment of user-centred care.

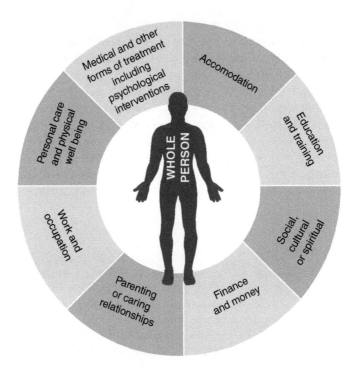

Figure 4.2 Whole-person approach

Source: Hafal, 2012, reproduced with kind permission

For example, in Wales, since the introduction of the Mental Health (Wales) Measure 2010, each care coordinator is required to discuss eight areas of people's lives in order to adopt a whole-person approach (see Figure 4.2).

Meaningful involvement in care starts with nurses ensuring that relevant and timely information is provided to service users. It is important that this is followed up by time with service users for people to discuss their queries and concerns. Care planning is an ongoing process and service users need to be involved at all stages of the discussion and decision making. This will occur in hospital and community settings (see example below).

EXAMPLE OF CARE PLANNING WITHIN A HOUSING ASSOCIATION SETTING

In the course of my work in sheltered housing, I experienced meaningful involvement in a different way. Here the work meant that you were exposed to people whose conditions were not always apparent on meeting them. Naturally many conditions develop over time, and as people relax or learn to accept your presence in their lives they open up and you begin to see conditions that may need to be referred on.

> The use of even the most basic care plan can provide the opportunity to help keep the relationship on a professional footing, while allowing staff to gain valuable information and trust. Part of your mission is to establish these 'multi-disciplinary' support teams for each resident. It will involve getting to know the family, medical contacts, spiritual contacts and social networks that people have. It is vital that residents in a sheltered housing setting have access to a professional advocate or friendly support worker. This facilitates people being involved in their care on an ongoing basis.
>
> *James*, practitioner

The National Institute for Mental Health in England and the Care Services Improvement Programme (NIMHE/CSIP) developed tools as part of the Making a Real Difference (2007) programme. The tools were intended to raise standards of involvement more widely in other organisations, and included:

- clarity
- inclusiveness
- equality of treatment
- positive attitudes
- good communication
- helpful information
- physical accessibility
- robust procedures and systems
- giving support
- providing resources
- meaningful involvement
- considering practical issues.

These tools relate to many aspects of user involvement, and if nurses focus on ensuring the above are present, this will promote good practice and promote involvement in joint care planning.

BENEFITS OF INVOLVEMENT IN CARE PLANNING: WORKING TOGETHER

The benefits of being involved in your own care are wide and varied. Many service users speak positively about the importance of having choices as part of the care planning process. Mental illness itself and the experience of living with it can have a huge impact on your dignity. During a period of mental ill health, people may have limited insight, or act in ways that are out of character. If individuals are able to influence their care and make choices, this will go some way to keeping their dignity intact, and may limit their feelings of powerlessness.

The care programme approach was introduced in England in the early 1990s, and its purpose was to ensure a system of care is in place for all individuals who require input from secondary mental health services. Essential elements are the appointment of a key worker who needs to remain in contact with the service user, and it is the key worker's role to monitor and coordinate care, and ensure regular reviews of that care.

Rethink highlights that care coordinators should fully involve service users in producing the care plan. This is important so that individuals know what support will be provided and who is responsible for ensuring that support is provided. It is good practice for care plans to state detail regarding what to do in a crisis, so that family and friends know who to contact in an urgent situation (including useful contact details). It is important that a review date is part of the care plan, so that it remains current and service users know when to expect a review of their care (Rethink, 2013). Service users can expect to have a copy of their care plan, and a copy should be sent to the GP and made available to family members, with the service user's consent.

Individuals who feel they have been fully involved in developing their care plans are far more likely to engage in services. One essential part of the mental health nurse's role, whether in a hospital or community setting, is to encourage this to occur.

It is worth noting that the term involvement appears in the care programme approach literature in the context of the involvement of the **multi-disciplinary team** and various staff roles. It is in the recovery literature that the term involvement refers more to the user themselves being involved in their own care and decision making.

It is essential that mental health staff from all sectors communicate effectively and regularly in order to ensure effective care provision. When service users are aware that members of the multi-disciplinary team communicate regularly with each other, there is increased confidence in service provision and a sense of joint working. Watch the language here:

Which of the following indicate meaningful user involvement in care planning?

a.   Simon participated in his care plan discussion.
b.   Simon adhered to the treatment policy.
c.   Simon was asked his opinion about the care plan.
d.   Simon talked through choices for his care plan and said he was now able to choose a treatment that he thought would help him towards recovery.

SHARED DECISION MAKING

Shared decision making is about the process of enabling service users to participate meaningfully in their own care by ensuring accessible information and choice (Adams et al., 2007). Taking advantage of clinicians' expert knowledge, shared decision making is then combined with the service user's values, circumstances and attitude to risk, and puts the individual in the driving seat so they can decide what is important to them (The Health Foundation, 2015). It is a big cultural shift from the traditional passive patient and expert professional model. It does mean that service users are more motivated to adhere to treatment plans, as they have been part of the care planning process and understand the thinking behind their care.

However, nurses need to challenge themselves and consider whether the service user really is in the driving seat, or if we are happy only if they are driving down the street we want them to (or the way services want them to go). Service users often create and suggest non-medical and non-psychological options for treatment. Suggestions made by service users need to be fully explored and discussed. We need to find ways forward together that allow for disagreement. As professionals, we need to question the usefulness of mental health services from the perspective of users themselves (Rogers & Pilgrim, 2010). If people do not find a **value** in services, then what is the point in their existence?

When service users are at the centre of decision-making processes concerning their own lives, they feel more empowered. It is important for individuals to see their right to choice respected, to be able to access information to make choices and to recognise that they have the same rights and responsibilities as others (Hafal, 2012). This may include **advance directives**, so others know how people want to be treated when they are unwell.

Some service users may not wish to be involved in their care planning processes. Professionals need to recognise and respect the wishes of individuals, and to be aware that these may change. The very nature of mental illness can have an influence on motivation, energy and activity levels. It is essential that service users, and their families, if people have consented to this, have useful and accessible information which relates to their care and treatment and how to access help. It is not uncommon for individuals to become more involved when their health improves.

REPRESENTATION: REFLECTING OTHERS' VIEWS

Whilst having service users involved in service planning and development is essential, it is worth considering how the service users involved are initially recruited. Any involvement may require certain knowledge, skills or experience, but there needs to be equity and fairness in order that a range of service users have the opportunity to be involved. Some service users have a representative type role, particularly if they are a service user representative from an organisation, charity or group. There may be mechanisms for users to go back and share information and to consult a wider group of individuals in order to obtain broader views.

Although service users may see themselves as ideally placed to represent the views of other users who may not be able to speak to staff candidly, McGowan highlights that knowledge of one's own difficulty does not translate as 'automatic insight into someone else's; and that using services equals knowing how to improve them' (McGowan, 2010). These issues are worth considering, as one or two service user representatives on a committee may simply be individuals who are not representing a wider service user community but simply their own views. This may be tokenistic, but it depends on the purpose of each particular involvement initiative. Clarity at the start of any project or meeting will help all those present to be clear about the nature of the involvement. There is a dilemma on how to obtain real representation, with one challenge being how to reach people who are least able to participate (Social Care Institute for Excellence, 2015). However, it is possible to involve hard-to-reach groups, and those who are seldom heard, by investing time and using methods that work for those groups.

There is a need to continually refresh user groups and to have ongoing strategies to recruit new service users. If there is a lack of mechanisms for linking with local user groups, those who have difficulty getting their voices heard may often be left out. The risk of having self-selected users may also mean that the the usual suspects are called on time and time again. Extending opportunities for the wider community to participate is important, with increased accessibility by using community venues. Equally, having a critical mass of service users will avoid tokenism.

User groups may be established with a particular aim, for example to ensure a user perspective in professional education programmes or to involve local people in a service improvement like setting up a new mental health treatment centre.

USER INVOLVEMENT IN MENTAL HEALTH SERVICE DEVELOPMENT

The saying 'Nothing about us without us' has been used to communicate the message that no policy or decision should be decided without the full participation of members of the group affected by the policy. This usually relates to marginalised groups and includes mental health service users and carers, whose voices have often not been heard.

The saying has its roots in Central European political traditions and came into use in the UK in the 1990s, often used within the disability rights movement. Mental health user groups and charities have fought hard during the past few decades to ensure the voices of service users are heard. For example, the National Involvement Partnership (2013) is clear about its mission which ensures user involvement remains current (see Figure 4.3).

THE NATIONAL INVOLVEMENT PARTNERSHIP

Our mission: to provide a platform that facilitates mental health service user and carer engagement wherever needed.

Our people: our network of over 11,000 people and groups across the country, which includes:

- old hands – experienced in engagement
- new hands – whose life experiences can be more current and more relevant
- diverse communities
- creative people, who may have developed, for instance, training or research.

Another tag line used in relation to participation is 'Having a voice, having a choice', which means the chance to have a voice when decisions are being made that affect you. This has links with the United Nations Convention on the Rights of the Child. The ethos and philosophy of involvement and participation share much in terms of values and principles, whether they are applied to health care settings, education or the voluntary sector. The National Children and Young People's Participation Standards in Wales highlights the importance of the following:

1. Information is easy for children and young people to understand.
2. It's your choice – you have enough information and time to make good choices.
3. No discrimination – every child and young person has the same chance to participate.
4. Respect – your opinion will be taken seriously.
5. You get something out of it – you will enjoy the experience.
6. Feedback – you will find out what difference your views have made.
7. Improving how we work – adults will ask you how they can improve how they work for the future.

Figure 4.3 The National Involvement Partnership

Whether service user involvement in mental health services is considered to be rhetoric or reality, it is worth noting the ongoing power differentials that exist in mental health services. Around half the people who are admitted to an inpatient setting in England are sectioned or detained under the Mental Health Act 1983; this Act of Parliament covers the care and treatment of people with mental health problems, with legislation as to how an individual can be admitted, detained and treated. For service users to know that they can be treated without their consent, effectively rendering people powerless, means that user involvement needs careful consideration in these circumstances. Some individuals feel they live with a constant threat that if they do not comply with certain treatments, they are likely to be subject to an assessment for a section of the legislation. This is particularly applicable to service users who are subject to **community treatment orders**.

Just as the early superintendents who ran Victorian mental asylums were seen as very powerful, so service users still have a sense that power exists today in mental health services, whether in hospital or community settings. It may be assumed that it was in the mid-1980s that mental health service user movements really started to become active. However, protests against the mental health system have occurred since the creation of mental hospitals 200 years ago (Campbell, 2005). Power can impact on the reality of service user involvement both in the individual's care and treatment and in user involvement in service planning and development. There is a sense that progress is slow in convincing managers and professionals that user involvement is a social and political right, not a privilege. Even though progress may be frustratingly slow at times, and involvement may seem like rhetoric, the democratisation of provision has political currency for all political parties, which is likely to continue.

Mental health service users have been encouraged by increasing numbers of active service users, and perhaps by the growing numbers of celebrities, politicians and public figures who are talking about their own mental health issues, which can help to de-stigmatise mental illness.

Branfield and Beresford's (2006: 1) report for the Joseph Rowntree Foundation, entitled *Making user involvement work*, contains the following quote, highlighting some of the 'them and us' issues:

> At first I didn't want to know other people who were disabled, I didn't want to be one of 'them', but gradually 'them' becomes 'we' and 'us' and you realise that talking and being with 'us' is where we get our strength. We can have a more powerful voice and perhaps we can make a difference.

'Them and us' often refers to two groups of people who perceive themselves as different, often because one has more power than the other. In the above quote, the service user does not wish to be considered one of them, but with time has changed. Equally, the 'them' and 'us' depends on how you identify your own position in relation to others. Reflecting back on Arnstein's ladder of participation, there is far more 'us' as a collaborative whole on the higher rungs:

> Sheffield Hearing Voices Group ... Is a weekly self-help support group open to anyone who experiences Paranoia or Hearing Voices. The facilitators are highly supportive and experience paranoia or voice hearing themselves.
>
> The strength of self-help groups is that you can speak to others who have 'been there', and you can find encouragement, reassurance, support and a listening ear. Group members say this group reduces isolation, and is an informal environment where people can share their fears and worries.

(Hearing Voices Network, 2016)

REFLECTION POINT 4.6

- What organisations or local groups have you visited where you have seen good examples of how people are properly involved?
- If you need guidance, ask a mentor/local colleague about a group that does involvement well and go and visit it.

EXAMPLES OF INVOLVEMENT IN MENTAL HEALTH SERVICE DEVELOPMENT

> When I moved to Swansea, my first experience of user participation was the Patient's Council and Swansea Network User Group. Both these groups are organised by a coordinator and consist of patients in hospital and in the community who have access to meaningful discussion with the authorities.
>
> The first campaign that I was involved with in 2001 was the Joseph Rowntree funded research into conditions in the local psychiatric hospital. Patients who had been discharged participated in questioning other patients and discharged patients on their opinion of hospital treatment and facilities. A few patients, including myself, made a television and radio appearance, and also contributed to articles in the local press. These exercises have gone a long way to help in making the substantial improvements in hospital services experienced today.
>
> **Ann, service user**

In 2010, Wales saw the agreement of the Mental Health (Wales) Measure, a piece of mental health legislation. Consultation was held by staff from the Welsh Assembly Government, covering changing of the Care Plan, individual involvement and the Independent Advocacy Scheme. From this, an All Wales Forum has been democratically formed with representatives of users and carers from all over Wales. A local forum has also been set up in each of the eight health authority areas, with the idea that important issues and developments should be discussed locally and then on a national basis to ensure that there is parity of services provided in all areas. These groups meet on a regular basis with Welsh Government staff and findings are fed back to the Welsh Government.

Last, but definitely not least, is what I consider to be one of the biggest breakthroughs in user and carer involvement – the direct participation of service users and carers in the training and development of nurses and social workers at Swansea University. The service user and carer involvement group is active on open days, at student selection events, in lessons, teaching delivery and programme evaluation.

USER INVOLVEMENT IN NURSE EDUCATION

Nurse education regulators in the UK now require programme managers to demonstrate how service users have been involved in the development, delivery and evaluation of nursing curricula. Currently, many universities have been challenged by the complexities of these activities, with few publishing guidelines on their successes, and limited guidance from education regulators.

Education staff have developed a range of methods in partnership with local individuals in order to involve users and carers. These include interviewing and assessing students, having users as mentors, involvement in programme planning, course validation, joint publications and conference presentations, as well as classroom teaching. Students have reported that users' stories are real and raw, but educators are clear that they do not want students to just enjoy user involvement; they also want to see students changed as a result, in terms of increased awareness and positive attitudes towards users and carers, in order to develop high quality nursing skills for practice. In terms of quality assurance, it is important that involvement activities are sustainable (Terry, 2013).

Service users and carers are an underutilised resource in nurse education, who can benefit from involvement with universities, just as universities benefit from them. Although the purpose of user involvement is to benefit student learning and increase students' self-awareness of the user perspective, users benefit from the experience too, reporting kudos from their involvement with local universities and increased confidence. Users and carers need their own identity in involvement activities, not the identity of a diagnosis, which serves to discriminate and engender hierarchical attitudes, mitigating against the true value of involvement.

REFLECTION POINT 4.7

What examples can you think of where meaningful service user involvement has been part of your nurse education programme?

It is worth noting that user involvement may be like a double-edged sword for some individuals. This can apply to user involvement in a range of settings. If users experience poor communication and a lack of respect, naturally this will have a negative impact, and by virtue will make further involvement unlikely. Involvement often requires a lot of giving. This includes giving time, sharing personal stories and experiences, and giving views which may relate to experiences of ill health that were extremely painful. Naturally, this giving has an impact, and means that involvement initiatives need to be well supported. The effort involved for some service users may relate to health issues, and people's vulnerability may be significant.

Service users often feel they can make a real difference, have a sense of feeling fulfilled and of being personally valued. In many ways, this is an active way of engineering social change, and it is not for the purpose of monetary reward (McKeown et al., 2014).

What does it take to be involved? When I stand in front of the class, I sometimes ask students 'what do you think it took for me to come here today? Do you think I just put my coat on and got the bus?' I tell them it involved an enormous effort, as I struggle with anxiety and depression and my confidence can be very low at times. I tell the students I pushed myself to come to the university so that they might hear my stories, and understand the importance of showing dignity to patients.

Tracy, service user

Effective user involvement needs the right people with the right attitude. The small things are very important and communication is key to effective involvement. If communication is misunderstood or absent, this can impact on users' perception significantly. A value base of working together, showing dignity and respect, and a strong commitment to partnership working, are essential.

REFLECTION POINT 4.8

What qualities do you have that would help facilitate meaningful user involvement?

OVERCOMING THE BARRIERS TO INVOLVEMENT

There are many barriers to meaningful user involvement, including issues relating to finance, representation, bureaucracy and understanding about the purpose of involvement.

Equally, those charged with ensuring that user involvement occurs commonly ask 'why won't service users get involved?', but on reflection a better question might be 'why would service users want to get involved?' (NHS England, 2015). Service users continue to debate their experiences of involvement, and wonder if their time and energies will bring about significant change. Notions that service user involvement may have a limited impact may deter involvement in the first place. Service users can indeed make a real impact, but for this to occur those working in mental health services need to accept and respond to the challenges of involvement far more than they have done so far (Centre for Mental Health, 2015).

Barriers to service users being meaningfully involved in their own care may be due to a range of factors. This may include negative staff attitudes, and likely power differentials between the user and mental health staff. Equally, service users being too unwell or not interested in involvement may impede such activities. Mental health nurses have an important role here in terms of facilitating involvement. Providing useful and accessible information in a timely manner can enable involvement to occur. Whilst individuals have to take empowerment for themselves, nurses can do a lot to support and encourage meaningful involvement in individual users' mental health care. This is likely to involve giving time, providing education and giving hope, as well as engaging relevant others who are important to service users regarding their ongoing care and treatment.

The benefits of service user involvement are widely recognised, and it is acknowledged that users possess a unique body of knowledge. Benefits of meaningful involvement include:

- Service users being recognised as experts in their experience, with a good knowledge of mental health services and of living with a mental health problem. No one else – no matter how well trained or qualified – can have had the same experience of the onset of mental illness, the same initial contact with services or the same journey through the mental health system.
- Many service user organisations have developed a range of **coping mechanisms** and survival strategies that help people manage their mental health problems. Many users can predict when they are about to become unwell and have a plan for **coping** in place. Service providers can use this expertise.
- Service users bring their own perspective on treatment and care and can prompt service providers and practitioners to re-evaluate their provision of services, challenge traditional assumptions and highlight the key priorities that users would like to see addressed.

- Service user involvement can be seen as providing a personally therapeutic experience and enabling people to feel that they are being listened to and that their contribution is being valued. Working collectively as part of a network of groups can help people increase their confidence and raise self-esteem. (Welsh Assembly Government, 2004)

> **"**
>
> Meaningful involvement for me is being able to take part in the activities of the user and carer group and making positive and beneficial contributions for the group's success. My expectations for the group would be to see the continuation of positive improvements in health services.
>
> I have found that since joining the group I have become more confident and self-assured and have regained some of my communication skills – a reward in itself. The group I belong to is really committed to making things better. People speak openly about their problems and their expectations are high.
>
> **Lucy, service user**
>
> **"**

Many service users find that they benefit from meaningful user involvement. This may include actively attending support groups or participating in a range of involvement activities. Lucy's cartoon in Figure 4.4 shows how talking to people and helping others has a positive impact on her mental health.

REFLECTION POINT 4.9

List 10 ways that meaningful user involvement can improve a service user's mental health.

User involvement activities vary widely, including users and academics or service staff jointly writing articles or co-researching. This book has been written with wide service user involvement from the early planning stage down to the content in each chapter. When asking service users what benefits they have gained from joint writing projects, individuals have said that such initiatives have been an important part of their recovery. Users who write about their experiences of mental health problems sometimes want others to feel that they are not alone, and have found it valid to use everyday language that is easily understood.

LISTENING IN DIFFERENT WAYS

In order to ensure user involvement is meaningful, it is essential that creative methods are used to ensure that significant involvement occurs. This may result in extra time and effort for those working in mental health services, but the benefits far outweigh the costs. This may involve holding listening events in voluntary organisations or gathering the views of people considered hard to reach.

Changes in technology mean that social media can provide an ideal platform for people to express views and ensure their voices are heard.

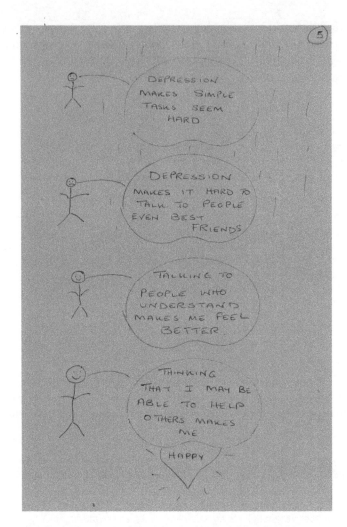

Figure 4.4 Lucy's cartoon about depression and how involvement helps

> People from all around the world who experience mental health difficulties are 'meeting' each other in social media. We're reading blogs written by each other. We're watching YouTube videos starring each other. We're listening to audio recorded by each other. We're talking to each other in Facebook groups, in comments sections of websites, on Twitter… Anywhere there is a space for people to share, speak and comment there is a space for people with mental health difficulties to run into each other…
>
> People like me could own language and ideas about mental health and it was possible for 'us' to define an identity that wasn't limited by what 'they' said we could and couldn't say. Loads of people with mental health difficulties never ran into anyone who experienced similar things to themselves unless they were lucky or currently in hospital or accessing some kind of care or support.

For many of us, our mental health difficulties have been misunderstood and in some cases shameful facts of our lives. Unless we were lucky and met people near us, in the past we have tended to communicate vertically with public services and charities providing us mental health support (evaluation, consultation). Social media lets us go horizontal, talking 'peer-to-peer' with others with similar experiences across the world.

Social media has created conditions where people who were previously isolated or marginalised can meet each other 'face-to-face' to share, debate, argue, build, destroy, criticise, praise, organise and develop. It's also created spaces where mental health difficulty isn't hidden.

Social media, then, is a space where we can learn from each other, debate with each other, band together and try to make change with each other and challenge the idea that who we are, what we want and what our lives mean should be defined by others.

For many of us social media at its best is a space where we meet with other like minds, discuss, share and learn, both about others and ourselves.

What's interesting is that social media is, still, somewhere there is a more level playing field between established 'professionals' and the rest of us. Some mental health bloggers have more readers than the trusts that provide them services. Some people with mental health difficulties on Twitter spark far larger debates than professionals in the same space.

Social media is still, for the time being, a place where we can find power we might not access in other ways and other places.

Mark Brown, 2015 talk on social media and mental health. Reproduced with permission.

FIND OUT MORE

BROWN (2015) THE BEST EFFING LONELY

Key messages for mental health nurses:

- Always involve people in their care.
- Involve people at all levels of service development and planning.
- Look for opportunities to increase meaningful user involvement.

Essential aspects of user involvement include changing ourselves to enable the participation of others, along with the development of more participatory processes in organisations. The **culture** of health services needs to change radically so that user involvement is valued in a wider context.

CONCLUSION

This chapter has provided an overview of meaningful user involvement and explored how involvement has changed over time. The importance of user involvement in care planning and the mental health nurse's role in this have been discussed, and whilst noting that not all service users wish to be involved, there are clear benefits to involvement. Being a partner in the care and treatment process or the changes and developments in mental health service delivery has started to change the power dynamics in services. Whether we consider that service users are now at the steering wheel and driving the involvement agenda, or whether they are simply offered a brief turn at the steering wheel occasionally, does depend on other individuals involved and the culture of services.

Involving service users in meaningful ways in the development of mental health services regarding both planning and delivery can be complex, and although user involvement is a familiar term, much rhetoric exists around involvement practices. Good practice is emerging, but the evidence is still minimal at present. The benefits of involving service users in nurse education is highlighted by many universities, students and service users, yet the impact of user involvement in health **profession** programmes is still not fully known. Barriers to user involvement are becoming more identifiable, which means that those involved can more actively negotiate solutions. This chapter has highlighted general principles that are essential in order to make involvement work well. Listening to service users in different ways is an important part of the present and future delivery of mental health services. Nurses need to be effectively engaged in listening and acting on what they hear in order to ensure involvement is meaningful for everyone involved.

CRITICAL DEBATE 4.1

- What role do mental health nurses have in meaningful service user involvement?
- Consider reasons why service users may wish to be involved and what can help this to occur meaningfully.
- Consider reasons why service users may choose not to be involved.
- What is the mental health nurse's role when people choose not to be involved?
- Consider what support you and your team need to offer to facilitate:
  - meaningful service user involvement in individualised care
  - meaningful service user involvement in mental health service development.

CHAPTER SUMMARY

This chapter has covered:

- What makes service user involvement meaningful
- The advantages and disadvantages of user involvement
- Ways that nursing students and mental health nurses can facilitate meaningful service user involvement
- Information about different ways that people can be involved in care and in service development
- Solutions to the challenges of service user involvement
- Challenges for you to think more about how people can be increasingly involved.

BUILD YOUR BIBLIOGRAPHY

Books

- Lloyd, M. (2012) *Practical care planning for personalised mental health care*. London: McGraw-Hill. This book is a useful resource which provides practical guidance and case studies on care planning.

- McKeown, M., Malihi-Shoja, L., Downe, S. & The Comensus Writing Collective (2010) *Service user and carer involvement in education for health and social care.* Oxford: Wiley-Blackwell. This book covers service user and carer involvement practices in the education of health and social care workers and was co-authored with service users and carers.
- Rogers, A. & Pilgrim, D. (2010) *A sociology of mental health and illness*, 4th edition. Buckingham: Open University Press. This book will help you understand the wider picture of the social, economic and political determinants of mental health issues. Chapter 11, 'Users of mental health services', is particularly relevant.

SAGE journal articles

Go to https://study.sagepub.com/essentialmentalhealth for further free online journal articles related to this chapter. If you are using the interactive ebook, simply click on the book icon in the margin to go straight to the resource.

FURTHER READING: JOURNAL ARTICLES

- Fothergill, A., Mitchell, B., Lipp, A., et al. (2012) Setting up a mental health service user research group: a process paper. *Journal of Research in Nursing, 18*(8), 746–759. This article reports on a collaboration set up by service users and nurses to develop a research group.
- Hodge, S. (2005) Participation, discourse and power: a case study in service user involvement. *Critical Social Policy, 25*(2), 64–179.
- Rose, D., Fleischmann, P. & Schofield, P. (2010) Perceptions of user involvement: a user-led study. *International Journal of Social Psychiatry, 56*(4), 389–401.

Weblinks

Go to https://study.sagepub.com/essentialmentalhealth for further weblinks related to this chapter. If you are using the interactive ebook, simply click on the book icon in the margin to go straight to the resource.

FURTHER READING: WEBLINKS

- Network for Mental Health: www.nsun.org.uk – this website aims to provide a platform to bring mental health service users and survivors together.
- NICE guidelines for service user experience in adult mental health: improving the experience of care for people using adult NHS mental health service: www.nice.org.uk/guidance/cg136
- Launchpad: http://launchpadncl.org.uk – a web resource by and for mental health service users.

ACE YOUR ASSESSMENT

Revise what you have learned by visiting https://study.sagepub.com/essentialmentalhealth. If you are using the interactive ebook, simply click on the tick icon to go straight to the resource.

ONLINE QUIZZES & ACTIVITY ANSWERS

- Test yourself with multiple-choice and short-answer questions and flashcards.

REFERENCES

Adams, J.R., Drake, R.E. & Wolford, G.L. (2007) Shared decision-making preferences of people with severe mental illness. *Psychiatric Services*, 58(9), 1219–1221. Available at: www.wpic.pitt.edu/education/CPSP/Reading/3%20%20V1B4%20Ses%203%20-%20Adams%20et%20al.pdf (accessed 03.08.17).

Arnstein, S.R. (1969) A ladder of citizen participation. *Journal of the American Planning Association*, 35(4), 216–224.

Brandon, D. (1991) *Innovation without Change? Consumer power in psychiatric services*. Basingstoke: Macmillan.

Branfield, F. & Beresford, P. (2006) *Making user involvement work: Supporting service user networking and knowledge*. York: Joseph Rowntree Foundation.

Brown, M. (2015) The best effing lonely: social media and #mentalhealth. *The New Mental Health*. Available at: http://thenewmentalhealth.org/?p=136 (accessed 03.08.17).

Campbell P. (1998) Listening to clients. In P. Barker, B. Davidson (eds), *Psychiatric nursing ethical strife*. London: Arnold.

Campbell, P. (2005) From little acorns: the mental health service user movement. In A. Bell & P. Lindley (eds) *Beyond the water towers: The unfinished revolution in mental health services 1985–2005*. London: The Sainsbury Centre for Mental Health.

Carr, S. (2007) Participation, power, conflict and change: theorizing dynamics of service user participation in the social care system of England and Wales. *Critical Social Policy*, 27(2): 266–276.

Centre for Mental Health (2015) *Mental health service user movement*. London: Centre for Mental Health.

Coldham, T. (2012) *A Review of Avon and Wiltshire Mental Health Partnership NHS Trust's Approach to Involvement*. London: NSUN.

Cooke, B. & Kothari, U. (2002) *Participation the new tyranny?* London: Zed Books.

Department of Health (DH) (2013) *The NHS Constitution: the NHS belongs to us all*. London: DH.

Hafal (2012) *A recovery approach to mental illness: A guide for students developed by people with a serious mental illness and their carers*. Neath: Hafal.

Hearing Voices Network (2016) *Sheffield Hearing Voices Group*. Available at: www.hearing-voices.org/groups/sheffield/ (accessed 20.9.17).

Hodge, S. (2005) Participation, discourse and power: a case study in service user involvement. *Critical Social Policy*, 25, 164–179.

Lawn, S. (2015) Integrating service user participation in mental health care: what will it take? *Int J Integr Care*, 15, e004. Available at: www.ncbi.nlm.nih.gov/pmc/articles/PMC4353213 (accessed 03.08.17).

Levin, E. (2004) *Involving Service Users and Carers in Social Work Education*. Resource Guide No. 2. London: Social Care Institute for Excellence.

Lloyd, M. (2010) *A practical guide to care planning in health and social care*. Maidenhead: Open University Press.

McGowan, J. (2010) John McGowan on service-user involvement. *Health Service Journal*, 27 May. Available at: www.hsj.co.uk/mental-health/john-mcgowan-on-service-user-involvement/5013865.article (accessed 03.08.17).

McKeown, M., Jones, F. & Wright, K.M. (2014) It's the talk! A study of involvement initiatives in secure mental health settings. *Health Expectations*, 19, 570–579.

Making a Real Difference (2007) *Valuing involvement: Good practice guidance for involving mental health service users and carers*. London: NIMHE/CSIP.

McLaughlin, H. (2009) What's in a name: 'client', 'patient', 'customer', 'consumer', 'expert by experience', 'service user' – what's next? *British Journal of Social Work*, 39(6), 1101–1117.

Mental Health Council of Australia (MHCA) (2011) *Consumer and carer experiences of stigma from mental health and other health professionals*. Canberra: MHCA.

Mind (2010) *The Mind guide to advocacy*. London: Mind.

National Institute for Health and Clinical Excellence (NICE) (2011) Service user experience in adult mental health: improving the experience of care for people using adult NHS mental health services. NICE (CG 136) guideline. Available at: www.nice.org.uk/guidance/cg136/resources/guidance-service-user-experience-in-adult-mental-health-improving-the-experience-of-care-for-people-using-adult-nhs-mental-health-services-pdf-35109513728197 (last accessed 22.11.17).

National Involvement Partnership (2013) *Nothing about us without us*. Available at: www.nsun.org.uk/assets/downloadableFiles/nip-leaflet-jan-20132.pdf (accessed 03.08.17).

National Survivor User Network (2014) The language of mental wellbeing. Available at: www.nsun.org.uk/assets/downloadableFiles/NIPTheLanguageofMentalWellbeing2.pdf (accessed 03.08.17).

NHS England (2015) *The NHS belongs to the people: a call to action*. Available at: www.england.nhs.uk/ourwork/patients (accessed 03.08.17).

Perkins, R. & Goddard, K. (2004) Reality out of the rhetoric: increasing user involvement in a mental health trust. *Mental Health Review Journal*, 9(1), 21–24.

Rethink (2013) *Factsheet: The care programme approach*. Available at: www.rethink.org/resources/c/care-programme-approach-cpafactsheet (accessed 03.08.17).

Rogers, A. & Pilgrim, D. (2010) *A sociology of mental health and illness*, 4th edition. Maidenhead: Open University Press.

Rush, B. (2004) Mental health service user involvement in England: lessons from history. *Journal of Psychiatric and Mental Health Nursing*, 11(3), 313–318.

Sayce, L., Kalathil, J. and Watson, E. (2012) *Caring with a difference: A study of the diverse needs and aspirations of families, friends and carers of people experiencing mental distress in Richmond*. London: Disabilities Rights UK and Richmond Borough Mind.

Scottish Government (2011) Patient Rights (Scotland) Act. Available at: www.legislation.gov.uk/asp/2011/5/pdfs/asp_20110005_en.pdf (accessed 31.10.17).

Shaw, S., Rosen, R. & Rumbold, B. (2011) *What is integrated care? An overview of integrated care in the NHS*. Research report. London: Nuffield Trust.

Social Care Institute for Excellence (2015) *Co-production in social care: What it is and how to do it*. SCIE Guide 51. Available at: www.scie.org.uk/publications/guides/guide51/ (accessed 20.09.17).

Terry, J. (2013) The pursuit of excellence in user involvement in nurse education: report from a travel scholarship. *Nurse Education in Practice*, 13, 202–206.

The Health Foundation (2015) *MAGIC: shared decision making*. Available at: www.health.org.uk/areas-of-work/programmes/shared-decision-making (accessed 03.08.17).

Time to Change (2013) Attitudes to mental illness 2012 research report: prepared for Time to Change. Available at: www.timetochange.org.uk/sites/default/files/121168%20Attributes%20to%20mental%20illness%202013%20report%20Annexes.pdf (accessed 28.11.17).

Toch, H. (1965) *The social psychology of social movements*. New York: Bobs Merrill.

Wa Munyi, C. (2012) Past and present perceptions towards disability: a historical perspective. *Disability Studies Quarterly*, 32(2) [online]. Available at: http://dsq-sds.org/article/view/3197/3068 (accessed 03.08.17).

Welsh Assembly Government (WAG) (2004) *Stronger in partnership: Involving service users in the design, planning, delivery and evaluation of mental health services in Wales*. Policy implementation guidance. Cardiff: WAG.

WORKING WITH FAMILIES AND CARERS

5

SIMON HALL AND MANDY REED

THIS CHAPTER COVERS

- Gaining an understanding of the range of emotions a carer can experience when a loved one becomes unwell
- Exploring confidentiality and ethical issues related to working with families and carers
- A consideration of the informal strategies that students and qualified nurses can offer to provide support and care for families and loved ones
- Identifying a range of assessment and psychoeducational tools that can help when working with carers
- The role of reflective practice when working with families and carers.

> It was a massive shock when my brother was diagnosed with psychosis. From the beginning there was so much information to understand, as well as coming to terms with how differently my brother was behaving. Once my brother was assigned a nurse it felt like a weight had been lifted, our family was no longer alone in trying to support my brother and deal with his diagnosis. Having a nurse involved in his care improved many aspects of all our lives. They were able to help us understand psychosis as a whole, including all the facts we needed to know about triggers, symptoms and treatment. Having an understanding of mental health felt like the first stage to my brother's recovery. Many stressful situations occurred due to family disagreements, with regards to my brother's care, but the nursing team encouraged us to have weekly meetings, where they were able to mediate the conversations and relieve the tension when conflict arose. The nurses also provided one to one time with myself and parents when we felt we needed reassurance. The support the nurses provided, to my brother and I, was phenomenal.
>
> **Katie, a service user's sibling on the importance of a
> nurse being involved in home care**

Visit **https://study.sagepub.com/essentialmentalhealth** to access a wealth of online resources for this chapter – watch out for the margin icons throughout the chapter. If you are using the interactive ebook, simply click on the margin icon to go straight to the resource.

> When I first met Katie's family it was with the local crisis team and we were trying to work together in coming up with a plan to avoid hospital admission, as it was clear that Katie's brother was not well and experiencing significant distressing symptoms of hallucinations with some delusional beliefs that had implications for all the family. After the initial acute phase we were able to reduce some of the distress for Katie's brother however, some symptoms remained as he believed someone was living in the attic and as a result of these thoughts he often investigated during the night, waking the whole family up. It was at this point we started formal family work with all the family present to look at solutions to the problem and create a safe space to discuss this issue and the other main issue around Katie's brother's peer group in the local community who enjoyed smoking cannabis. It was important to focus on the positives of such a strong family bond and create an environment adaptable to change, especially as it became apparent that medication would only reduce the symptoms and not eradicate them.
>
> **Simon, mental health nurse**

INTRODUCTION

The Office for National Statistics (2002; Linden, 2007) states that there are over 1.5 million people providing unpaid care for a relative or friend with a mental health **illness**, with more than half of these people providing over 20 hours per week of psychological and hands-on support and 55% stating that their health and social life have been greatly affected by their caring roles (Askey et al., 2009; Repper et al., 2008; Simpson & Benn, 2007). It is suggested by Goodwin and Happell (2007) that informal carers provide three times the amount of care of that of the average mental health nurse, providing an estimated 104 hours a week to their loved one. These high levels of care give emphasis to the idea that the 'real' experts of how to care best for their loved ones are informal **carers** (Gray et al., 2008; Shiers et al., 2009).

One of the most traumatic times for loved ones is the first time their loved one becomes unwell. Families experience and describe a significant loss of control and feelings of sadness and guilt (Reed et al., 2010). It can be really hard for families to contact the police and mental health services in this kind of a crisis; feelings of failure and betrayal can be overwhelming and delay them seeking help and support. Families are often unaware of their right to be involved in decisions about their loved one's care (Worthington et al., 2013; RCP, 2015); they may then be left wondering if they have made the right decision (Reed et al., 2010).

Most carers subsequently assume the caring role for their loved ones living with a serious mental illness (SMI) following an **acute** episode of care (from hospital-based care to community), despite having insufficient knowledge and being unprepared to assume such caring responsibilities (LUCAS KU Leuven/EUFAMI, 2015).

National policy and guidance stress the importance of health professionals working collaboratively with **service users**, families and carers (DH, 2014; NICE, 2015; Worthington et al., 2013). As many as 70% of young people experiencing a first episode of **psychosis** (FEP) either live with or maintain connections with close family members (Addington & Burnett, 2004). It is therefore an intrinsic aspect of our role as mental health nurses to collaborate with families and carers to share the care of their loved one as soon and as practicably as is possible. This chapter will explore the carer journey and the ways you can help, both as a student and for when you qualify.

WHO IS A CARER?

When you speak and work with family members, they are often hesitant about being described as a carer, seeing themselves first and foremost as mum, dad, partner, sibling, and each may have different needs (Sin et al., 2015; Smith et al., 2007). Regardless, the term 'carer' is typically used by services and policymakers, and is readily understood. Wray and Braine (2016) suggest that the terms carer and caregiver can be used interchangeably; in this chapter, we will be using the term carer to refer to anyone undertaking the significant role of providing care for another who may be emotionally, practically and financially dependent on them.

REFLECTION POINT 5.1

- Who amongst your family and friends knows you best?
- Who within your family and friends might best be suited to support you if you became unwell?
- Would one person support you better in some situations and another person in others?

STRESS, RESILIENCE AND GRIEF

Mental health nurses can help support families and carers by exploring some of the reasons discussed above. One important theory is Zubin and Spring's (1977) stress vulnerability model, which can be used to create a shared understanding of stress and its impact on families. It can also explain why some members of the family appear to cope better than other members of the family (Turton, 2015).

Heru and Drury (2011) argue that although there is an increase in stress for families, it can be a rewarding process if resilience is developed within the family. To promote family resilience, nurses need to expand their role by assisting families to enhance their **coping mechanisms**, providing methods to support their loved ones whilst maintaining their own wellbeing (Yeager et al., 2013). One way we can do this as professionals is to work with families by helping them to identify their unique stressors and promote the development of positive **coping** skills to decrease these.

Bishop and Greeff (2015) found that if carers could be helped to become more 'in control' of their lives, this then enabled them to cope better with challenging circumstances. Another important consideration is a family's spirituality and how it may empower a family's resilience or, in some circumstances, could make care planning around this more complicated. Shah et al. (2010) looked at the effects of **culture** and religion in relation to caregiving, identifying positive aspects such as improved resilience and greater access to social support, but be mindful that Green et al. (2010) identified that certain cultures can experience higher rates of **stigma** and shame than others.

USEFUL INTERVENTIONS AND STRATEGIES

Always be prepared to listen to a carer. This will support your ongoing assessments and care planning:

- Undertake individual assessments to develop an understanding of the impact of caring.
- Offer tailored information either through leaflets, signposting to online resources or attending local support groups.

Useful **assessment tools** when working with families and carers are:

- carers assessment – all carers are entitled to an assessment of their needs – your local electronic record system will have this built into it
- general health questionnaire (GHQ) – this is a really useful and quick self-reported questionnaire that can identify stress, physical health concerns and low **mood** in a carer
- timelines – these can help to identify family strengths and positive coping strategies in previous adverse circumstances
- genograms/sociograms – these explore interpersonal relationships and family systems
- family questionnaire – this self-report measure considers the frequency and impact of a range of behaviours within the family home and their coping strategies
- knowledge about **schizophrenia**/psychosis interview – this looks at diagnosis, symptomology, aetiology, medication, course and prognosis and management
- relative assessment interview – this comes in two versions, one for people who have been in mental health services for some time and the other for first episode psychosis (FEP). It is completed separately for each carer.

CASE STUDY:
PSYCHOSIS

(Fuller detail about the range of possible assessment tools can be found in Barrowclough & Tarrier, 1992; Smith et al., 2007; Withnell & Murphy, 2012.)

To truly appreciate the impact of a loved one experiencing mental illness, it is important that mental health nurses consider a carer's sense of grief and loss for their loved one (Boss, 1999; Parkes & Prigerson, 2010). A key model to help us understand this process is Worden's (2009) task of 'normal' mourning; this has been adapted with regards to the experience and **recovery** of carers. The first task for a carer is to accept the reality of the mental health problem affecting the individual and the loss of the person the carer used to know; the second is experiencing the sadness, fear and other emotions that this loss brings; third, the carer adjusts to an **environment** in which the individual may have different goals and expectations, and is able to move forward with their own recovery and life (Reed et al., 2010).

REFLECTION POINT 5.2

- Think about a loss you may have had in your own life (for example, a favourite pet, a grandparent or a friend), how it affected you and what/who helped you at the time.
- Who would you turn to for supervision and support now if you are affected by another person's loss when out on placement?

Read this account from a sibling on the issues around caring and what it felt like:

When I was in my early 20's I 'lost' my sister. My sister did not die – she was very much alive, but she became unwell with what turned out to be a severe mental illness. I was thrown into supporting her alongside my parents – we had no language for what was happening to us so it was impossible to explain to anyone else what we were experiencing. None of us had experienced exceptional losses so we could not acknowledge that we were experiencing a massive loss; but without the funeral.

(Continued)

No sibling has the same relationship with another sibling. Although I was involved with my sister's challenging behaviour I was never acknowledged as such by services. It was hard to work out what was happening to me – no one realised that I had 'lost' a sibling. I realised that I would have to work this out for myself in some way. Some years later, when a family friend commented that 'it has taken you a long time to come to terms with your situation' I was astonished. It made me realise that no one really understands the process that has to be worked out by each and every one of us. It still makes me feel angry today.

Eleanor, a sibling: the complexities of being a sibling

REFLECTION POINT 5.3

- Emotional tips – being with and being alongside are some of the most valued skills mental health nurses display (Gunasekara et al., 2013).
- Sometimes there are no answers to the inevitable 'Why me? Why now?' questions that carers ask. As mental health nurses, we have to be able to tolerate strong emotions in the people we care for and to validate their feelings and maintain/hold the hope.

MAKING A DIFFERENCE 5.1

Confidentiality

Rowe (2012) found that confidentiality is a widely established barrier when working with families and carers. Furthermore, a study by Wilson et al. (2015) found that 56.3% of informal carers have experienced difficulties obtaining information from mental health professions, which was attributed to a lack of regard as a carer by the mental health team, the unavailability of staff and a lack of patient consent. Professionals must regularly revisit information sharing with the service user throughout their care journey, and encourage the service user to involve their carers. It is also important to explain to carers what is happening and why, so that they can understand the benefit of confidentiality when building a trusting and effective working relationship (Bellesheim, 2016).

Families can feel that confidentiality is a shield that workers feel they can hide behind and can find themselves feeling they have to fight for information (Wainwright et al., 2015). However, this should not be the case - NICE (2014) guidance recognises that despite issues of confidentiality being complex, the involvement of families should be encouraged and revisited regularly. Workers should create a culture of listening to families as often as they want to share information about their loved ones, which does not break service user confidentiality (Smith et al., 2007). This is done by emphasising the importance of collaborative working with all parties involved throughout the entire care pathway, as opposed to focusing on the individual's right to confidentiality (Cree et al., 2015; Worthington et al., 2013).

Recent evidence suggests that families can hold valuable information and their input may lead to better outcomes for their loved ones (Eassom et al., 2014). The 'Triangle of Care' promotes an alliance between service users, families and professionals (Worthington et al., 2013) and adopting a collaborative approach to care, we can increase opportunities and positive outcomes for service users (Worthington et al., 2013). Confidentiality must not become a barrier to this process and we must consider including carers and families in the care process when we can.

MAGGIE AND GUY'S STORY

Maggie phones the local intensive support team in desperation over concern for her son who has been experiencing an increase in his distressing and intrusive thoughts for several months. As a family, they had been trying to access home support for many weeks to no avail, despite having been offered it during a brief inpatient admission as part of a discharge package. Currently, even an urgent outpatient appointment with the psychiatrist has not been organised, and no one seems to know why or when it might happen. Guy is having episodes most days when he becomes overwhelmed by his thoughts and has become increasingly hopeless about his future; Maggie is really worried he may try to end his life and spends most of her time ensuring Guy is not left on his own at home. On the phone, she describes her concerns and admits that her mood and mental health are deteriorating as a result of the strain of looking after Guy. The duty nurse, Pam, on the other end of the phone (who has never met either of them) suggests Maggie spends time practising deep breathing exercises to help her cope and that she tells Guy that 'there is light at the end of the tunnel'. Pam also says she will pass on the message about the appointment and that 'no doubt someone will get back to her soon' with a date, but if Guy hasn't heard anything in another week to phone the team again.

CRITICAL THINKING STOP POINT 5.1

- How do you imagine Maggie received these suggestions?
- Do you think they were appropriate in the circumstances?
- If not, why not? What policy and theory underpin your thoughts?
- Can you think of anything else the nurse could have said and why?

INTERVENTIONS YOU CAN EMPLOY AS A STUDENT TO SUPPORT CARERS AND SERVICE USERS

Mental health nurses have various options open to them when considering psychoeducation in their care planning. Psychoeducation refers to any planned intervention that looks at a care provision in a holistic way, whilst also providing information, support and coping strategies to carers and their loved ones (Economou, 2015). Psychoeducation interventions can reduce incidents of admission and relapse, and improve treatment compliance (Prasko et al., 2011; Reed et al., 2010). Evidence suggests that psychoeducation alongside appropriate medication has better long-term results for service users (Kreyenbuhl et al., 2009). However, to improve positive outcomes, families need greater access to education and information, including social, emotional and economic support (French et al., 2010). Providing no support may lead to increased internalised stigmatisation, resulting in the service user feeling disempowered, withdrawing or having an increased risk of relapse (Topor et al., 2006).

INFORMAL INTERVENTIONS FOR CARERS

The following list is a summary of the range of practical interventions you will be able to employ as a student nurse when working with carers (it is then followed by some sound advice from a sibling, Eleanor, to help us all):

- exploration of distress and provision of emotional support
- exploration of contexts related to client's symptoms/problems
- initial carers' assessment (and signposting on to carers' services)
- involving the family in care planning and reviews wherever and whenever possible
- provision of information about the appropriate mental health issue and the kind of services they can expect to receive for themselves and their loved one
- encouraging realistic expectations and helping the family to maintain a sense of hope
- tips and suggestions to enhance coping strategies; this can include encouraging realistic expectations
- enhancing their ability to anticipate and solve problems and develop coping skills
- identifying early warning of relapse and agreeing a plan of action
- liaison and advocacy with mental health and other services
- helping the family to be reflective, explore options, reach a shared understanding, deal with strong feelings (e.g. anger, guilt) and encourage a sense of personal agency.

Eleanor's sister has schizophrenia. Here are Eleanor's tips for working collaboratively with families and for coping as a student nurse:

1. First and foremost, take time to listen to the family member; they will have important information to share and will really value the gift of time to tell their story. Remember, you can always listen, even if you do not have permission at that point in time to share information about their loved one in return.
2. Stress that it is important for them to not blame their son, daughter, sibling, parent or themselves for the illness. Emphasise the modern knowledge that psychosis is NOT caused by the relatives and help to overcome any possible family stigma.
3. As a student be mindful that family members may express very different coping mechanisms and that this can cause additional stress. Above all, try to suspend your judgement when hearing or witnessing something by a family member and remember to consider the intention behind an action, not the action itself.
4. Try to gently encourage and support them to return to or take up a new pastime/interest and maintain social networks.

CONCLUSION

In essence, by combining the strategies and tips suggested for working collaboratively with carers, there is much you can do as a student nurse and beyond to promote best practice. A fundamental assumption to take away from this chapter is that families generally want to be involved and can make many positive contributions in helping us as professionals to meet the care needs of their loved ones. Your role as a mental health nurse is to have **open dialogue** with families, looking at various ways to support them and the person being cared for.

CHAPTER SUMMARY

This chapter has covered:

* The range of emotions a carer can experience when a loved one becomes unwell, with a focus around 'resilience' and 'grief'
* The importance of confidentiality and ethical issues relating to working with families and carers, and ways to maintain a dialogue with carers throughout the recovery journey
* A range of useful assessment tools that can help when working with carers in practice
* Important informal strategies that you can use in providing support and care for families and loved ones.

BUILD YOUR BIBLIOGRAPHY

Book chapters

* Burbach, F., Fadden, G. & Smith, J. (2010) Family interventions for first-episode psychosis. In P. French, J. Smith, D. Shiers, M. Reed & M. Rayne (eds) *Promoting recovery in early psychosis: A practice manual.* Oxford: Wiley-Blackwell. This chapter looks at formal family interventions for first episode psychosis. It explores issues relating to the implementing of family interventions in the context of family-orientated EI services, providing service examples from two NHS EI service contexts.
* Withnell, N. & Murphy, N. (2012) The role of education in family intervention. In N. Withnell and N. Murphy (eds) *Family interventions in mental health* (chapter 11). Maidenhead: Open University Press. This chapter outlines an overview of the different types of education that carers have found useful. It also provides information on when education for carers is best used and tips on how to find educational resources.
* Wilson, C. (2017) Supporting the families of people with dementia. In N. Withnell and N. Murphy (eds) *Caring for people with dementia: A shared approach* (chapter 8). London: SAGE. This is a chapter that not only provides some useful advice for this specialist group that we were unable to go into in any detail in this chapter, but it also has some good activities that promote reflective practice.

SAGE journal articles

Go to https://study.sagepub.com/essentialmentalhealth for further free online journal articles related to this chapter. If you are using the interactive ebook, simply click on the book icon in the margin to go straight to the resource.

FURTHER READING: JOURNAL ARTICLES

* Kartalova-O'Doherty, Y. & Tedstone Doherty, D. (2009) Satisfied carers of persons with enduring mental illness: who and why? *International Journal of Social Psychiatry*, 55(3), 257-271.

- Lawn, S. & McMahon, J. (2014) The importance of relationship in understanding the experiences of spouse mental health carers. *Qualitative Health Research*, *24*(2), 254-266.
- Parker, R., Leggatt, M. & Crowe, J. (2010) Public interest and private concern: the role of family carers for people suffering mental illness in the twenty first century. *Australasian Psychiatry*, *18*(2), 163-166.

Weblinks

FURTHER
READING:
WEBLINKS

Go to https://study.sagepub.com/essentialmentalhealth for further weblinks related to this chapter. If you are using the interactive ebook, simply click on the book icon in the margin to go straight to the resource.

- Carers UK: www.carersuk.org – this is a useful website designed for carers by carers, offering practical advice and support.
- Caring for Mental Health Survey: www.caringformentalhealth.org – this is a website dedicated to some recent research around carers' experiences from an international perspective.
- Rethink: www.rethink.org – this is a website that hosts a major charity that supports all involved with mental illness; there is a specific tab which holds information for carers and families that is particularly useful.
- The Carers Trust: https://professionals.carers.org – this website offers a wide range of resources and information for anyone who works with carers; it includes a link to the 'Triangle of Care'.

ACE YOUR ASSESSMENT

ONLINE
QUIZZES &
ACTIVITY
ANSWERS

Revise what you have learned by visiting https://study.sagepub.com/essentialmentalhealth. If you are using the interactive ebook, simply click on the tick icon to go straight to the resource.

- Test yourself with multiple-choice and short-answer questions and flashcards.

REFERENCES

Addington, J. & Burnett, P. (2004) Working with families in the early stages of psychosis. In P. McGorry & J. Gleeson (eds) *Psychological interventions in early psychosis: A practical treatment handbook*. Chichester: Wiley.

Askey, R., Holmshaw, J., Gamble, C., et al. (2009) What do carers of people with psychosis need from mental health services? Exploring views of carers, service users and professionals. *Journal of Family Therapy*, *31*, 310–331.

Barrowclough, C. & Tarrier, N. (1992) *Families of schizophrenic patients: Cognitive behavioural intervention*. London: Nelson Thornes.

Bellesheim, K.R. (2016) Ethical challenges and legal issues for mental health professionals working with family caregivers of individuals with serious mental illness. *Ethics & Behaviour*, *26*(7), 607–620.

Bishop, M. & Greeff, A.P. (2015) Resilience in families in which a member has been diagnosed with schizophrenia. *Journal of Psychiatric and Mental Health Nursing*, *22*(7), 463–471.

Boss, P. (1999) *Ambiguous loss. Learning to live with unresolved grief*. Cambridge, MA: Harvard University Press.

Cree, L., Brooks, H., Berzins, K., et al. (2015) Carers' experiences of involvement in care planning: a qualitative exploration of the facilitators and barriers to engagement with mental health services. *BMC Psychiatry*, *15*(1), 1–11.

Department of Health (DH) (2014) *Carers strategy: Second national action plan 2014 – 2016*. Available at: www.gov.uk/government/uploads/system/uploads/attachment_data/file/368478/Carers_Strategy_-_Second_National_Action_Plan_2014_-_2016.pdf (accessed 03.08.17).

Eassom, E., Giacco, D., Dirik, A., et al. (2014) Implementing family involvement in the treatment of patients with psychosis: a systematic review of facilitating and hindering factors. *BMJ Open*, *4*(10), e006108.

Economou, M.P. (2015) Psychoeducation: a multifaceted intervention. *International Journal of Mental Health*, *44*(4), 259–262.

French, P., Smith, J., Shiers, D., et al. (2010) *Promoting recovery in early psychosis: A practice manual*. Chichester: Wiley-Blackwell.

Goodwin, V. & Happell, B. (2007) Consumer and carer participation in mental health care: the carer's perspective. Part 1 – the importance of respect and collaboration. *Issues in Mental Health Nursing*, *28*(6), 607–623.

Gray, B., Robinson, C., Seddon, D. et al. (2008) 'Confidentiality smokescreens' and carers for people with mental health problems: the perspectives of professionals. *Health & Social Care in the Community*, *16*(4), 378–387.

Green, R., Smith, G. & Patel, I. (2010) Using family work to support an Asian man coping with psychosis. *Mental Health Practice*, *13*(9), 30–36.

Gunasekara, I., Pentland, T., Rogers, T., et al. (2014) What makes an excellent mental health nurse? A pragmatic inquiry initiated and conducted by people with lived experience of service use. *International Journal of Mental Health Nursing 23*(2), 101–109.

Heru, A. & Drury, L. (2011) Developing family resilience in chronic psychiatric illnesses. *Medicine and Health Rhode Island*, *94*(2), 45–46.

Kreyenbuhl, J., Nossel, R. & Dixon, L.B. (2009) Disengagement from mental health treatment among individuals with schizophrenia and strategies for facilitating connections to care: a review of the literature. *Schizophrenia Bulletin*, *35*(4), 696–703.

Linden, D. (2007) *5 key facts for carers*. London: Princess Royal Trust for Carers.

LUCAS KU Leuven/EUFAMI (2015) *Caring for Carers Survey: Experiences of family caregivers of persons with severe mental illness*. Available at: www.caringformentalhealth.org (accessed 16.09.17).

National Institute for Health and Care Excellence (2014) Psychosis and schizophrenia in adults: prevention and management. NICE guideline (CG 178). Available at: www.nice.org.uk/guidance/cg178 (accessed 03.08.17).

National Institute for Health and Care Excellence (2015) Psychosis and schizophrenia in adults. NICE quality standard 80. Available at: www.nice.org.uk/guidance/qs80/chapter/quality-statement-6-assessing-physical-health (accessed 03.08.17).

Office for National Statistics (ONS) (2002) *Carers 2000 general household survey*. London: TSO.

Parkes, C.M. & Prigerson, H.G. (2010) *Bereavement: Studies of grief in adult life*, 4th edition. London: Penguin.

Prasko, J., Vrbova, V., Latalova, L., et al. (2011) Psychoeducation for psychotic patients. *Biomedical Papers of the Medical Faculty of the University Palacký, Olomouc, Czechoslovakia, 155*(4), 385.

Reed, M., Peters, S. & Banks, L. (2010) Sharing the care with families. In P. French, J. Smith, D. Shiers, M. Reed & M. Rayne (eds) *Promoting recovery in early psychosis: A practice manual*. Oxford: Wiley-Blackwell.

Repper, J., Nolan, M., Grant, G., et al. (2008) *Family carers on the margins: Experiences of assessment in mental health*. London: National Coordinating Centre for the Service Delivery and Organisation (NCCSDO) research programme.

Royal College of Psychiatrists (2015) *Carers and confidentiality*. Available at: www.rcpsych.ac. uk/healthadvice/partnersincarecampaign/carersinconfidentiality.aspx (accessed 03.08.17).

Rowe, J. (2012) Great expectations: a systematic review of the literature on the role of family carers in severe mental illness, and their relationships and engagement with professionals. *Journal of Psychiatric and Mental Health Nursing, 19*(1), 70–82.

Simpson, A. & Benn, L. (2007) *Scoping exercise to inform the development of a national mental health carer support curriculum*. London: City University.

Shah, A., Wadoo, O. & Latoo, J. (2010) Psychological distress in carers of people with mental disorders. *British Journal of Medical Practitioners, 3*(3), a327.

Shiers, D., Rosen, A. & Shiers, A. (2009) Beyond early intervention: can we adopt alternative narratives like 'woodshedding' as pathways to recovery in schizophrenia? *Early Intervention in Psychiatry, 3*, 163–171.

Sin, J., Jordan, C.D., Barley, E.A., et al. (2015) Psychoeducation for siblings of people with severe mental illness. *Cochrane Database of Systematic Reviews, 5*, CD010540.

Smith, G., Gregory, K. & Higgs, A. (2007) *An integrated approach to family work for psychosis: A manual for family workers*. London: Jessica Kingsley.

Topor, A., Borg, M., Mezzina, R., et al. (2006) Others: the role of family, friends and professionals in the recovery process. *American Journal of Psychiatric Rehabilitation, 9*(1), 17–37.

Turton, W. (2015) An introduction to psychosocial interventions. In S. Walker (ed.) *Psychosocial interventions in mental health nursing*. London: Sage.

Wainwright, L.D., Glentworth, D., Haddock, G., et al. (2015) What do relatives experience when supporting someone in early psychosis? *Psychology and Psychotherapy: Theory, Research, and Practice, 88*, 105–119.

Wilson, L.S., Pillay, D., Kelly, B.D., et al. (2015) Mental health professionals and information sharing: carer perspectives. *Irish Journal of Medical Science, 184*(4), 781–790.

Withnell, N. & Murphy, N. (2012) *Family interventions in mental health*. Maidenhead: Open University Press.

Worden, W.J. (2009) *Grief counselling and grief therapy: A handbook for the mental health practitioner*, 4th edition. New York: Springer.

Worthington, A., Rooney, P. & Hannan, R. (2013) *The Triangle of Care: Carers included – A guide to best practice in mental health care in England*, 2nd edition. London: Carers Trust. Available at: https://professionals.carers.org/sites/default/files/triangle_of_care_2016_latest_version.pdf (accessed 03.08.17).

Wray, J. & Braine, M.E. (2016) Supporting families and carers. *British Journal of Nursing, 25*(9), 474.

Yeager, K., Cutler, D., Svendsen, D., et al. (2013) *Modern community mental health: An interdisciplinary approach*. New York: Oxford University Press.

Zubin, J. & Spring, B. (1977) Vulnerability: a new view of schizophrenia. *Journal of Abnormal Psychology, 86*(2), 103–126.

DIVERSITY ISSUES WITHIN MENTAL HEALTH CARE

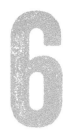

TOMMY DICKINSON, AMRITA MULLAN, RACHEL LYON, LAUREN WALKER, DONNA TAYLOR AND JESS BRADLEY

THIS CHAPTER COVERS

- The importance of recognising the specific mental health needs of disabled people and individuals from a diverse range of cultures, religions, genders and sexualities
- The ways in which patients may vary in their beliefs about the health care system and their attitudes about seeking appropriate care, especially mental health care
- The importance of reflecting on your values and attitudes towards disabled people and individuals from different cultures, religions, genders and sexualities
- Solution-focused interventions to enhance the experience of patients who may be disabled or from a diverse range of cultures, religions, genders and sexualities.

It is pertinent that people from all cultures, religions, genders, sexualities and minority ethnic groups are involved in decision making about the kinds of services they need, and how we make services accessible and appropriate to meet their individual needs, so that their priorities and values inform the process.

Ramsey Quilliam, retired mental health nurse

Visit **https://study.sagepub.com/essentialmentalhealth** to access a wealth of online resources for this chapter – watch out for the margin icons throughout the chapter. If you are using the interactive ebook, simply click on the margin icon to go straight to the resource.

I was off work a lot when [she] was ill, and what they do then is they make you see Staff Health. And I had this wonderful doctor, and she actually gave me this form to fill in, 'Do you think you're depressed?'

Yes, yes, yes, all the way down.

And she looked at me, she said, 'My goodness, you've ticked a lot! Come in!' And she said, 'Why do you think you're depressed?'

And I immediately came out with it – 'My girlfriend's dying.'

And she was so lovely – she came out and hugged me. Oh, she was so lovely. And she said, 'Tell me all about it.'

And of course, I was crying my eyes out. And she said, 'Right, you're not to go back to work; I'm signing you off now, with reactive depression. And you're not to go back to work at all, you go home and look after her.'

And that was lovely, then. What a wonderful woman.

And eventually, she [her girlfriend] just got worse and worse and worse […] she was crying out with pain […] And then she said, 'I think I need to go to hospital.' […] she was lying on the stretcher, and she said, 'I am going for the angels.' Oh, it was awful. It was just terrible. And the Sister was lovely, because she said, 'Well, who are you?' and I said, 'I'm her relationship, we're a gay couple'. And she put her arm round me, she was a lovely Sister, lovely, put her arm round me and everything, and took her up to the ward. She died a few hours later.

Paaie Clague (cited in Traies, 2014)

Commentary: There are two moments in this story at which Paaie felt she had to 'come out' – first to the occupational health doctor and then to the ward sister. Paaie's life had been lived 'in the closet'; her experience in the Army had made her extremely secretive about her sexual orientation. She was never out at work; her social circle consisted entirely of other lesbians. It was only in these two moments of extreme need that she let her guard down, and on both occasions, as you have seen, she met with the unconditional compassion she desperately needed.

INTRODUCTION

Mental health nursing has a chequered history in dealing with diversity (Dickinson, 2015; McFarland-Icke, 1999). However, characteristics such as racial and cultural backgrounds, disabilities, genders, religious beliefs and sexual **orientations** open up complementary ways of perceiving, thinking and acting that enrich our understanding of mental health and **recovery**. In the diverse society that we live in today, mental health nurses are expected to recognise diversity in their practice and actively tackle oppression. Indeed, respect for diversity is a well-established tenet of mental health nursing practice. People can be situated in ways that invite multiple oppressions, and these can interact to magnify detriment and discrimination. The notion of intersectionality helps to make sense of this and is a key strand of critical thinking represented in the emergent field of **Mad Studies** (LeFrançois et al., 2013).

In this chapter, you will identify the components of disability, sexuality, gender, **ethnicity**, **culture** and religion that can **affect** the **therapeutic relationship**; and learn how you can incorporate this knowledge to promote an inclusive **environment** and provide culturally competent care.

EQUALITY AND DIVERSITY

Whilst the terms 'equality' and 'diversity' are sometimes used interchangeably, they are not the same. Equality is about 'creating a fairer society, where everyone can participate and has the opportunity to fulfil their potential' (DH, 2004). By striving to eliminate prejudice and discrimination within mental health care, services can deliver personal, fair and diverse care, thus making it more accountable to the patients it serves and tackling discrimination in the workplace (Hunt, 2004).

In short, diversity literally means difference. Diversity aims to recognise, respect and **value** people's differences to contribute and realise their full potential by promoting an inclusive culture for all staff and patients. It is about acknowledging individual as well as group differences, treating people as individuals and placing positive value on diversity in the community and in the workforce. It is paramount that group and individual diversity needs are met and considered in order for mental health services to create an inclusive culture for all staff and patients. Indeed, if mental health nurses are to take a holistic approach, they need to make a commitment to equality through the recognition of diversity.

EQUALITY LEGISLATION

Legislation governing equality in England, Wales and Scotland was streamlined into a single piece of law, known as the Equality Act 2010, in an effort to simplify and strengthen existing law. This Act prohibits discrimination, to help achieve equal opportunities across all aspects of society and does so by specifying 'protected characteristics'. The nine protected characteristics are: age; disability; gender reassignment; marriage and civil partnership; pregnancy and maternity; **race**; religion and belief; sex; and sexual orientation. Under the Equality Act, individuals are afforded protection against discrimination, harassment and victimisation. However, in addition to its protective function, the Equality Act endeavours to promote equality to groups of people who may be disadvantaged or under-represented, or have particular needs, but must be applied in a way that is proportionate to the aim.

Comparatively, the existing equality protection in Northern Ireland remains unconsolidated and, as a result, provides less comprehensive and enforceable rights with uneven and diverse application (Northern Ireland Assembly, 2011). As such, Northern Ireland continues to retain the Equal Pay Act 1970; Sex Discrimination Act 1976; Disability Discrimination Act 1998; Race Relations Order 1997; Northern Ireland Act 1998; Fair Employment Treatment Order 1998; Employment Equality (Sexual Orientation) Regulations 2003; and Employment (Age) Regulations 2006.

Whilst the UK's Equality Act 2010 seeks to address previous deficiencies in equality law, these remain pervasive in Northern Ireland's law. Primarily, the complexity of the equality law in Northern Ireland has led to difficulties for those seeking to exercise their rights, as well as those endeavouring to comply with its provisions and poor consistency in its application. Moreover, the arguably outdated legislation of Northern Ireland fails to keep abreast of new forms of discrimination, therefore offering little or no protection, and may ultimately breach standards within international human rights conventions (Equality Commission for Northern Ireland, 2014).

BLACK AND MINORITY ETHNIC GROUPS

In recent times, England and Wales ethnic makeup has become increasingly diverse, with rising numbers identifying with minority ethnic groups (Office for National Statistics, 2012). Whilst the majority ethnic group remained White British, the 2011 Census showed the UK's population comprised 2.2% mixed/multiple ethnic groups; 7.5% Asian/Asian British; 3.3% Black/African/Caribbean/Black British and 1% other ethnic groups. A similar pattern emerged from the data of the Scottish census, with the African, Caribbean or Black groups representing 1%; Asian groups 3%; mixed or multiple ethnic groups 0.4%; and the White population holding the largest percentage at 96% (Scottish Government, 2011). In Northern Ireland, additional ethnic groups were identified, however the White population remained the greatest at 98.21%; Chinese 0.35%; Irish Traveller 0.07%; Indian 0.34%; Pakistani 0.06%; Bangladeshi 0.03%; other Asian 0.28%; Black Caribbean 0.02%; Black African 0.13%; Black other 0.05%; Mixed 0.335; and other populations represent 0.13% (Northern Ireland Statistics & Research Agency, 2011). This diversity enriches our society but also brings with it challenges for health care providers, health care systems and policymakers, to ensure that mental health services are appropriate for and relevant to a multicultural society.

Table 6.1 Culture, race and ethnicity

Concept	Characterised by	Perceived as	Assumed to be	In reality
Culture	Behaviour, attitudes, etc.	Social, changeable	Passed down by parents, parent substitutes	Variable and changeable blueprint for living
Race	Physical appearance	Physical, permanent	Genetically determined	Socially constructed
Ethnicity	Sense of belonging	Psychosocial, partially changeable	How people see themselves in terms of background and parentage	Culture-race, mixture

Source: adapted from Fernando, 2010

CULTURAL COMPETENCE

An individual's values, beliefs and behaviours are influenced by factors including race, ethnicity, language, age, socio-economic status and occupation (Kramer et al., 2002). It is imperative that a health care system integrates these factors into the delivery of its services, to ensure it meets its legal, moral and ethical obligation, to provide care that is both person-centred and culturally competent (Belfast Trust, 2014). On an individual level, mental health nurses have had a legal and professional duty to promote equality in accordance with the Race Relations (Amendment) Act 2000 (now subsumed under the new Equalities Act). A culturally competent service helps to improve health outcomes and quality of care and reduces racial and ethnic disparities; and a culturally competent professional provides care which is safe, effective, timely, equitable and individual (Betancourt et al., 2005).

Cultural competence is considered an ongoing process which is developed over time (Campinha-Bacote, 2002). The model in Figure 6.1 highlights the stages by which cultural competence is acquired, allowing mental health nurses to work effectively with black and minority ethnic (BME) groups.

BLACK AND MINORITY ETHNIC ISSUES IN MENTAL HEALTH

It is widely documented that health disparities exist between black and minority ethnic (BME) groups and the majority white population, with BME people suffering from increased morbidity and reduced life expectancy, and experiencing greater difficulty accessing health care. This disparity also extends to mental health, with increased rates of mental ill health and poorer experience within mental health services and treatment outcomes (Owen & Khalil, 2007).

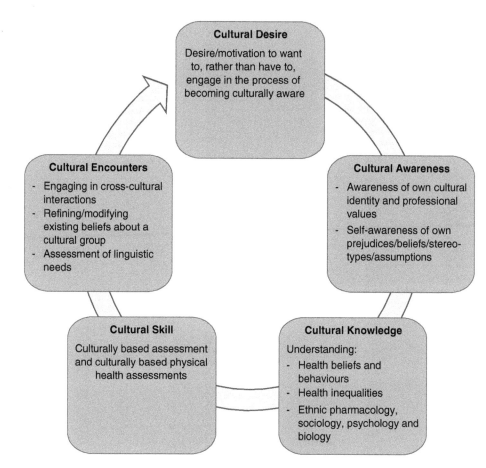

Figure 6.1 Culturally based physical and mental health assessments

Source: adapted from Campinha-Bacote, 2002

Rates and routes of admission

Although there is an impetus to reduce hospital admissions, it is important to consider the routes of admission into mental health services as these may vary among societies and may be reflective of the cultural appropriateness, attractiveness, attitudes towards services and an individual's previous experience (Goldberg, 1999).

In England, it is well documented that African-Caribbean men are 3–13 times more likely to be admitted to mental health hospitals than their White counterparts (Davies et al., 1996; Van Os et al., 1996). This has resulted in a disproportionate representation of those from black communities in the mental health system. However, focus has moved away from their over-representation to the pathway in which they arrive there. It has been found that Black people, in comparison to White people, are more likely to experience 'an aversive pathway into mental health services', with a greater number of compulsory detentions under the Mental Health Act 1983 [as amended] in England and Wales, greater involvement in legal and forensic settings, and increased rates of transfer to medium- and high-security settings (National Association for the Care and Resettlement of Offenders, 2007: 3). These patterns are also reflected amongst Black women who are three times more likely to be admitted to a forensic unit than White women (Maden et al., 1992).

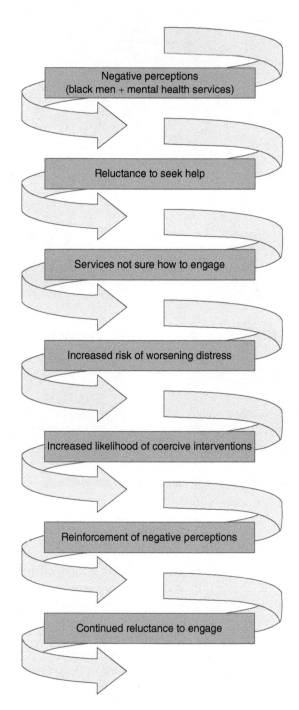

Figure 6.2   Spiral of oppression

Source: Trivedi, 2002

Issues faced by BME groups in mental health do not stand alone but have a close relationship to one another. Although perceptions of Black patients will be discussed in more detail later, the association of increased risk and fear of danger amongst Black people has led to an increased likelihood that these patients will be detained by the police under Section 136 of the Mental Health Act 1983 [as amended] in England and Wales and be taken to a **place of safety** (Braine, 1997).

The disproportionate rates of compulsory detention amongst Black people has been found to be independent of psychiatric diagnosis, total number of admissions a year, marital status, employment, sex, age and type of accommodation (Davies et al., 1996). Possible explanations for Black people entering services involuntarily have included mental health services being inaccessible or inappropriate to this community (Davies et al., 1996). Arguably, the way Black people have contact with mental health services creates an aversive experience of them, leading to services being viewed as antitherapeutic, thereby creating a delay in seeking help, which ultimately leads to an increased likelihood of compulsory admission (Moodley & Perkins, 1991). Figure 6.2 demonstrates Trivedi's (2002) 'spiral of oppression', whereby Black people do not trust mental health services, and those who work within them hold a sense of fear towards these patients, which leads to poor engagement on both sides.

CASE STUDY:
PARANOID
SCHIZOPHRENIA

DIAGNOSIS OF SCHIZOPHRENIA

Research shows that people from BME groups are more likely to be diagnosed with mental health problems, despite differing opinion about whether the prevalence of mental health problems in these groups is any higher than the majority White population (DH, 2005; CQC, 2009). More specifically, it is widely documented that African-Caribbean patients are more likely to be diagnosed with severe mental **illness**, in particular **schizophrenia** (Coid et al., 2000; Davies et al., 1996). Additionally, the inquiry into the death of David 'Rocky' Bennett, along with other issues, highlighted that African-Caribbeans are more likely than other ethnic groups to be diagnosed with drug-induced **psychosis**. In this way, Black people are considered to suffer 'double jeopardy' (Fernando, 2002). These findings contrast with lower rates of psychosis among the majority White population and conflicting results in Asian populations.

American psychiatrists document that the disparities in the diagnosis of schizophrenia between racial groups is explained by the White psychiatrists' lack of understanding and subsequent inability to properly evaluate the feelings and behaviour of Black people as a result of mutual mistrust and hostility (St Clair, 1951). Inevitably this will lead to diagnostic difficulties including atypical **syndromes** being misdiagnosed as schizophrenia (Littlewood & Lipsedge, 1981). These findings are not unique to the USA, but are also reflected in the results of UK studies. Specifically, Bhugra et al. (1997) concluded, the incidence of schizophrenia is higher in males of all ages but only in females under the age of 30. Research appears to focus heavily on African-Caribbeans, however King et al. (1994) argue that this is misleading as all BME groups are vulnerable.

'BIG, BLACK AND DANGEROUS'

The death of David 'Rocky' Bennett, who died following prolonged restraint and the earlier deaths of Orville Blackwood, Michael Martin and Joseph Watts in Broadmoor Hospital, brought about discussion regarding institutional racism in UK health care (McKeown & Stowell-Smith, 2001). In both inquiries it was found that professionals drew on stereotypes of black patients as 'aggressive,' which was further heightened by a diagnosis of schizophrenia and subsequently generated a fear of violence amongst staff. These perceptions are supported by research and extend to other ethnic minority groups, with clinicians over-predicting violence amongst members of these communities and under-predicting violence in White majority groups (Hicks, 2004). Yet research shows no correlation between race and actual assaultive behaviour (Hoptman et al., 1999).

Institutional racism in this respect manifests itself not in direct racism but what is termed the colour blind and culture blind approach (Fernando, 2002). Here, mental health practitioners are unaware of their own bias and ignore the existence of racism in the wider society, resulting in patients' race being unrecognised and their self-perception, social opportunities, rights and life experiences invalidated (Fernando, 2002). This leads to culturally blind practice where health related behaviours, variations in beliefs associated with illness and treatment preferences are misinterpreted or not considered (Engebretson et al., 2008). Although superficially this may be perceived as an attempt to avoid discrimination, it assumes homogeneity amongst patients and subsequently leads to a failure to provide individualised care.

An over-prediction of dangerousness, cultural ignorance and stereotypical views coupled with the **stigma** and **anxiety** associated with mental illness, influences the delivery of mental health care, in particular towards African-Caribbean patients. The perception of heightened risk translates to an increased likelihood of African-Caribbean patients receiving more coercive treatments including the use of manual restraint, seclusion and rapid tranquilisation (Hicks, 2004). This is further supported by the David Bennett inquiry, which found that nurses more easily initiated restrictive practice as a result of perceptions held about this group of patients. It is therefore unsurprising that Black and ethnic minorities are less likely to receive psychotherapy in comparison to their White counterparts. The increased use of coercive treatment towards Black patients has been found to remain on discharge from detention, where the use of restrictive community orders is more likely to be enforced (CQC, 2009).

MEDICATION

As mentioned earlier, psychological therapies are less available to BME groups, with perceptions held that members of these groups are unable to articulate their feelings as effectively as their White majority counterparts (Royal College of Nursing, 2004). This discriminatory practice severely disadvantages BME groups and leads to these communities receiving medication as the primary form of treatment (Fernando, 2002; McKenzie et al., 2001). As a result, there is an increased likelihood of BME patients receiving **antipsychotic** medication, higher doses and more frequently depot formulations, of which this disparity is even more pronounced amongst Black patients (Kuno & Rothbard, 2002). This finding is partly supported by Lloyd and Moodley (1992), who concluded, whilst there was no significant difference in doses of antipsychotic medication between Black and White patients, Black patients were more likely to receive depot antipsychotic and at markedly higher doses. Additionally, the David Bennett inquiry suspected the prescription of poly-medication was more likely amongst members of Black communities when compared to White patients, as they were perceived to be more dangerous and a nuisance (DH, 2005).

CULTURAL COMPETENCY IN PRACTICE

If a patient's cultural, social, and religious needs are not considered in the delivery of care, this may affect their reactions and exacerbate symptoms. It is therefore crucial that patient care is delivered in accordance with their needs. Although not an exhaustive list, Table 6.2 contains some of the barriers BME groups may encounter when accessing mental health services and the steps that can be taken to overcome these in clinical practice.

Table 6.2 Overcoming barriers to services in clinical practice

Barrier(s)	In practice
Language	Ask about your patient's proficiency of English and consider the use of an interpreter Find out the correct pronunciation of their name and how they prefer to be addressed Avoid the use of jargon or complex clinical language
Lack of information regarding available services	Provide information leaflets in your patient's native language, if appropriate
Stigma and fear of mental ill-health and social rejection	Promote mental health for all, working with individuals and communities to overcome discrimination and promote social inclusion (National Institute for Mental Health in England, 2003)
Not registered with a GP	Be aware of the different sources of support and help-seeking patterns
Reluctance to accept western medication	Be aware that health beliefs about psychiatry may be different across cultures. Therefore, it is important to find out how your patient perceives their mental illness. Always remain aware that you are nursing someone from a different culture. Therefore, they may put different interpretations on events and feelings
Isolation and lack of social/family support	Signpost individuals to appropriate BME groups
Misunderstanding leading to misdiagnosis	Allocate longer periods of time for assessments where an interpreter is being used. Summarise frequently throughout assessments to check your understanding
Generalisations and assumptions	Ensure your care plans detail each patient's ethnic origin and cultural needs

Source: adapted from Belfast Trust, 2014

CRITICAL THINKING STOP POINT 6.1

- Write a 'cultural biography' that reflects how your own culture has influenced and shaped your beliefs about mental health and mental illness.
- Discuss your cultural biography with your mentor and record your discussion and reflections for your portfolio.

CASE STUDY 6.1

Adina is an 18-year-old female and is admitted under Section 2 of the Mental Health Act 1983 [as amended] (England and Wales), to an acute mental health, mixed-sex ward and has a longstanding history of anxiety. As part of the admission process, information is gathered regarding Adina's religious and cultural needs. Adina informs staff that she is a strict Orthodox Jew, she speaks limited

(Continued)

English and her preferred language is Hebrew, maintains a Kosher diet and on the Sabbath she observes the rule that she will not 'work'. The admitting nurse is unsure of what this entails and asks Adina to explain what it means. Adina informs the nurse that from sunset on Friday to sunset on Saturday this religious injunction prohibits engaging in tasks which initiate the flow of electricity, such as turning on a light switch, writing, and carrying items. The nurse needs to develop a care plan to ensure other members of the nursing team are aware of and know how to meet this need.

Questions

- What aspects of care should be considered in the initial care plan to meet Adina's religious needs and how could these be addressed in clinical practice?
- How would you develop this care plan during Adina's admission and are there any other considerations you may need to take into account?

As a nurse with experience in a variety of clinical settings, I have found that person centred planning and understanding diversity should never be underestimated when trying to engage individuals to participate in occupational activity. When working on a forensic unit, the weekends were always quiet and patients were often at a loose end, which was not always beneficial to their wellbeing or recovery. I suggested having a 'world day' every Sunday in which the patients were encouraged to select a country. Once they had selected a country, they would be given a variety of different tasks that related to that country; whether that was to plan a menu, impart some knowledge about the country (e.g. fun facts, a phrase, history) or play music originating from the selected country, etc. It turned out to be quite successful in that both patients and staff were equally enthusiastic about taking part. It also created an opportunity to learn about different cultures in a fun and informal manner, as all individuals were freely contributing or learning information without feeling they were being 'assessed' or 'judged' by their peers or clinicians.

Donna Taylor, learning disability nurse

WOMEN'S MENTAL HEALTH

Women's experience of mental health differs from men's for both biological and social reasons. The area of women's mental health is relatively new and considerably more research is required to develop better understanding of and treatments for many of the mental illnesses experienced by women (Castle et al., 2006). Women's health is inextricably linked to their status in society; it benefits from equality and suffers from discrimination. Various feminist inspired critics have highlighted and challenged inequities for women within psychiatric services (Chesler, 1972; Millett, 1990; Ussher 1991). Today, the status and wellbeing of countless millions of women worldwide remain tragically low (WHO, 1998).

Approximately twice the proportion of women as men are diagnosed as having mental health problems (Green et al., 2002). Women are more likely than men to experience abuse, be in poverty and be lone parents, to **self-harm** and suffer from anxiety and/or **depression**, and to attempt suicide.

However, they are more likely to seek talking therapies and benefit from self-help (Kermode et al., 2007). Eating **disorders** and **body image** are issues with great relevance to women's lives (Hudson et al., 2007). While it seems that eating disorders are more prevalent amongst women, it may be that help seeking and openness about these disorders is lower amongst men.

Women are more likely than men to be in a caregiving role and the sedation caused by many psychiatric drugs makes looking after children/dependent adults difficult. Side-effects in general may be experienced as worse by women than men. Possible reasons for women experiencing a greater side-effect profile, as a result of antipsychotic medication, include the length of time such medication is stored in adipose tissue, more comorbid illnesses which increase the likelihood of drug interactions, and a higher prevalence of immune reactions (Castle et al., 2006).

PERINATAL MENTAL HEALTH

Women's mental health may have a consequential effect on their reproductive health – for example, oestrogen and progesterone influence **mood** and emotions. Phases of women's lives, including puberty, childbirth and menopause, are factors that may increase their risk of developing mental illness. More specifically, so too are miscarriage and termination, the phase of menstrual cycle, use of hormonal contraception, pregnancy, the postpartum period, breastfeeding or weaning, infertility treatment, hysterectomy and perimenopause.

The majority of women with severe mental illness (SMI) are mothers (Diaz-Caneja and Johnson, 2004). Women with SMI are substantially more likely to have child caring responsibilities than their male peers and women with bipolar disorder are at significantly greater risk of developing puerperal psychosis (Frisch & Frisch, 2009). Fear of losing custody of children colours interaction with mental health services. Women with SMI feel they are assumed to be inherently poor parents. Mothers receive little continuing support with parenting; instead, help may arrive only at times of crisis and is not always what the mothers would want. Custody loss is frequent – only 20% of mothers with SMI still have full custody of their children (Joseph et al., 1999). Women talk about the fulfilling aspects of motherhood and its role as an incentive to stay or get well (Antai-Otong, 2008). However, having children makes it difficult for mothers to adhere to medication and use mental health services, which may be perceived as non-concordance. Furthermore, the need to wake up during the night to attend to their children's needs may decrease the mother's ability to adhere to a medication regime.

MEETING WOMEN'S NEEDS

Short and Donna (2007) argue that current mental health service provision fails to adequately address the specific needs of women and can re-traumatise the women in its care. Women with mental ill health need treatment that is, first, tailored to women and, second, individualised. Women need to feel safe on wards and in the community, that staff respect them for who they are and that services are meeting their specific needs. Some women may benefit from women-only spaces and culturally appropriate staff/staff attitudes.

Women should have access to psychological therapies, as it has been shown that they do well with talking therapies, group therapy and self-help. Complementary therapies such as aromatherapy and reflexology are also often highly valued by women, although the evidence base for these is sparse (Short & Donna, 2007). Psychological treatments can also help women to cope with the emotional numbing which may be experienced as a result of taking antipsychotic medication. Finally, mental health services rarely, if ever, provide crèches so mothers may miss appointments. Those interviewed in a study by Caneja & Johnson (2004) said they would like respite for children of mothers with a mental illness, family support workers and support groups. The Drayton Park Crisis House (Killaspy et al., 2000) was seen by three of Caneja's research participants as a positive alternative to inpatient care. Children were able to stay with their mother in residential care for up to four weeks rather than being separated from them and placed with family or foster **carers**.

MAKING A DIFFERENCE 6.1

Being sexually abused by my uncle for most of my childhood I was naturally very scared of men. When I self-harmed on the acute ward sometimes I was restrained, invariably by men. This brought my traumatic history to the fore and cumulated in a vicious cycle of me wanting to harm myself further. It was only when I was moved into a specialist women's unit, which had a high proportion of female staff, that I began to feel more secure. I worked with my Named Nurse to develop a care plan around my advance directive that if my self-harming became so severe that for my safety I needed to be restrained, it would only be female staff that restrained me. As a result of this my desire to self-harm reduced and I was eventually discharged. I now have a female community psychiatric nurse visit me at home. In my opinion, having accessed the specialist women's service was paramount to my journey to recovery.

Eunys Vorgel Kelly, mental health survivor

CRITICAL THINKING STOP POINT 6.2

The nurse should be aware of certain cultural considerations specifically relevant to women. For example, some older South Asian women can be softly spoken and reluctant to express direct opinions; and some Asian women avoid shaking hands with one another or with men.

DISABLED PEOPLE'S MENTAL HEALTH

Disabled people are much more likely to experience poverty and social isolation than their non-disabled counterparts. These factors are positively correlated to mental health problems and, as such, it is likely that disabled people are disproportionately represented within the client base of mental health services. This may be particularly the case for learning impaired people (Cooper et al., 2007) and people who have recently acquired an impairment.

Table 6.3 shows two competing models of disability – the medical model and the social model. An example to demonstrate the difference between the two models would be the case of a wheelchair user who is unable to access a building because the building has steps. The medical model places the disabling factor in the fact that the person cannot walk up steps. The social model places the disabling factor in the lack of level access. The social model was first developed by Oliver (1990) and has since become the preferred model of disabled people's organisations in the UK on the pragmatic basis that reducing barriers to access has a greater potential to improve the lives of disabled people than seeking

Table 6.3   The medical versus the social model of disability

Model	Understanding of disability	Language used to address patient
Medical	Sees disability as a medical problem which resides within the individual	'Person with a disability'
Social	Sees disability as a social problem which resides in the barriers (physical, social, attitudinal) which prevent disabled people from being included in all aspects of life	'Disabled person'

Source: adapted from Goodley, 2011

out individual cures or fixes. When dealing with disabled patients, it is best practice to identify any barriers to accessing the service and seek to reduce them.

There can be many barriers for disabled people accessing treatment within a mental health setting, which vary depending on impairment. Giving the patient time in advance to prepare for the meeting with as much information as possible (the length, venue and topics covered), and asking what you can do to help meet their access needs in advance, are useful. You should also make sure you look at any relevant files, such as speech and language reports, in advance. Meeting people's access needs might involve 'physical' things like changing venues to a place that might better meet their needs, or rearranging furniture so that wheelchairs or other equipment can fit. It might mean allocating more time to the meeting if you need to discuss extra issues around accessibility or if the patient might need more time to absorb any information. It could involve providing written material in another format, or inviting an interpreter, family member, friend or personal assistant (carer) along to support them. Remember that if another person is coming in to support the patient, questions should be directed at the patient alone. It could also mean changing how you interact with the patient, using plain English if communication might be an issue, or asking more follow-up questions to check understanding.

Many people with learning impairments may exhibit behaviours such as echoing what others have said, overactivity or a very active imagination, which can be completely normal for them but pathologised as echolalia, **hypomania**, or **hallucinations** or **delusions** within a mental health context (Hardy et al., 2010). As such, it is important to build a picture of what constitutes 'normal' behaviour on a case-by-case basis. This should take into account that neurodivergent people (those displaying atypical patterns of thought) have different normalities to neurotypical people, that many people may have undiagnosed learning impairments, and that, conversely, behaviour that seems normal for a neurotypical person may be a signifier of distress in a neurodivergent person. The Royal College of Nursing has produced best practice guidance on working with patients with learning impairments in a mental health setting (see Hardy et al., 2010).

CRITICAL THINKING STOP POINT 6.3

Values and beliefs

A values and beliefs exercise is a versatile and meaningful way of exploring your values and beliefs. It can be used to help you create an individual and shared purpose for practice or care. Answer the following questions individually and then share your responses with your fellow nursing students:

(Continued)

- Recall times when you have been so absorbed in what you were doing that you hardly noticed the time. What were you doing?
- Think about the things that you find meaningful. What do you think of? Include ideals, feelings and activities.
- What are the five most important to you? Prioritise them.
- What is important to you as a future registered nurse?
- What do you feel is most important to accomplish with your patients?
- What matters most to you when you are NOT nursing?

LESBIAN, GAY, BISEXUAL AND TRANS MENTAL HEALTH

FENWAY
HEALTH

The **lesbian**, gay, **bisexual** and **trans** (LGBT) community is diverse (see Table 6.4 for a description of common LGBT identities). Whilst the L, G, B and T are often grouped together as an acronym that suggests homogeneity, each letter represents a wide range of people of different races, ages, socio-economic status, ethnicities and identities. Nevertheless, what binds them together as social and gender minorities are their shared experiences of discrimination and stigma, the challenge of living at the intersection of many cultural backgrounds and trying to be part of each, and, particularly with respect to health care, a long history of discrimination and lack of awareness of health needs by health professionals (see Fenway Health, http://fenwayhealth.org/). For example, between the 1930s and the 1970s some members of the LGBT community received aversion therapy: chemical and electrical treatment within psychiatric hospitals, in an attempt to 'cure' them of their 'sexual deviations'. Chemical aversion therapy involved using emetics to produce nausea and vomiting in the patient while showing him pictures of naked men, in the hope that he would come to associate the two. In electrical aversion therapy, the patient would be asked to watch pictures of men in various states of undress, whereupon electrical shocks would be administered if he got an erection above a certain size. Men convicted of homosexual offences[1] were given a choice of going to prison or undergoing treatment. Thinking it would be an easier option, many made the calamitous decision to undergo the treatment (Dickinson, 2015).

This has resulted in LGBT people sharing a common set of challenges in accessing culturally competent health services and achieving the highest possible level of health. Indeed, LGBT people have higher incidences of mental health problems than their heterosexual counterparts as a result of living in a homophobic society, which can lead individuals to experience 'minority stress' (Almeida et al., 2009). Minority stress is the psychological consequences of harassment and stigmatisation that members of minority groups may face. It is important to note that minority stress is a significant factor in mental health and wellbeing. Being LGBT places one outside of societal norms around gender and sexuality, thus positioning one as 'different from the norm'; an inevitably stressful experience which can be an influential contributing factor in becoming mentally distressed (Mayer, 2003).

Indeed, LGBT people have higher rates of self-harm (King et al., 2008), suicide/suicidal ideation (Haas et al., 2010; Mayock et al., 2008) and substance use (Buffin et al., 2012) than their heterosexual/ **cisgender** counterparts. Moreover, 49% of lesbian and bisexual women and 34% of gay and bisexual men do not feel able to be 'out' to any health care providers (Guasp & Taylor, 2012). This means that health care providers often miss out on important contextual factors, which may impact on a patient's care.

---

[1]Sex between men was illegal in England and Wales until the Sexual Offences Act became law in 1967, decriminalising sex between two consenting male adults over the age of 21 in private. Men in Scotland, Northern Ireland, Guernsey, Jersey and the Isle of Man had to wait until 1980, 1982, 1983, 1990 and 1993 respectively.

Table 6.4 Common LGBT identities

Bisexual: A person who is sexually and/or romantically attracted to women and men. You may see this shortened to bi.

Cis/cisgender: A cis person is someone who does identify with the gender that they were assigned at birth, i.e. a person who is not trans.

Gay man: A man who is sexually and/or romantically attracted to other men.

Intersexed person: An intersexed person (old word = hermaphrodite) is someone who has physical characteristics that differ from the typical male or female arrangements. They are most likely to be intermediate between the sexes, having some male and some female characteristics, or to have under-developed sex characteristics. Around 1 in 2000 people is identified as intersexed at birth. They may have chromosomal or hormonal differences - if an intersexed person is identified at birth, doctors usually test chromosomes and hormones to help them advise parents which gender to bring their baby up as. The notion of intersex complicates the legal insistence on a two-option (male/female) model. The system does not allow for sex or gender expressions other than male or female, although, for many people, their sex is not so clear-cut.

Lesbian: A woman who is sexually and/or romantically attracted to other women.

Non-binary: A person who identifies outside the gender binary, i.e. a person who identifies as neither a man nor a woman. Genderqueer, androgyne and gender fluid are non-binary gender identities you might hear used.

Pansexual: A person who has the capability of attraction to others, regardless of their gender identity or biological sex. A pansexual could be sexually and/or romantically attracted to someone who is male, female, transgender, intersex or genderqueer.

Trans: A trans person is someone who does not identify with the gender that they were assigned at birth. Trans (sometimes written trans*) is an umbrella term to describe a wide range of identities. Some trans people suffer from gender dysphoria, a sense of intense discomfort caused by the mismatch between their physical sex and their gender identity. This may cause them to seek out medical interventions such as hormones or surgery.

Transgender: Usually this refers to a trans person who socially and/or medically transitions from one binary gender to another. You may also hear the term transsexual used which implies a greater focus on medical transition which some consider to be pathologising.

Transitioning: The process of changing the way one's gender is lived publicly. Transitioning may involve changes in clothing and grooming, a name change, change of gender on identity documents, hormonal treatment and surgery.

As such, it is imperative to create an environment where LGBT patients feel comfortable discussing their sexuality and identity within a clinical environment.

There are several ways in which to make LGBT patients feel more comfortable in a clinical environment. LGBT patients often search for subtle cues in the environment to determine acceptance. This can include 'physical' cues, such as displaying a non-discrimination statement addressing equality issues such as homophobia, transphobia and biphobia where it can be seen publically, and providing LGBT-specific health promotion literature within waiting rooms and on notice boards (Eliason & Schope, 2001).

In consultations, it is important to stress that discussions of sexuality with clinical staff remain confidential and will be dealt with sensitively. This means that clinicians should not assume that patients are heterosexual or cisgendered, or that their relationships take a particular form (i.e. marriage), and same-sex partners should be treated as any other close family member.

When patients disclose their sexual orientation, clinicians should be mindful of adopting an appropriate response. This may include briefly thanking the patient for disclosing the information, confirming that it will be kept confidential and signposting them to any relevant LGBT-specific services, if appropriate.

If you are the first person that the patient has told, you may wish to talk more in depth about the issue and what support they may need, always letting the patient take the lead. Clinicians should be mindful not to ignore this information – the patient will have disclosed their sexuality because they either feel it is relevant to their care or because it is an important part of their identity.

Clinicians should also be mindful in attributing patients' mental health problems as being 'caused by' their sexuality or identity. Whilst the LGBT community has higher prevalence rates for mental health problems than the cisgender and heterosexual community, it is not an innate part of being LGBT (Dalloway & Dickinson, 2014). Rather, it is often a symptom of living in a homophobic, transphobic and biphobic society. The patient may also feel that their sexuality is irrelevant to their mental health, and this should be respected.

Finally, it is important to create a safe environment for LGBT people. Staff in inpatient settings should be mindful of the safety and security of LGBT individuals, who may be subjected to negative comments or behaviour related to their LGBT identity from other patients. It is pertinent to challenge homophobia, transphobia and biphobia on the ward and in the wider clinical environment. It is important to do this without 'outing' the patient as LGBT, i.e. by saying, 'this behaviour is inappropriate' or 'you are disturbing other patients'.

TRANS MENTAL HEALTH

Whilst on placement with an A&E liaison team we undertook a risk assessment on a trans woman who had taken an overdose. The Registered Nurse who was supervising me explained that the patient was trans, however he referred to her using the incorrect pronoun. The patient was clearly uncomfortable with this and she later explained to me that similar attitudes in her local area had caused her to become isolated and low in mood. When writing up her notes, the nurse asked why I referred to her as female rather than male, explaining that in his opinion, she was physically male and, therefore, would use a different pronoun. I stressed the importance that she identified as a female and, therefore, I would be referring to her using the pronoun that she preferred. I later spoke to my mentor about the situation, stressing the importance that we recognise people's individual choice (NMC Code, 2015), which I did not feel the other nurse was doing with this patient. It is important in situations like this to speak with your mentor to help resolve the issue and prevent future harm to patients.

Rachel Lyon, mental health nursing student

According to the Trans Mental Health Study (N = 991), 66% of trans people use mental health services for reasons other than to access gender transition treatments (McNeil et al., 2012). When undergoing transition-related treatment, many trans people feel that being open about any mental health problems can complicate their access to treatment, with some trans individuals having their gender treatment delayed or even denied on grounds that they have accessed mental health services (Webb et al., 2014). Moreover, trans people are often denied access to mental health treatment as they can be seen as 'too complicated', or their mental health problems are viewed as related to their trans status. As such, trans people are less likely to access help with mental health problems and are disproportionately represented in crisis services (McNeil et al., 2012).

WHAT'S THE EVIDENCE? 6.1

WHAT'S THE
EVIDENCE?
6.1 ARTICLES

Read the following articles (available at https://study.sagepub.com/ essential mental health):

Dickinson, T., Cook, M., Hallett, C. & Playle, J. (2014)
Dickinson, T., Cook, M., Playle, J. & Hallett, C. (2012)
Simpson, P., Horne, M., Brown Wilson, C., Brown, L., Dickinson, T. & Torkington, K. (2017)
Simpson, P., Horne, M., Brown, L.E., Dickinson, T. & Brown Wilson, C. (2016)

Now consider the questions below:

1. For LGBT people, who may remember that homosexuality and cross-gender transvestism were classified as mental illnesses and routinely (and largely unsuccessfully) 'treated' with barbaric aversion therapy until the 1980s, how do you think this may affect their perception of mental health services?
2. If you were instructed by a senior nurse or medical officer to undertake a clinical intervention that you did not agree with, for whatever reason, what would you do and why?
3. You are working in a nursing home and one of the residents, with mental capacity, wants to continue having a sexual/intimate relationship with his same-sex partner. What are your thoughts on this?
4. What factors may impede on his ability to maintain a sexual/intimate relationship with his partner within a nursing home environment?
5. How could you work around some of these environmental factors?

CASE STUDY 6.2

Onnee, aged 57, is a trans woman with a diagnosis of posterior cortical atrophy (PCA), also known as Benson's syndrome. This is a rare degenerative condition in which damage occurs at the back (posterior region) of the brain. Onnee was admitted to a specialist nursing home that provides nursing intervention for younger people with dementia. On admission, the team was unsure which gender unit to place her on, so they placed her on the male unit. This has caused great distress to Onnee and some of the male patients have been noted to mock her. Staff on the unit are also struggling with this and are addressing her with incorrect pronouns, which is very upsetting for Onnee. She wants to use the female bathroom, but other female patients are complaining about this. Therefore, she is currently using the disabled toilet.

Questions

- How would you deal with the transphobic behaviour on the unit?
- Which gender unit do you think Onnee should be on?

CRITICAL DEBATE 6.1

Now that you have worked through this chapter and considered some of the issues, why not deliberate the following questions with your fellow nursing students:

1. How would valuing diversity enhance mental health nursing practice?
2. If someone from another culture, religion or sexuality, or a person who identifies outside the gender binary, is admitted to your mental health setting, is it not up to that person to adjust?
3. What specific actions could you take in a mental health setting that would show that you acknowledge and appreciate diversity?

CONCLUSION

This chapter has explored the components of disability, sexuality, gender, ethnicity, culture and religion that can affect the therapeutic relationship. It is paramount that mental health nurses recognise that these unique characteristics within their patients open up complementary ways of perceiving, thinking and acting that enrich our understanding of mental health. Mental health nurses are generally striving to provide patient-centred and high quality care in often challenging, stressful and frustrating environments. Patients should receive a holistic assessment that endeavours to promote health and considers the unique characteristics among those with a mental illness to foster a state of mental, social and emotional wellbeing for all. Creating an environment or displaying an attitude that does not value and embrace these characteristics may curtail patients' recovery. If mental health nurses are to provide culturally competent care, they must recognise and respect diversity and actively tackle oppression.

CHAPTER SUMMARY

This chapter has covered the following ideas:

- Respect for diversity is a well-established tenet of mental health nursing practice and helps to promote recovery.
- Mental health nurses must recognise and respect diversity and actively tackle oppression.
- Unhelpful practices and pejorative attitudes towards diversity can obstruct recovery.
- Each patient is unique, with different social, biological and psychological factors that may influence their response to stress and ill health.
- Knowledge of various cultural patterns and variances helps the nurse begin to relate to patients of different ethnic and cultural backgrounds.
- To provide competent nursing care, nurses must be alert to, and knowledgeable regarding, factors that may impact on the care of patients. This includes issues related to gender, disability, sexuality, culture and ethnicity.

BUILD YOUR BIBLIOGRAPHY

Books

- Dickinson, T. (2015) *'Curing queers': Mental nurses and their patients, 1935–1974*. Manchester: Manchester University Press. 'This book should be read by everyone with an interest in mental health care and by all who recognise their democratic responsibility to ensure that those in need are assisted and neither deceived nor abused.' *Peter Nolan, Professor of Mental Health Nursing (Emeritus), Staffordshire University*

- Leininger, M.M. & McFarland, M.R. (2006) *Culture care diversity and universality: A worldwide nursing theory.* Boston, MA: Jones and Bartlett Publishers. This book aims to support nurses who would like to develop their skills in providing culturally competent practice.
- Zeeman, L., Aranda, K. & Grant, A. (2014) *Queering health: Critical challenges to normative health and healthcare.* Monmouth: PCCS Books. For those looking to provide insight into equality and diversity in their nursing practice, then this book does just that in a way that will inspire.

SAGE journal articles

Go to https://study.sagepub.com/essentialmentalhealth for further free online journal articles related to this chapter. If you are using the interactive ebook, simply click on the book icon in the margin to go straight to the resource.

FURTHER
READING:
JOURNAL
ARTICLES

- Bains, J. (2005) Race, culture and psychiatry: a history of transcultural psychiatry. *History of Psychiatry, 16*(2), 139-154.
- Jimenez, M.A. (1997) Gender and psychiatry: psychiatric conceptions of mental disorders in women, 1960-1994. *Affilia, 12*(2), 154-175.
- Mildenberger, F. (2007) Kraepelin and the 'urnings': male homosexuality in psychiatric discourse. *History of Psychiatry, 18*(3), 321-335.

Weblinks

Go to https://study.sagepub.com/essentialmentalhealth for further weblinks related to this chapter. If you are using the interactive ebook, simply click on the book icon in the margin to go straight to the resource.

FURTHER
READING:
WEBLINKS

- The Royal College of Nursing (RCN) has produced suicide prevention guidance for trans young people. See, e.g., Dockerty, C. & Guerra, L. (2015) Preventing suicide among trans young people: A toolkit for nurses. Available at: www.suicideinfo.Ca/wp-content/uploads/2015/09/Preventing-Suicide-among-Trans-Young-People_oa.pdf
- The RCN has also produced a suicide prevention kit for lesbian, gay and bisexual young people. See, e.g., Guerra, L. (2015) Preventing suicide among lesbian, gay, and bisexual young people: A toolkit for nurses. Available at: www.gov.uk/government/uploads/system/uploads/attachment_data/file/412427/LGB_Suicide_Prevention_Toolkit_FINAL.pdf
- Transcultural C.A.R.E. Associates have produced some online resources regarding transcultural health care practice. Available at: http://transculturalcare.net/

——— ACE YOUR ASSESSMENT ———

Revise what you have learned by visiting https://study.sagepub.com/essentialmentalhealth. If you are using the interactive ebook, simply click on the tick icon to go straight to the resource.

ONLINE
QUIZZES &
ACTIVITY
ANSWERS

- Test yourself with multiple-choice and short-answer questions and flashcards.

REFERENCES

Almeida, J., Johnson, R.M., Corliss, H.L., Molnar, B.E. & Azrael, D. (2009) Emotional distress among LGBT youth: the influence of perceived discrimination based on sexual orientation. *Journal of Youth and Adolescence, 38*(7), 1001–1014.

Antai-Otong, D. (2008) *Psychiatric nursing: Biological and behavioral concepts.* 2nd edtn. New York: Thompson Delmar Learning.

Belfast Trust (2014) *Ethnic minorities mental health toolkit: A guide for practitioners.* Available at: www.belfasttrust.hscni.net/pdf/BME_Cultural_Awareness_Document_sml.pdf (accessed 02.08.15).

Betancourt, J.R., Green, A.R., Carillo, J.E., et al. (2005) Cultural competence and health disparities: key perspectives and trends. *Health Affairs, 24*(2), 499–505.

Bhugra, D., Leff, J., Mallett, R., et al. (1997) Incidence and outcome of schizophrenia in Whites, African-Caribbeans and Asians in London. *Psychological Medicine, 27,* 791–798.

Braine, D. (1997) *Black people and sectioning: The black experience of detention under the civil section of the Mental Health Act.* London: Little Rock Publishing.

Buffin, J., Roy, A., Williams, H. et al. (2012) *Part of the picture: lesbian, gay, and bisexual people's alcohol and drug use in England (2009–2011).* Available at http://lgbt.foundation/policy-research/part-of-the-picture (accessed August 2015).

Campinha-Bacote, J. (2002) The process of cultural competence in the delivery of healthcare services: a model of care. *Journal of Transcultural Nursing, 13*(93), 181–184.

Caneja, D. & Johnson, S. (2004) The views and experiences of severely mentally ill mothers: a qualitative study. *Social Psychiatry and Epidemiology, 36*(6),472–482.

Care Quality Commission (CQC) (2009) *Count me in 2009: the National Mental Health and Learning Disability Ethnicity Census.* London: CQC/National Health Mental Health Development Unit.

Castle, D., Kulkarni, J. & Abel, K.M. (eds) (2006) *Mood and anxiety disorders in women.* Cambridge: Cambridge University Press.

Chesler, P. (1972) *Women and madness.* New York: Doubleday.

Coid, J., Kahtan, N., Gault, S. et al. (2000) Ethnic differences in admission to secure forensic psychiatry services. *British Journal of Psychiatry, 177,* 241–247.

Cooper, S.A., Smiley, E., Morrison, J., et al. (2007) Mental ill-health in adults with intellectual disabilities: prevalence and associated factors. *The British Journal of Psychiatry, 190*(1), 27–35.

Dalloway, L. & Dickinson, T. (2014) It's all in the mind. *Gay Times,* June.

Davies, S., Thornicroft, G., Leese, M., et al. (1996) Ethnic difference in risk of compulsory psychiatric admission among representative cases of psychosis in London. *British Medical Journal, 312,* 533–537.

Department of Health (DH) (2004) *Breaking through: Building a diverse leadership workforce.* London: The Stationery Office.

Department of Health (DH) (2005) *Delivering race equality in mental health care: An action plan for reform inside and outside services.* London: DH.

Diaz-Caneja, A. & Johnson, S. (2004) The views and experiences of severely mentally ill mothers. *Social psychiatry and psychiatric epidemiology, 39*(6), 472-482.

Dickinson, T. (2015) *'Curing queers': Mental nurses and their patients, 1935–1974.* Manchester: University of Manchester Press.

Dickinson, T., Cook, M., Hallett, C. & Playle, J. (2014) Nurses and subordination: a historical study of mental nurses' perceptions on administering aversion therapy for 'sexual deviations'. *Nursing Inquiry,* 21(4), 283–293.

Dickinson, T., Cook, M., Playle, J. & Hallett, C. (2012) 'Queer' treatments: giving a voice to former patients who received treatments for their 'sexual deviations'. *Journal of Clinical Nursing*, 21(9), 1345–1354.

Dockerty, C. & Guerra, L. (2015) Preventing suicide among trans young people: A toolkit for nurses. Available at: www.gov.uk/government/uploads/system/uploads/attachment_data/file/417707/Trans_suicide_Prevention_Toolkit_Final_26032015.pdf (accessed 02.08.15).

Eliason, M.J. & Schope, R. (2001) Does 'don't ask don't tell' apply to health care? Lesbian, gay, and bisexual people's disclosure to health care providers. *Journal of the Gay and Lesbian Medical Association*, 5(4), 125–134.

Engebretson, J., Mahoney, J. & Carison, E.D. (2008) Cultural competence in the era of evidence-based practice. *Journal of Professional Nursing*, 24(3), 172–178.

Equality Commission for Northern Ireland (2014) *Gaps in law between Great Britain and Northern Ireland*. Available at: www.equalityni.org/ECNI/media/ECNI/Publications/Delivering%20Equality/Gaps-in-Equality-Law-in-GB-and-NI-March-2014.pdf (accessed 28.02.16).

Fernando, S.J.M. (2002) *Mental Health, Race and Culture*, 2nd edition. Basingstoke: Palgrave.

Fernando, S.J.M. (2010) *Mental Health, Race and Culture*, 3rd edition. Basingstoke: Palgrave.

Frisch, N.C. & Frisch, L.E. (2009) *Psychiatric mental health nursing*. New York: Thomson Delmar Learning.

Goldberg, D. (1999) Cultural aspects of mental disorder in primary care. In D. Bhugra and V. Bhal (eds) *Ethnicity: An agenda for mental health*. London: Gaskell. pp. 23–28.

Goodley, D. (2011) *Disability studies: An interdisciplinary introduction*. London: Sage.

Green, G., Bradby, H., Chan, A., et al. (2002) Is the English National Health Service meeting the needs of mentally distressed Chinese women? *Journal of health services research & policy*, 7(4), 216–221.

Guasp, A. & Taylor, J. (2012) *Experiences of healthcare: Stonewall health briefing*. Available at: www.stonewall.org.uk/sites/default/files/Experiences_of_Healthcare_Stonewall_Health_Briefing__2012__.pdf (accessed 02.08.15).

Guerra, L. (2015) Preventing suicide among lesbian, gay, and bisexual young people: A toolkit for nurses. Available at: www.gov.uk/government/uploads/system/uploads/attachment_data/file/412427/LGB_Suicide_Prevention_Toolkit_FINAL.pdf (accessed 02.08.15).

Haas, A.P., Eliason, M., Mays, V.M., et al. (2010) Suicide and suicide risk in lesbian, gay, bisexual, and transgender populations: review and recommendations. *Journal of Homosexuality*, 58(1), 10–51.

Hardy, S., Chaplin, E. & Woodward, P. (2010) *Mental health nursing of people with learning disabilities: RCN guidance*. Available at: www.rcn.org.uk/__data/assets/pdf_file/0006/78765/003184.pdf (accessed 02.08.15).

Hicks, J.W. (2004) Ethnicity, race, and forensic psychiatry: are we color blind? *Journal of the American Academy of Psychiatry and the Law*, 32, 21–33.

Hoptman, M.J., Yates, K.F., Patalinjug, M.B., et al. (1999) Clinical prediction of assaultive behaviour among male psychiatric patients at a maximum security forensic facility. *Psychiatric Services*, 50(11), 1461–1466.

Hudson, J.I., Hiripi, E., Pope, H.G., et al. (2007) The prevalence and correlates of eating disorders in the National Comorbidity Survey Replication. *Biological psychiatry*, 61(3), 348–358.

Hunt, B. (2004) Recent equality legislation in the UK. *Nursing ethics*, 11(4), 411–413.

Joseph, J.G., Joshi, S.V., Lewin, A.B., et al. (1999) Characteristics and perceived needs of mothers with serious mental illness. *Psychiatric Services*, 50(10), 1357–1359.

Kermode, M., Herrman, H., Arole, R., et al. (2007) Empowerment of women and mental health promotion: a qualitative study in rural Maharashtra, India. *BMC public health*, 7(1), 225.

Killaspy, H., Dalton, J., McNicholas, S. et al. (2000) Drayton Park, an alternative to hospital admission for women in acute mental health crisis. Psychiatric Bulletin, 24(3), pp.101–104.

King, M., Coker, E., Leavey, G., et al. (1994) Incidence of psychotic illness in London: comparison of ethnic groups. *British Medical Journal, 309*, 1115–1119.

King, M., Semlyen, J., Tai, S.S., Killaspy, H., et al. (2008) A systematic review of mental disorder, suicide, and deliberate self-harm in lesbian, gay and bisexual people. *BMC Psychiatry, 8*, 70.

Kramer, E.J., Kwong, K., Lee, E., et al. (2002) Cultural factors influencing the mental health of Asian Americans. *Western Journal of Medicine, 176*(4), 227–231.

Kuno, E. & Rothbard, A.B. (2002) Racial disparities in antipsychotic prescription patterns for patients with schizophrenia. *American Journal of Psychiatry, 159*, 567–572.

LeFrançois, B., Menzies, R. & Reaume, G. (eds) (2013) *Mad matters: A critical reader in Canadian mad studies*. Toronto: Canadian Scholars Press.

Littlewood, R. & Lipsedge, M. (1981) Some social and phenomenological characteristics of psychotic immigrants. *Psychological Medicine, 11*, 289–302.

Lloyd, K. & Moodley, P. (1992) Psychotrophic medication and ethnicity: an inpatient survey. *Social Psychiatry and Psychiatric Epidemiology, 27*, 95–101.

Maden, A., Swinton, M. & Gunn, M. (1992) The ethnic origin of women serving a prison sentence. *British Journal of Criminology, 32*(2), 218–221.

Mayer, I.H. (2003) Prejudice, social stress, and mental health in lesbian, gay, and bisexual populations: conceptual issues and research evidence. *Psychological Bulletin, 129*(5), 674–697.

Mayock, P., Bryan, A., Carr, N. et al. (2008) *Supporting LGBT lives: A study of mental health and well-being*. Dublin: Gay and Lesbian Equality Network.

McFarland-Icke, B.R. (1999) *Nurses in Nazi Germany: A moral choice in history*. Princeton, NJ: Princeton University Press.

McKenzie, K., Samele, C., Van Horn, E., et al. (2001) Comparison of the outcome of the treatment of psychosis for people of Caribbean origin living in the UK and British Whites: report from the UK 700 trial. *British Journal of Psychiatry, 178*, 160–165.

McKeown, M. & Stowell-Smith, M. (2001) 'Big, black and dangerous'?: the vexed question of race in forensic care. In Landsberg, G. & Smiley, A. (eds) *Forensic mental health: working with offenders with mental illness*. New Jersey: Civic Research Institute.

McNeil, J., Bailey, L., Ellis, S., et al. (2012) *Trans mental health study*. Available at: www.scottishtrans. org/wp-content/uploads/2013/03/trans_mh_study.pdf (accessed 02.08.15).

Millett, K. (1990) *The loony-bin trip*. New York: Simon and Schuster.

Moodley, P. & Perkins, R.E. (1991) Routes to psychiatric inpatient care in an inner London borough. *Social Psychiatry and Psychiatric Epidemiology, 26*, 47–51.

National Association for the Care and Resettlement of Offenders (2007) *Black communities, mental health and the criminal justice system*. Available at: www.ohrn.nhs.uk/resource/policy/ Nacroblackcommunities.pdf (accessed 17.08.15).

National Institute for Mental Health in England (2003) *Inside outside: Improving mental health services for black and minority ethnic communities in England*. Available at: http://webarchive. nationalarchives.gov.uk/20130107105354/http:/www.dh.gov.uk/prod_consum_dh/groups/dh_ digitalassets/@dh/@en/documents/digitalasset/dh_4019452.pdf (accessed 01.08.15).

Northern Ireland Assembly (2011) *Equality and human rights legislation in Northern Ireland: A review*. Available at: www.niassembly.gov.uk/globalassets/documents/raise/publications/2011/ ofmdfm/7511.pdf (accessed 28.02.16).

Northern Ireland Statistics & Research Agency (2011) *Key statistics for Northern Ireland*. Available at: www.nisra.gov.uk/Census/key_stats_bulletin_2011.pdf (accessed 28 February 2016).

Office for National Statistics (ONS) (2012) *Ethnicity and national identity in England and Wales 2011*. Available at: www.ons.gov.uk/ons/dcp171776_290558.pdf (accessed 01.08.15).

Oliver, M. (1990) *The politics of disablement: Critical texts in social work and the welfare state*. London: Macmillan.

Owen, S. & Khalil, E. (2007) Addressing diversity in mental health care: a review of guidance documents. *International Journal of Nursing Studies*, *44*(3), 467–478.

Royal College of Nursing (2004) *Transcultural health care practice: An educational resource for nurses and health care practitioners*. Available at: www.rcn.org.uk/development/learning/transcultural_health/transcultural (accessed 12.08.15).

Scottish Government, *The (2011) Summary ethnic group demographics*. Available at: www.gov.scot/Topics/People/Equality/Equalities/DataGrid/Ethnicity/EthPopMig (accessed 28 February 2016).

Simpson, P., Horne, M., Brown Wilson, C., Brown, L., Dickinson, T. & Torkington, K. (2017) Older care home residents and sexual/intimate citizenship. *Ageing and Society*. 37, 243–265.

Simpson, P., Horne, M., Brown, L.E., Dickinson, T. & Brown Wilson, C. (2016) Sexuality and intimacy among care home residents. *Nursing Times*, 112(10), 14–16.

St Clair, H.E. (1951) Psychiatric interview experience with negroes. *American Journal of Psychiatry*, *108*, 113–19.

Traies, J. (2014) *Intimate fears: Old lesbians talking about the future*. Unpublished paper delivered at Critical Diversities conference, 11 July, London South Bank University.

Trivedi, P. (2002) Racism, social exclusion and mental health: a black service user's perspective .' *In* K. Bhui (ed). *Racism and Mental Health: Prejudice and Suffering*. London: Jessica Kingsley.

Ussher, J. M. (1991) *Women's madness: Misogyny or mental illness?* Amherst, MA: University of Massachusetts Press.

Van Os J., Castle, D.J., Takei, N., et al. (1996) Psychotic illness in ethnic minorities: clarifications from the 1991 census. *Psychological Medicine*, *26*, 203–208.

Webb, L.A., Bradley, J. & Williams-Schultz, G. (2014) *Falling through the cracks: Non-binary people's experiences of transition related health*. Available at: www.actionfortranshealth.org.uk (accessed 02.08.15).

World Health Organization (1998) *Life in the 21st century: A vision for all*. Geneva: World Health Organization.

ORGANISATIONS AND SETTINGS FOR MENTAL HEALTH CARE

7

JOE FORSTER, SARAH LOUGHRAN, ROB MACDONALD AND IAN CALLAGHAN

THIS CHAPTER COVERS

- The community as the basis for mental health care
- Transition to the least restrictive service
- The pathway to recovery.

"

We live in an era in which we recognise the value of good design, and are seeking ever better ways to achieve it. As a student nurse in the 1970s, the last days of the asylums, I lived in a nurses' home in the hospital grounds. With cafeteria, laundry, social club, library, even a part-time bank branch and of course my workplace on site, there was hardly any need to ever leave the campus. The sense of everything being provided and regulated meant that institutionalisation was a reality for many of the staff as much as for the patients. Things seemed resistant to change, though many improvements were won. I discovered a new way of organising care by moving to a primary-nurse-led unit where decisions about the service were based on clinical need without the use of formal ward management hierarchies. This taught me to look for what was really needed without preconceptions about what should be provided or how.

Gradually, I heard that many of those patients we believed required long-term locked wards in that first asylum had resettled into ordinary housing with community support. As well as reorientation to a community-based model of service, I found myself involved with new approaches to care, including co-production and co-design, and developing awareness of how interactions at work meet my own needs for validation and self-worth. And when I received talking treatment myself, accessed by visiting a clinic while living in my own home, it underlined that there is no 'them' and 'us'; it's just 'us' – we are all searching to bring meaning and wellbeing into our lives.

Joe Forster, mental health nurse

"

Visit **https://study.sagepub.com/essentialmentalhealth** to access a wealth of online resources for this chapter – watch out for the margin icons throughout the chapter. If you are using the interactive ebook, simply click on the margin icon to go straight to the resource.

"

For me, physical and psychological space are not separable. With a lifelong bipolar affective disorder I have experienced several mental health facilities. The threshold between the unit and outside is invariably first experienced during an episode on the threshold of sanity and the inner insane world, perhaps arriving handcuffed in a police car. One unit, forty miles from home as an emergency admission, was relatively new with internal courtyards, an interior street with some daylight, and colour – yellow – had been used inside. Going outdoors was restricted but eventually allowed as my recovery developed. My bedroom just had a view onto grey gravel, no plants or greenery, and seemed a solitary, cellular space. The shared dining room and queueing for medication felt clinical and undignified, and at that time, the lounge and TV room were used for smoking. Not greatly attracted by line dancing or basic art, I found I really had nothing to do. Another unit nearer home looked like a fortress with inner courtyards occasionally opened for patients, windowless meeting and dining rooms, no relationship to gardens or landscape, dark and almost colourless furniture. The immediate perception is of fear. Observation is kept into the room, in the shower, in the kitchen. At first I stayed close to to my room where a robin who came to my window sill became my companion. Gradually I spent time in the 'street' walking and pacing, washing clothes, walking to the exits only to be halted by a member of staff. Towards the end of my treatment nurses took me to a garden centre for seeds to plant back in the hospital. I found a nearby pale stone church and clambered up the bell tower to find the ringers; it was springtime and the yellow daffodils were in bloom.

It's always good to ask why things are the way they are. My ideal space would look over a garden with an oak tree and a pine tree. There has to be a window with a view; perhaps there is in the near distance an inviting garden seat in the sun. My interior space can be personalised with books, posters and sculptures. A radio and the sound of voices and music are important. Anti-ligature should be understated and talking therapy would be predominant. The hospital is a place of entrances and exits, secured locations and gateways to the seasons outside and sanctuary within. Here I am sitting in the window seat of a coffee bar. The music is in the background, the lighting gentle and the colours warm. Pictures on the wall are of places that I know. People are strolling on their way on the pavement outside.

Dr Rob MacDonald, service user

"

INTRODUCTION

Person-centred care respects the integrity of each individual, part of which means respecting the location to which they belong – their home and its integration with their family and community. In our **service user** box above, Dr Rob MacDonald contrasts his prior experience of hospital design with his ideal space. Many of his wishes have now been incorporated in hospital buildings designed with his input, with an understanding that experts by experience can improve the way services work and the quality of their outcomes. His priority throughout is remaining connected with and returning to the landscape, the community and ordinary life. As a student and a nurse, you may work in a variety of different organisations, places and settings; they are all part of the community, and integration with that community, rather than separation from it, is what is important.

THE COMMUNITY AS THE BASIS FOR MENTAL HEALTH CARE

CASE STUDY:
DESIGN IN
MENTAL
HEALTH
NETWORK

Most mental health care takes place away from specialist buildings and may not even be readily recognised as such. We promote our own mental health and that of others by connecting with one another, keeping active, being in the moment, learning, and participating in community life (Aked et al., 2008). When we need help, we may turn to family, friends or other groups. When structured or professional intervention is required, we may access it through a school, an employer or a self-help group. Specialist settings for more formal support include the general practitioner surgery, health centre, outpatient department and hospital, although it may often be delivered by professionals visiting service users at home.

The ability of our **environment** to provide space to access health promotion, structured help and formal support should be thought of on many layers, each having facets from the specific to the global (Lawrence, 2011). Individual housing that is free from damp and overcrowding, safe neighbourhoods with adequate transport and facilities, and worldwide regulation of pollution, energy and water supply are incorporated in the physical, material context. Social considerations include the security of employment and housing tenure, access to a system of health and social care, and freedom from civil or international conflict. Culturally, autonomy in our own life, integration of our ethnic and social group with society at large, and the migration of populations have an influence.

WHAT'S THE EVIDENCE? 7.1

A salutogenic approach has been suggested to apply the idea that buildings and neighbourhoods can be planned and designed not only to avoid causing harm (such as through so-called 'sick-building syndrome' or overcrowding), but also to promote wellbeing through social cohesion, personal control and ergonomic, aesthetic, restorative design. This provides the framework for a growing body of research to guide the architecture of health care in the future (Dilani, 2015).

CASE STUDY 7.1

Halton Autistic Family Support Group (HAFS)

As an example of active community participation, HAFS provides services run by and for families coping with autistic spectrum disorder. As they themselves put it, 'HAFS provides services to the whole family unit for families for Halton who have a child or young adult with a condition within the broad range of autistic spectrum disorders. HAFS is unique in this respect as most support groups either cater for the affected person or parents. One of the first things you'll notice at our meetings is the friendly and caring atmosphere. You are NOT alone anymore'. Through volunteering, fundraising, grants and accessing available resources, HAFS provides a range of services to ensure every child reaches their full potential, from support group meetings, social events, trips and activities to specialist advice - including representation at hearings and appeals - on accessing formal health and social care, education and benefits.

HAFS employs a full-time, salaried development manager and sessional staff to support activities. However, HAFS is not able to receive direct statutory funding as that would require compromising its 'family first' ethos by signing up to the commissioners' 'children first' principle. While hoping to eventually build a new, innovative autism centre of excellence, HAFS has a high street shop as its premises and hires a local play centre for larger group activities. Spaces within the premises are delineated for different purposes, with its charity goods fundraising shop forming a welcoming, visible entrance. Shelving partitions lead off to a flexible meeting and activity area with kitchen, toilets and office accessed from it. HAFS families have moulded both their service and their building to meet their own needs. (www.hafs.org.uk)

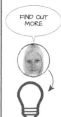

FIND OUT MORE

HAFS

CRITICAL THINKING STOP POINT 7.1

Should government funding be provided to user-led services even when their model of care has some different principles to accepted best practice?

Go to http://study.sagepub.com/essentialmentalhealth to find a suggested answer to this question.

CRITICAL THINKING STOP POINT 7.1 ANSWER

TRANSITION TO THE LEAST RESTRICTIVE SERVICE

When care moves from ordinary life in the community to specialist settings, the concept of **recovery** suggests we should think in terms of transition rather than placement. In this way, home and the community continue to be the focus of belonging for the service user, whose priority is to remain integrated with them rather than to adapt to a separate environment.

Transition between settings may involve varying levels of security and supervision, while therapeutic care is constant in all settings. Physical security – having a protected perimeter and the use of barriers to misconduct (such as locked doors) – is provided by the building and equipment, and may be supplemented by the procedural security of policies governing activity within the unit. Relational security arises from the quality of relationships enabling knowledge, awareness and **collaboration** to manage risks (Craissati & Taylor, 2014). These types of security may fluctuate, as, for example, a service user in their own home might be closely supervised by family members and visiting staff at a time of crisis while retaining their own front door key (higher relational security but lower physical security), while a service user in a prison health care centre during a stable time might only have routine interactions with staff (higher physical security but lower relational security).

Standards and guidance require that people receive services in the least restrictive and stigmatising environment possible (NICE, 2014). This makes flexibility of approach necessary as a service might accommodate people at different stages of their need for security, or those in transition to another level. Relational security can be individualised by collaboration between service users and staff, while physical features can be co-designed to be unobtrusive and adaptable. For example, it is increasingly common for access to the outdoors to be provided without the need for locked doors, supervision or unsightly fencing by internal courtyards enclosed by the building itself (Shaw, 2015). However, the impact on **self-harm** by lowering or removing so-called ligature points only partly manages such risks, and relationships and therapy remain the key (Hall, 2015).

> It is difficult to compare different areas because illnesses and challenges are different. I feel people don't always know where they fit in, however they still know what is expected. In wards, people are usually working towards shared outcomes with a more united feel. One ward was white, bright and clean with natural light and an impression of space and freedom, but more like a hotel than a home. Communal areas were open plan, so noise could be an issue, however there were prayer rooms if you wanted time for reflection and patients had their own private rooms. It was easy to find your way around, with a garden in the centre. I found the greenery calming, though it could have had more seating to enjoy the peace and quiet. The dining room felt like a school canteen, quite demoralising.
>
> Another hospital was less modern, and the brightly coloured walls were less clinical but sometimes over-stimulating. There was less space and more concrete outside. Every room came off one corridor which had no windows. It felt darker and less hopeful. Shared dormitories felt a lot less private and made finding a quieter environment difficult. High ceilings and the dining room gave a more homely feel, like an old house, and seemed more relaxed. The room used for creative activities overlooked greenery but was also used for meetings which limited time for both. Visitors were always treated with respect and on the whole so were patients, who were always listened to. Most patients don't want to be there and look forward to leaving. If leave is stopped or unable to be facilitated, explaining honestly and taking collaborative steps are appreciated. Tension appears to arise through frustration and lack of activity. There was always a clear model of care and consistency managing risk.
>
> **Sarah Loughran, student nurse**

CRITICAL THINKING STOP POINT 7.2

In what ways did Sarah experience the environment in the same way that a service user, visitor or carer might?

Go to http://study.sagepub.com/essentialmentalhealth to find a suggested answer to this question.

CRITICAL THINKING STOP POINT 7.2 ANSWER

Taken as a whole, the health care system has more buildings, property and infrastructure (the 'estate') than any other sector in the UK, and is the construction industry's biggest client. The Department of Health challenged a consortium of construction companies to find ways to give better **value** for money, greater energy efficiency and more effective buildings. A series of collaborative initiatives have been set up and one, called ProCure21+, identified a system of repeatable components which need not be re-designed afresh for every new building, including those basic room layouts which work best in practice. It draws an analogy with the modern motor car where the same engine, chassis and components might be used across vehicles, even from different manufacturers, to efficiently produce models which still differ greatly in their accessories and extras, styling and target market. To co-design the mental health care bedroom, the DH commissioned the service-user-run Mental Fight Club to hold workshops to work with them to identify the issues and ascertain solutions (ProCure21+, 2015).

WHAT'S THE EVIDENCE? 7.2

Research shows that when integration with the community is maintained, by views outside, accessible entrances and contact with family and friends, health outcomes are improved. However, there are too many design variables to test every combination, and no one solution fits all situations (Codhinoto et al., 2008), so grey evidence from experts by experience, post-occupancy evaluation and service review is an important contribution to the co-design of both services and facilities.

Nurses at all levels can contribute alongside other stakeholders, both in local **co-production** and in higher-level strategy and regulation. One student describes his experience as a Care Quality Commission (CQC) team member, beside professionals and service user experts by experience, during a statutory inspection of the **acute** inpatient, psychiatric intensive care and crisis home treatment services of an NHS trust. Despite feeling somewhat inadequate amongst such experienced people, he was welcomed and told that 'as a student, [he] would have a unique perspective and an unblemished view of mental health care services', and taking part left him feeling empowered to confidently question practice. Reception was mixed, with some staff members openly hostile and negative and others approachable and receptive. One welcomed the student inspector, saying 'if I'm doing something wrong, then I would rather know about it so I make sure I do it right' (Foster, 2015).

CASE STUDY 7.2

Cheshire and Merseyside Suicide Reduction Network (Champs, 2015)

Suicide prevention has been a government priority for some time. Current national strategy emphasises the importance of organisations working together and aspiring to bold goals. One regional response to this is the Cheshire and Merseyside public health collaboration for a zero-suicide vision and strategy. Overseen by local government public health, a network of organisations and stakeholders has been formed to guide and mobilise action to prevent suicide. This entails each organisation playing its part and collaborating with others in ways which fit in with the wider initiative. The NHS mental health care provider trusts in the region have signed up to the strategy objective to introduce the 'Perfect Care' model developed in the USA to eliminate suicide among service users by transforming care, arguing that accepting any lower target is settling for failure for those people affected by poor outcomes. (www.no-more.co.uk)

NO-MORE

CRITICAL THINKING STOP POINT 7.3

CHECK YOUR ANSWERS

Should organisations set targets for perfect care and ideal outcomes, and to be the best in their field?

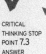

Go to http://study.sagepub.com/essentialmentalhealth to find a suggested answer to this question.

CRITICAL THINKING STOP POINT 7.3 ANSWER

Brave aspirations and collaborative working can improve health care outcomes. However, successive governments have been criticised for frequent top-down, bureaucratic restructuring that has distracted from innovation and improvement (Ham et al., 2015). By ensuring we ourselves and others are involved in co-production, design and strategy, we can help prioritise innovation over reorganisation. This means working with different agencies who may be involved as service provider, building owner and facilities manager in a particular setting, alongside the multi-agency nature of the holistic provision of the service. Each of these agencies might be a public sector body such as an NHS provider trust, a commercial business such as a construction or facilities management company, a charity working with people on their own terms, a social enterprise using business methods for community benefit, or a voluntary interest group seeking to advance a cause. Co-production would provide the means for their different organisational **cultures** to focus on the same core purpose.

CRITICAL THINKING STOP POINT 7.4

If we are to be genuinely innovative in organising our health care, how can we challenge our expectations by looking further afield for inspiration? For example, innovations from a similar culture such as the USA may have actually been achieved in services for voluntary patients with insurance plans rather than reflecting the UK public sector model (Hackman, 2015), while we could learn from developing countries where, unencumbered by the baggage of our extensive and sometimes centralised infrastructure, new approaches are built around the strengths of communities with little funding (Crisp, 2010).

THE PATHWAY TO RECOVERY

MAKING A DIFFERENCE 7.1

When I was admitted during a catastrophic crisis in my life, it was to a secure inpatient unit and I lost hope of ever getting better. This unit was as isolated as I felt, far away from work, family and friends (all of which I had lost anyway), with only a bus to the nearest town every two hours. The ward could only be reached through one locked door after another, and then being in a seclusion suite meant yet another door locked behind you. I was a handful at first, I had difficult relationships with those around me, and, while the security of the environment was there to keep me and others safe, I did not have a clear idea about what I was there to achieve.

But even in those difficult circumstances I found social engagement is possible. This gave me the hope and optimism to say 'Recovery is possible from seclusion to social inclusion' and to feel that I could rebuild my life, starting by taking responsibility for what had happened before. When I became a service user representative while still in hospital, I began making a difference which could benefit myself and other people. After hospital this led to my appointment as National Service User Lead for Recovery and Outcomes, and my involvement in the national conference, the network of nine Regional Recovery and Outcomes Groups and the National Service User Achievement Awards, which all promote the involvement of service users in their recovery. At the national charity Rethink Mental Illness I work to influence strategy and campaigns, and as a peer-review team member for the Royal College of Psychiatrists, I go to units around the country to promote good standards of design and practice.

I appreciate those staff who were able to 'Be kinder than necessary; everyone you meet is fighting some kind of battle'. They stuck with me, even when resources were stretched, sometimes meaning cancelled activities and little time to build good relationships.

Ian Callaghan, Recovery and Outcomes Manager, Rethink Mental Illness (www.rethink.org)

RETHINK

In our 'Making a difference' box, Ian Callaghan describes his journey through secure care to becoming a national authority on the delivery of recovery. Now a manager, writer and campaigner, he is a keynote speaker and award winner at events in the UK and overseas. He influences mental health care strategy and practice through his positions working with NHS England, the Royal College of Psychiatrists and Rethink Mental **Illness**. His work, commitment and energy have promoted the implementation of new ideas on service user involvement, recovery and quality, particularly in secure care (McNicoll, 2014).

On placement in a secure unit, although they weren't treating me like a child I sometimes felt like one as students were only cleared to hold certain keys. Unable to open the gate in the middle of the ward, I'd have to ask to be let through it if I was on the wrong side. I was able to discuss this feeling with other staff, and patients also made good-natured jokes about it: 'Can you let me in ... oh wait, you can't'. I expected to do less as it was very secure, but managed to do more and my mentor helped me get involved in care planning.

On an acute ward, smoking was banned so patients would temporarily quit for a few weeks. Shared dormitory bays could mean an acutely psychotic person sharing with a recovering person who might find the situation difficult.

Patricia, mental health nursing student

CRITICAL THINKING STOP POINT 7.5

Should outdoor smoking areas be provided, or should patients be prevented from smoking while in hospital?

CRITICAL
THINKING STOP
POINT 7.5
ANSWER

The notion of recovery has some resonance with the concept of normalisation (Wolfensburger, 1985). After a series of scandals exposing degrading and inhumane conditions in the large hospitals for people with learning disability which were the legacy of the asylum system, in a process which was mirrored in institutions for those with mental illness, an accelerated programme of closure and community care was put in place (Taylor & Taylor, 1989). Instead of separate facilities provided by the institution in order that the person may be removed from the community, it was envisaged that they would return to the community and use the ordinary, everyday amenities that were enjoyed by everyone, living 'an ordinary life'. The service would be reorientated to provide whatever support was needed to enable this, no matter how challenging (King's Fund Centre, 1980). Thus, while an institution in which a swimming pool was provided (though few if any were) might superficially seem to offer a degree of relative luxury, a service in an ordinary house which planned and implemented sufficient care to enable visiting the local baths would be infinitely preferable.

Services can support recovery when they are designed around the home and community, organised to make use of and strengthen social networks. A human scale is important and can be achieved by legible landscapes and buildings with rational relationships to each other (Shaw, 2015).

CASE STUDY 7.3

Mental Fight Club (2016)

Named after the spiritually exalting clarity of Ben Okri's poem 'Mental Fight' (itself titled in homage to Blake's hymn *Jerusalem*) and the confusing, dark world of the David Fincher movie *Fight Club*, in an expression of the bipolar fusion of opposing worlds, Mental Fight Club was set up by service user Sarah Wheeler. An initial series of performances of the poem sparked regular meetings with a creative exploration of themes of wellbeing, and the formation of the weekly all-day Dragon Café. Here, a varied programme of performances and creative activities is provided alongside a wholefood menu and alternative therapies. Further support takes place online in the form of podcasting and blogging. A large team of volunteer patrons gains confidence and skills in a non-threatening atmosphere and, in running the service themselves, achieve a purpose beyond the artificial creation of activity for its own sake. Mental Fight Club bridges the transition between formal services and community integration, and runs its Dragon Café drop-in service with the simple aim that patrons should leave feeling better than when they arrived. (www.mentalfightclub.com)

MENTAL
FIGHT
CHARITY

CRITICAL THINKING STOP POINT 7.6

How can staff members support service user organisations like Mental Fight Club without becoming over-involved or controlling?

Go to https://study.sagepub.com/essentialmentalhealth to find a suggested answer to this question.

CRITICAL DEBATE 7.1

Badly designed buildings can waste up to 25% of the cost of running the service by inefficient performance (MIND, 2006). Involving a building's end-users enables an effective design response to service requirements, saving money and improving quality and outcomes. However, the cost and challenges of that involvement can be a barrier. What arguments can be used to support the involvement of stakeholders in designing their buildings and services?

CRITICAL
DEBATE 7.1
ANSWER

CRITICAL DEBATE 7.2

Expressed emotion (EE) consists of criticism, hostility and emotional over-involvement towards a person with a mental health problem. High EE in families is strongly associated with poor outcomes, and the same has been shown within staffed settings (Berry et al., 2010). A sensitively designed milieu based on trust and tolerance, without the need for obtrusive barriers, regulations or intrusive supervision, might mirror low EE and improve outcomes. Could the EE effect therefore be applicable to the organisational and built environment?

CHALLENGING CONCEPTS 7.1

Some service users may be detained against their wishes or belive they are surviving abuse rather than using a service or resent the restrictions of the setting. Yet it is essential they are engaged in the design and production of their service and remain integrated with their community. Other agencies involved in designing and providing the service may need us to build the bridges that will hold hope, reach a shared understanding and maintain engagement in those challenging circumstances.

CHAPTER SUMMARY

In this chapter, we have learned how the organisation of services and the settings in which they are delivered should:

- Empower and strengthen communities by being integrated with them.
- Improve the quality of the physical environment and social milieu.
- Enable each of us to be effective in our role as a member of our community, a part of the service workforce or someone affected by our own or our family and friends' mental health issues.

By recognising these roles and environments, we can determine the ways in which we each fit into the process of procuring the best quality outcomes.

BUILD YOUR BIBLIOGRAPHY

Books

- Campling, P., Davies, S. & Farquharson, G. (2004) *From toxic institutions to therapeutic environments: Residential settings in mental health services.* London: Gaskell. The creation of therapeutic social environments in mental health care settings.
- Crisp, N. (2010) *Turning the world upside down: The search for global health in the 21st century.* London: CRC Press. A new approach to thinking about our cultural baggage and how we might side-step it to learn new ways to provide health care.
- Chrysikou, E. (2014) *Architecture for psychiatric environments and therapeutic spaces.* Amsterdam: IOS Press. Exploring theories of therapeutic design and the evidence base to support them.

SAGE journal articles

FURTHER
READING:
JOURNAL
ARTICLES

Go to https://study.sagepub.com/essentialmentalhealth for further free online journal articles related to this chapter. If you are using the interactive ebook, simply click on the book icon in the margin to go straight to the resource.

- Na, Y., Palikhe, S., Lim, C. & Kim, S. (2015) Health performance and cost management model for sustainable healthy buildings. *Indoor and Built Environment, 25*(5): 799-808.
- *Quah, S.R. (2017) Partnership: the missing link in the process of de-institutionalization of mental health care. International Journal of Health Services, 47*(3): 532-549.
- Sadler, B.L., DuBose, J. & Zimring, C. (2008) The business case for building better hospitals through evidence-based design. *Health Environments Research & Design Journal, 1*(3): 22-39.

Weblinks

FURTHER
READING:
WEBLINKS

Go to https://study.sagepub.com/essentialmentalhealth for further weblinks related to this chapter. If you are using the interactive ebook, simply click on the book icon in the margin to go straight to the resource.

- www.dimhn.org – a social enterprise network joining service users with designers and the construction industry.
- www.kingsfund.org.uk – a think tank monitoring the impact of health policy.
- www.merseycare.nhs.uk – an NHS trust working towards co-production to achieve bold aspirations.

Video

VIDEO LINK
CHAPTER 7

- www.theguardian.com/membership/video/2015/jan/21/future-nhs-mental-health-services-video – a panel discussion on the future of UK mental health services.

ACE YOUR ASSESSMENT

ONLINE
QUIZZES &
ACTIVITY
ANSWERS

Revise what you have learned by visiting https://study.sagepub.com/essentialmentalhealth. If you are using the interactive ebook, simply click on the tick icon to go straight to the resource.

- Test yourself with multiple-choice and short-answer questions and flashcards.

REFERENCES

Aked, J., Marks, N., Cordon, C., et al. (2008) *Five ways to wellbeing.* London: New Economics Foundation.

Berry, K., Barrowclough, C. & Haddock, G. (2010) The role of expressed emotion in relationships between psychiatric staff and people with a diagnosis of psychosis: a review of the literature. *Schizophrenia Bulletin, 37*(5): 958–972.

Champs (2015) *No more: Zero suicide.* Bromborough, Cheshire: Champs Public Health Collaborative.

Codhinoto, R., Tzortzopoulos, P., Kagioglu, M., et al. (2008) *The effects of the built environment on health outcomes.* Salford: HaCIRIC.

Craissati, J. & Taylor, P. (2014) Forensic mental health services in the United Kingdom and Ireland. In J. Gunn & P. Taylor (eds) *Forensic psychiatry: Clinical, legal and ethical issues.* London: CRC Press.

Crisp, N. (2010) *Turning the world upside down: The search for global health in the 21st century*. London: CRC Press.

Dilani, A. (2015) The beneficial health outcomes of salutogenic design. *World Health Design*, June, 18–35.

Foster, A. (2015) When the inspectors call. *Mental Health Practice, 18*(8): 11.

Hackman, R. (2015) Detroit tackles suicide taboos head on. Available at: www.theguardian.com/society/2015/feb/18/detroit-suicide-taboo-depression-screening-mental-health-henry-ford (accessed 01.16).

Hall, C. (2015) Joint standards progressing. *The Network*, April, 17–20.

Ham, C., Baird, B., Gregory, S., et al. (2015) *The NHS and the coalition government*. London: The King's Fund.

King's Fund Centre (1980) *An Ordinary Life: Comprehensive locally-based residential services for mentally-handicapped people*. London: The King's Fund.

Lawrence, R.J. (2011) Health begins at home. In A. Capon (ed.) *Healthy city design*. Stockholm: International Academy for Design and Health.

McNicoll, A. (2014) *'I'll never forget the social worker who stuck with me when I was at my lowest'*. Available at: www.communitycare.co.uk/2014/10/20/still-remember-social-worker-stuck-lowest (accessed 01.16).

Mental Fight Club (2016) *The story of Mental Fight Club*. Available at: www.mentalfightclub.com (accessed 01.16).

MIND (2006) *Building solutions*. London: MIND.

National Institute for Health and Care Excellence (2014) Psychoris and Schizophrenia in adults: prevention and management. NICE guideline (CG178). Available at: *www.nice.org.uk/guidance/cg178* (accessed 01.16).

ProCure21+ (2015) *Standardisation*. Available at: www.procure21plus.nhs.uk/standardisation (accessed 01.16).

Shaw, C. (2015) Clock view captures public imagination. *The Network*, October, 13–16.

Taylor, J. & Taylor, D. (1989) *Mental health in the 1990s: From custody to care?* London: Office of Health Economics.

Wolfensberger, W. (1985) Social role valorization: a new insight, and a new term, for normalization. *Australian Association for the Mentally Retarded Journal, 9*(1): 4–11.

THE POLICY CONTEXT FOR CONTEMPORARY MENTAL HEALTH CARE

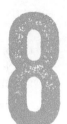

BEN HANNIGAN, BETHAN EDWARDS, IAN HULATT AND ALAN MEUDELL

THIS CHAPTER COVERS

- Understanding policy
- Mental health policy to 2017
- Prospects for the future
- Analysis of policy and its impact combined with service user reflections and activities.

Visit **https://study.sagepub.com/essentialmentalhealth** to access a wealth of online resources for this chapter – watch out for the margin icons throughout the chapter. If you are using the interactive ebook, simply click on the margin icon to go straight to the resource.

INTRODUCTION

Some readers may question the relevance of a chapter titled *Policy* in a book of this type. Chapters on working in interprofessional teams, promoting **recovery** and providing skilled psychosocial interventions might appear altogether more obvious in a textbook titled *Essentials of Mental Health Nursing*. Policy, however, shapes the world in which people live, work and receive services. One way of demonstrating this is to consider how policy **affects** the life of you, the reader. If you happen to be a student mental health nurse in England commencing your education before the 2017–18 academic year, it is unlikely that you will have needed to pay tuition fees for your programme of study. You may have friends studying other subjects and have observed that the situation is very different for them. Like students of history, physics and most other subjects, students of mental health nursing beginning their education from autumn 2017 onwards in English universities will be expected to take out loans to pay their tuition. Why is this so? The answer is because policymakers have made decisions, and these decisions have consequences. Perhaps you are a student learning to become a mental health nurse whilst also caring for young children. You may be receiving help with the costs of your childcare and be in receipt of child benefit. Again, these are matters of policy, just as are a multitude of other things: the nursing curriculum you are following; the curriculum in the school your children go to; the tax you pay on the goods and services you purchase; the targets set for the hospitals you have placements in or that you use when you need their help. Policy, in other words, affects all of us. Because of this we need to know more about it. And, as mental health nurses, we need particularly to know about policy as this is directed at the organisation of mental health care and the lives of people using services.

UNDERSTANDING POLICY

If you were sceptical initially about studying policy, you may now be a little more convinced of its importance and its impact. But what is 'policy' exactly, how is it made and what shapes the direction it takes? Buse et al. (2012) write that policy is about decisions, made by people with authority and responsibility in a given area. This could be for health, housing, education, international affairs, or for something else entirely. Buse and colleagues add that policy is also made at different levels and by people located in different types of institution. For example, the World Health Organization (WHO) plays an important role in the development of policy for health systems at a global level, establishing a direction and aspirations for individual nations. Interested readers are referred to the WHO's mental health web pages (which can be found at www.who.int/mental_health/en) and to its *Comprehensive Mental Health Action Plan 2013–2020* (WHO, 2013) specifically. This establishes four key objectives for the current period, set in a broader human rights framework. One of these objectives, to give an example, is for countries to provide 'comprehensive, integrated and responsive mental health and social care services in community-based settings' (WHO, 2013: 14–16). At the international level, the European Commission also makes policy, directed at the improvement of health across the member states of the European Union (EU). Readers are referred to the Commission's mental health pages (http://ec.europa.eu/health/mental_health/policy_en) and asked to consider the **values** and goals contained in the EU's current *Joint Action for Mental Health and Wellbeing* (www.mentalhealthandwellbeing.eu).

 WHO HEALTH POLICY

 EUROPEAN COMMISSION

 EU JOINT ACTION

At national level, in the UK public policy for health is made separately by governments within the four countries. We say more about mental health policy convergence and divergence a little later in this chapter, but at this stage it is enough to remember that health systems and policy vary in important ways across England, Wales, Scotland and Northern Ireland. These reflect differing sets of ideas and priorities found amongst government-level policymakers. Policies affecting nurses are also made by professional and regulatory bodies (for example, by the Nursing and Midwifery Council (NMC), the

Royal College of Nursing, and Unite). The NMC's authority to publish a Code for nurses and midwives, and to hold registrants to this, is an example which shows how important this institution is. At a more immediate level, policies are made by local organisations and institutions such as NHS trusts or health boards, and on an even smaller scale by individual teams or services. These, too, help shape the work that nurses and others do.

In all these cases, it is important to consider who has responsibility for policy, along with how policy is made, why and with what ends in sight. Policy always reflects particular values and assumptions, and policy for the health service is certainly no exception. As Buse et al. (2012) observe, policy is closely connected to politics and to power, and is often open to dispute and contest. Consider how, in the run-up to any Westminster or devolved government election in the UK, the NHS invariably becomes a major battleground for politicians. Examples of health service debates which have taken place over recent decades include the level of public expenditure (raised through taxes) which could, or should, be spent on the NHS, the relative role of private care providers and the suitability of mechanisms to **drive** up quality and/or efficiency. In the mental health context, think about how specific national policies have been made (and have been picked up and implemented at local level) because of a changing political agenda and circumstances. The 'care programme approach', for example, was introduced in the early 1990s as a formal system for the coordination of care because of concerns over people with mental health difficulties being discharged from hospital with no support and without anyone taking responsibility for them (Simpson et al., 2003).

> Most of the time, policy feels like something made by people in power suits sitting in a boardroom, playing buzzword bingo: offering everything, giving nothing and frequently failing to do the former. People creating policy are far removed from the experiences and consequences their policies have upon the person who's going into their sixth month on a psychiatric intensive care unit or from the person crippled with agoraphobia who hasn't left the house in five years. I would like to see the day when policy is truly created by service users and carers.
>
> **Owain, service user**

Where **service users** and **carers** have been involved in making policy, it has usually been in a room where they are outnumbered by professionals to a degree where they have little or no influence. Also, it is legislation which drives policy and here the public have even less say. Of course, there are high-profile events which have led to the public driving legislation, for instance Megan's Law.

Whether policy is made at global, national or local level, the impression we may have given so far is that policy is made 'out there', and (through some top-down mechanism) extends to influence the work that people do and the services that people receive. This may be an over-simplification. The relationships between policy, services and practice are actually very complex. Not all national-level public policy is uniformly implemented in all places. Policies may interact in contradictory ways, triggering unintended consequences. At the local level, policy may be 'felt' in all manner of different ways. For some scholars of policy, a better way of thinking about the relationships between policy and practice is to take a bottom-up, rather than a top-down, view. The US policy analyst Lipsky argued that, from the position of the person on the receiving end of public services, 'policy' is what is implemented by people working on the front line (Lipsky, 1980). This means that policy is not what is published by national governments, but is what 'street-level bureaucrats' (to use Lipsky's term) do in their day-to-day practice. This is an important **insight**: policy shapes, but does not entirely dictate, the actions of professionals. From the felt perspective of the service users, policy is what practitioners do, and do not do.

> I can't remember ever seeing a policy when I was last in hospital, but I remember my daily life being constantly shaped by the hospital's policies. I'd wake up at 8am, because that's when it was 'meds time'. I'd have five scheduled meals/snacks during the day, always at the wrong time. Everything I ate was recorded on a food diary because that was what was done for people with an eating disorder. When my blood pressure went really low, I'd have my 'obs' taken every hour, sometimes more than that, because that was the procedure. I couldn't see my friends when I wanted, because visiting time was at 5pm and then at 7pm. At night I'd be woken every hour with a nurse shining a torch in my face.
>
> After a while I spoke to the ward manager about my wake up time, because I suffer from hypersomnia, and waking up at 8am was making me so tired that I would have to sleep in the afternoon, missing OT sessions. With her agreement, my medication time was changed, so I had my medication when I naturally woke up. We also talked about meal times and she agreed that my lunch could be kept in the ward kitchen, so I could eat it when I felt hungry at 2pm. She was willing to be flexible to the way my life is at home, which was so important. So long as I agreed to eat what was on my meal planner for the day and alerted someone to when I was eating, she was happy to make my stay more personalised.
>
> **Rhiannon, service user**

Critical thinking stop point 8.1 is an opportunity for you to think about the consequences of this line of analysis.

CRITICAL THINKING STOP POINT 8.1

One message we want to convey in the opening section of this chapter is that, from the perspective of the person on the receiving end, policy is what is implemented by staff working in face-to-face services. Another is that policies do not always pull in the same direction, creating tensions and contradictions. In this exercise, first think about your current practice workplace or your most recent clinical placement. What, in general, are the policies to be found there? Perhaps there is a file or folder with lots of local policies contained within. What are these about, are they all implemented and how do they relate to policy on a larger scale? Are you inspired, or bored, when you read these? Then, in order to make some links from the local to the national: what local written policies, strategies or value statements are there about promoting 'recovery'? What local policies are there regarding the use of coercive powers (such as those enshrined, for England and Wales, in the Mental Health Act 1983 as amended in 2007)? What local policies are there about medication

(Continued)

administration? How do these policy and value statements intertwine, and what tensions might there be? Think about actual day-to-day practice in your workplace or placement area, and put yourself in the shoes of someone using this service. How far does care feel recovery-oriented? What, if any, are the gaps between recovery-focused care, as this is documented in policy, and care as it is actually experienced? What conclusions do you draw from this exercise about the relationship between policy as it is written down and policy as it is demonstrated in everyday practice?

MENTAL HEALTH POLICY TO 2017

Hopefully, the service user voices and Critical thinking stop point 8.1 will have alerted you to the importance of making connections between policy at national and local levels, and at the level of everyday practice. In order that you understand the large-scale contours of policy, we now turn our attention to the detail of mental health policy as this has unfolded over recent years, but as you read this section we encourage you to continue linking policy and action at the national, local and face-to-face levels.

A first observation to make is that the mental health field is not one which national policymakers have always paid much attention to. For many years, mental health services were concentrated in hospitals and rarely attracted the gaze of government. This has changed. Community mental health care has its origins in the middle of the 20th century (Hannigan & Allen, 2006), and policies directed at this emerged in the decades following. For example, in the 1970s the White Paper *Better Services for the Mentally Ill* (Department of Health and Social Security, 1975) introduced for the first time the idea of the interprofessional community mental health team (CMHT), through which comprehensive care might be provided to all people living within defined geographical localities.

It was not until the late 1990s that mental health became a UK policymaking priority. This happened under the New Labour government led first by Prime Minister Tony Blair. Across all parts of the UK (but particularly in England), over the following years a raft of new policies transformed services (Hannigan & Coffey, 2011). These were initially directed at challenging perceived failures in community care, including the claim that services had neglected to meet the combined health and social care needs of people with severe and long-term mental health difficulties discharged from hospital. Specific policies for England at this time included a ten-year mental health plan (Department of Health, 1999) and a major reorganisation of community services which saw the introduction of new types of team providing crisis care and home treatment, early intervention and assertive outreach (Department of Health, 2001). Policy then took aim at restrictive working practices and the boundaries between professional groups, including doctors, nurses, social workers and others. A new Mental Health Act for England and Wales was introduced, controversially introducing **community treatment orders**. This also replaced the role of 'approved social worker' with that of 'approved mental health professional' (AMHP) (Coffey and Hannigan, 2013) and introduced the role of **'responsible clinician'** (Mental Health Act 2007). In the face of some resistance at the time this legislation was made, it allowed suitably prepared nurses (and other professionals) in possession of clear competencies to fulfil roles during 'sectioning' and compulsory treatment which only social workers and psychiatrists had hitherto been able to do. Policy for mental health has since expanded to take in the promotion of positive mental health and wellbeing (Hannigan & Coffey, 2011).

It is important to remember that this is also the period in which power to make social policy passed from the UK government in Westminster to new, nationally devolved, authorities. In addition to England, new policies for mental health appeared in other countries of the UK, and significant differences in emphasis emerged. In Wales, the newly devolved government was (at first) less concerned with the top-down reorganisation of services and more interested in promoting the values which it believed should underpin mental health care across the country. In an early post-devolution strategy document, these were described as including the idea that mental ill health should be considered in relation to its socio-economic determinants, and that services should tackle **stigma** and promote recovery (National Assembly for Wales, 2001). Doubt was cast, in this strategy, on the value of assertive community treatment teams, in contrast to the position developing in England. In Wales, mental health services for people of working age were twice given a national service framework, or a blueprint for how care and treatment should be organised in all parts of the nation (Welsh Assembly Government, 2002, 2005), and then a ten-year plan (Welsh Government, 2012). By 2010 Welsh policymakers had also introduced a new law mandating for: the provision of **primary mental health** care; statutory care and treatment planning and care coordination for people using specialist mental health services; advocacy in hospital; and the right for a reassessment of needs for people recently discharged (Mental Health (Wales) Measure 2010). This was introduced with cross-party support and followed extensive consultation with service users, carers, representatives from charities and professional bodies. The Measure was a landmark moment, shifting power in favour of people living with mental health difficulties who now had new, legally enshrined, rights. The issue now is how well it is being implemented, with test cases awaited to establish in law its level of success.

> The introduction of the Mental Health Measure in Wales has been a good thing for me; it means that if I am discharged from services I can ask for an assessment without first having to go to my GP to be referred. This gives me a safety net if I start to become unwell again, something I didn't have before the Measure. It also means it is my decision to be assessed and not reliant on going through a number of hoops first.
>
> **Huw, service user**

In Scotland, where the authority to make law independent from Westminster is longstanding, in the mental health field the Scottish Government introduced a new mental health legal framework (Mental Health (Care and Treatment) (Scotland) Act 2003) through a process which avoided many of the fierce debates seen in England (Cairney, 2009). For example, embedded in Scottish legislation was a commitment to the principle of reciprocity. Policymakers were clear in stating that, when society insists on compulsory treatment for **mental disorder**, in return the individual can expect to receive ongoing high-quality care. In Scotland, efforts were also put into the development of approaches and tools to promote recovery (for more information, see www.scottishrecovery.net), and most recently into a new ten-year strategy which includes emphases on prevention and early intervention, access and physical wellbeing (Scottish Government, 2017). In Northern Ireland, recent mental health policy has developed in the context of the end of the Troubles, beginning with a high-level commission known as the Bamford Review (www.health-ni.gov.uk/articles/bamford-review-mental-health-and-learning-disability). With high rates of mental ill health across the country, policy in Northern Ireland has now progressed to the creation of a country-wide service framework emphasising care across the life span (Department of Health, Social Services and Public Safety (DHSSPS), 2011) and a strategy (as other parts of the UK have) to tackle suicide (DHSSPS, 2012), with plans for this to be updated.

THE BAMFORD
REVIEW

CRITICAL THINKING STOP POINT 8.2

FIND OUT
MORE

CRISIS CARE
CONCORDAT

This exercise is designed to help you close the gap between national policy and policy at the local level, through reflecting on the emergence of one of the centrepieces of the former Labour government's mental health policy: crisis resolution and home treatment teams. In the context (at that time) of a largely non-UK evidence base (Hannigan, 2013), these appeared in large numbers across many parts of the UK in the early years of the new century, with the aim of providing alternatives to hospital admission (Johnson & Thornicroft, 2008). Across the four countries, England led in the creation of a national crisis care concordat, outlining how different organisations should work together (www.crisiscareconcordat.org.uk). Speak to people in the area you work in (or in which you have your clinical placements) to consider these questions: when were crisis resolution and home treatment teams set up? What was the local thinking behind them, what evidence was used to inform their establishment, and what impact have they had? How were, and are, they staffed? How were, and are, they integrated with other parts of the local mental health system, and what is the service user journey into, through and out of them?

You might want to extend this type of local analysis to consider other types of community team, and indeed the overall shape of the local system in which you work. In the early part of the century, teams providing assertive community treatment also appeared. Are there teams of this type in the area you work in now? Or have they disappeared, with the work they once did being brought back into locality-based interprofessional community mental health teams? What's the local story?

> Having had an eating disorder which I have relapsed and recovered from many times over the last 15 years, I was really glad when the Eating Disorders Framework for Wales was introduced in 2009. It meant for the first time I received support from a specialist eating disorder service when I relapsed again in 2012. They supported me along with my CPN [community psychiatric nurse] in the community and provided specialist input to the staff team on the ward when I was an inpatient. Before 2009, specialist eating disorder services for severe and enduring eating disorders were not provided across Wales, but the framework made this a requirement for every health board. I only wish I had had this service and expertise a long time ago.
>
> Rhiannon, service user

TIME TO
CHANGE

By 2010, New Labour had been voted out of government and had been replaced by a Conservative/ Liberal Democrat coalition which stayed in power until 2015. During this time, mental health stayed towards the top of the health and social policy agenda, thanks largely to the interests of the Liberal Democrats. *No Health without Mental Health* (Department of Health, 2011) took a life-course approach to the promotion of mental health and wellbeing. It emphasised the importance (amongst other things) of tackling stigma and inequalities through initiatives such as *Time to Change* (see www.time-to-change.org.uk), and raised the priority of improving the physical health of people living with mental health problems. In England, continued support was also promised for the Improving Access to Psychological Therapies (IAPT) programme. This was an initiative commenced under the previous government and designed to improve the timeliness and effectiveness of talking therapies for people with commoner mental health difficulties, often offered through primary care services.

In NHS England, a new way of funding mental health services appeared through the introduction of what was initially termed 'payment by results'. This involved the 'clustering' of groups of people and the linking of these groups to costed packages of care. With the impact of this still working its way through the English mental health system, early concerns expressed by some include the crudeness of the 'clusters' and the poor fit between them and the needs of the real people being served by mental health practitioners (Royal College of Psychiatrists, 2014). Anecdotal evidence from service users is that this approach may lead to the time-limiting of care and treatment, and to limitations on the availability of some interventions.

The idea of 'parity of esteem' was also introduced under the coalition government, becoming enshrined in the Health and Social Care Act 2012. This referred to the idea that standards of care for people with mental health difficulties should be just as exacting as standards of care for people with physical health needs. As one expression of this policy, new targets on improving access to mental health services in England were introduced, along with maximum waiting list times for people referred for specialist care and treatment (Department of Health, 2014). However, the coalition government was also committed to reducing public expenditure following the global economic crisis from 2008 onwards. In the face of public commitments to parity of esteem, evidence mounted that mental health services were being denied much-needed resources, with many of the investments made in the late 1990s and early 2000s being withdrawn. Using all the available evidence, including the government's own data and data unearthed through a series of Freedom of Information requests made by the BBC and the journal *Community Care*, Docherty and Thornicroft (2015) showed how health and social care resources for people with mental health difficulties were in sharp decline, leading to a growing gap between those in need of help and those actually receiving it.

CRITICAL THINKING STOP POINT 8.3

Evidence is growing that the shape of mental health services is changing as resources made available for health and social care diminish. Speak to service managers and senior professionals in the area in which you work or have your placements, and find out what is happening. How are decisions being made? How are teams and services being reconfigured or cut altogether? What impact is this having on the lives of people using services, and on staff?

PROSPECTS FOR THE FUTURE

Towards the tail-end of the coalition government in Westminster, work began on a new strategy for the NHS in England as a whole, under the title *Five Year Forward View* (NHS England, 2014). This has a number of distinct elements. One is that greater emphasis needs to be placed on public health and prevention, in order that action now reduces rates of chronic and preventable **illness** in the future. Where New Labour introduced national frameworks to uniformly raise standards across the whole country, the *Five Year Forward View* sees a greater place for flexibility in order that services reflect local contexts. It also looks ahead to a health (and social) care system in which services are much more finely tailored to individual needs, and are better coordinated. One aim here is that people with coexisting mental health and physical health difficulties are helped in ways which are much more joined up. This aspiration is far from novel, however, and success this time around is likely to depend on a whole host of factors, including how staff communicate across organisational and professional boundaries, the adequacy of information technology systems, and so forth.

As part of the wider programme of work associated with the *Five Year Forward View*, a taskforce was established in spring 2015 to develop a five-year strategy for the improvement of mental health across the life course. The taskforce was chaired by Paul Farmer from the national charity Mind, and reported in 2016 in a document which made a strong case for investing in: accessible, round-the-clock, community-focused care; a better-integrated approach to meeting mental and physical health care needs; and a focus on mental health promotion and ill health prevention, including for children and young people (The Mental Health Taskforce, 2016). Like many other, predecessor, documents, the *Five Year Forward View for Mental Health* also placed an emphasis on services promoting recovery in a personalised way.

Meanwhile, debate has been taking place within the nursing field on future preparation for practice and on the work of mental health nurses specifically. A team led by Lord Willis published its *Shape of Caring* review with 62 recommendations gathered under eight themes (Health Education England, 2015). These include the idea of new models of nursing preparation, by adding (for example) a fourth, preceptorship, year and by reviewing the existing four fields. These proposals have triggered commentary and critique. Some have expressed concern over the erosion of mental health nursing as a distinct, pre-registration, sphere of practice (Coffey et al., 2015). Others have argued that the *Shape of Caring* failed to address the organisation and content of mental health nursing work (McKeown & White, 2015).

CRITICAL THINKING STOP POINT 8.4

In this exercise, we ask you to reflect on the challenges and opportunities for mental health services as the themes for the next five years (in England, at least) begin to emerge. What are the prospects for tackling the root causes of mental ill health at a time when public services continue to be reined in?

CONCLUSION

One message this chapter has attempted to convey is that policy is not somehow 'out there', removed from the world of everyday practice in which most nurses are engaged. From the felt perspective of the person with mental health needs, policy is revealed via the types of interaction they have with services and the people working in them. To give an example: government exhortations that care should be more co-produced, recovery-oriented and collaborative mean nothing unless services are set up to make this happen, and nurses (and others) act in ways which reflect these aspirations.

A second key message from this chapter is that policy for health and social care is constantly developing and remains in a state of flux. This happens in response to new challenges and also to ideological shifts reflecting changes in government at national level. The detail of what is current in mental health policy outlined in this chapter will, inevitably, become out of date very quickly. Future policy will mould the types of services which are provided, the groups of people whose care is prioritised and the work that nurses do. It will lead to changes in the education of practitioners, and perhaps to changes in the composition of the workforce. A task for mental health nurses is both to keep in touch and to seek opportunities to influence, at all levels, from the local to the national. This is because, as this chapter has demonstrated, policy shapes the system in which nurses work.

CHAPTER SUMMARY

This chapter has covered:

- How policy is made and by whom
- The shape of past and present policy for mental health services across the UK
- Emerging themes for policy in the future.

BUILD YOUR BIBLIOGRAPHY

Books

- Buse, K., Mays, N. & Walt, G. (2012) *Making health policy*, 2nd edition. Maidenhead: Open University Press. This is a good, general, text on health policy.
- Glasby, J. & Tew, J. (2015) *Mental health policy and practice*, 3rd edition. Basingstoke: Macmillan. This popular book, aimed at all people interested in mental health care, is now in its third edition.
- Hulatt, I. (ed.) (2014) *Mental health policy for nurses*. London: Sage. This accessible edited book is aimed at nurses from student level onwards.

SAGE journal articles

Go to https://study.sagepub.com/essentialmentalhealth for further free online journal articles related to this chapter. If you are using the interactive ebook, simply click on the book icon in the margin to go straight to the resource.

FURTHER READING: JOURNAL ARTICLES

- Callaghan, J.E.M., Fellin, L.C. & Warner-Gale, F. (2017) A critical analysis of child and adolescent mental health services policy in England. *Clinical Child Psychology and Psychiatry*, 22(1), 109–127.
- Long, V. (2016) 'Heading up a blind alley'? Scottish psychiatric hospitals in the era of deinstitutionalization. *History of Psychiatry*, 28(1), 115–128.
- Patel, V. (2014) Why mental health matters to global health. *Transcultural Psychiatry*, 51(6), 777–789.

Weblinks

Go to https://study.sagepub.com/essentialmentalhealth for further weblinks related to this chapter. If you are using the interactive ebook, simply click on the book icon in the margin to go straight to the resource.

FURTHER READING: WEBLINKS

- www.who.int/mental_health/en – the World Health Organization's mental health website.
- www.gov.uk/government/organisations/department-of-health; www.gov.scot/Topics/Health; www.health-ni.gov.uk; http://gov.wales/topics/health/?lang=en – these are the websites for health policy across the governments of the UK.

ACE YOUR ASSESSMENT

Revise what you have learned by visiting https://study.sagepub.com/essentialmentalhealth. If you are using the interactive ebook, simply click on the tick icon to go straight to the resource.

- Test yourself with multiple-choice and short-answer questions and flashcards.

REFERENCES

Buse, K., Mays, N. & Walt, G. (2012) *Making health policy*, 2nd edition. Maidenhead: Open University Press.

Cairney, P. (2009) The 'British policy style' and mental health: beyond the headlines. *Journal of Social Policy*, *38*, 671–688.

Coffey, M. & Hannigan, B. (2013) New roles for nurses as approved mental health professionals in England and Wales: a discussion paper. *International Journal of Nursing Studies*, *50*, 1423–1430.

Coffey, M., Pryjmachuk, S. & Duxbury, J. (2015) The shape of caring review: what does it mean for mental health nursing? *Journal of Psychiatric and Mental Health Nursing*, *22*, 738–741.

Department of Health (1999) *A national service framework for mental health*. London: DH.

Department of Health (2001) *The mental health policy implementation guide*. London: DH.

Department of Health (2011) *No health without mental health: a cross-government mental health outcomes strategy for people of all ages. Supporting document: the economic case for improving efficiency and quality in mental health*. London: DH.

Department of Health (2014) *Closing the gap: priorities for essential change in mental health*. London: DH.

Department of Health and Social Security (DHSS) (1975) *Better services for the mentally ill*. London: HMSO.

Department of Health, Social Services and Public Safety (2011) *Service framework for mental health and wellbeing*. Belfast: DHSSPS.

Department of Health, Social Services and Public Safety (2012) *Protect life: A shared vision*. Belfast: DHSSPS.

Docherty, M. & Thornicroft, G. (2015) Specialist mental health services in England in 2014: overview of funding, access and levels of care. *International Journal of Mental Health Systems*, *9*(1), 34.

Hannigan, B. (2013) Connections and consequences in complex systems: insights from a case study of the emergence and local impact of crisis resolution and home treatment services. *Social Science & Medicine*, *93*, 212–219.

Hannigan, B. & Allen, D. (2006) Complexity and change in the United Kingdom's system of mental health care. *Social Theory & Health*, *4*, 244–263.

Hannigan, B. & Coffey, M. (2011) Where the wicked problems are: the case of mental health. *Health Policy*, *101*, 220–227.

Health Education England (2015) *Raising the bar: Shape of caring – a review of the future education and training of registered nurses and care assistants*. Leeds: Health Education England.

Johnson, S. & Thornicroft, G. (2008) The development of crisis resolution and home treatment teams. In S. Johnson, J. Needle, J. Bindman & G. Thornicroft (eds) *Crisis resolution and home treatment in mental health*. Cambridge: Cambridge University Press.

Lipsky, M. (1980) *Street-level bureaucracy: Dilemmas of the individual in public services*. New York: Russell Sage Foundation.

McKeown, M. & White, J. (2015) The future of mental health nursing: are we barking up the wrong tree? *Journal of Psychiatric and Mental Health Nursing, 22,* 724–730.

National Assembly For Wales (2001) *Adult mental health services for Wales: Equity, empowerment, effectiveness, efficiency.* Cardiff: National Assembly for Wales.

NHS England (2014) *Five year forward view.* London: NHS England.

Royal College of Psychiatrists (2014) Royal College of Psychiatrists' statement on mental health payment systems (formerly Payment by Results). London: RCP.

Scottish Government (2017) *Mental health strategy: 2017–2027.* Edinburgh: Scottish Government.

Simpson, A., Miller, C. & Bowers, L. (2003) Case management models and the care programme approach: how to make the CPA effective and credible. *Journal of Psychiatric and Mental Health Nursing, 10,* 472–483.

The Mental Health Taskforce (2016) *The five year forward view for mental health: A report from the independent mental health taskforce to the NHS in England.* London: NHS England.

Welsh Assembly Government (2002) *Adult mental health services: A national service framework for Wales.* Cardiff: WAG.

Welsh Assembly Government (2005) *Raising the standard: The revised adult mental health national service framework and an action plan for Wales.* Cardiff: WAG.

Welsh Government (2012) *Together for mental health: A strategy for mental health and wellbeing in Wales.* Cardiff: Welsh Government.

World Health Organization (2013) *Mental health action plan 2013–2020.* Geneva: WHO.

MADNESS AND THE LAW

BOB SAPEY

9

THIS CHAPTER COVERS

- Understandings of 'madness'
- The politics of mental health
- Citizenship and the law
- From lunacy to mental health
- The reformation of the Mental Health Act (MHA)
- Community treatment orders
- The Maastricht approach
- Dangerousness and the law.

INTRODUCTION

It is imperative that mental health nurses understand the law, as applied to mental health, and, in particular, whichever Mental Health Act/legislative instrument applies in their national context (see the Appendix at the end of the book for further information). This chapter discusses how current **mental health law** in England and Wales came into being and, as a result, will help you to understand the underpinning and historical concepts behind the Mental Health Act as it is today. It will also consider how the use of the powers bestowed on mental health clinicians bring about profound and life-changing experiences. Controversial issues are raised to enable you to deconstruct your own views, learn from the perspectives of others and consider these within a legal, ethical and professional framework.

SEE ALSO
APPENDIX

THE POLITICS OF MENTAL HEALTH LEGISLATION

Our health services are regulated by laws that set minimum standards of practice and qualification to practise, that regulate the funding and entitlement to services and, in the case of mental health services, also authorise courts and professionals to detain and treat people against their will. This deprivation of liberty and compulsory treatment are justified by beliefs such as the following:

- people affected by mental illnesses may not know what is in their best interest, so it is necessary to give others the authority to make decisions on their behalf
- patients may decline treatments because they dislike their side-effects or they fail to understand their necessity, so there needs to be provision for compulsory treatment
- when people are mentally ill, they may lose touch with reality to such an extent that they become a danger to themselves or others, so mental health laws are needed to detain, constrain and protect them
- psychiatry needs to be afforded the authority to manage mental health services as its medical understanding of madness is deemed superior to other explanations.

The belief that madness is a form of **illness** has led to **medical treatments** that have included:

- surgically destroying connections in the frontal lobes of the brain with an instrument inserted through the patient's eye socket
- deliberately causing people to undergo convulsions by passing electricity through their brains
- deliberately causing people to go into a coma by overdosing them with insulin
- binding people in wet sheets that would gradually warm and then become so hot that patients would scream in pain
- torturing patients by prescribing and forcibly administering neuroleptic drugs that 'cause trembling, shivering and contractions, but mainly make the subject apathetic and dull his intelligence' (UNCHR, 1986: 29). This remains the standard treatment for people experiencing **psychosis**, despite being deemed to be a form of torture by the United Nations since 1986.

CRITICAL DEBATE 9.1

How is it that so many societies, particularly throughout the developed world, have such laws for dealing with mental health?

Why, in a world where we have international human rights laws, are nation states permitted to authorise the detention and torture of people believed to be ill?

CRITICAL
DEBATE 9.1
ANSWER

For me, one of the clearest discussions of these issues is offered by Clive Unsworth in his 1987 book, *The Politics of Mental Health Legislation*. One of the important points he makes is that mental health laws not only give authority to psychiatry to decide how patients should be treated and to do so coercively, they also limit that authority and in so doing protect the sane. From the 18th century and the era of the enlightenment, new groups of rich people were created who challenged the traditional power of the ruling classes, the aristocracy and the church. A new contract between people and the state emerged in which all people should enjoy freedom, autonomy and responsibility – people became legal subjects and governments would only be allowed to act within constitutional limits. At the same time, the authority of psychiatrists increased with their claim to a scientific understanding of madness and to be able to safeguard the rest of society from those perceived as insane and dangerous. Having replaced traditional power with legitimate representative authority, governments felt it necessary to ensure that psychiatry did not pose a threat to the liberty of the sane; rather, individuals should be left alone to make their own decisions on how to lead their lives.

However, the right to determine one's own actions was not considered to be absolute; rather, there may be limits to the status of being a legal subject and these limits would need to be defined. Paupers and criminals were deemed to forfeit that status, while others, notably children and people of 'unsound mind', were deemed to lack the capacity to accept the responsibility that accompanies the rights of freedom and autonomy. People of unsound mind became partial legal subjects, free when deemed to be well, but also in need of care when ill. Their residual rights and their need for care became the subject of mental health legislation, initially the 1890 Lunacy Act, then the 1930 Mental Treatment Act, the 1959 Mental Health Act, and finally the 1983 Mental Health Act with its subsequent amendments through the 2007 Mental Health Act.

FROM LUNACY TO MENTAL HEALTH

Prior to the 1959 Mental Health Act, the main way in which people would be committed to an asylum would be through the courts. A magistrate, often at the request of a doctor and a person's relatives, would make the orders. Many people were institutionalised for life due to their unacceptable social behaviour. Others would be locked up from childhood because they had learning difficulties.

The shift from '**lunacy**' through 'mental treatment' to 'mental health' in the way legislation was constructed represented change both in attitudes and in practice. The 1959 Mental Health Act put doctors in charge of deciding if someone should be detained. Social workers might also be involved as mental welfare officers, though this was treated more as an administrative, rather than a skilled, task. It was necessary for the local authority to ensure that there were sufficient people to administrate the detention process being conducted by the psychiatrists. In one authority, ambulance drivers were appointed so as to streamline the process – they were usually called to take the patient to the asylum. One of the features of the way the 1959 Act worked was that people were frequently admitted under section 29, an emergency order that only required one doctor. This might be the psychiatrist or a GP, but, either way, this section was used because it was convenient.

THE REFORMATION OF THE MENTAL HEALTH ACT

CASE STUDY:
THE ACUTE
WARD

Following the Winterwerp v The Netherlands case in the European Court of Human Rights in 1979, the UK government set about looking at the need for reform of this Act. MIND was closely involved throughout the development of the Bill and the new 1983 Mental Health Act was hailed as a significant step towards prioritising the rights of people experiencing mental distress. The rights of appeal to hospital managers, to tribunals and to the **Mental Health Act Commission** were embedded in the Act and all patients were to be informed of these rights. It became a routine part of nursing duties during admission.

The 1983 Act also created the role of 'approved social worker'. This was to be for qualified social workers only and they had to undertake some form of post-qualifying course and examination. The public sector union NALGO took industrial action at the time to protest about the impact this would have on unqualified social workers and on others who would have to undertake exams. However, the Act soon became firmly established and social workers began to professionalise and to have some impact on psychiatric practice. The 1980s was also a time of many people being discharged from hospital to be cared for in the community, and it is often looked on as a time of optimism.

However, about a decade later, politicians and trade unions opposed to the closure of psychiatric hospitals, along with significant parts of the tabloid press, began to talk about the dangerousness of community care. As fears grew, it became difficult for psychiatrists, nurses or social workers to take risks. In 1997, the New Labour government proposed to replace the 1983 Act with one that would allow psychiatrists to lock up people with so-called **personality disorders** indefinitely, so as to prevent them being violent toward others. The impact of this proposal was to create an alliance of almost every group representing professionals and patients. This mental health alliance continued to oppose the government's proposals until they were changed.

The 2007 Mental Health Act has amended the 1983 Act in some significant ways – in particular, the role of approved social worker was replaced by the approved mental health professional who could also be a nurse or occupational therapist, though to date most are still social workers. Responsible clinicians could be psychologists rather than doctors. The Act also changed the definition of **mental disorder**, simplifying it to 'any disorder or disability of the mind'. In particular, the government did not like the existence of psychopathic disorder, which most psychiatrists viewed as untreatable by medicine. To the government, this was seen as a loophole, as a way of psychiatry refusing to detain dangerous people.

COMMUNITY TREATMENT ORDERS

The Act also introduced **community treatment orders**, by which people could be forced to take medication as a condition of discharge from hospital. While this has led to more people being discharged, in its first full year of use it resulted in a 30% increase in the numbers of people being detained in hospital, with the National Health Service's own researchers suggesting that psychiatrists and social workers had been filling beds (NHS Information Centre, 2010). With the subsequent cuts to hospital provision under the 2010–15 coalition government, this trend was interrupted, but it is still worth noting how professionals responded to the availability of vacant beds in hospitals.

CRITICAL DEBATE 9.2

How is the legal regulation of mental health nursing affected by different perspectives:

- The legal perspective?
- The social perspective?
- The professional perspective?

What makes them different?

CRITICAL
DEBATE 9.2
ANSWER

The tension between 'legalism' and professionalism was played out through these Acts as the balance of protection of the rights of citizens and the autonomy of the professionals changed. The law curtails the authority of psychiatry which might otherwise extend its reach. Kathleen Jones, who termed the idea of legalism, described three competing approaches to legislation:

1. Medical: with the emphasis on physical treatment
2. Social: with its emphasis on human relations
3. Legal: with an emphasis on procedure and aiming at the protection of individual liberty. (Unsworth, 1987: 19)

Legalism in Kathleen Jones's view is the development of complex legal safeguards to prevent sane people from being detained and/or treated. The law grows ever more complex in order to ensure that only the 'insane' are actually subjected to psychiatric control. The Rosenhan (1973) experiment in 1973 showed just how vulnerable sane people can be to detention and treatment by psychiatrists. Joanna Moncrieff (2010: 376) makes the point that:

> what the Rosenhan experiment tells us, and why it caused the consternation it did, is that in ordinary practice, psychiatric diagnoses are applied to whoever presents themselves or is presented to psychiatric services, unless a good case can be made that they should be dealt with by another institution.

Unsworth (1987) suggests that the main functions of mental health legislation are:

- the regulation of mental health practices
- the division of labour in the mental health system
- inhibiting and restricting the power of psychiatry.

The regulation of mental health practices may limit the authority of doctors to treat people without consent, but it mandates their medicalised, psychiatric expertise. The division of labour in the mental health system places psychiatrists at the top of the hierarchy, and it gives roles to psychology, nursing and social work. But legislation also accords a role to families, especially through the role of the nearest relative. Most notably, the nearest relative can request the discharge of a detained patient and object to their detention and compulsory treatment under the Mental Health Act.

The function of inhibiting and restricting the power of psychiatry is essentially a restriction on the authority of the state and its capacity to exercise this through psychiatry. Unsworth argues that where the state uses soft approaches to social control, such as psychiatry, this type of check is more essential than might otherwise be the case. This can certainly be seen in some of the debates and tensions regarding mental health and human rights.

Two significant human rights afforded to all of us are the right to liberty and the right to be free from torture. However, both of these are often absent for many people experiencing mental distress. Sections 2 and 3 of the 1983 Mental Health Act allow psychiatrists and approved mental health professionals (AMHPs) to detain people and to treat them without their consent if they are 'suffering from a mental disorder' and if detention and treatment are considered to be in the interests of their health or safety, or to protect someone else. The 1983 Act was intended to ensure that detention and treatment are carried out within clear procedures by competent professionals. The European Court of Human Rights had ruled in 1979 in Winterwerp v The Netherlands that detention must not be arbitrary, and Article 5 of the European Convention on Human Rights, to which the UK signed up in 1951 and which was later enshrined in English law through the 1998 Human Rights Act, requires the respect of people's 'liberty and security'. However, the Convention makes certain exceptions to the right of liberty, including where people are deemed to be of 'unsound mind'. Thus, people experiencing mental distress can be denied the protection of European and British human rights legislation if they are deemed to be of unsound mind by an authorised person, namely a psychiatrist. But the concept of unsound mind is not an exact one. In the Winterwerp v The Netherlands ruling, the European Court of Human Rights also said that the Convention on Human Rights:

> does not state what is to be understood by the words 'persons of unsound mind'. This term is not one that can be given a definitive interpretation ... it is a term whose meaning is continually evolving as research in psychiatry progresses, an increasing flexibility in treatment is developing and society's attitude to mental illness changes. (Winterwerp v The Netherlands, para. 37)

Beauchamp and Childress (2013) remind us that we should do no harm (non-maleficence) and also that we have a code of justice: give to people their right or due. As a consequence of this and our code of practice (NMC, 2015), we do our very best to try to alleviate the pain and suffering of the individual and to respect their choices. Consider Case study 9.1 in light of this, and also the law:

CASE STUDY 9.1

Jade is 22. She is an informal patient on a mental health assessment ward. Until now, she would have described herself as a 'survivor'. A survivor of abuse, a survivor of a major depressive illness and also a survivor of psychiatric services. However, she has been in hospital more than she has been out in the last four years. When in hospital, she feels intimidated and robbed of her privacy and at home she feels lonely, desperate and unable to cope. She drinks to create a haze in which life is bearable, but finds that this also seems to take away a sense of restraint. She is ashamed of who she has become and, despite many attempts to kill herself, feels that she can't even do that properly.

Jade is in hospital again. You are working a night shift and sat by her bedroom door observing her sleep. You go to check on her and she asks you to sit with her. She is crying, saying that she just cannot bear the rest of life if it is going to be like the last four years. She pleads with you to turn your back so that she can leave the hospital to kill herself. She feels that being in hospital is cruel as it is making her continue living a life that is torture. She promises that no one will ever know that it was you that let her out and shows you a note that she has pre-rewritten to say that she pretended to be asleep so that she could sneak off when you nipped to the loo. She says, in a very calm and considered fashion, that it really would be the kindest thing for you to do.

What would you do?

You see her pain; you want to relieve her suffering. You feel helpless. Many people more experienced than you have tried and failed.

You would be acting illegally if you were to help her to leave, as that would, effectively, be helping her to kill herself – in other words, it would be 'assisted suicide' (Smith, 2010). This is not mental health legislation; it is the 1961 Suicide Act.

WHAT IS ASSISTED SUICIDE?

Assisted suicide is when someone deliberately assists or encourages another person to kill themselves and is illegal under English law (Suicide Act 1961). It is a criminal offence in England and Wales to: 'aid, abet, counsel or procure the suicide of another or an attempt of another to commit suicide' (Suicide Act 1961).

Would you detain her using 'nurses' holding power'?

HOW CAN MENTAL HEALTH LAW BE CHANGED?

The European Convention on Human Rights' (ECHR) ruling that 'unsound mind' cannot be defined and should evolve with changing knowledge and attitudes is important as it does mean that mental health law can be changed over time by policy and practice. Most significantly, in 2006 the United Nations Convention on the Rights of Persons with Disabilities (CRPD) appears to make significant changes to the position of people with mental health issues. Article 12 states that all people with disabilities should 'enjoy legal capacity on an equal basis with others in all aspects of life'. This suggests that the concept of unsound mind as a term to exclude people as legal subjects is no longer valid.

Furthermore, Article 14 of the CRPD states that people should never lose their liberty on the basis of a disability, putting the legality of the 1983 Mental Health Act into question. The first ground for detention, as I have noted earlier, is that someone is suffering from a mental disorder. George Szmukler (2010) has argued that mental health legislation is essentially discriminatory. He argues that while mental health laws are aimed at reducing danger, they only target people experiencing mental distress which excludes the majority of dangerous people. If we were serious about targeting dangerousness, we might want laws aimed at detaining young men in city centres on Friday and Saturday nights, rather than people who are experiencing severe mental distress.

The CRPD has also been significant in highlighting some of the negative aspects of affording authority to psychiatry, because of its medical model of practice. In 2008 Manfred Nowak, the special rapporteur to the UN Human Rights Committee, reported to the General Assembly of the United Nations on his *review of the torture framework in relation to persons with disabilities*. In his report, Nowak wrote:

> Inside institutions, as well as in the context of forced outpatient treatment, psychiatric medication, including neuroleptics and other mind-altering drugs, may be administered to persons with mental disabilities without their free and informed consent or against their will, under coercion, or as a form of punishment. The administration in detention and psychiatric institutions of drugs, including neuroleptics that cause trembling, shivering and contractions and make the subject apathetic and dull his or her intelligence, has been recognized as a form of torture. (Nowak, 2008: para. 63)

If treating people with neuroleptics without their informed consent is torture, then it is contrary to Article 3 of the European Convention on Human Rights and to Section 134 of the 1988 Criminal Justice Act. Nowak was quoting from an earlier report in February 1986 from a previous special rapporteur (UNCHR, 1986), meaning that the use of neuroleptics without informed consent has been considered a form of torture by the United Nations for over a quarter of a century, during which time it has remained common practice within western psychiatry. However, Robert Johns says that in the case of Grare v France (1993) the European Court of Human Rights refused to accept that the side-effects of medicines might constitute torture, although he did argue that,

> it may be worth noting that, in this case, the treatment in question did not have permanent and foreseeable adverse effects, but was simply something considered disagreeable and unacceptable to the service user. It remains to be seen how the courts would view other kinds of treatment. (Johns, 2004: 255)

This is quite different to the view taken in Alaska where, in 2006, the Supreme Court agreed

> that the right to be free from unwanted psychotropic medications was 'fundamental' under the Alaska Constitution and ... that 'the truly intrusive nature of psychotropic drugs may be best understood by appreciating that they are literally intended to alter the mind. Recognizing that purpose, many states have equated the intrusiveness of psychotropic medication with the intrusiveness of electroconvulsive therapy and psychosurgery. (Gottstein, 2008: 56)

More recently, the European Court of Human Rights (X v Finland, 2012) has agreed that forcibly treating people when they have been detained for assessment is a breach of human rights. While this does not interfere with the operation of Section 3 of the 1983 Act under which people are admitted for 6 or 12 months for treatment, it does put into question the legality of forcibly treating people under Section 2, when they will have been admitted for a period of 28 days for assessment.

ALTERNATIVE APPROACHES

Our legislation creates the mental health system as we know it, so much so that it is difficult to imagine a system that might exist without the current legal framework, but it is important that we try to do so. There are alternative approaches being used more successfully than the pharmaceutically dominated treatments that form the mainstream of psychiatry, for instance the **Maastricht approach** to voice hearing and **open dialogue**.

The first of these is an approach that has led to the development of the Hearing Voices Network throughout the world. It is called the Maastricht approach as it was at Maastricht University that Marius Romme, who pioneered a new way of thinking about voice hearing, was working. This approach re-imagines the meaning and causes of the **auditory hallucinations** that are normally regarded as symptoms of illness such as **schizophrenia** and bipolar disorder. Rather than being symptoms of an illness, hearing voices has been found to be a normal psychological and emotional response to extreme trauma, especially childhood trauma associated with abuse. Rather than medicating people with neuroleptics to suppress their **hallucinations**, Romme and his colleagues have developed ways of helping people to understand and cope with their voices. The voices may not disappear, but they can be made less damaging. This is a social psychiatric approach in which people get support from a wide range of professionals and from other voice hearers. There are nearly 200 hearing voice groups around the UK, mostly provided by voice hearers.

The Maastricht approach to understanding voices casts doubt on the validity of conventional medical explanations of psychosis, so much so that some argue it may undermine the very credibility of psychiatry's claim to understand and explain madness (Moskowitz & Corstens, 2007). I have also argued (Sapey, 2013) that, as a consequence, approved mental health professionals should question the authority of psychiatrists to recommend detaining people with psychosis under the Mental Health Act, and that their duty is to seek alternative treatments.

One such alternative is Open Dialogue, which is the mainstream approach to the treatment of psychosis used in Western Lapland in Finland. On its website (at http://opendialogueapproach. co.uk), Open Dialogue UK describes it as having 'drawn on a number of theoretical models, including systemic **family therapy**, dialogical theory and social constructionism'. It typically involves the therapeutic team working with the patient and their family as a group and in their own homes to help them develop a dialogue at times of crisis. What is remarkable about this approach, according to Daniel Mackler (2014), is that it appears to be so successful in responding to first episodes of

OPEN DIALOGUE

psychosis that diagnoses of schizophrenia are about 15% of the rate elsewhere in Finland, Europe and the USA.

Neither of these two approaches would be effective if they were forced on people; indeed, by their very nature they involve **therapeutic relationships** that must be entered into freely. As with other non-mental health services, both would require legislation to ensure they were funded to become mainstream services and they may require legislation to set standards of practice, though with **peer support** this must differ significantly from professionalised services. What they would not require is a mental health act that enforces treatment.

DANGEROUSNESS

CRITICAL DEBATE 9.3

Consider the media headline: 'A man who was arrested for slashing a policeman with a knife has been detained under the Mental Health Act':

- What is your first response?
- Do you think that your response differs from that of the general population?
- Should it differ? If so, why?

✓

CRITICAL
DEBATE 9.3
ANSWER

Let us consider the broader question of dangerousness. Wind back the clock to before the man (above) attacked the police office. What would happen if we deemed him as being dangerous, because he had said that he hated the police and were going to make them suffer, but hadn't actually attacked the police office at that time? He is invited to be admitted to hospital, but he refuses to enter into treatment. Szmukler et al. (2010) argue that to ensure consistency with other health conditions, we need a fusion of mental health and mental capacity laws (Mental Capacity Act 2005), so that if someone is incapable of making a decision, they would then be dealt with as lacking capacity. But if someone is not lacking capacity, yet is a danger to others, they should be dealt with in the same way as other dangerous people. This has similarities to the arguments of the mental health alliance, that dangerousness should not be made a health issue for political or professional gain.

It can also be argued that when people do commit acts of violence, in part as a response to hearing voices, that rather than demonstrating the need to suppress those voices, it illustrates the failure of the dominant pharmacological psychiatry. Indeed, if such a person had received alternative help to enable them to cope with and control their voices, if they had been regarded as a vulnerable human being in need of support rather than as a 'schizophrenic' in need of compulsory containment, they may never have reached the point of desperation that led to violence.

Mental health legislation reflects social and political attitudes towards mental distress. **Professions**, the government and people experiencing distress have historically competed and continue to do so, to have legislation changed in their favour. This is ongoing and I hope I have demonstrated the importance of understanding mental health legislation as a construct. This opens up the potential to imagine change and to be part of that process, although, depending on your view of the issues, you might argue for more or less **coercion**!

CRITICAL DEBATE 9.4

- When we detain people in hospital, and we justify this on the basis that they are a danger to themselves and others, in what ways can such coercion and paternalism be commensurate with an espoused ethos of recovery?
- What might the impact of detention be for service users and the mental health workforce?
- Who, indeed, are the 'users' of services in such a context: the primary patients or the public at large?
- Is it possible to conceive of forms of mental health legislation that do not justify compulsion and coercion?

CRITICAL DEBATE 9.4 ANSWER

CONCLUSION

This chapter has taken a rather discursive position, deconstructing practice in the UK around the use of mental health law. There is a good deal of historical information that allows us to see our current practice in the context of what has gone before. Similarly, we are asked to consider the human rights of people with mental health problems, both in hospital and in the community.

CHAPTER SUMMARY

If you read this chapter and work through the debates suggested, you will be able to:

- Describe the historical developments that have led to our current systems
- Describe and critique how the deprivation of liberty and compulsory treatment are justified in the 'best interests' of the person and others
- Acquire a critical and enquiring position about the impact of detaining somebody in hospital against their will
- Demonstrate an awareness of the roles of the multi-disciplinary team, for example psychiatrist, social worker and nurse.

BUILD YOUR BIBLIOGRAPHY

Books

- Barber, P., Brown, R. & Martin, D. (2012) *Mental health law in England and Wales: A guide for mental health professionals*, 3rd edition. London: SAGE.
- Jones, M.A. (2014) *Mental Health Act manual*. London: Sweet & Maxwell.
- Mandelstam, M. (2019) *Safeguarding vulnerable adults and the law*. London: Jessica Kingsley.

SAGE journal articles

Go to https://study.sagepub.com/essentialmentalhealth for further free online journal articles related to this chapter. If you are using the interactive ebook, simply click on the book icon in the margin to go straight to the resource.

FURTHER READING: JOURNAL ARTICLES

- Bingley, W. (1984) Book review: legal rights and mental health care. *Medico-Legal Journal, 52*(1), 70-71.
- Prins, H. (2001) Whither mental health legislation? (Locking up the disturbed and the deviant). *Medicine, Science and the Law, 41*(3), 241-249.
- Rosenman, S. (1994) Mental health law: an idea whose time has passed. *Australian and New Zealand Journal of Psychiatry, 28*(4), 560-565.

Weblinks

FURTHER READING: WEBLINKS

Go to https://study.sagepub.com/essentialmentalhealth for further weblinks related to this chapter. If you are using the interactive ebook, simply click on the book icon in the margin to go straight to the resource.

- MIND: www.mind.org.uk/information-support/legal-rights/mental-health-act-1983/#.WBtDKoUufZA
- NHS Choices: www.nhs.uk/NHSEngland/AboutNHSservices/mental-health-services-explained/Pages/TheMentalHealthAct.aspx
- World Health Organization (WHO): www.who.int/mental_health/media/en/75.pdf – ten basic principles of mental health care law

——————— ACE YOUR ASSESSMENT ———————

ONLINE QUIZZES & ACTIVITY ANSWERS

Revise what you have learned by visiting https://study.sagepub.com/essentialmentalhealth. If you are using the interactive ebook, simply click on the tick icon to go straight to the resource.

- Test yourself with multiple-choice and short-answer questions and flashcards.

REFERENCES

Beauchamp, T.L. & Childress, J.F. (2013) *Principles of Biomedical Ethics*, 7th edition. Oxford: Oxford University Press.

Gottstein, J. (2008) Involuntary commitment and forced psychiatric drugging in the trial courts: rights violations as a matter of course. *Alaska Law Review, 25*(1), 51–106.

Johns, R. (2004) Of unsound mind? Mental health social work and the European Convention on Human Rights. *Practice, 16*(4), 247–259.

Mackler, D. (2014) *OPEN DIALOGUE: An alternative Finnish approach to healing psychosis*. Available at: https://youtu.be/HDVhZHJagfQ (accessed 05.08.17).

Mental Capacity Act 2005. Available at: www.legislation.gov.uk/ukpga/2005/9/contents (accessed 01.12.17).

Moncrieff, J. (2010) Psychiatric diagnosis as a political device. *Social Theory & Health, 8*(4), 370–382.

Moskowitz, A. & Corstens, D. (2007) Auditory hallucinations: psychotic symptom or dissociative experience? *Trauma and Serious Mental Illness, 6*(2/3), 35–63.

NHS Information Centre (2010) *Inpatients formally detained in hospitals under the Mental Health Act 1983 and patients subject to supervised community treatment: annual figures, England 2009/10.* London: NHS Information Centre.

Nowak, M. (2008) *Interim report of the special rapporteur on torture and other cruel, inhuman or degrading treatment or punishment*. New York: United Nations.

Nursing & Midwifery Council (NMC) (2015) *NMC Code*. London: NMC. Available at: www.nmc.org.uk/standards/code (accessed 10/08/17).

Rosenhan, D. (1973) On being sane in insane places. *Science, 179*(4070), 250–258.

Sapey, B. (2013) Compounding the trauma: the coercive treatment of voice hearers. *European Journal of Social Work, 16*(3), 375–390.

Smith, S.W. (2010) Assisted suicide and the law: what every nurse should know. *British Journal of Nursing, 19*(13), 858–859.

Suicide Act (1961) www.legislation.gov.uk/ukpga/Eliz2/9-10/60 (accessed 03.11.16).

Szmukler, G. (2010) *How mental health legislation discriminates unfairly against people with mental illness.* Gresham College lecture, 15 November. Available at: www.gresham.ac.uk/lectures-and-events/how-mental-health-law-discriminates-unfairly-against-people-with-mental-illness (accessed 05.08.17).

Szmukler, G., Daw, R. & Dawson, J. (2010) A model law fusing incapacity and mental health legislation. *Journal of Mental Health Law.* Special Issue, *20*, 11–22.

United Nations Commission on Human Rights (UNCHR) (1986) Torture and Other Cruel, Inhuman or Degrading Treatment or Punishment Report by the special rapporteur, Mr P. Kooijmans, appointed pursuant to Commission on Human Rights resolution 1985/33. E/CN.4/1986/15. Available at: http://ap.oh.chr.org/documents/E/CHR/resolutions/E_CN.4_RES_1985_33.pdf (accessed 26.11.17).

Unsworth, C. (1987) *The politics of mental health legislation.* Oxford: Oxford University Press.

Winterwerp v Netherlands 6301/73 (1979) ECHR 4

X v Finland 34806/04 (2012) ECHR 4

INDEPENDENT ADVOCACY IN MENTAL HEALTH CARE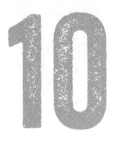

JULIE RIDLEY, STEPHANIE DE LA HAYE, JUNE SADD, KAREN NEWBIGGING AND KAREN MACHIN

THIS CHAPTER COVERS

- What is meant by 'independent advocacy' and how this differs from professionals' advocacy role or 'best interest' advocacy
- The legal duty or obligation of mental health professionals, including nurses, to support patients' and service users' right to independent advocacy
- The value of Independent Mental Health Advocate (IMHA) services for patients and service users detained or in the community under mental health law, including how advocacy can support recovery
- How nurses and other mental health professionals can and should promote and support independent advocacy in ward and community settings.

When an Advocate was appointed to the young people's unit in 2010, the team had reservations; we had always seen ourselves as advocates for young people, taking pride in decisions made in the best interests of the patient. One of the hurdles to overcome was hostility from staff towards an unknown role: most knew about advocacy in a broad sense but perceived them as interfering. Our first Advocate had no prior experience with mental health issues. So it all seemed very challenging. The advocacy service offered training to staff and the unit provided sessions around mental health to the Advocate. In the early days, medical and nursing staff saw the Advocate as adversarial and she saw them as hostile. However, due to a shared conviction about vulnerable young people's right to advocacy that is independent of the NHS, we had to make this work.

The Advocate offered young people something nursing staff couldn't: an independent ear. It was important to successful acceptance of advocacy on the unit to have a staff champion, as were regular three-way meetings between the champion, Advocate, and myself as manager to tackle emerging misunderstandings. Now the advocacy service is an essential part of young people's admission to the unit and to staff induction. Although it's been a lot of work on both sides, we are seeing the benefits. Our discharge questionnaire asks – 'did you feel listened to while in hospital?' – and I think the reason for so many positive responses is because young people now have a choice to speak to the advocacy service.

Carol Fry, modern matron

Visit **https://study.sagepub.com/essentialmentalhealth** to access a wealth of online resources for this chapter – watch out for the margin icons throughout the chapter. If you are using the interactive ebook, simply click on the margin icon to go straight to the resource.

'Advocacy' may have little meaning to us as patients and service users, especially at times when we are in distress. At times of needing an advocate we are invariably in situations of care and/ or control; situations in which we believe our decisions can be impacted by what we perceive as an excessive amount of power. The feelings experienced by patients and service users come from a place of extreme vulnerability. We desperately need information and support, even though we might appear to reject it, including information and support to access advocacy.

Service users and patients seek support to challenge decisions about their care and/or treatment and about social solutions including housing and welfare. Can you provide advocacy if you are working for the organisation being challenged? As an employee you are compromised because of your accountability to the organisation; you are biased however much you try not to be. For nurses, advocacy is an extension to the caring role and will be part of the job description but there is also a need to 'advocate for advocacy', a vital role for those on the frontline of services. You are after all supporting us in our journey and so are well placed to inform and signpost. Service users can feel very isolated and having an advocate alongside can help move us from this dark place, and we need you to enable this. Enabling is a skilled process and we need you to be the bridge between independent advocacy and service users.

June Sadd, survivor

INTRODUCTION

'Advocacy' has been defined as 'the process of identifying with and representing a person's views and concerns, in order to secure enhanced rights and entitlement, undertaken by someone who has little or no conflict of interest' (Henderson & Pochin, 2001: 1). 'Independent advocacy' involves a partnership between an unpaid volunteer or a member of the community (citizen advocate) or a professional paid **advocate** and a person who may be feeling vulnerable, isolated or disempowered (Newbigging et al., 2015). This chapter is about mental health advocacy and, in particular, the statutory right to advocacy for people detained in hospital or on a **community treatment order** (CTO) under the Mental Health Act in England and Wales (hereafter referred to as '**compulsion**'); the **value** of independent advocacy to patients and **service users**; and why it is important for you as a future mental health nurse to understand and be supportive of independent advocacy. We make reference to different types of advocacy but mainly focus on Independent Mental Health Advocacy (IMHA) services in England and Wales under the 2007 Amendment to the 1983 Mental Health Act. The chapter draws unashamedly on the authors' recent work in this area, including the largest national participatory research study of IMHA services in England, academic articles, a co-produced book and practice resources produced in partnership with the Social Care Institute for Excellence (SCIE).

Whilst independent advocacy is available in Scotland and Northern Ireland, the arrangements in these jurisdictions differ. The Mental Health (Care & Treatment) (Scotland) Act 2003 recognised the importance of independent advocacy in supporting people to 'have their own voice heard in decisions made about their health and wellbeing' and enshrined the right of access to independent advocacy for people with a '**mental disorder**' (section 259). In Northern Ireland, the government recognises the role of advocacy in **safeguarding** people's rights and promoting increased choice and control over their lives, but there is no specialist statutory mental health advocate role as such (The Regulation and Quality Improvement Authority, 2012). As a student nurse, you will need to understand the advocacy role and work with independent advocates in a range of settings, both in hospital and in the community and under different legal contexts.

Being a key part of the frontline mental health team, you need to have an awareness and understanding of the patient's experience of detention and to recognise why independent advocacy is needed, as well as appreciating the potential of advocacy to support user/patient participation, autonomy and **recovery**. In this chapter, we encourage you to think through the tensions within the nursing **profession's** own claims to an advocacy role, and also to consider why it is important not simply to rely on family **carers** as proxy representatives of the patient/service user view. The chapter also reflects on how advocacy can make a difference to the care team.

CRITICAL THINKING STOP POINT 10.1

What do these accounts tell you about the concept of 'advocacy' and what is important for it to be effective? Throughout this chapter, reflect on your own stance about advocacy as part of the nurse job description and 'independent advocacy' as provided by independent sector organisations.

WHY INDEPENDENT ADVOCACY IS NEEDED

As the service user voice at the start of this chapter suggested, being compulsorily admitted to a psychiatric ward is often disempowering and impacts on a person's self-esteem, health, relationships, employment and community life (Sibitz et al., 2011). There is much debate about compulsion and how it is founded on stigmatised conceptions of people with mental health problems, how the experience can result in the person feeling stigmatised long after they have left hospital, and how it can contradict recovery practice (Repper & Perkins, 2014: Newbigging et al., 2015). Most countries have a legal basis for compulsion, and although widespread variation in rates has been noted, many European countries report increasing rates of compulsion (Kallert et al., 2005). Furthermore, there is some evidence to indicate that the use of coerced medication is more common in the UK than in other European countries, where alternative forms of restraint are used (Jarrett et al., 2008). This needs to be placed within the context of the United Nations Convention on the Rights of Persons with Disabilities (UNCRPD), which represents a significant shift towards protecting the autonomy of people experiencing mental distress (Craigie, 2015).

Whilst the majority of accounts are undoubtedly negative, given that compulsion means legally treating someone against their will, the research uncovers both negative and positive experiences. While some people experience compulsion as unhelpful, disempowering and humiliating, others experience it as supportive and helpful (Johansson & Lundman, 2002; Ridley, 2014). Good services clearly provide helpful support and are recovery-focused, but many people still experience psychiatric wards as frightening places, such that those in crisis describe them as traumatising and impersonal, and seek to avoid them at all costs (Mind, 2011). As involuntary patients, people often have little say over their treatment plan, which can include forced medication, physical restraint and seclusion, all of which might result in problematic relationships with staff as well as sparking incidents of **aggression** (Duxbury & Whittington, 2005). Advocacy is thus grounded in the recognition that there are major power disparities between services and the people using those services (Brandon et al., 1995).

Even when individuals understand what is happening to them and the restrictions of the legal section they are kept in hospital under, they may be uncertain about the length of time they will be detained in hospital and may be unaware of their legal rights (Ridley, 2014). Some will also be acutely distressed or experiencing sedation at the time of admission. Holding conflicting views with the clinical team about what is the most **appropriate treatment**, combined with a power imbalance between service users and mental health professionals, can impede the development of a trusting relationship and, ultimately, can **affect** the person's recovery. Feelings of powerlessness and a lack of control are an almost universal experience of compulsion, despite the majority of people recognising their mental health was poor prior to admission (Katsakou et al., 2012).

Advocacy then provides a mechanism, through supporting service users to voice their opinions, for ensuring that vulnerable people can get their voices heard and have their rights protected. As this patient in an **acute** ward commented about the experience of having an advocate:

> I felt more empowered, I felt more able to get the right outcomes, with somebody there who was on my side. She made me feel like, yes I can deal with these issues that I wasn't getting anything, any help with. She made me feel empowered basically. (Newbigging et al., 2012: 194)

At its core, advocacy seeks to empower people to have greater control and choices in their relationship with health and social care services. Statutory advocacy (IMHA, Independent Mental Capacity Advocate (IMCA), Deprivation of Liberty or DoLs) and other forms of advocacy (e.g. generic mental health, citizen or volunteer advocacy, self-advocacy) are available to people with mental health problems in a range of hospital, residential and community contexts, and, as a student nurse or qualified nurse, you may encounter one or more of these types of independent advocacy. What we are specifically concerned with in this chapter is IMHA. Recovery-orientated services are, by definition, based on dialogue and partnership. There is clearly a place for independent advocacy in facilitating such dialogue, as one professional reflects:

> The essence of our job is to have a meaningful dialogue with our service users. Some service users may not have English as their first language, they may have a learning disability, they may be very unwell – it's fantastic from my point of view that an advocate helps the staff have a dialogue with a patient. So we should always see that as a huge opportunity, as a huge benefit. (Matron, NHS Foundation Trust) (SCIE/UCLan film)

Independent advocacy can enable shared decision making to take place; it can promote the least restrictive alternatives so that people can hold onto what is important in their lives when in a mental health crisis; and advocacy can help increase the accountability of mental health services to service users. When detained against their will, people are likely to feel that they have no rights and that they have to battle for everything. The impact of having their voice heard can shift this power imbalance and enable staff and patients/service users to work constructively together. Thus, advocacy is a fundamental part of a recovery-focused service (Machin & Newbigging, 2016).

MAKING A DIFFERENCE 10.1

'It only began to change when along came a light (advocate)'

Being sectioned in hospital is a very lonely, frightening experience. You're desperately hoping and searching for help, information, some clarity over your situation. In my experience of this dark place, it only began to change when along came a light (advocate). I had no idea what an advocate was, let alone how much they could help me. Upon meeting the advocate it became very clear, very quickly, this wasn't just another member of staff. This person listened to me: this person LISTENED. I became

(Continued)

a name, a human being again, not just a section. We spoke at length about my situation and how we could go about improving it. The advocate spoke to me like a person, open and honest, nothing was guarded or sugar coated. I asked a question, I got a straight answer, good or bad, it was the information I was craving. From then on, every ward round or meeting with the doctor, I'd take the advocate. The advocate asked a question on my behalf, usually getting a positive result or feedback. Me asking that same question, I'd get a 'we'll discuss it as a team and get back to you'; the advocate asked and it's done. Through my time in hospital the advocate became a tool to speed up the process of getting out, asking about my therapy or medication. A good advocate becomes your mouthpiece, asking the questions you need answering, getting you the results you need. My experience of hospital is a place where information doesn't flow to and from the right people, the advocate unblocks this process. By introducing common sense and a dose of reality (in a very unreal situation), you know where you stand, you know what's happening. Working together with my advocate sped up the process of everything I needed, reducing medication, increasing leave, and eventually getting discharged. (Kris Chastey, Foreword, in Newbigging et al., 2015: 8)

INDEPENDENT MENTAL HEALTH ADVOCACY (IMHA)

The development of independent advocacy has happened alongside an increasing emphasis in health and social policy on patient and public involvement (NHSE, 2017); greater user choice and control (DH, 2007); and safeguarding the rights of vulnerable people. Advocacy increases the accountability of services to patients and service users in that it helps staff understand the experience of being detained and ensures patients and service users are involved in decision making. In a mental health context, advocacy is part of wider developments to democratise psychiatry. Its beginnings have been traced back to petitioners in the 17th century seeking more humane treatment of inpatients in so-called mad-houses or asylums (see Chapter 3 in Newbigging et al., 2015). Most recently, a legal right to advocacy was established with the creation of the IMHA role under the 2007 Mental Health (Amendment) Act and implemented in England and Wales in 2009.

But what has IMHA got to do with you as a nurse? An IMHA is a type of independent advocate with a particular role and responsibilities under **mental health law** in England and Wales. People detained under the Mental Health Act have a *right* to this type of advocate, and it is the overall responsibility of the hospital and clinicians and part of your job role to ensure they receive information about it. This includes asking an IMHA to visit a patient who lacks the capacity to decide whether or not to instruct an advocate so that they can explain what they can offer (DoH, 2015). The following people are eligible for IMHA, irrespective of their age. In the Act, they are referred to as 'qualifying patients' and this includes patients who are:

- detained under the 1983 Act
- liable to be detained under the Act, even if not actually detained, including those who are currently on leave of absence from hospital or absent without leave
- conditionally discharged restricted patients
- subject to guardianship
- subject to community treatment orders (CTOs)
- other patients (informal patients) being considered for a treatment to which section 57 applies (specific treatments such as psychosurgery); or they are under 18 and being considered for electroconvulsive therapy (ECT) or any other treatment to which section 58A applies. (DH, 2015)

As the Mental Health Act 1983 Code of Practice (DH, 2015: 54) states IMHA services provide an additional safeguard for patients subject to the Act. IMHAs operate within the framework of the law to ensure that qualifying patients are given and understand information relating to the section of the MH Act they are kept in hospital under or are subject to in the community, and that they understand the legal rights and safeguards they have. They support qualifying patients to exercise these rights through helping them to participate in decision-making about their care and treatment. The Independent Mental Capacity Advocate (IMCA) introduced under the Mental Capacity Act 2005 and designed to safeguard the interests of people who lack capacity to make specific decisions (including where they live and about serious medical treatment options), is sometimes confused with IMHA. In theory, where a person is deemed to be lacking in capacity and is subject to both the Mental Capacity Act 2005 and the Mental Health Act, they would be entitled to support from both an IMCA and an IMHA, and may even have rights under the Deprivation of Liberty (DoLS) provisions (Dept. of Health, 2015). In general though, the Mental Health Act has tended to 'trump' the Mental Capacity Act in such situations. (Herlihy & Holloway, 2009: 479)

Since 2009, hospitals in England and Wales and their staff, including nurses, have had a duty to provide qualifying patients with oral and written information about their right to an IMHA, and to promote this right actively. Research, however, has found that this is not always happening and also that there is a lack of awareness and understanding about IMHA amongst professionals in mental health services, including forensic mental health services, as well as amongst service users (Hakim & Pollard, 2011; Newbigging et al., 2012; Palmer et al., 2012). It is worth noting that arrangements for IMHA are different in Wales, where all inpatients, including those not subject to the MH Act, are entitled to access an IMHA (Welsh Government, 2011). This had been identified as good practice (National Institute for Health and Clinical Excellence, 2011) and a recommendation has been made to government that access should be on an opt-out rather than an opt-in basis (House of Commons Health Select Committee, 2013). Not only is it professionals' duty to promote and raise awareness of the right to an IMHA, they must also ensure that IMHAs are able to meet with patients in private, can attend meetings about patients' care, and they must facilitate access to mental health notes as appropriate. A service manager explains:

> It is a statutory right for service users to have access to an IMHA whenever they arrive on a ward for inpatient treatments or are offered treatments in the community under a community treatment order. A service user has the right to access an IMHA, they should be given information by a nurse on how to access the service ... It is a statutory right now for patients to be able to access their clinical notes via the IMHA, it's obviously very important for staff to realise that. (Community service manager, NHS Foundation Trust) (SCIE/UCLAN film)

Our research on IMHA found wide variation not only in the uptake of advocacy across geographical areas but amongst different groups of qualifying patients (Newbigging et al., 2012). Five groups were particularly underserved by advocacy – people from Black, Asian and minority ethnic (BAME) communities; people with learning difficulties; older people with **dementia**; people with hearing impairments or who are D/deaf; and young people under 18 years of age. A recurring theme was that those who are likely to need advocacy the most have poorest access, in other words they are being disadvantaged in accessing IMHA. The reasons qualifying patients gave for not accessing IMHA services included not knowing about them and not understanding the IMHA role. This underlines the importance, when promoting advocacy, of nurses being aware of the needs of those who are further marginalised because of their **ethnicity**, gender, sexuality, age, physical disability or learning disability.

WHAT'S THE EVIDENCE? 10.1

Research on statutory advocacy

WHAT'S THE
EVIDENCE
10.1 ARTICLES

The following resources are available via https://study.sagepub.com/ essentialmentalhealth and provide further information on statutory advocacy in England:
Newbigging, K., Ridley, J., McKeown, M., et al. (2012)
Townsley, R. & Laing, A. (2011)

CAN NURSES BE ADVOCATES?

For some time, it has been claimed that advocacy is part of the role of professionals like nurses and social workers (Dalrymple & Boylan, 2013). Codes of professional **ethics** state that nurses should act as advocates, though arguments against this were, for instance, raised by the **survivor**/service user and professional voices at the start of this chapter. Nurse education is faced with the challenge of preparing nurses in a complex context (Altun & Ersoy, 2003). Our research on the quality of IMHA services (Newbigging et al., 2012) identified that many nurses believed themselves to be the patients' advocate. As a result, some ward staff view independent advocacy and the IMHA role as superfluous and may be reluctant to facilitate access to advocacy services or to take the steps necessary to ensure IMHAs are involved in key meetings. Others, however, have a well-developed understanding of how their role differs and can coexist alongside the independent advocacy role, and will take extra steps to promote advocacy services and create a welcoming **environment** for advocates on the ward:

> From our point of view it's fantastic that an advocate helps the staff to have a dialogue with a patient. So we should always see advocacy as a huge opportunity; and as a huge benefit. (Nurse, in Altun & Ersoy, 2003)

Research has concluded that professionals' understanding of advocacy influences and shapes their attitude to and relationship with independent advocacy, and the extent to which they are prepared to promote it to patients and service users. The main point of contention has been confusion and misunderstanding around what nurses' role should be in advocating for patients, and the role of independent advocacy delivered by independent sector advocacy organisations, especially when nurses feel that they are best placed to know patients well:

> I mean I'd see myself as being an advocate and I have done on many occasions, like, you know, especially around complaints. If patients make complaints I'd seek to rectify the complaints in the first instance if they were, you know, locally resolvable. (Modern matron, Secure Services, in Newbigging et al., 2012: 104)
>
> A relationship between a nurse and a patient is quite close, that's what we try to make it therapeutic. We try and really understand their emotions and their needs. Sometimes it's difficult to separate other things from that because you become close with that person, now an Advocate doesn't have that emotional bond with the patient because they don't spend that length of time and they're not trained to do that. (Staff nurse, acute ward, in Newbigging et al., 2012: 105)

In a study of student nurses' views of what mental health nursing looks like, the mental health nurse was seen as an advocate because they were understood to be able to present the patient's case in ward rounds (Rungapadiachy et al., 2004). On this interpretation, advocacy implies speaking on behalf of the patient, especially if the latter feels unable to do so. One participant explained: 'sometimes when a patient had an adverse reaction to his or her medication it was usually the nurse who informs the doctor and suggests to the doctor that the patient's medication be reviewed'. It is also interesting to note that mental health nurses found advocating on behalf of the patient frustrating because of the lack of cooperation from some consultants. Some were also perceived to advocate on behalf of doctors by persuading patients to take their medication.

Informal discussions with student nurses at an academic institution in England found many did feel they were part of the advocacy pathway alongside independent advocacy. Around half of the 22 first-year nursing students did not know what IMHA was, but all had ideas of how they could advocate on behalf of a patient in a ward context, and advocating for the best interests of patients was an important element of what they thought was part of the mental health nurse's role (de la Haye, 2015). As one said:

I feel, when qualified as a nurse I play a vital role as a professional advocate within the staff/patient relationship. And as a nurse I have a closer relationship with the patient and so can make more time for them.

CAN FAMILY AND FRIENDS BE ADVOCATES?

The introduction of community treatment orders (CTOs) in mental health law in the UK places a further responsibility on family and friends who are supporting individuals as unpaid carers, and in some cases it has done so without providing any extra support for them or the people they support. However, while advocacy services specifically for carers are very limited, they do benefit indirectly from advocacy for the person they support. Knowing there is someone else who has a more complete knowledge about services and the person's rights can be reassuring for the whole family.

Family and friends may want to act as advocates on aspects of a person's care, such as helping them to secure accommodation or aftercare. Indeed, services may rely on carers to provide this support as resources are increasingly stretched. But there may be other areas which cause significant friction within their relationships, including the suitability of hospital care or the relevance of medication, or sensitive topics which haven't been discussed within the family, such as sexuality or substance use – all of which should challenge the assumption by services that carers can act independently for the patient or service user. During a crisis, a person may be suspicious of a relative's motives. A minority of families may include a hidden history of abuse, and in some cases abusive relationships will be known about. Further, some families might not feel able to say they cannot provide support. In these instances, carers may act from what they perceive to be the 'best interests' of the person concerned, which may not necessarily be the same as what the person wants. So while a family member may have acted at some point as the person's advocate, and staff may view them in this capacity, this does not replace the person's right to access an independent advocate.

Clearly, family and friends also need to be informed about forms of statutory advocacy such as IMHA even where it may not directly apply to them. Family members often say they would value this information early, before a crisis, emphasising that during a crisis it may feel too late, with so many other things to consider. They suggest that people who are in crisis may be unable to understand information about advocacy, and that carers or nearest relatives can play an important role in ensuring that the person is aware of the availability of advocacy services, and can reinforce information about the role of advocates and how to access one.

CRITICAL THINKING STOP POINT 10.2

Identify the strengths and limitations of family carers acting as the patient or service user's advocate. Can you think of any circumstances where a family carer has advocated for the patient or service user? What were the challenges and how did this impact on the patient's/service user's access to independent advocacy?

HELPFUL FOR ASSIGNMENTS!

CASE STUDY:
CARE
QUALITY
COMMISSION

A MODEL TO UNDERSTAND PRACTICE

Organisational **culture** and routine practice will have a direct bearing on whether or not the potential of advocacy can be realised within a particular health care context. Studies have highlighted that advocates seek to have constructive relationships with mental health professionals whilst remaining independent in order to achieve better outcomes (Carver & Morrison, 2005). However, this is not always possible and staff can be hostile or negatively disposed towards advocacy. This is often grounded in a misunderstanding of the role and concerns about the implications of advocating for the individual's perspective, which may be perceived by professionals as being in conflict with his or her 'best interests'. From our IMHA study, we identified two key components of the relationship – understanding of the advocacy role, and disposition or attitude towards advocacy. We used these to develop a model which assesses the nature and quality of the relationship and how this impacts on service users' experience of advocacy (Newbigging et al., 2012; McKeown et al., 2014) (see Figure 10.1).

Constructive working relationships between professionals and advocates reflect both a good understanding of the role of advocacy and a positive disposition towards it. In this scenario, nurses view the challenge that advocates pose in a positive way, as deepening their understanding and increasing their accountability to qualifying patients. One ward manager captures this:

> She's [the advocate] quite integral to what we're doing but her independence is so important. What she made clear to me is her role is advocating for what the patient is asking and articulating even where it might not actually be to the patient's benefit, I.e. that's she's saying what they've asked. Now it might be that she tries to help them with that and to work that out and we have a number of conversations now about that. So what we tend to do is when patients have got particular problems, we'll sit down all three of us together so it's really direct, we're able to resolve things you know properly. No matter what I do, the patient's always going to see me as a Ward Manager, whether they like me, don't like me, I'm a nurse you can't take that away and I manage the ward. I think having an Advocate that's able and committed, then you've got immense possibilities for progressing things that you might have struggled with. (unpublished data, Newbigging et al., 2012)

In this situation, there is understanding of the potential conflict of interest in the professional's role with that of the person concerned and the advocate is experienced as enabling effective negotiation between potentially conflicting standpoints. In developing good working relationships with professionals, advocates may compromise their independence or give the impression to patients and service users that they are part of the clinical team (Carver & Morrison, 2005). This is captured in the top left-hand quadrant of our model in Figure 10.1.

Described as 'enmeshed relationships', professionals are grounded in a positive disposition to advocacy but lack an appreciation of the necessity of its independence. It is, therefore, important that

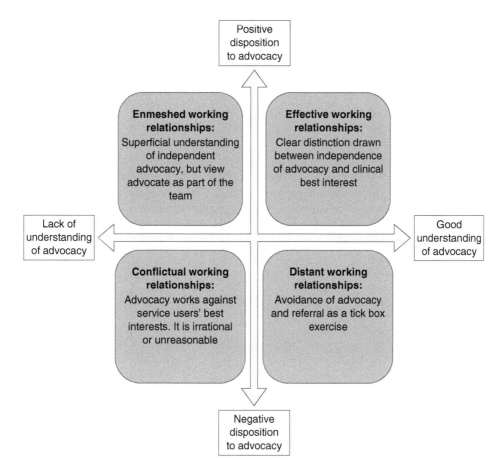

Figure 10.1 A model for the relationship between mental health professionals and advocates

both mental health professionals and advocates keep effective boundaries in order to maintain the independence of advocacy.

Maintaining these boundaries requires a reciprocal respect for the confidentiality of the information shared between the three parties, and requires that the focus on the role of the advocate in promoting rights and strengthening participation in decision making is sustained. In some instances, for example, a professional may direct their comments to the advocate rather than the person concerned, failing to recognise the fundamental purpose of advocacy.

There can be highly conflictual relationships between professionals and advocates, where professionals have a good understanding of the role but are negatively disposed towards it, viewing it as a challenge to their professionalism:

> I've been called into a room where the advocate has gone through the list of the patient's grievances so to speak in quite an abrupt manner. And I've said 'yes we sorted that yesterday, yes they're getting that tomorrow,' you know, I've just stood there and I suppose in a way I've resented the implication that we haven't addressed those issues. (Nurse, in Newbigging et al., 2012: 178)

This stance may reflect a pervasive paternalistic approach that is symptomatic of a wider organisational culture that lacks a positive approach to self-determination, or the role of nurses in compulsion and their sensitivity to potential criticism. It may, however, also reflect concerns about the quality or approach of the IMHA or the advocacy service. We noted, for example, concerns about the availability of IMHAs, which reflect capacity issues and, ultimately, the effectiveness of the **commissioning** of IMHA services and the level of investment in them.

Perhaps hardest to comprehend is that depicted in the lower-left quadrant of Figure 10.1, where professionals' understanding of the advocacy role is poor and their attitude to advocacy is negative. In this scenario, there is a lack of effort to ensure that qualifying patients are made aware of their right to an advocate, to facilitate access to an IMHA and to take care to ensure that the IMHA has a private space to meet with service users or that key meetings are scheduled to enable the IMHA to attend if necessary. Thus, referral becomes a tick-box exercise that can be reported to managers, but quickly evidences the fact that a genuine commitment to the rights of qualifying patients, and the importance of service users having a voice, is seriously lacking. That this is the case in practice in some settings is evidenced by the Care Quality Commission review which identified variations in practice such that detained patients are not always aware of their rights nor routinely involved in decisions about their care and treatment (CQC, 2015).

CRITICAL THINKING STOP POINT 10.3

Applying the model to practice

We offer this model as a framework for nurses and other mental health professionals to reflect on their practice and the culture of the organisation. We invite you now to locate yourself and your organisation in the quadrant that best describes your relationship and that of your service (e.g. the ward on which you work) with advocacy. Where you place yourself and your service may be different but the question remains the same: what steps need to be taken to ensure and maintain a positive relationship with independent advocacy?

CRITICAL DEBATE 10.1

The Nursing Code (Nursing & Midwifery Council (NMC), 2015) includes the following sections:

> 2.1 **Work in partnership with people** to make sure you deliver care effectively.
>
> 2.3 Encourage and **empower people** to share decisions about their treatment and care.
>
> 3.4 **Act as an advocate** for the vulnerable, challenging poor practice and discriminatory attitudes and behaviour relating to their care.
>
> 4.1 Balance the **need to act in the best interests** of people at all times with the requirement to **respect a person's right to accept or refuse treatment.**

How do you translate this into effective practice? What kind of relationship with independent advocacy would support this approach?

CHAPTER SUMMARY

This chapter has covered the following ideas:

- Independent advocacy has the potential to support the self-empowerment of patients and service users, to improve the dialogue between professionals and service users, and to result in recovery-focused outcomes.
- When service users seek support to challenge decisions about their care and/or treatment, it is important that people advocating for and with them are independent of the mental health service provider.
- While nurses might hold the belief that they are the patient's or service user's advocate, the strong potential for conflict of interest has to be acknowledged in mental health nursing.
- There are differences between advocating for someone's 'best interests' and advocating on their behalf that need to be recognised by nurses in how they think about their own role, and in how they relate to independent advocates on the ward.
- Implementation of a specific form of advocacy in England and Wales – the Independent Mental Health Advocate (IMHA) under the Mental Health Act 2007 – placed a legal duty on hospital staff and others to promote people's right to independent advocacy by facilitating access to IMHA services and supporting advocates on the ward.
- Regardless of whether or not service users have support from family or friends who may act as their advocate at times, those who are qualifying patients under the Mental Health Act have a right to access IMHA and must be made aware of this. The potential for conflicting interests and views between the person and their family should be recognised by services.
- Understanding of advocacy and disposition towards advocacy are key dimensions determining whether or not the relationship between professionals and advocates is constructive and effective.

BUILD YOUR BIBLIOGRAPHY

Books

- Macadam, A., Watt, R. & Greig, R. (2014) *The impact of advocacy for people who use social care services*. London: NIHR School for Social Care Research. Not specifically mental health focused, this text usefully reviews research on the benefits of independent advocacy for service users.
- Machin, K. & Newbigging, K. (2016) *Advocacy: A stepping stone to recovery*. London: Centre for Mental Health & Mental Health Network, NHS Confederation. This article describes the use of advocacy to support recovery-focused services.
- Newbigging, K., Ridley, J., McKeown, M., et al. (2015) *Independent mental health advocacy: The right to be heard – Context, values and good practice*. London: Jessica Kingsley. Provides an up-to-date review of critical issues with independent mental health advocacy.

SAGE journal articles

- Go to https://study.sagepub.com/essentialmentalhealth for further free online journal articles related to this chapter. If you are using the interactive ebook, simply click on the book icon in the margin to go straight to the resource.

FURTHER
READING:
JOURNAL
ARTICLES

- Martin, G. (1998) Communication breakdown or ideal speech situation: the problem of nurse advocacy. *Nursing Ethics, 5*, 147-157.
- Watson, C. & O'Connor, T. (2017) Legislating for advocacy: the case of whistleblowing. *Nursing Ethics, 24*(3), 305-312.

Other journal articals

- Hewitt, J. (2001) A critical review of the arguments debating the role of the nurse advocate. *Journal of Advanced Nursing, 37*(5), 439-445.

Weblinks

FURTHER
READING:
WEBLINKS

Go to https://study.sagepub.com/essentialmentalhealth for further weblinks related to this chapter. If you are using the interactive ebook, simply click on the book icon in the margin to go straight to the resource.

- Carers UK (2014) *Being heard: a guide to selfadvocacy for carers*: www.carersuk.org/help-and-advice/get-resources/being-heard-a-self-advocacy-toolkit-for-carers-uk – link to *Carers Scotland* and a helpful resource in relation to carers and advocacy.
- Social Care Institute for Excellence (SCIE): www.scie.org.uk/independent-mental-health-advocacy – link to 12 good practice resources for service users, professionals, commissioners and advocacy services. See, in particular, *At a glance briefing: Understanding IMHA for mental health staff*, Social Care TV films for staff and *Improving equality of access to IMHA*. These all identify the benefits of advocacy for service users.
- SCIE: www.scie.org.uk/care-act-2014/advocacy-services/commissioning-independent-advocacy/inclusion-empowerment-human-rights/types.asp – link to resources in relation to the Care Act 2015 providing information about independent advocacy.

────────── ACE YOUR ASSESSMENT ──────────

ONLINE
QUIZZES &
ACTIVITY
ANSWERS

Revise what you have learned by visiting https://study.sagepub.com/essentialmentalhealth. If you are using the interactive ebook, simply click on the tick icon to go straight to the resource.

- Test yourself with multiple-choice and short-answer questions and flashcards.

REFERENCES

Altun, I. & Ersoy, N. (2003) Undertaking the role of patient advocate: a longitudinal study of nursing students. *Nurse Ethics, 10*(5): 462–471.

Brandon, D., Brandon, A. & Brandon, T. (1995) *Advocacy: Power to people with disabilities*. Birmingham: Venture.

Care Quality Commission (2015) *Monitoring the Mental Health Act in 2013/14*. Newcastle: CQC. Available at: www.cqc.org.uk/sites/default/files/monitoring_the_mha_2013-14_report_web_0303.pdf.pdf (accessed 08.03.15).

Carver, N. & Morrison, J. (2005) Advocacy in practice: the experiences of independent advocates on UK mental health wards. *Journal of Psychiatric and Mental Health Nursing, 12*(1), 75–84.

Craigie, J. (2015) A fine balance: reconsidering patient autonomy in light of the UN convention on the rights of persons with disabilities. *Bioethics*, *29*(6), 398–405.

Dalrymple, J. & Boylan, J. (2013) *Effective advocacy in social work*. London: Sage.

De La Haye, S.J. (2015) Unpublished discussion with nursing students. Sheffield Hallam University.

Department of Health (DH) (2007) *Choice matters 2007–08: putting patients in control*. London: DH Available at: http://webarchive.nationalarchives.gov.uk/20080817163612/http://www.dh.gov. uk/en/Publicationsandstatistics/Publications/PublicationsPolicyAndGuidance/DH_076331 (accessed 01.10.17).

Department of Health (DH) (2015) *Mental Health 1983 Code of Practice*. Available at: www.gov.uk/ government/uploads/system/uploads/attachment_data/file/395494/mh-code.pdf (accessed 05.08.17).

Duxbury, J. & Whittington, R. (2005) Causes and management of patient aggression and violence: staff and patient perspectives. *Journal of Advanced Nursing*, *50*(5), 469–478.

Hakim, R. & Pollard, T. (2011) *Independent mental health advocacy: Briefing paper 3*. London: Mental Health Alliance. Available at www.mentalhealthalliance.org.uk/resources/Independent_Mental_ Health_Advocacy_report.pdf (accessed 15.04.16).

Henderson, R. & Pochin, M. (2001) *A right result? Advocacy, justice and empowerment*. Bristol: Policy Press.

Herlihy, D.P. & Holloway, F. (2009) The Mental Health Act and the Mental Capacity Act: untangling the relationship. *Psychiatry*, *8*(12), 478–480.

House of Commons Health Select Committee (2013) Post-legislative scrutiny of the Mental Health Act 2007. Available at: www.parliament.uk/business/committees/committees-a-z/commons-select/ health-committee/news/13-08-14-mha2007cs (accessed 5 August 2017).

Jarrett, M., Bowers, L. & Simpson, A. (2008) Coerced medication in psychiatric inpatient care: literature review. *Journal of Advanced Nursing*, *64*(6), 538–548.

Johansson, I.M. & Lundman, B. (2002) Patients' experience of involuntary psychiatric care: good opportunities and great losses. *Journal of Psychiatric and Mental Health Nursing*, *9*(6), 639–647.

Kallert, T.W., Glöckner, M., Onchev, G., et al. (2005) The EUNOMIA project on coercion in psychiatry: study design and preliminary data. *World Psychiatry*, *4*(3), 168–172.

Katsakou, C., Rose, D., Amos, T., et al. (2012) Psychiatric patients' views on why their involuntary hospitalisation was right or wrong: a qualitative study. *Social Psychiatry and Psychiatric Epidemiology*, *47*(7), 1169–1179.

Machin, K. & Newbigging, K. (2016) *Advocacy: A stepping stone to recovery*. London: Centre for Mental Health & Mental Health Network, NHS Confederation.

McKeown, M., Ridley, J., Newbigging, K., et al. (2014) Conflict of roles: a conflict of ideas? The unsettled relations between care team staff and independent mental health advocates. *International Journal of Mental Health Nursing*, *23*(5), 398–408.

MIND (2011) *Listening to experience: An independent inquiry into acute and crisis mental health care*. London: MIND.

National Institute for Health and Clinical Excellence (NICE) (2011) Service user experience in adult mental health: improving the experience of care for people using adult NHS mental health services. NICE Guideline (CG136). Available at: http://guidance.nice.org.uk/CG136/ NICEGuidance/pdf/English (accessed 23 March 2014).

Newbigging, K., Ridley, J., McKeown, M., et al. (2012) *The Right to be heard: Review of the quality of IMHA services*. Report for the Department of Health. Preston: University of Central Lancashire.

Newbigging, K., Ridley, J., McKeown, M., et al. (2015b) *Independent mental health advocacy: The right to be heard – Context, values and good practice*. London: Jessica Kingsley.

NHSE (2017) *Patient and public participation policy*. Leeds: NHSE.

Nursing & Midwifery Council (NMC) (2015) *The code: Professional standards of practice and behaviour for nurses and midwives*. Available at: www.nmc-uk.org/code (accessed 28.01.16).

Palmer, D., Nixon, J., Reynolds, S., et al. (2012) Getting to know you: reflections on a specialist independent mental health advocacy service for Bexley and Bromley residents in forensic settings. *Mental Health Review Journal*, *17*(1), 5–13.

Repper, J. & Perkins, R. (2014) The elephant on the table. *Mental Health and Social Inclusion*, *18*(4). Available at: www.emeraldinsight.com/doi/full/10.1108/MHSI-09-2014-0032 (accessed 05.08.17).

Ridley, J. (2014) The experiences of service users. In S. Matthews, P. O'Hare and J. Hemmington (eds) *Approved mental health practice: Essential themes for students and practitioners*. Basingstoke: Palgrave Macmillan.

Rungapadiachy, D.M., Madill, A. & Gough, B. (2004) Mental health student nurses' perception of the role of the mental health nurse. *Journal of Psychiatric and Mental Health Nursing*, *11*, 714–724.

Sibitz, I., Scheutz, A., Lakeman, R., et al. (2011) Impact of coercive measures on life stories: qualitative study. *British Journal of Psychiatry*, *199*(3), 239–244.

The Regulation and Quality Improvement Authority (2012) *Provision of advocacy services in mental health and learning disability inpatient facilities in Northern Ireland*. Available at: www.rqia.org.uk/cms_resources/Advocacy_Report_final%20report.pdf (accessed 15.04.2016).

Townsley, R. & Laing, A. (2011) *Effective relationships, better outcomes: Mapping the impact of the independent mental capacity advocate service in England (1 April 2009 to 31 March 2010)*. London: Social Care Institute for Excellence.

Welsh Government (2011) *Delivering the independent mental health advocacy service in Wales*. Available at: http://gov.wales/docs/dhss/publications/111222advocacyen.pdf (accessed 15.04.16).

THE ETHICAL MENTAL HEALTH NURSE

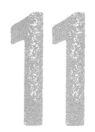

KAREN M. WRIGHT AND ALAN ARMSTRONG

THIS CHAPTER COVERS

- What are ethics? What are values?
- Why should mental health nurses understand morals and ethics?
- How do ethics relate to 'values-based' mental health practice?
- What are the principles of values-based practice?
- How can I use these theories and philosophies to make an ethical (or morally) good decision?

"

Karen Wright is a mental health nurse who still practises alongside her academic post. The case study presented in this chapter (*Anna*) is created from experiences on a specialist eating disorder unit and reflects the daily dilemmas encountered by nursing staff working within such services today. Additionally, *Jane* initially had a therapeutic relationship with Karen when she was a community psychiatric nurse circa 2000 (when covering for Jane's care coordinator who is referred to here as 'Adam'). Jane moved away and recently contacted Karen about her subsequent recovery journey, so relates her previous experience which she remembers extremely clearly, despite the passage of years and change of roles.

"

"

What I will say is that having never tried to think about my experiences from a nursing perspective before, I now have a great deal more respect for the mental health 'triers'!

I was referred by my GP with first episode psychoses in January 2000 when I was 32 and a museum curator (decorative art). When I left Preston in 2002 I had a diagnosis of schizophrenia (paranoid) which was later changed to 'schizoaffective disorder, depressive' in 2005 in Wycombe where I still live. From 2007 to the present date I've been fantastically lucky to have the same CPN who has brought me a long way – especially in building a trusting relationship – and who I also like and respect.

Jane, service user (Jane's voice can be heard specifically in relation to her search for a prognosis)

"

INTRODUCTION

We each enter nursing with our sense of what is right and wrong, and what some people would refer to as our 'ethical compass'. Many use the two terms **'values'** and **'ethics'** interchangeably, and, although they are different, we require both to make decisions that are in the best interest of ourselves and those we work with or care for. Effectively, we define 'ethics' as 'dealing with what is good or bad, right or wrong' (Barker, 2011: 3). For the mental health nurse, it's important that we make 'good' and 'right' decisions, and this chapter will seek to explore what that means for our practice. We can learn how to *do* nursing, but learning how to *be* a nurse requires us to reflect on who we are and how we use ourselves and how our underpinning values show themselves to those who we work with and those in our care (Armstrong, 2006).

'Education without values, as useful as it is, seems rather to make man a more clever devil.' – C.S. Lewis

WHAT ARE ETHICS?

Singer (1994: 3) says that 'ethics is about how we ought to live'. Nursing ethics are, therefore, how we are to nurse. Ethics and your ethical values underpin everything that you do and some extraordinary philosophers have had a good deal to say about it for some hundreds of years. In this chapter, we attempt not to baffle you with philosophy, but to provide explanation and exploration of these concepts to enable you to utilise these to help you make 'good' decisions as well as 'evidence-based' decisions. In short, ethical thinking enables us to behave in a 'good' or 'moral' way.

WHAT ARE VALUES?

Values, on the other hand, are what are important to you and how you see the world. So, when we talk about **'values-based practice'** in nursing, we mean those values that align with being an ethical, professional and caring nurse. Such values may include honesty, candour and trustworthiness (Armstrong, 2007). Dworkin (1993, cited in Galeza, 2014) also uses the term 'moral values' to describe beliefs we hold about morality; besides morality, we commonly hold values about many different aspects of life including politics and religion.

PERSONAL MORALS

Here we are concerned with the use of 'morals/ethics' in the personal sense – for example, students express their personal beliefs about ethical issues and their beliefs concern the way we should act, the way we should conduct ourselves and the way we should be towards others. Our personal morals usually develop from informal sources of moral education including our parents, schoolteachers and university tutors! Sources of moral education can also include our friends, peers, work colleagues, the media and religious figures. Such sources help to inform our 'intuitive' moral judgement and help us to make decisions. In fact, Allmark (1992) suggests that nurses make most ethical decisions using their intuition.

Most of us have views on these ethical issues without having formally studied ethics, and ethicists refer to these views as 'common-sense ethics' (Hanssen & Alpers, 2010). Some people are able to provide reasons in support of their common-sense ethical views, whilst others aren't able to provide any reasons for their common-sense ethical views. Instead, they might say, for example, 'I simply *know* it is wrong to steal'. 'Knowing' it's (morally) wrong to steal is an example of a moral intuition and, in our everyday ethical lives, we often appeal to these sorts of moral intuitions.

Another common example is murder; some people say that no reason is required to support their view that murder is morally wrong. Such personal morals/ethics express a person's view on what is morally right/wrong and morally good/bad.

GROUP MORALS

This usage concerns the morals/ethics of a group of people; examples include professional groups such as nurses and doctors and other non-health care examples, such as sportsmen and charity workers. Group ethics include formal statements, rules and regulations, which serve to guide and place certain limits on one's conduct. Members of the group are expected to comply with these statements, rules and regulations – for instance, nurses must comply with the NMC Code (NMC, 2015).

WHY NURSES SHOULD UNDERSTAND MORALS AND ETHICS

Nurses have a professional duty to understand ethics and a professional and legal duty to practise in an ethical manner. Hence, we study ethics in order to comply with professional and group ethics, such as the NMC (2015) Code and current legislation, such as the Human Rights Act 1998 and the Mental Capacity Act 2005. However, a stronger reason to study and understand ethics lies in one's self-development – in nursing, we usually refer to this as 'personal and professional development' (PPD or PDP). In ethics, we refer to one's moral agency and to the notion of human **flourishing**, i.e. ideas concerning how we can live successful lives. It could be said that the *strongest reason* for nurses to study, comprehend and apply ethics is the 'helping' relationship between nurse and patient being rooted in one's sense of morality, e.g. duty, obligation and virtue.

We don't exist in isolation, although ethics is sometimes taught as if we do. As individuals, we each have a uniqueness and an independence. But we also have an interconnectedness with others. To be a morally *good* nurse, to make ethically *right* and *sound* decisions, and to work morally well within a **multi-disciplinary team** (MDT), requires that we have an insightful understanding of the interconnectedness of each other. This in part means that we need to know our own values and the values of others including our patients.

VALUES AS MORAL MOTIVES

A motive is a reason for doing something. Moral values play an important role in influencing our decisions and guiding our actions (Yeo et al., 2010). Therefore, our moral values serve as important moral motives; for example, in the statement – 'It's morally right to give money to charity' – the underpinning moral values might include kindness, compassion and justice.

VALUE SETS AND VALUE SYSTEMS

Compared with the numerous beliefs we typically have, we tend to have only a narrow value set. Once organised and prioritised, we can then call this our value system. Values can be hierarchal and dynamic, i.e. they can change through the life span. Our value systems will therefore contain different values, some more important than others; this is one reason why we might wish to organise and prioritise our value set, e.g. through the process known as 'values clarification'. Our value systems are learned through experience, observation and socialisation (e.g. Settelmaier & Nigam, 2007).

MORAL/ETHICAL THEORY

CASE STUDY: COMMUNITY MENTAL HEALTH NURSE

Moral theories – also known as ethical theory or ethical frameworks – form part of normative ethics: that part of ethics dealing with norms and values. The two central questions of western normative ethics are:

1. How *should* people *act*?
2. How *should* people *be*?

Ethicists develop moral theories in part to provide us with *action guidance* on the above complex questions. Moral theory is a particular part of ethics; it's possible to study ethics without studying moral theory. The two central questions have been at the heart of western ethics for over 2500 years. These are deep philosophical questions with no clear answers. (Eastern ethical traditions are incredibly interesting, e.g. Buddhism and its emphasis on compassion. But here we limit our focus to the ethics of the West, e.g. the UK, the EU and the USA.) The idea of 'action guidance' may sound complex, but in essence it means helping people make decisions and take action by giving them some form of help or guidance. This kind of guidance is usually given verbally, i.e. in the words used between people during conversations. Another common phrase for action guidance is 'moral prescription'; advising people on the course of action they should take is a crucial aspect of moral education.

MORAL THEORY AND OBLIGATION

Several moral theories are based on the notion of *moral obligation* and *moral duty* (for degree level studies, we see obligation and duty as equivalent). Such theories can be referred to as *obligation-based (OB) moral theories*. Ethicists who believe in OB theories hold that *living an ethical life* is fundamentally concerned with *abiding by a life of obligation and duty*. Obligations are exerted on us by various external sources, for instance legal obligations are drawn from the law and professional obligations arise from professional bodies such as the NMC and can be found in the NMC Code (2015). Moral obligations are exerted on us from ethicists, cultural and religious values and norms, and both formal and non-formal sources of moral education, such as parents, school teachers, peers, friends and university tutors.

Now that we have considered the underpinning philosophy and theory of ethics, albeit briefly, we will turn to how we apply ethical principles to our practice. We will consider the theory and apply it to 'Anna', a young woman with anorexia in a specialist eating **disorder** unit (SEDU).

THE FOUR PRINCIPLES APPROACH TO NURSING ETHICS

Beauchamp and Childress (2013) conceived a principle-based moral framework known as the 'four principles' approach. It sets forth four moral principles: Respect for autonomy, Beneficence, Non-Maleficence and Justice, which nurses can use to aid their moral thinking. This is an influential principle-based moral framework, which has become heavily influential in western ethical decision making and ethics education. We will consider these four principles, in turn, reflecting on their relevance for mental health nursing:

Respect for autonomy: autonomy, or 'self-determination', refers to the right to live one's own life and to make one's own decisions. 'Respect for autonomy' is the nurse's obligation to respect a patient's 'rights of autonomy'. Being 'autonomous' requires one to have the capacity to understand information and the risks and benefits of proposed treatment/care. As nurses, we have a responsibility to enable people to make informed choices and to have a degree of self-determination with regard to their **care plan**. In Case study 11.1, we consider 'Anna' (a pseudonym).

CASE STUDY 11.1

Anna

Anna is a voluntary patient in a specialist eating disorder unit (inpatient). At 5'2' (1.55m) and weighing only 70lbs (31.7kg) her BMI is 12.8. She is visibly emaciated. She is 18 years old and was diagnosed at age 16 as having anorexia nervosa after she collapsed following an audition for a dance academy. She disputes the diagnosis and attributes her collapse to exhaustion due to the intensive dance training, rehearsing and lack of sleep.

Anna agreed to her admission informally because her psychiatrist became so concerned about her that he discussed possible detention in hospital under mental health legislation. At that time, Anna's BMI was 11.2. She has been in hospital for three months; she is desperate to be discharged but fears she will be detained against her will if she attempts to leave. She does not want to eat the food put in front of her and rejects it at every mealtime. She wants to go home.

CRITICAL THINKING STOP POINT 11.1

- What would happen if we enabled Anna to be autonomous?
- What is in Anna's 'best interest'?

WHAT'S THE EVIDENCE? 11.1

Silber (2011) suggests that most hospitalised patients with *anorexia nervosa* receive some form of treatment against their will. Most ethical discussions on the topic focus on the conflict between respect for patients' autonomy and the wish to save lives (George, 1997; Vandereycken, 2006).

Nurses are thus accused of being 'paternalistic' when they become protective of patients whom they see as vulnerable. Paternalism is an institutional construction that overrules the preferences, decisions or actions of a patient in support of their overall treatment and evokes an oppressive fostering of dependence (Breier-Mackie, 2006; Christensen & Hewitt-Taylor, 2006).

Beneficence: the obligation to do good for patients and the obligation to promote patients' well-being. For example, if a patient has a headache, you are morally obliged to do something to benefit the patient. Like most ideas in ethics, the idea of 'doing good' is impossible to measure. It's also subjective and deeply personal (e.g. patient-centred care). As nurses, we care for patients; 'caring for' clearly involves doing some beneficent actions. Some distinctions can be drawn between 'caring for' someone (which suggests a duty-based motive, i.e. an obligation) and 'caring about' and also 'caring with', which both suggest a more mutual, values-based relationship, such as one based on compassion.

So, let's consider 'Anna' again. She does not come to the dining room herself, as some of the patients do. It always takes a nurse to go to her room and try to coax her into coming for her meal. Once at the table, she looks terrified; she takes only tiny mouthfuls and clearly cannot bear to have the food in her mouth. Staff will sit with her for 45 minutes, but usually end up giving her a meal replacement drink, which means another 45 minutes sitting with her and persuading her to drink it. Anna begs to be allowed to leave her food; she cries and screams at the nurse, who sits with her, that she is ruining her life.

CRITICAL THINKING STOP POINT 11.2

What can the nurse do that is beneficent and helps Anna to feel 'cared for' despite the difficulties she is experiencing in the dining room?

Non-maleficence:[1] the obligation to refrain from intentionally harming others and the obligation to prevent others from being harmed. The 'intentionally' is important – early in the history of medical ethics, circa 1900, this principle was understood to literally mean 'do not harm' and it is still today the cornerstone of medical ethics education found in the maxim (or rule) 'first, do no harm'. But, unfortunately, in Anna's case, she might suggest that we do cause degrees of harm in that she feels **anxiety**, turmoil, misery and distress as a result of the care she is provided with. So, one key aspect of this principle is that we weigh the foreseeable harms against the intended benefits. We should then aim to maximise the benefits and minimise the intentional harms. This is a 'stringent', perhaps almost impossible, principle to adhere to in some situations; it's one thing to minimise the intentional harms for your patient, but we are similarly obliged to do this for others too.

Clearly, there is a link between beneficence and non-maleficence and the actions that these two principles will motivate and require. 'Beneficence' is a positive moral obligation, i.e. acting beneficently requires one to take action to bring about benefits and goods.

'Non-maleficence' is a negative moral obligation, i.e. acting non-maleficently may mean doing nothing. For some, the principle of non-maleficence is seen to be morally weightier than beneficence – recall that the cornerstone of medical ethics education is the slogan 'first do no harm', not 'first, do good'.

---

[1] 'Non' = no; 'mal' = harm; literally – 'no harm'.

Justice: there are two types of justice to be considered here: distributive and retributive. In terms of distributive justice, how, morally speaking, should we distribute scarce health care resources? Distributive justice involves such important ethical issues as fairness, desert and entitlement. This is one of the main moral principles at work when there are inequalities in accessing health care.

One of the most notable resources, which often seems scarce, is time. How one nurse organises and manages her time: for example, at a simple level, how much time she spends with a patient; how teams of nurses do this, and how we all do this – are fundamentally moral questions concerning fairness, equality and equity.

Anna revisited: Anna has been given an additional 100 calories for her tea, as her 'meal plan' has been increasing slowly over the last week because she has gained a little weight. She has been offered a 'thick and creamy yoghurt' for her dessert and is aghast. She sees no justification for making her eat more. She has gained weight and now perceives this additional food to be unnecessary. There are nine patients in the dining room, all struggling to eat, all wishing that they could leave the room and hating the 'refeeding regime' that is part of their care plans. There are three members of staff. Anna has been crying loudly, she's been screaming at the nurses that it's unfair and has had her head on the table hitting the table top beside her. A nurse has been sat beside her comforting her and doing their best to de-escalate the situation. Jodie, a patient on the next table, is fed up. She gets up and tries to walk out, saying 'OK, so I have eaten my thick and creamy [expletive] yoghurt, so why is it that little Miss Anna gets all the [expletive] attention and I get less attention for complying!?'

CRITICAL THINKING STOP POINT 11.3

Is it fair and just that Anna gets more time and attention than Jodie?

DEONTOLOGY

The word 'deontology' is derived from the Greek 'deon', meaning duty. You will have heard the word 'duty' many times, as the NMC Code refers to the nurse's duty of care many times (NMC, 2015), thus nursing is frequently considered to be deontological. Deontological moral theories are act-centred theories that can be based on moral obligations, moral principles and moral rights.

Nurses experience a vast range of moral obligations, moral principles and moral rights, which tend to relate to different types of deontology, each type appealing to a different moral concept:

Example 1: Act x is right if it accords with veracity [the obligation to tell the truth].

Example 2: Act x is right if it accords with fairness [the moral principle].

Deontological moral theories appeal to 'morally important features' that occur at the same time as or before the act; therefore, deontological moral theories are characterised as 'backward looking'. Examples of 'morally important features' are: motives, intentions, divine commands and intuitions:

> Example 3: Act x is right if it's prescribed by a god [a divine command].

> Example 4: Act x is wrong because it disrespects the person's autonomous wishes [a moral right].

Deontological moral theories place great importance on the intrinsic nature of the act. That is, are some acts in and of themselves morally right? Are some acts in and of themselves morally wrong? For example, irrespective of the consequences, should a nurse lie to a patient? A famous deontological slogan is 'The end doesn't always justify the means'. In other words, good [bad] outcomes alone are not sufficient to make an act morally right [or wrong].

CONSEQUENTIALISM

Consequentialist moral theories are concerned with assessing the consequences/outcomes of actions and omissions (e.g. Pettit, 1991; Hooker, 2000). Broadly speaking, a typical consequentialist holds that an action/omission is morally right if it produces good consequences. For example:

1. It's morally right to feed Anna because this will produce a good outcome, i.e. it will promote her nutritional status and help to prevent malnutrition. Broadly speaking, a typical consequentialist holds that an action/omission is morally wrong if it produces bad consequences.
2. It's morally wrong not to feed Anna because this will produce a bad outcome, i.e. her nutritional status will deteriorate further and she will be malnourished.

Some consequentialists, for example Goodin (1991), argue that we should carry out the action that will produce better consequences than any other action.

Utilitarianism is a radical (extreme) form of a consequentialist theory (Goodin, 1991). A utilitarian holds that acting ethically is about maximising the best consequences for the majority of people. Two common slogans which relate to utilitarianism are:

1. 'the greatest happiness for the greatest number'; and
2. 'the end justifies the means'.

The merits of consequentialist theories are often seen to include the idea that they serve to promote the majority of people's interests, and such theories support some of our common-sense intuitions, for instance that pleasure ought to be maximised and pain minimised; and that the value of 1000 people's lives is more important than the value of one person's life. Moral intuitions form an important and common source of knowledge in many people's ethical decision making. Unlike their critical rejection in science, the important role played by moral intuitions isn't rejected in ethics simply because there is no empirical evidence to support them.

Classical utilitarianism argues that consequences are the only important thing in morality. Classical utilitarianism also argues that everyone's interests should be judged impartially – this criticism is known as the 'nearest and dearest objection'.

In our daily lives, we give considerable thought to the outcomes of our actions and this is also true in nursing. Specifically, in nursing, we think a lot about the outcomes of interventions, treatments and care. In nursing, we strive hard to promote patients' interests, and trying to promote someone's interests is an example of consequentialist thinking (e.g. DH, 2010; NMC, 2015).

The idea of best interest is an important idea in modern health care. Best interest, as an idea, is grounded in obligation ethics, specifically beneficence (Edwards, 2009). Striving hard to promote a patient's best interest is an important feature of consequentialism.

MORAL PROBLEMS AND DILEMMAS

Within nursing practice, there are many moral problems and moral dilemmas. Both moral problems and dilemmas arise from moral and ethical issues. Moral problems can be resolved, i.e. one morally 'correct' option is apparent – 'correct' meaning 'morally preferable' to all parties involved in the decision, such as patient, relatives, nurses, doctors. Ethicists talk about moral problems being 'resolvable' and they mean that each person's interests are promoted or respected or at least not overridden.

Let's consider this in relation to Jane. This was Jane's first episode of psychosis. She was working as a museum curator, a job she loved and was good at, she had her own home which she was renovating sympathetically according to its Victorian style and her future should have been bright. It wasn't too long before she was given the frightening diagnosis of 'schizophrenia' and, understandably, she was anxious to know how this was going to progress, what her chances of a full recovery were and, effectively, her 'prognosis'. Jane could not get a straight answer and ultimately concluded:

> One obvious reason why professionals find discussing prognosis difficult is because they simply don't know.

So, she sought to understand, but became even further baffled:

> It was 'I'm not ill ... I'm not ill' ad nauseam for years. I accept it now - just about. I don't know how nurses manage this one as it must unintentionally invalidate a lot of what they are trying to communicate. It must have been very discouraging and boring for Adam and then others to have to go round in circles endlessly trying to get me to accept I was ill while trying not to discourage me, or alarm me to the point of total withdrawal.

> But on the other hand reassurance never worked terribly well for me either, so it was a no win situation. I would then minimise my problems, feel guilty about not being well, thought it was something I was doing wrong and could overcome in some magical unspecified fashion combined with a good dose of willpower. Totally believing in people who announce you can overcome your mental illness by positive mental attitude, long walks and fish oil is probably not a good idea, and in fact some of them get so much airtime they can actually be rather dangerous. For me it was a pointless endeavour anyway, but there's still misguided hopefulness within me that somehow, one day ... The end result was a sense of failure and despair, and the cycle of self-hatred, and desire to hurt and punish myself by not taking medication repeated itself over and over again.

CRITICAL THINKING STOP POINT 11.4

- Think about this using a deontological approach: do we have a duty, as nurses, to tell the truth, to be candid and honest?
- Think about this using a utilitarian approach: could we have done something to prevent Jane from feeling such a sense of failure and despair? For example, would telling her that medication was the only way forward have prevented her subsequent misery?
- How do we promote a person's autonomy in a situation like this? Jane wanted to be self-determining, but this included avoiding the medication that could have made a difference to her symptoms, but also had unwanted side-effects.

The deliberation of such situations always involves a careful consideration of many different kinds of knowledge, such as empirical and moral. It includes an assessment of one's moral values and beliefs. When one 'deliberates', one hopes to reach a decision; deliberation is therefore an example of problem solving. Professional codes such as the NMC (2015) can oversimplify moral requirements, i.e. the moral dilemma is not 'solved' by 'applying' the Code. Professional codes, such as the NMC, are grounded in shared values and are based on firm moral and professional rules.

Issues of morality and ethics become profoundly important when reflecting upon recent service failings, such as the Mid Staffordshire Hospital and Winterbourne View scandals. Roberts and Ion (2014) pose the legitimate question, how can nurses find themselves caught up in such palpable anomalies of practice? They refer to the writings of Hannah Arendt who considered the similar question of how did ordinary German citizens become accommodated to the horrors of Nazism? For, Arendt, the answers to such questions recognised evil as banal, with people fairly quickly becoming habituated to a new order of things. In the health care context, this behoves nurses to be continually vigilant to changes of circumstances that default to a 'new normal' way of working, if this is to the detriment of care.

CRITICAL DEBATE 11.1

Kant argued that 'we have no obligation to sacrifice our true needs, those satisfactions which are essential to our happiness, in order to promote the well-being of others' (Gregor, 1963: 105).

Kant's theory is an example of a deontological moral theory, which, as we have seen, does not concern itself with the rightness or wrongness of actions, nor with their consequences, but on whether or not they fulfil our duty.

Many of the tasks of mental health nursing care are unpleasant, but we do them because we believe that it will be for the benefit of others. We also have a profound 'duty of care' which drives us to provide interventions, even when it is difficult for us to do so. Examples of this include applying restraint to a psychotic and violent person who would otherwise harm themselves or others, or coaxing a distressed woman with anorexia to eat despite her sobs and obvious discomfort.

Hence, does the above statement not conflict with the nurses' moral duty to conduct the interventions mentioned here?

CONCLUSION

This chapter has attempted to provide a whistle-stop tour of some of the underpinning theory and philosophy which are foundational to values-based practice. Ultimately, we hope that you have gained an understanding of how our ethical frameworks and code of conduct were developed. Fundamentally, we hope that gaining **insight** into what is 'right', 'good' and 'just' will assist you to make good decisions which are in the best interest of those you care for, and yourselves.

'Educating the mind without educating the heart is no education at all.' (Aristotle)

CHAPTER SUMMARY

After reading this chapter, you should:

*   Know what are ethics and what are values
*   Recognise the utility of constructing an ethical argument for practice, especially if there is a dilemma about what to do for the best
*   Understand how ethics relate to 'values-based' mental health practice, and how this relates to the NMC Code
*   Be able to provide an ethical rationale for a decision.

BUILD YOUR BIBLIOGRAPHY

Books

*   Barker, P. (ed.) (2011) *Mental health ethics*. Abingdon, Oxon: Routledge. This book provides an overview of traditional and contemporary ethical perspectives in an accessible way.
*   Beauchamp, T.L. & Childress, J.F. (2013) *Principles of biomedical ethics*, 7th edition. Oxford: Oxford University Press. You cannot study ethics without hearing about Beauchamp & Childress, which has become the 'go to' book for medical ethics.
*   Edwards, S.D. (2009) *Nursing ethics: A principle based approach*, 2nd edition. Basingstoke: Palgrave Macmillan. This book is a concise text that seems disproportionately inclusive for its size.
*   Singer, P. (ed.) (1994) *Ethics*. Oxford: Oxford University Press.

SAGE journal articles

Go to https://study.sagepub.com/essentialmentalhealth for further free online journal articles related to this chapter. If you are using the interactive ebook, simply click on the book icon in the margin to go straight to the resource.

FURTHER READING: JOURNAL ARTICLES

*   Abma, T. & Widdershoven, G. (2006) Moral deliberation in psychiatric nursing practice. *Nursing Ethics*, 13(5), 546-557.
*   Granerud, A. & Severinsson, E. (2003) Preserving integrity: experiences of people with mental health problems living in their own home in a new neighbourhood. *Nursing Ethics*, 10(6), 602-613.
*   Moe, C., Kvig, E.I., Brinchmann, B., et al. (2013) 'Working behind the scenes': an ethical view of mental health nursing and first-episode psychosis. *Nursing Ethics*, 20(5), 517-527.

Weblinks

Go to https://study.sagepub.com/essentialmentalhealth for further weblinks related to this chapter. If you are using the interactive ebook, simply click on the book icon in the margin to go straight to the resource.

FURTHER READING: WEBLINKS

*   Mental Health Law Online: www.mentalhealthlaw.co.uk - an internet resource on mental health law and mental capacity law for England and Wales.

- Nursing and Midwifery Council: www.nmc.org.uk
- The Royal College of Psychiatrists (2014) CR186. Good Psychiatric Practice: Code of Ethics: www.rcpsych.ac.uk/usefulresources/publications/collegereports/cr/cr186.aspx

GREAT FOR
REVISION!

ONLINE
QUIZZES &
ACTIVITY
ANSWERS

——————— ACE YOUR ASSESSMENT ———————

Revise what you have learned by visiting https://study.sagepub.com/essentialmentalhealth. If you are using the interactive ebook, simply click on the tick icon to go straight to the resource.

- Test yourself with multiple-choice and short-answer questions and flashcards.

REFERENCES

Allmark, P. (1992) The ethical enterprise of nursing. *Journal of Advanced Nursing, 17*(1), 16–20.

Armstrong, A.E. (2006) Towards a strong virtue ethics for nursing practice. *Nursing Philosophy, 7*(3), 110–124.

Armstrong, A.E. (2007) *Nursing ethics: A virtue-based approach.* Basingstoke: Palgrave Macmillan.

Barker, P. (ed.) (2011) *Mental health ethics.* Abingdon, Oxon: Routledge.

Beauchamp, T.L. & Childress, J.F. (2013) *Principles of biomedical ethics,* 7th edition. Oxford: Oxford University Press.

Breier-Mackie, S. (2006) Medical ethics and nursing ethics: is there really any difference? *Gastroenterology Nursing, 29*(2), 182–183.

Christensen, M. & Hewitt-Taylor, J. (2006) Modern nursing: empowerment in nursing – paternalism or maternalism? *British Journal of Nursing, 15*(13), 695–699.

Department of Health (DH) (2010) *Essence of care.* London: DH.

Edwards, S.D. (2009) *Nursing ethics: A principle-based approach.* Basingstoke & New York: Palgrave Macmillan.

Galeza, D. (2014) Dworkin's argument on abortion. *The King's Student Law Review, 5*(2), 33–51.

George, L. (1997) The psychological characteristics of patients suffering from anorexia nervosa and the nurse's role in creating a therapeutic relationship. *Journal of Advanced Nursing, 26,* 899–908.

Goodin, R. (1991) Utility and the good. In P. Singer (ed.) *A companion to ethics.* Cambridge: Blackwell.

Gregor, M.J. (1963) *Laws of freedom.* New York: Barnes and Noble.

Hanssen, I. & Alpers, L. (2010) Utilitarian and common-sense morality discussions in intercultural nursing practice. *Nursing Ethics, 17*(2).

Hooker, B. (2000) *Ideal code, real world: A rule-consequentialist theory of morality.* Oxford & New York: Clarendon Press/Oxford University Press.

Nursing and Midwifery Council (NMC) (2015) *The code: Standards of conduct, performance, and ethics for nurses and midwives.* London: NMC.

Pettit, P. (1991) Consequentialism. In P. Singer (ed.) *A companion to ethics.* Cambridge: Blackwell.

Roberts, M. & Ion, R. (2014) A critical consideration of systemic moral catastrophe in modern health care systems: a big idea from an Arendtian perspective. *Nurse Education Today, 34*(5), 673–675.

Settelmaier, E. & Nigam, M. (2007) *Where did you get your values and beliefs?* In J. Hawley (ed.) *Ethics in clinical practice: An interprofessional approach.* Edinburgh: Pearson Education.

Silber, T.J. (2011) Treatment of anorexia nervosa against the patient's will: ethical considerations. *Adolescent Medicine: State of the Art Reviews, 22*(2), 283–288.

Singer, P. (ed.) (1994) *Ethics.* Oxford: Oxford University Press.

Vandereycken, W. (2006) Dealing with denial in anorexia nervosa. *Eating Disorders Review, 17*(6), 1–4.

Yeo, M., Moorhouse, A., Kahn P. & Rodney, P. (eds) (2010) *Concepts and cases in nursing ethics,* 3rd edition. Peterborough, ON: Broadview Press.

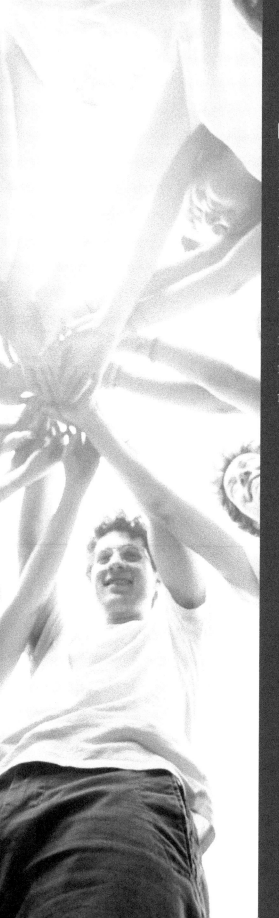

PSYCHIATRIC UNDERSTANDINGS OF MENTAL HEALTH

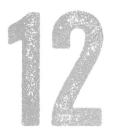

DUNCAN DOUBLE

THIS CHAPTER COVERS

- The concept that mental health work is interdisciplinary and not just medical.
- The controversy about whether mental health problems should be understood as 'illness'.
- The differences between psychiatry and the rest of medicine.
- The belief that psychiatrists, like other mental health practitioners, need to be patient-centred in practice.
- Evidence that the effectiveness of psychiatric treatments is biased.

"

The orthodox medical approach to the problem of interpreting and treating mental disorders regards mental illness as brain disease. Psychiatrists find it difficult to give up this belief. Challenges to this orthodoxy have been dismissed as 'anti-psychiatry' and seen as disreputable. I have directly experienced this through being seen as an anti-psychiatrist myself. I was suspended for six months by my NHS Trust from October 2000.

Following investigation, I was told I needed retraining and would be sent for further education in organic psychiatry. It was indicated that my philosophy about psychiatry may need to be examined and my scepticism about the use of medication challenged.

None of these things happened and I am still practicing as an NHS psychiatrist seventeen years later! I am not an anti-psychiatrist. However, I think the view that one adopts about the nature of mental illness does matter. Most psychiatrists are pragmatic and look at psychosocial as well as biological aspects when assessing a patient. They don't necessarily just focus on medication in treatment. I do not want to polarise debate in the mental health field.

Duncan Double, psychiatrist (2004)

"

Looking back on my psychiatric 'career', the things that made the most difference were being listened to and treated as an individual with hopes and fears. Yet this rarely happened in the turmoil of repeated detentions, forced treatment and oppressive observation. There was kindness but infused with an expectation that you would comply. Disagreement was seen as a lack of insight or denial. If you did something 'bad' like running away, taking an overdose, refusing medication, you were scolded, even 'punished' – leave cancelled, special observations imposed, extra medication given. At times I did need to be kept safe but what I wanted more than anything was to control my own destiny, and for mental health professionals to support me in this. Rarely did anyone say 'why is this happening?' or 'what can we do differently?'

In any walk of life uncertainty about change and difference tends to translate into a bias – often unrecognised – that maintains the status quo. Mental health practitioners who speak up about concerns or voice alternative views on mental health issues can face ridicule, exclusion, even disciplinary action and referral to professional regulators. Yet we need people to question, listen, and reflect if we are to change the culture of mental health services to one based on respectful relationships and open dialogue. Given the imbalance of power that still characterises mental health services, we need people working in them, including those in leadership positions, to find the strength and humility to make this a reality.

Kay Sheldon, former non-executive director of the Care Quality Commission

INTRODUCTION

You do not need to worry that this chapter will mislead you about psychiatric understandings of mental health. Although it may be written from an uncommon psychiatric perspective, most psychiatrists would not object to any of its content. It is a legitimate way of understanding mental **illness** and its treatment from a psychiatric point of view. It has been written to help you appreciate the perspective of psychiatrists as a mental health nurse. Psychiatry is a branch of medicine. Some may see this statement as a truism. Why would there be any reason to question it? After all, patients present to doctors with psychological symptoms and also with physical symptoms that may have a psychological origin. People may express concern to doctors about the mental state of patients. If a patient requires detention under mental health legislation, the support of two medical recommendations is required. How can mental health work not involve doctors?

Yet mental health work is an interdisciplinary activity and other professionals besides doctors combine to provide a service. Much of professional work requires mere common sense and is generic, not specifically requiring any medical or other disciplinary expertise. Doctors do not have a monopoly on mental health assessment and treatment. They train and qualify as doctors before specialising in psychiatry, but other disciplines, such as nursing, also provide the opportunity to specialise in the mental health field.

Also, psychiatric practice is controversial. For example, Peter Kinderman (2014) has argued that mental health care should actually be non-medical, as it is not treating 'illness' as we understand it. From his point of view, doctors should concentrate on the biological aspects of mental health care and this should be seen as a minority activity within the field as most psychiatric presentations are psychosocial, not biomedical, in origin. By contrast, Peter Sedgwick (1982) would have regarded Kinderman's position as 'psycho-medical dualism' because psychosocial approaches should not be separated too much from medicine. Sedgwick adopted a unitary concept of illness, beneath which are subsumed both physical and mental aspects (Cresswell & Spandler, 2009). Conceptual conflict exists about the nature of mental illness and this is as much of an issue for psychiatrists as it is for specialists from other disciplines.

Even if we accept that psychiatry is a medical specialty, there are some differences between psychiatry and the rest of medicine. The 19th century saw the development of the anatomoclinical method in medicine, linking clinical signs with physical pathology. This approach produced remarkable progress in medicine in general and we now try to explain physical illness as caused by its pathology. Its success with psychiatry was more limited. Essentially, what it amounted to was the recognition that **dementia** paralytica was a late consequence of syphilis; that senile dementia had a physical cause such as Alzheimer's **disease**; that there could be focal abnormalities in the brain; and that learning disability could also have physical causes. However, most psychopathology is functional, in the sense that there are no structural abnormalities in the brain (Double, 2006).

Furthermore, psychiatric practice should be patient-centred, like other mental health work, rather than focus too much on brain abnormalities. From this perspective, psychiatric assessment explores patients' main reasons for consultation, their concerns and their need for information (Stewart et al., 2003). It seeks an integrated, holistic understanding of the person, including emotional needs and life issues. Proper psychiatric treatment finds common ground with patients about what the problem is and mutual agreement on how to manage problems.

Modern psychiatry has its origins in the state provision of asylums in the 19th century. Outpatient psychiatry and community care developed in the 20th century, making the traditional asylum increasingly irrelevant. Of course, some patients still need inpatient treatment, including assessment and treatment under **mental health law**. Psychiatry has always tended to assume that mental illness is a brain **disorder**, with an emphasis on physical treatment. Historically, this has led to examples of overzealous physical treatment (Double, 2011; also see Case Study 12.1). This situation arises because of a bias towards overestimating the effectiveness of psychiatric treatment, including medication, and this state of affairs persists in modern practice. This chapter, instead, takes a critical look at the integration of mind and brain, acknowledging the limitations of **psychotropic medication** in particular. The primary focus of mental health work, including psychiatry, should be on understanding the patient as a person.

In this chapter, you are going to learn about psychiatry as a medical specialty. All disciplinary contributions, including nursing, should be democratically valued in mental health work and the psychiatric perspective should not necessarily be dominant. You will appreciate that mental health practice needs to have an integrated conceptual understanding of mind and brain. You will also understand that physical symptoms can have a psychological origin. In other words, complete psychosomatic understanding is important for all mental health practitioners, including nurses. Such understanding is also particularly vital for doctors who are not always as good as they should be at identifying the psychological origins of patients' symptoms. This situation will be demonstrated with some examples.

CRITICAL THINKING STOP POINT 12.1

Do you think mental illness is a brain disease?

Mental health nurses do not need to be philosophers but they do need to appreciate that there is a problem with the relationship between mind and brain. Think about whether your thoughts, feelings and behaviour are due to your brain. Why should these biological processes be any different, or not, for someone seen as mentally ill?

CHECK YOUR ANSWERS

CRITICAL THINKING STOP POINT 12.1 ANSWER

CASE STUDY 12.1

Flawed pioneer of biological psychiatry

Bayard Taylor Holmes (1852–1924) was a Chicago physician and surgeon, whose son was diagnosed with dementia praecox aged 17. Holmes was devastated by his son's illness and vowed to use his scientific expertise to find a cause and cure for dementia praecox (the precursor name for schizophrenia).

He came to believe that caecal stasis led to the production of ergot-like toxic amines that poisoned many organs in the body, including the brain, leading to dementia praecox (Noll, 2011). The solution was appendicostomy or caecostomy and daily irrigations of the caecum. This theory was congruent with popular theories of autointoxication at the time. For example, Emil Kraepelin, the originator of the concept of dementia praecox, speculated that the sex glands were the source of toxins that poisoned the brain in dementia praecox. In fact, Kraepelin was unusual in blaming the sex glands rather than the intestines for autointoxication.

The first patient Holmes operated on was his son, but unfortunately he died four days later. This didn't stop him and colleagues operating on a further 21 patients. Only one other patient died from complications of his surgery. This story needs to be set in the context of Andrew Scull's (2005) book about Henry Cotton, who operated on 645 patients by removing what he considered to be hidden infections in various parts of the body, particularly teeth and tonsils; 25–30% of Cotton's patients died, particularly from colectomy.

THE PATIENT PERSPECTIVE ON MENTAL HEALTH PRACTICE

Gail Hornstein (2011) has collated a bibliography of first-person narratives of madness in English. Patients have always written about their experiences of mental illness and their **recovery** from it. Some see themselves as **survivors** of the psychiatric system, because treatment can become abusive and may have been imposed on them against their will. Hornstein's (2009) book, *Agnes's Jacket*, tells the story of the seamstress Agnes Richter, who, in a Victorian-era German asylum, stitched a mysterious autobiographical text into every inch of the jacket created from her institutional uniform. The book provides a critical analysis of the madness narrative genre. Mental illness may often be more understandable than the biomedical explanations given by psychiatry.

The first section of Hornstein's bibliography lists personal accounts of madness by survivors themselves. Many of these accounts were written some time ago, and not just by people in the modern **service user** movement in psychiatry, which has developed since the 1970s (Crossley, 2006). There were precursors, such as the mental hygiene movement. The concept of 'mental hygiene' can be difficult to understand because of the way the term 'hygiene' is associated with cleanliness. However, the meaning refers to the conditions and practices that help to maintain mental health, and these days we use the term 'mental health' in much the same sense as 'mental hygiene'. Adolf Meyer, Professor of Psychiatry at Johns Hopkins University at the beginning of the 20th century, originally suggested the term to Clifford Beers, when Beers went to discuss his autobiography *A mind that found itself* (1908). In this book, Beers described his mistreatment by staff in a psychiatric hospital, including physical abuse and degrading treatment for his manic-depressive illness from which he eventually recovered. He acknowledged the seriousness of his condition, as well as highlighting the brutal practices that may have hindered his recovery. The philosopher and psychologist, William James, encouraged Beers to publish his book.

> Having at last got round to your MS, I have read it with very great interest and admiration for both its style and its temper. I hope you will finish it and publish it. It is the best written out case that I have seen; and you no doubt have put your finger on the weak spots of our treatment of the insane, and suggested the right line of remedy...
>
> You were doubtless a pretty intolerable character when the maniacal condition came on you and you were bossing the universe. Not only ordinary tact, but a genius for diplomacy must have been needed for avoiding rows with you; but you were certainly wrongly treated nonetheless: and the spiteful Assistant M.D. at ____ deserves to have his name published. Your report is full of instructiveness for doctors and attendants alike.
>
> (Letter from William James to Clifford Beers about the manuscript *A Mind that Found Itself*)

Beers wanted to campaign for psychiatric reform and in May 1908 organised a meeting to set up the Connecticut Society for Mental Hygiene. Beers became secretary in the USA of the National Committee for Mental Hygiene, a voluntary agency for which he raised millions of dollars. The International Committee for Mental Hygiene was formed in 1919 and its name was changed in 1947 to the World Federation for Mental Health, an organisation that still exists today. Beers had to work closely with establishment psychiatrists, perhaps preventing the mental hygiene movement becoming the user movement, as we understand it today.

Failings in the mental health system are not only in the past. For example, Diana Rose spent most of 1999 in **acute** psychiatric care. She described the story of that year in an article in *OpenMind* (2000). What she portrayed is the 'sharp end' of psychiatry: control and restraint, forced injections, ECT, close observations and seclusion. Nurses are particularly involved in this aspect of psychiatric practice in inpatient wards.

The point Rose makes in the article is primarily about communication. For example, she explained what it was like relating to nurses in the secure unit of the hospital. Their main task seemed to be recording 30-minute checks of the whereabouts of patients. Rose says there was little personal interaction. The atmosphere was not much better on the acute ward, where she says she only got attention if she caused trouble. As she improved towards discharge, she was bored and care seemed bureaucratic and negative.

Rose does not mean to imply that the staff were terrible people. However, in their role as nurses they seemed 'too busy' to be helpful. Communication between fellow patients often seemed better than that between patients and staff. Her conclusion was that the **culture** of psychiatry has to change so that people are not treated as 'cases' or instances of categories, but as people with hopes, fears and aspirations.

CRITICAL THINKING STOP POINT 12.2

Is your practice as a nurse ethical?

Thinking about the above section on the patient perspective, would you describe your practice as a nurse as ethical? If so, think of some examples where you have put this into practice. If not, think about what some of the hindrances to proper ethical practice have been.

CRITICAL
THINKING
STOP
POINT 12.2
ANSWER

PSYCHIATRIC PERSPECTIVES ON MENTAL HEALTH PRACTICE

Psychiatrists have become concerned over recent years that their role may be taken over by other non-medical professionals. There was a policy called New Ways of Working (Department of Health, 2007) that encouraged all **multi-disciplinary team** members to focus on their skills rather than their status. It was recognised that expertise within the team may well mean that consultation with a psychiatrist is not always needed. This policy led to a reaction for a remedicalised psychiatry (Harrison et al., 2012), which suggested psychiatrists should focus on 'what doctors do best' and practise a brain-based medicine of the mind. There were problems with New Ways of Working and policy has now moved on to promote professional expertise (Department of Health, 2010). This should operate in partnership with patient expertise. However, the policy never justified the implication that psychiatry should be unconcerned about psychosocial factors. In fact, the personal dimension is the primary element of mental health practice (Bracken et al., 2012).

We should welcome other professionals taking on consultant roles, including being **responsible clinicians** under the Mental Health Act in England and Wales. However limited in practice this development has been so far, it is happening in other areas of medicine besides psychiatry. It offers more choice to a patient to be able to see a consultant from another profession, such as nursing or clinical psychology. Other professions should be encouraged to take on the responsibility that has traditionally been undertaken by the doctor. This includes non-medical prescribing. Non-medical professionals have always had a central role in managing patients in hospital. This continues to be the case with care coordination in the community.

None of this discussion means that medical training is not of **value** for psychiatry. This is because many physical complaints have a psychogenic origin and a medical training should allow doctors to place such cases in perspective. In fact, as argued by Fulford (1989), psychiatry could be seen as the pre-eminent medical speciality because practice is so obviously determined by values. This may be more hidden in the rest of medicine but a focus on the patient as person is inevitably central. Psychosomatic presentations are so common that they are essential to medical practice, so psychiatry should be seen as a proper form of medical practice. In Germany, for example, psychosomatic medicine has developed as a separate specialty. There may not be too much advantage much of the time in having a medical training for most mental health work, but at least psychiatrists should understand mental health problems in their overall medical context.

MEDICALLY UNEXPLAINED SYMPTOMS

These days, the term 'medically unexplained symptoms' tends to be used as a label for symptoms for which doctors cannot find a physical cause. Its meaning is little different from similar terms used previously, such as functional, hysterical, psychosomatic and somatoform disorders. Doctors, perhaps particularly in general practice, are confronted with a diverse range of symptoms that do not necessarily conform to neat textbook descriptions of physical diagnoses. General practitioners (GPs) operate in a clinical setting of low actual disease prevalence and deal with a high incidence of non-specific symptoms. It has been estimated that as many as 70–90% of general practice presentations are without serious physical disorder (Barsky, 1981). Medically unexplained symptoms are also common in secondary hospital care. About 50% of patients meet such criteria across a range of outpatient clinics, with medically unexplained symptoms being the most common diagnosis in some specialities (Nimnuan et al., 2001). Physical disease is overdiagnosed and psychogenic symptoms are commonly over-investigated by doctors to exclude a physical cause.

Psychiatric disorders are also under-recognised in general practice and medical practice in general. Research suggests that GPs fail to diagnose up to half of cases of **depression** or **anxiety** on initial presentation (Goldberg & Huxley, 1992). Over the longer term, this figure may not be as high or as clinically important as this initial impression may suggest. Some depressed patients are given a diagnosis at subsequent consultations or recover without a GP's diagnosis. However, there is still a significant minority of patients (14% in this study) with a diagnosis of persistent depression that is undetected (Kessler et al., 2002). The failure of detection of depression is commonly presumed to arise because of a lack of psychological mindedness amongst doctors. In general, doctors value objective evidence of disease more than subjective experience. This tendency creates a bias towards the over-diagnosis of physical disease.

More or less any physical symptom can be mimicked by psychiatric disorder. For example, non-cardiac chest pain is very common and often chronic (Bass & Mayou, 2002). Patients who perceive themselves to be at risk of ischaemic heart disease, maybe because of a family history, are particularly vulnerable. Such pain is usually mild and transient but, in some cases, symptoms continue and are disabling.

Doctors need to undertake a full history and examination to differentiate cardiac from non-cardiac pain. The cardinal symptom of cardiac ischaemia is the pain known as angina pectoris. Characteristically, it is a tight sensation in the centre of the chest, provoked by exertion and lasting only a few minutes. The chance of pain being cardiac in origin is very low if going uphill does not cause pain, and the pain occurs commonly at rest and lasts longer than 5 minutes.

Patients presenting to doctors with non-cardiac emotional pain do not generally show conspicuous signs of anxiety or depression. Distressing events, perhaps particularly those signifying loss, threat and rejection, may precipitate the symptoms. Explanation and treatment of the psychological problems may be beneficial.

CASE STUDY 12.2

Effort syndrome

Psychological trauma casualties of the Second World War who complained of breathlessness, palpitations, chest pain, giddiness, fainting attacks and fatigue, with their symptoms in the main related to exercise, were recognised as having effort syndrome. Most patients thought they had heart disease. Maxwell Jones, a psychiatrist, was part of a team from the Maudsley Hospital in London that went to Mill Hill Emergency Hospital in 1942. An effort syndrome unit was set up under the joint directorship of Jones and a cardiologist. The emphasis lay in the application of sociological and psychological concepts to treatment. As the understanding of individual symptoms developed, it became clear that effort syndrome was a psychosomatic complaint. Information was given to patients in a discussion format about the physiological mechanisms involved in the production of symptoms. The educational approach was found to affect the patients' attitude to their symptoms, even if the symptoms did not necessarily disappear. Patients began using the discussion groups to raise problems bearing on ward life. This was one of the origins of the therapeutic community in psychiatry.

As another example, one of the commonest gastrointestinal disorders is bowel habit disturbed by diarrhoea or constipation occurring alone, or alternating, associated with abdominal pain for which no organic cause can be found. This presentation is commonly diagnosed as irritable bowel **syndrome** (IBS) (Ford & Talley, 2012). Other symptoms such as the relief of pain or discomfort by defecation, or abdominal bloating, are considered supportive of the diagnosis. The syndrome occurs more commonly in women, usually between the ages of 20 and 40 years. Patients may appear anxious but otherwise generally seem well. Psychological disorder is more common in patients with IBS than those without IBS.

Again, doctors need to undertake a full history and examination of the patient to make the diagnosis, which should be reached using symptom-based clinical criteria, rather than excluding underlying organic disease by exhaustive investigation. Longitudinal follow-up in patients with a positive diagnosis of IBS suggests that the development of subsequent organic disease is rare. Diagnostic testing should be reserved for those with lower gastrointestinal alarm symptoms, such as those developing symptoms for the first time over the age of 50 years, or those with weight loss, rectal bleeding or an abdominal mass.

Reassurance may be beneficial, especially as there is sometimes an underlying fear of cancer. In fact, an effective and empathetic doctor–patient relationship has been found to be associated with increased patient satisfaction and reduced consultations. Dietary changes, including increased roughage, may help. Antispasmodic medication has been found to be more effective than placebo in treating symptoms.

WHAT'S THE EVIDENCE? 12.1

Resources for patients with irritable bowel syndrome

WEBLINK: NHS IBS

WEBLINK: IBS NETWORK

The NHS Choices website has a webpage on irritable bowel syndrome (www.nhs.uk/conditions/irritable-bowel-syndrome/pages/introduction.aspx) which provides information and gives some real-life examples. One patient, Geoff Lyon, shares his story of severe IBS since early childhood (www.nursingtimes.net/clinical-archive/gastroenterology/irritable-bowel-syndrome/1994694.article). He runs a self-help group for the IBS Network (www.theibsnetwork.org), which is the national charity for irritable bowel syndrome.

MIND-BRAIN INTEGRATION

CHALLENGING CONCEPTS 12.1

Is mental illness a brain disease?

- Minds are enabled by but not reducible to brains.
- Science can include the study of the person.
- Psychiatry can be practised without taking the step of faith of believing that mental illness is due to a brain abnormality.
- Mental illness shows *through* the brain but not necessarily *in* the brain.
- Psychiatric diagnosis is not about finding an entity of some kind, but about providing understanding.

Philosophers have always grappled with the mind–brain problem. Mental states, such as our thoughts, feelings and actions, are non-physical. The question is how these relate to our brain, which is a physical entity. Of course, the brain is the origin of **cognition**, **affect** and behaviour. But minds are enabled by and not reducible to brains. Mental health practitioners don't need to be philosophers but they do need to realise that there is an issue in this respect.

Related to this issue, brain-based study is seen as scientific. Should the study of human nature also be seen as scientific? Mental health practitioners need to recognise that there is an issue about the breadth of definition of science. The wider definition is not just physics and chemistry, nor even the use of experimental techniques. It is about the application of rigour to observing, documenting, comparing and ordering data. As far as psychiatry is concerned, science can either be seen as including the study of the person or restricted to neuroscience as the only scientific method and solution.

Adopting the position of mind–brain integration is different from seeing the brain as the cause of mental illness. There may be apparent advantages in taking the latter position. The difficulty of dealing with the uncertainty of human action may seem to be avoided. Dealing with disturbed people is not easy. The temptation is to retreat into an objectification of those identified as mentally ill by focusing on their brain abnormalities.

I don't want to be misunderstood. Of course, I'm not saying that mental illness has nothing to do with the brain. In fact, it's a tautology to say that mental illness is due to the brain. The thoughts, feelings and behaviour of people who are not mentally ill are due to their brain. We have an integrated understanding of their mental and brain activities. In the same way, we should have an integrated understanding of the mental and brain activities of people who are mentally ill. Mental illness must show through the brain but may not necessarily be present in the form of an abnormality in the brain.

Not all psychiatrists take the step of faith of believing that mental illness is due to a brain abnormality. There has always been a minority view that takes more of a sociopsychobiological rather than a biomedical point of view. This has implications for both diagnosis and treatment.

Psychiatric diagnosis needs to be recognised for what it is. In the words of Eleanor Longden (2013), 'The important question in psychiatry isn't "what's wrong with you?" but "what happened to you?"' A single-word psychiatric diagnosis will be unreliable, even using operational criteria, because of the meaningful nature of psychiatric assessment. Psychiatric diagnosis is not about finding an entity of some kind, but about providing understanding. We should not be surprised that the wishful aspirations of DSM-5 to include the genetic markers and pathognomic neurobiological findings of **mental disorders** have failed.

LIMITATIONS OF PSYCHIATRIC TREATMENT

We also need to be more sceptical about treatments, such as medication. The use of medication, including psychotropic medication, in society is ubiquitous. Some people come to a consultation with a doctor seeking medication for their mental health problems, although not all consultations with doctors seem necessarily to be motivated by the aim of acquiring a prescription (Little et al., 2001). Nonetheless, the placebo effect may be powerful. Countless ailments throughout history have seemingly been relieved by medicines and other medical interventions because sufferers and their doctors have believed in them.

Discontinuation problems from medication are very common, if only because of what medication may come to mean to people. Adopting the view that one suffers from a biochemically based emotional illness is an identity-altering view of reality. People, therefore, may form attachments to their medications more because of what they mean to them than what they actually do. Any change threatens an equilibrium related to a complex set of meanings that their medications may have acquired. It is, therefore, not surprising that there may be a negative placebo, or nocebo, effect from stopping medication.

Randomised clinical trials (RCTs) were introduced to try and eliminate expectancy effects. However, there are still methodological problems with RCTs, not just because of poor quality research. The most methodically rigorous trials are associated with less treatment benefit than poor quality trials (Jüni et al., 2001). Conclusions in trials may be affected by idiosyncratic factors, such as whether they are funded by for-profit organisations, commonly drug companies, making the results more positive because of a biased interpretation of trial data (Als-Nielsen et al., 2003).

Results of RCTs are not always as clear-cut as may be assumed. For example, antidepressants are not always effective and there is a considerable placebo response, making the difference between active and placebo treatment in clinical trials much smaller than most people realise (Kirsch, 2009). In fact, one third of the published RCTs of approved antidepressants are negative for efficacy (Thase, 1999).

Even the best quality trials may still not completely eliminate bias. In particular, they are not as double-blind as is commonly assumed. Trials need to be double-blind, meaning that both patients and assessors are unaware of whether they are receiving active or placebo treatment, because otherwise expectations can affect the outcome. If not blinded, any improvement may merely be due to the placebo effect.

There is evidence from short-term antidepressant trials that blindness can be breached. When patients are asked whether they have been put onto a placebo or an active antidepressant, it is found that they can guess correctly better than would be predicted by chance (Even et al., 2000). Patients and doctors may be cued in to whether patients are taking active or placebo medication by a variety of means. Patients in clinical trials are naturally curious to ascertain whether they are in the active or the placebo group, and may, for example, notice that the placebo tablets they have been taking taste different from medication to which they have previously become accustomed. Active medication may produce side-effects that distinguish it from inert medication.

The degree to which patients are unblinded can be correlated with an apparent antidepressant effect. In other words, unblinding is significant and means that any positive result could be due to the placebo effect. Statistically positive results in some trials may, therefore, merely be the consequence of an amplified placebo effect made apparent because of unblinding. The problem is that the results of 'double-blind' studies tend to be automatically accepted as scientifically valid. A misleading self-deception is encouraged that trials can be conducted completely double-blind and the role of expectancies is thereby underestimated.

WHAT'S THE EVIDENCE? 12.2

Are antidepressants effective?

- Statistically significant results are found in most randomised controlled trials of antidepressants, but not all.
- The difference in outcome, on average, in clinical trials between active and placebo treatment is much smaller than generally realised.
- A good proportion of patients are not helped by antidepressants, even in the clinical trials.
- Patients are able to break the blind in clinical trials which means that expectancy effects are not completely eliminated.
- It is possible that the found statistically significant difference is due to placebo amplification because of unblinding (see blog post by Irving Kirsch at www.huffingtonpost.com/irving-kirsch-phd/antidepressants-the-emper_b_442205.html).

WEBLINK:
IRVING KIRSCH

Patients show a preference for psychological therapy over medication in the ratio of 3:1 (McHugh et al., 2013). Psychological therapy trials, though, have different methodological problems from drug trials. The basic difference is that they cannot be conducted double-blind because patients are always aware of whether they have received the psychological therapy under investigation or an alternative control intervention, which may merely be continuing on a waiting list.

Trials of psychotherapy do show a significant effect size on average (Lambert & Ogles, 2010). However, there are issues about the adequacy of control groups. Psychotherapy may be statistically and clinically beneficial compared to no treatment control conditions and improvement due to spontaneous remission, but its effects may be largely non-specific. There are common factors in psychotherapy, such as expectation for improvement, persuasion, warmth and attention, understanding and encouragement. It has been difficult to find significant differences in the outcomes between different therapies, which has been called the Dodo Bird effect: 'Everyone has won and all must have prizes' (Luborsky et al., 1975: 995).

USEFUL FOR
ASSIGNMENTS!

The Improving Access to Psychological Therapies (IAPT) programme has been introduced on the basis of claims that psychological therapy, particularly cognitive behavioural therapy (CBT), is highly effective and will save money by reducing disability benefits and increasing tax receipts (Layard & Clark, 2015). However, the programme was not set up using randomised controlled trials. Improvements may be due to natural recovery and self-fulfilling expectancy effects.

CASE STUDY:
COGNITIVE
BEHAVIOURAL
THERAPY

WHAT'S THE EVIDENCE? 12.3

Is psychotherapy effective?

- Psychotherapy trials cannot be conducted double-blind.
- Significant effect sizes can be demonstrated in clinical trials.
- There is still a question about whether psychotherapy is better than placebo because of the issue of the adequacy of control groups.
- Non-specific factors may contribute to an improvement in trials.
- Improvements demonstrated in the IAPT programme may be due to expectancy effects.

CHALLENGING CONCEPTS 12.2

Democratic mental health practice

- High quality care can only be provided through a partnership of patient and professional expertise.
- Psychiatrists' fear that their role is being taken over by other non-medical professionals does not justify a remedicalised psychiatry.
- Other professions should be encouraged to take on the responsibility that has traditionally been undertaken by the doctor.
- A medical training is beneficial for mental health practice as many patients go to their doctor with physical complaints whose origins are psychosocial.

CONCLUSION

Biomedical attitudes should not dominate practice (Challenging Concepts Box 12.2). Psychiatric diagnosis is about providing understanding, not about discovering an entity of some kind, for example with presumed biological correlates. Evidenced-based medicine requires scepticism about psychiatric treatments such as medication. Mental health nurses need to be able to engage with these issues as much as any other discipline within the mental health field.

———— CHAPTER SUMMARY ————

In this chapter, you have seen that:

- Psychiatry is a medical speciality
- Psychiatry requires a focus on the patient perspective
- Much mental health work does not require specific disciplinary expertise
- Patients can complain of physical symptoms that have a psychosocial origin
- Mental health practice functions within the problem of the relationship between mind and brain, making practice controversial
- The evidence about the effectiveness of psychiatric treatment is open to interpretation.

———— BUILD YOUR BIBLIOGRAPHY ————

Books

There are many textbooks of psychiatry. They all have a different style. It is worth looking at one such psychiatric textbook at least, for example:

- Cowen, Harrison & Burns (2012) *Shorter Oxford textbook of psychiatry*, 6th edition. Oxford: Oxford University Press.
- Bracken, P. & Thomas, P. (2005) *Postpsychiatry: Mental health in a postmodern world*. Oxford: Oxford University Press. This is an early critical psychiatry text.
- Double, D.B. (ed.) (2006) *Critical psychiatry: The limits of madness*. Basingstoke: Palgrave Macmillan. This book presents critical psychiatry proposals for a more ethical basis for practice with a blueprint for transforming services in alliance with service users.

- Tyrer & Steiner (2009) *Models for mental disorder: Conceptual models in psychiatry*, 4th edition. Chichester: Wiley. This book describes the different theoretical approaches for understanding mental illness.

SAGE journal articles

Go to https://study.sagepub.com/essentialmentalhealth for further free online journal articles related to this chapter. If you are using the interactive ebook, simply click on the book icon in the margin to go straight to the resource.

FURTHER READING: JOURNAL ARTICLES

- Double, D.B. (2002) The history of anti-psychiatry: an essay review. *History of Psychiatry*, *13*(50), 231–236.
- Hopton, J. (2006) The future of critical psychiatry. *Critical Social Policy*, *26*(1), 57–73.
- Kerr, L.K. (2009) Essay review: the humanities reforming psychiatry. *Theory & Psychology*, *19*(3), 431–438.

Weblinks

Go to https://study.sagepub.com/essentialmentalhealth for further weblinks related to this chapter. If you are using the interactive ebook, simply click on the book icon in the margin to go straight to the resource.

FURTHER READING: WEBLINKS

- There is considerable debate on the internet about psychiatry. The Critical Psychiatry Network (www.criticalpsychiatry.co.uk) was formed in Bradford in 1999. It is a small group of psychiatrists that provides a network to develop a critique of the contemporary psychiatric system. My own critical psychiatry blog (www.criticalpsychiatry.blogspot.co.uk) encourages critical comment and debate about psychiatry. Also look at some websites written to provide information and support for patients, such as those by Mind, the mental health charity (www.mind.org.uk).

———— ACE YOUR ASSESSMENT ————

Revise what you have learned by visiting https://study.sagepub.com/essentialmentalhealth. If you are using the interactive ebook, simply click on the tick icon to go straight to the resource.

ONLINE QUIZZES & ACTIVITY ANSWERS

- Test yourself with multiple-choice and short-answer questions and flashcards.

REFERENCES

Als-Nielsen, B., Chen, W., Gluud, C. et al. (2003) Association of funding and conclusions in randomized drug trials. JAMA, *290*, 921–928.

Barsky, A.J. (1981) Hidden reasons why some patients visit doctors. *Annals of Internal Medicine*, *94*, 492–498.

Bass, C. & Mayou, R. (2002) Chest pain. *BMJ*, *325*, 588–591.

Beers, C. (1908) *The mind that found itself*. New York: Longmont, Green & Co.

Bracken, P., Thomas, P., Timimi, S., et al. (2012) Psychiatry beyond the current paradigm. *British Journal of Psychiatry*, *201*, 430–434.

Cresswell, M. & Spandler, H. (2009) Psychopolitics: Peter Sedgwick's legacy for the politics of mental health. *Social Theory and Health*, *7*, 129–147.

Crossley, N. (2006) *Contesting psychiatry: Social movements in mental health*. London: Routledge.

Department of Health (DH) (2007) *Mental health: New ways of working for everyone*. London: DH.

Department of Health (2010) *Responsibility and accountability best practice guide: Moving on from New Ways of Working to a creative, capable workforce*. London: DH.

Double, D.B. (2004) Suspension of doctors: medical suspensions may have ideological nature. BMJ, *328*,709–710.

Double, D.B. (ed.) (2006) *Critical psychiatry: The limits of madness*. Basingstoke: Palgrave Macmillan.

Double, D.B. (2011) The professional context: the psychiatrist. In P. Barker (ed.) *Mental health ethics: The human context*. Abingdon: Routledge.

Even, C., Siobud-Dorocant, E. & Dardennes, R.M. (2000) Critical approach to antidepressant trials: blindness protection is necessary, feasible and measurable. *British Journal of Psychiatry, 177*, 47–51.

Ford, A.C. & Talley, N.J. (2012) Irritable bowel syndrome. BMJ, *345*, e5836.

Fulford, K.W.M. (1989) *Moral theory and medical practice*. Cambridge: Cambridge University Press.

Goldberg, D. & Huxley, P. (1992) *Common mental disorders*. London: Routledge.

Harrison, P., Bullmore, E., Jones, P., et al. (2012) *The future of psychiatry: Apothecaries – a cautionary tale*. Eletter. Available at: http://bjp.rcpsych.org/content/199/6/439.e-letters#the-future-of-psychiatry-apothecaries---a-cautionary-tale (accessed 7 August 2017).

Hornstein, G.A. (2009) *Agnes's jacket: A psychologist's search for the meanings of madness*. New York: Rodale.

Hornstein, G.A. (2011) Bibliography of first-person narratives of madness in English, 5th edition. Available at www.gailhornstein.com/files/Bibliography_of_First_Person_Narratives_of_Madness_5th_edition.pdf (accessed 13.12.15).

Jüni, P., Altman, D.G. & Egger, M. (2001) Assessing the quality of controlled clinical trials. BMJ, *323*, 42–46.

Kessler, D., Bennewith, O., Lewis, G. et al. (2002) Detection of depression and anxiety in primary care: follow up study. BMJ, *325*, 1016–1017.

Kinderman, P. (2014) *A prescription for psychiatry: Why we need a whole new approach to mental health and wellbeing*. Basingstoke: Palgrave Macmillan.

Kirsch, I. (2009) *The Emperor's new drugs: Exploding the antidepressant myth*. London: The Bodley Head.

Lambert, M.J. & Ogles, B.M. (2010) The efficacy and effectiveness of psychotherapy. In: Lamber, M.J. (ed.) *Bergin and Garfield's handbook of psychotherapy and behavior change*, 5th edition. New York: John Wiley & Sons.

Layard, R. & Clark, D.M. (2015) *Thrive: The power of evidence-based psychological therapies*. Harmondsworth: Penguin.

Little, P., Everitt, H., Williamson, I., et al. (2001) Preferences of patients for patient centred approach to consultation in primary care: observational study. BMJ, *322*, 468–472.

Longden, E. (2013) *The voices in my head*. TED talk. Available at: www.ted.com/talks/eleanor_longden_the_voices_in_my_head (accessed 20.03.16).

Luborsky, L., Singer, B. & Luborsky, L. (1975) Comparative studies of psychotherapies: Is it true that 'everyone has won and all must have prizes'? *Archives of General Psychiatry, 32*, 995–1008.

McHugh, R.K., Whitton, S.W., Peckham, A.D. et al. (2013) Patient preference for psychological vs. pharmacological treatment of psychiatric disorders: a meta-analytic review. *Journal of Clinical Psychiatry, 74*, 595–602.

Nimnuan, C., Hotopf, M. & Wessely, S. (2001) Medically unexplained symptoms: an epidemiological study in seven specialities. *Journal of Psychosomatic Research, 51*, 361–367.

Noll, R. (2011) *American madness: The rise and fall of dementia praecox*. Cambridge, MA: Harvard University Press.

Rose, D. (2000) A year of care. *OpenMind, 106*(Nov/Dec). Available at: www.critpsynet.freeuk.com/Rose3.htm (accessed 13.12.15).

Scull, A. (2005) *Madhouse: A tragic tale of megalomania and modern medicine*. New Haven, CT: Yale University Press.

Sedgwick, P. (1982) *Psychopolitics*. London: Pluto.

Stewart, M., Brown, J.B., Weston, W.W., et al. (2003) *Patient centred-medicine: Transforming the clinical method*, 2nd edition. Abingdon: Radcliffe Medical Press.

Thase, M. (1999) How should efficacy be evaluated in randomized clinical trials of treatments for depression? *Journal of Clinical Psychiatry, 60*(suppl. 4), 23–31.

SOCIOLOGICAL UNDERSTANDINGS OF MENTAL HEALTH

13

DAVID PILGRIM AND MICK McKEOWN

THIS CHAPTER COVERS

- The contribution of sociological knowledge to understanding mental health care
- The language of mental health and how it can be contested
- Distinctions between theories of social causation, social construction and social realism
- The implications for social change.

It started early when I felt different. I always felt like a square peg in a round hole, everyone was always better than me. An uncle said I had a face only a mother could love. Yes, ugly I felt – it carried on – stupid – why couldn't I tell the time or read like the other kids? But I got through life and became a mum. One baby after another plus a husband to contend with – it was like looking after three children. I was exhausted as my first child never slept. So, with the tiredness I couldn't stop crying. I went to the doctors – he put it down to post-natal depression and prescribed antidepressants. I had never been on medication before – wow this made me feel worse and even more tired and gave me really vivid bad dreams, and that was only the start of things to come. Eventually I reached such a low point I was suicidal.

Trying to look after two small children became increasingly more difficult. This showed to me that medical practitioners don't understand people's problems as they haven't got the time to listen or consider what else is going on in their life. For example, people might experience distressing issues such as domestic violence or alcohol and drug problems. In the long run this has led me to be more interested in social understandings of mental health rather than a simple medical model.

Because of this and other dissatisfaction with mental health services I have joined in with groups that have campaigned for better services. I now consider myself to be a community activist, and get involved in lots of opportunities where I have the ability to help others, including supporting research at the local university. I am interested in how poverty and austerity adversely affect mental health in families and neighbourhoods, and the voluntary sector group I work in has itself suffered cuts to its budget. This is unfortunate as I think community activism and research can help people to feel better if they get involved. Sadly, now even volunteering can be penalised by the benefits system.

(Continued)

Visit **https://study.sagepub.com/essentialmentalhealth** to access a wealth of online resources for this chapter - watch out for the margin icons throughout the chapter. If you are using the interactive ebook, simply click on the margin icon to go straight to the resource.

I really dislike labelling and stigma. In my experience, people are afraid of mental health as they can't see it, and so people in mental distress can try and hide this. To this day I don't even like the term mental health. For years I've walked the walk of mental health, and this is certainly not on lovely soft grass; more like a gravelly path with no shoes on and the dust being kicked up in your face. However, now I feel like there is no stopping me. I still have my ups and downs, we all have our vulnerabilities, but I feel I am now able to make a real difference. My research work has taken me across the country to other universities like Oxford and Leeds, opening up new horizons and new pathways: a lot less gravelly and dusty.

Mo Thomas, service user

Most mental health problems have at least some social component to them and my feeling is that for many people the things that happened to them are more likely to seriously affect their mental health, than genetics. Sexual abuse, physical abuse, poverty, deprivation, racism, all these and many, many more are often crucial factors in the development of mental health problems.

Psychiatry often finds it easier to medicate troublesome behaviours than spend time understanding why they occur, and the financial and physical resources to deal with people in other ways than medicating them are usually absent. Despite laudable recent attempts to combat it, the stigma associated with mental health problems remains powerfully present and the undesirable side-effects of psychiatric medications are something that often helps to make people easily identifiable as being different to wider society.

An understanding of social issues is invaluable for nurses and should be a core part of nurse education. My disenchantment with the prevalence of the medical model in psychiatry was a major factor for me in moving away from acute psychiatry to work with drug users where better resourcing meant that a realistic social model could be more prominent.

Jon Derricott, mental health nurse

In order to build trust and to understand an individual you also need to understand where they came from, their relationships, their culture and their beliefs. They all have different backgrounds, and these affect who they are and how they view their treatment. It also changes the way that they view us. I always make a point of asking not just about them, but also about their family and things that are important to them. That way, they know how important they are to me, as a person, not just a patient.

Gemma McDermott, student nurse

INTRODUCTION

This chapter deals with the range of sociological understandings of mental **disorder**, and also considers the lesser scrutinised topic by sociologists of positive mental health and wellbeing. Given the contested aspects of psychiatry and mental health services and the affinities for alternative provision or different ways of making sense of human experiences, sociological theories hold appeal in adding to a more plural range of understandings. Sociology aims to make sense of society or phenomena within it in social terms: that is, with regard to social factors and in consideration of social relations between people, groups and institutions. There is no single, overarching sociological theory; rather, there are a number of perspectives which emphasise different ideologies or dimensions of society. Many of the most notable critiques of bio-psychiatry have emanated from a sociological perspective. Indeed, a social model of mental distress has been suggested as a conceptual alternative to a pathologising psychiatric knowledge base (Beresford, 2002).

Nurses and other disciplines can share in contesting psychiatric dominance and orthodoxy, and sociological ideas can prove to be useful in this regard. Similarly, the very nature of nurses' work and how this is organised is amenable to sociological **insights**. The disciplinary **ambivalence** about **mental disorder** reflects that of others such as psychology. On the one hand, some researchers have focused on causes and on the other meanings, with some trying to balance the two. Thus, three sociological positions will be summarised: social causationism, social constructivism and social realism.

THE SOCIAL CAUSES OF MENTAL DISORDERS

Since the 19th century, an interest in the social causes of mental disorder can be traced to the observations of those in charge of asylums and in the theorisations about the traumatic effects of warfare. These observations were not inherently sociological in ambition but they gave confidence to subsequent formal developments, for example in Durkheim's work on suicide and later in the 'ecological wing' of the Chicago School of sociology.

A working assumption of social causationists is that the disorders described by psychiatry are real and that the role of empirical sociology is to trace the relevant antecedent or maintaining social forces that make a whole or partial contribution to etiology. Thus, causationism entails a realist paradigm, which can be compared with the others. A particular focus of social causationists has been to trace the impact of social disadvantage. For example, it is clear that in mental as well as physical health there is a clear class gradient. Poor people are more at risk of developing a mental disorder than rich people (with some exceptions to this rule, such as diagnoses like bipolar disorder and obsessive-compulsive **personality** disorder).

Although social class is the strongest predictor of mental ill health, others are implicated as well. For example, women are at greater risk of being diagnosed with a mental disorder than men. Most of this is accounted for by the diagnosis of **depression** in primary care; men are more prevalent in detained psychiatric populations. This could mean that women are distressed more than men because of gender oppression but other hypotheses are possible (for example, women present more readily in primary care consultations). Also, women are admitted to psychiatric hospital at the same frequency as men but the latter are kept longer and so have a higher point prevalence of residence. It could be that decisions about women and men with similar mental health problems focus not on symptoms per se but on risk calculations (with men being deemed to be more risky).

The advantage of sociologically informed psychiatric **epidemiology** is that it provides the sort of scientific confidence associated with objectivism and empiricism. However, there are four main disadvantages of this sociological contribution:

- Pre-empirical conceptual problems associated with psychiatric knowledge are either not acknowledged or are evaded; for example, in the work of George Brown and his colleagues (Brown, 1959; Brown & Harris, 2012). That is, the concept validity of psychiatric diagnoses has been criticised by many inside and outside of sociology, but this type of sociological work takes the validity of diagnosis for granted.
- Psychiatric epidemiology investigates correlations between mental **illness** and antecedent variables but correlations are not necessarily indicative of causal relationships.
- Epidemiology cannot illuminate the lived experience of mental health problems or the variety of meanings attributed to them by patients and significant others.
- Medical epidemiology attempts to map the distributions of causes of **disease**, not merely the cases of disease. Because most of psychiatric illness is described as 'functional' (i.e. it has no known biological marker and its cause or causes are either not known or contested), psychiatric epidemiology cannot fulfill the general expectation of mapping causes.

THE SOCIAL CONSTRUCTION OF MENTAL DISORDERS

The ecological wing of the Chicago School was noted above but its other wing, rooted in the work of Weber and Mead, was articulated as 'symbolic interactionism'. From this perspective, people are always engaged in meaning-making activity, making sense of the world through negotiating the symbols and **culture** present in everyday life. If meanings are exchanged between individuals and groups in society, then, logically, this principle should apply to mental disorder as well. Indeed, after the Second World War this interactionist view became popular first in the work of Goffman (1959) and then in labelling theory, also called 'social reaction theory' (see Scheff, 1966). The importance of the exchange of meanings and the concepts used by lay people and professionals have been an important starting point not only for this current of symbolic interactionism but appears as well in modified form in later versions of radical constructivism and critical realism (Brown, 1995). Examples of each will be given to illustrate this point.

Symbolic interactionism

This current of thought from the Chicago School of sociology has been important in two main ways for our understanding of mental disorder. The first relates to professional mental health work and its preferred understandings of its own tasks and knowledge base. This is exemplified in Goffman's (1961) essays in the book *Asylums*, in which he describes how psychologically deviant people are turned into patients and how the very weak knowledge base of psychiatry coexists with a very powerful cultural mandate for social control. For Goffman, significant others and psychiatric professionals exert power to impose 'degradation rituals' and the patient is subjected to a 'betrayal funnel'. Later work suggested that Goffman over-stated this onsite set of negotiations and underplayed decisions already made in the lay arena, with psychiatrists largely rubber stamping decisions already made there (Coulter, 1973).

Radical constructivism

This perspective largely describes the theories of a group of sociologists who have adopted the work on madness by Michel Foucault (e.g. 1965, 1980). For radical constructivists, mental disorder is a by-product of psychiatric activity and the focus of sociological investigation is the deconstruction of that activity. This approach does not make a distinction between action and ideas or praxis and ideology, instead there is a focus on the unity of 'discursive practices'. Effectively, madness is socially constructed; the ways we talk and think about mental health are what actually bring things into being. After Foucault's original interest in the emergence of psychiatric ideas, later radical constructivists were concerned with deconstructing the following changes occuring during the 20th century:

- Psychiatry as a professional enterprise is no longer restricted only to the asylum.
- Its practices are no longer only associated with coercive social control.
- Large bands of the population have been induced into an individualised state of psychological mindedness about their existence, via the media and education.
- Following on from the last two points, voluntary relationships involving lengthy conversations about the self are now sought out by the public and deployed by professionals (versions of counselling and psychotherapy).

SOCIAL REALISM

Some realists have taken a middle position between radical constructivism and social causationism. This work has been linked philosophically with critical realism and empirically with general systems theory, and has been associated with some developments of the 'biopsychosocial model' of mental health work. The emphasis within social realism is on real social forces (like the social causationists) but also on a sceptical view of professional knowledge (like the radical constructivists). For social realists, it is not reality that is socially constructed but our understanding of reality. Thus, it is possible to argue that social factors determine psychological deviance (madness and misery), while remaining sceptical of the knowledge use to describe it (a form of weak rather than radical constructivism). Another reflection of critical realist philosophy in this third sociological approach is that social realists accept that all human action, including that of patients and those around them, reflects human agency under conditions of constraint. We are both determined and determining beings. Social realists, therefore, are able to accommodate the perspective and intentions of all of these social actors as well as the biological, psychological and **social determinants** of that action.

For social realists, social reality does not mechanistically determine people's actions, nor is social reality simplistically constructed by human agency. Society can be transformed or reproduced by intentional human action, but society has existence prior to the lives of people. The material conditions of reality *constrain* action but do not in any simple way *determine* it. In the mental health context, social realists see causes, or 'generative mechanisms', of mental ill health as possibly social, psychological or biological, compatible with affinities for so-called biopsychosocial models. However, social realists are also highly critical of most deployments of such models for over-emphasising the biology due to the professional and epistemological dominance of psychiatry (Pilgrim, 2013). Certain mental health nurses have taken up critical realist perspectives to inform nursing research and evaluation (McEvoy & Richards, 2003).

Sociological perspectives demand that considerations of mental health and illness regard a double significance of the social. First, there is ample evidence that social determinants are the cause of what we know as mental illness. Second, that beyond thinking about cause, constructivist theories highlight the social dimensions of knowledge, language and power and how we can consider the constructed nature of what we mean by mental illness. These standpoints can be both compatible and incommensurable. Arguably, however, there is a need to consider both causation and meaning in developing a full understanding of mental health and illness.

MENTAL HEALTH: A CONTESTABLE NOTION

The very terminology of mental health can be confusing and mental health can mean different things to different people. There are three broad ways in which the term mental health is used. First, the language of 'mental health' is used to indicate a positive state of psychological wellbeing. Second, mental health is a prefix for services, to denote that sector of health care services that supports people who use these services, designated in the third usage, where mental health is a prefix for problems. This denotes the opposite of mental health – a negative state of psychological wellbeing.

To some extent, the general usage of the language of mental health and mental health services can be understood on the basis of its acceptability to different groups of people rather than any definitional precision (Pilgrim, 2005). The descriptor 'psychiatric services', though widely used and reflecting the relative dominance of psychiatry, does not really do justice to the range of professional disciplines which make up modern multi-disciplinary teams. Mental illness services might actually be a more accurate label, given the extent of medicalisation, but is arguably unpalatable and stigmatising and too narrow for the range of problems and needs served. Hence, mental health services may be the least problematic way of describing services, or even euphemistic, and does not escape problems arising from critical scrutiny of the notion 'mental health'.

Contemporary health policies reflect a positive notion of mental health, and matters of social **value** and productivity have been explicitly linked to indices and expectations of happiness. The economist Richard Layard (2010) has been prominent in setting this agenda that has included the substantial policy of Improving Access to Psychological Therapies (IAPT) and, more latterly, the contentious linking of psychological assessment and support to work capability and benefits entitlements (Thomas, 2016).

CONTESTING PSYCHIATRIC LEGITIMACY

CASE STUDY:
SUE

In this book and elsewhere, various criticisms of psychiatry have been marshalled to make a case for transformative change that, at the very least, is concerned with a more plural care and treatment offering. In this way, sociological and other critique has seriously challenged biomedical reductionism and highlighted the gap between policy rhetoric that privileges holistic approaches and the actuality of fairly homogenous, if not monoglot, risk-averse, coercive services (Read, 2005; Vassilev & Pilgrim, 2007). Similarly, despite much fanfare regarding systems for supporting **service user** voice and involvement, this operates within cultural and organisational constraints and has yet to result in profound transformational change (Hodge, 2005, 2009).

For critical commentators, the illusion of empowerment and co-option of potentially emancipatory practices into mainstream structures represents a new tyranny, reflecting the role of mental health services in wider systems of social control (Cooke & Kothari, 2002). From a similar perspective, seemingly progressive notions such as **recovery**, first instigated by service user activists, have become neutered of their radical potential through assimilation into the mainstream (Harper & Speed, 2012; Pilgrim & McCranie, 2013). All of this is compounded by a parallel turn in society, the exaggeration of risk consciousness in social and public policy arenas, and most obviously in mental health services (Lupton, 1999). This combination of factors results in ever-increasing numbers of people subject to the compulsory powers of **mental health law** alongside more subtle processes of control elsewhere, and justifies policies replete with problems for progressively minded practitioners and service users alike.

Hence, contemporary services do not escape the sort of criticisms voiced by the likes of Goffman (1961) and Foucault (1965), who highlighted systematic processes by which patients endure mortification at the hands of service systems and the myriad ways by which psychiatry is as much about serving government and governance as ameliorating mental distress (Slemon et al., 2017; see also

Rose, 1990). From the time they were writing in the 1960s, these authors' concerns were taken up by a wide-ranging **anti-psychiatry** movement, conjoined with radical practitioners such as Ronnie Laing and David Cooper that inspired certain alternatives to mainstream psychiatry (Chapman, 2016; Proctor, 2016). To some extent, the anti-psychiatry movement has not gone away, with critical calls remaining for either the complete abolition of mental health services as we know them or a slow strategy of attrition (Burstow, 2015). Also emerging in this period, reacting to dissatisfaction with services and to some extent intertwined with the establishment of specific alternative forms of care, was a vociferous service user/**survivor** movement making similar calls for change (Crossley, 2006; Spandler, 2006). Latterly, this has culminated in service users themselves making a case for a range of alternatives outside of the mainstream, supported by user-led research and knowledge production (Russo & Sweeney, 2016).

Taken as a whole, the range of criticisms of psychiatry can be seen to call into question its very legitimacy. Associated occupational groups, such as mental health nursing, are similarly enmeshed in a crisis of legitimacy, exacerbated by their close proximity to service users and their key role in the face-to-face administration of the psychiatric enterprise and mechanisms of **coercion** (McKeown & White, 2015). Coppock and Hopton (2002), respectively, radical social work and mental health nursing practitioners, suggested that the legitimacy shortcomings of psychiatry do not necessarily trump the faith that the public has in medicine and psychiatry, and hence deference to its power. For these authors, this acquiescence in psychiatric monopoly on the part of the public may be due to insufficient knowledge of mental health to object to (Pilgrim, 1992), socialisation processes (Ingleby, 1983) or approval of psychiatric intervention because of a disinclination to assume the support role (De Swaan, 1990). Simple criticism of this state of affairs does nothing on its own to change anything.

Perhaps for as long as there has been organised psychiatric institutions, there has been some semblance of resistance to psychiatric power. Since the 1970s, people who have experienced the mental health system have formed organised groups, often styling themselves as survivors. These groupings mirror the activities of other civil rights movements and have been referred to as new **social movements**, in contrast to so-called old social movements such as the labour movement (Brown & Zavetoski, 2005; Crossley, 2006; Rogers & Pilgrim, 1991). A distinction is highlighted between different forms of organising, with newer social movements having affinity for looser structures, distributed democracy and shared roles, whilst older movements are criticised for the ossification of democratic processes and inflexible bureaucracies (Habermas, 1981). Others have argued that criticism of different organising models is less important than an imperative to forge political alliances between movements. Arguably, recent trade union renewal initiatives promise a shift away from an exclusive focus on the workplace to organising in communities, raising the potential for alliances change-seeking between the mental health workforce and service user movements (McKeown et al., 2014). Substantive change demands ideas for action and it is to some of these that we now turn.

PETER SEDGWICK: PROTO-CRITICAL REALIST?

There has been recent interest in the ideas of radical critic, Peter Sedgwick, who pointed out the limitations of a too simple anti-psychiatry and made a persuasive argument for a way forward that would embrace effective alternative forms of care (Spandler et al., 2016). Sedgwick sadly took his own life shortly after the publication of his most famous work, *Psychopolitics* (1982). With hindsight, Sedgwick's analysis of mental health services and society at large arguably consists of an early application of critical realist ideas to this context (Pilgrim, 2016). For Sedgwick (1982), the mental illness concept is easily debunked, with bio-psychiatry having the same flaws as broader bio-medicine in neglecting more holistic conceptualisations and collapsing into biological reductionism; most obviously seen in mind–body distinctions (Cresswell & Spandler, 2009, 2016).

Thus, one of the most telling criticisms of psychiatric orthodoxy is the role it plays in maintaining an unhelpful conceptual and practical demarcation between physical and mental health. Sedgwick makes the rather obvious, but often neglected, logical point that this is a problem for all medical knowledge and practice, not unique to psychiatry. A consequence of this can be that critics of simple medical models can make an error of their own – throwing out the baby of all biological relevance with the bathwater of biological reductionism. In other words, the quest for non-medical explanations and social causes and meanings need not deny any relevance to biological theories or associated medical interventions. Instead, more sophisticated analyses are required.

Rather than dismiss mental illness as a concept, however, Sedgwick suggests that it best functions in enabling a claim on resources, including health, social and welfare support, which might be undermined if psychiatry was to be abolished without necessary alternative provision. Hence, Sedgwick argued for building cross-sectional alliances for social change, ideally between activists in the health workforce and service user movements and a corollary politics of mental health to inform and support these efforts. So, from this perspective, mental distress is real and requires a state-wide, organised response, but the form that this takes ought to consist of a plural range of alternatives, being quite different from simplistic bio-psychiatry (Spandler, 2014).

Taking a lead from Sedgwick, cross-sectional alliances can be seen as a way forward. Sedgwick saw such alliances as necessary for the basis of the dialogue required between relevant groups (workers, service users and **carers**) to bring into being alternative forms of care and the systems to support them. Borrowing from anarchism, the Marxist Sedgwick favoured a process of prefigurative communication, whereby the people involved in seeking change attempt to model the world they would like to see in the course of trying to achieve it. If there is to be a forging of alliances to help transform mental health services and construct alternatives, then an important question remains over whether all parties would agree this is a worthwhile goal and take part. Radical service users and survivors, who would need to be involved, may not care to participate because of a lack of trust, born out of a history of harm experienced at the hands of services. Staff who don't see anything wrong with present services may also be reluctant to join a political alliance calling for radical change. Spandler and McKeown (2017) have argued that a necessary first step for forming constructive alliances would be the establishment of grassroots truth and reconciliation processes, which could begin to build trust and heal the harm that has been experienced by service users or staff in the system.

CONCLUSION

Adopting a social realist position is useful for developing analyses of psychiatry that can present meaningful insights into prevailing problems and also serve up solutions that are concerned with action for change. A summary of the relevance and implications of applying critical realist ideas to the mental health context suggests a healthy scepticism is required for concepts more often than not taken for granted (Rogers & Pilgrim, 2014):

- Whatever we call it, madness or distress has existed throughout history and across different societies and is determined by many factors, known and unknown.
- Notions of distress and madness can be distinguished in terms of our ability to understand them independently of societal norms. Distress such as **anxiety**, sadness or fear is reasonably consistently known across different contexts or even species. Designated forms of madness however are less conceptually stable, and are typically defined in terms of deviance from norms; and these normative concerns can change substantially over time or across different societies.

- Notions of positive mental health incorporate assumptions about meaning and **mood** that are also normative.
- Judgements about health or illness must implicitly be social, and these need to be recognised as value judgements. A good way of reminding ourselves of this is to acknowledge that the language and terminology of mental disorder have to imply there is also an 'ordered' state which the 'disordered' state deviates from.

Rogers and Pilgrim (2014) present three main arguments informed by social understandings and relevant to critical debates regarding mental health. First, psychological deviance represents a set of problems in need of a remedy. Thus, a good society should concern itself with the amelioration or prevention of madness or mental distress and this ought to involve social measures such as those designed to reduce **inequality** or tackle various perceived social problems. Second, society should be selective about which forms of deviance it is most concerned about, and intervene accordingly. To some extent, this position is informed by an assumption that certain human experiences, such as those defined as major mental disorder, warrant such **classification** and subsequent intervention. Alternately, other forms of distress are best thought of as ordinary misery, exist on a continuum and require social policies designed to maximise collective wellbeing or happiness. Third, misery and madness just exist, are meaningful in their own right and it is not necessarily the business of the state to organise interventions grounded in assumptions of normalcy or attempt to contain people who live through these diverse forms of human experience.

The third argument resonates with the perspectives taken up by certain anti-psychiatrists combining existentialist and Marxist ideas, such as David Cooper (1968) or the post-structuralist informed post-psychiatry movement (Bracken & Thomas, 2001). Latterly, the emergent field of **Mad Studies**, allied with contemporary anti-psychiatrists, also shares common ground with this viewpoint (e.g. LeFrançois et al., 2013; Burstow et al., 2014).

Rogers and Pilgrim (2014) note that the availability of these different perspectives renders any attempt to think rationally about public health or social policy fraught with potential problems. The competing arguments are variously eugenic, paternalistic or libertarian and as such are together incompatible for organising society. The undercurrents of these tensions can be seen in various recent policies regarding social inclusion and **stigma** prevention, perhaps pointing to reasons why these initiatives often fail or perpetually reproduce the very perceived social failing they are purportedly designed to address.

CRITICAL THINKING STOP POINT 13.1

What do you think is the value of sociological understandings of mental health?

Think about the concluding arguments for understanding mental health and health care measures in society. Which do you prefer? How might mental health services be organised differently if they were to follow the implications of your preferred perspective?

CRITICAL
THINKING
STOP
POINT 13.1
ANSWER

CHAPTER SUMMARY

This chapter has covered:

- Discussion of the contribution of key sociological theories to making sense of mental health/distress and mental health care

- Critique of services and key concepts from social perspectives
- Identification with social realism as a productive theoretical basis for critique of bio-psychiatry and a foundation for seeking transformative change.

BUILD YOUR BIBLIOGRAPHY

Books

- Archer, M., Bhaskar, R., Collier, A., et al. (2013) *Critical realism: Essential readings*. London: Routledge. A reasonably accessible collection of writing on critical realism.
- Coppock, V. & Hopton, J. (2002) *Critical perspectives on mental health*. London: Routledge. An excellent earlier review of critical ideas written by practitioner academics from social work and nursing backgrounds.
- Rogers, A. & Pilgrim, D. (2014) *A sociology of mental health and illness*, 5th edition. Maidenhead: Open University Press/McGraw-Hill Education. A comprehensive coverage of sociological and other critical ideas for understanding mental health. Takes up a social realist perspective in more depth.

SAGE journal articles

FURTHER
READING:
JOURNAL
ARTICLES

Go to https://study.sagepub.com/essentialmentalhealth for further free online journal articles related to this chapter. If you are using the interactive ebook, simply click on the book icon in the margin to go straight to the resource.

- Aneshensel, C.S. (2015) Sociological inquiry into mental health: the legacy of Leonard I. Pearlin. *Journal of Health and Social Behavior, 56*(2), 166–178.
- Brown, P. (1984) Marxism, social psychology, and the sociology of mental health. *International Journal of Health Services, 14*(2), 237–264.
- Watson, D.P. (2012) The evolving understanding of recovery: what does the sociology of mental health have to offer? *Humanity & Society, 36*(4), 290–308.

Weblinks

FURTHER
READING:
WEBLINKS

Go to https://study.sagepub.com/essentialmentalhealth for further weblinks related to this chapter. If you are using the interactive ebook, simply click on the book icon in the margin to go straight to the resource.

- British Sociological Association Sociology of Mental Health Study Group: www.britsoc.co.uk/groups/medical-sociology-groups/sociology-of-mental-health-study-group
- Mad Studies website: https://madstudies2014.wordpress.com
- Mental Health History Timeline: http://studymore.org.uk/mhhtim.htm – detailing service user/survivor movement history, compiled by Andrew Roberts.

ACE YOUR ASSESSMENT

ONLINE
QUIZZES &
ACTIVITY
ANSWERS

Revise what you have learned by visiting https://study.sagepub.com/essentialmentalhealth. If you are using the interactive ebook, simply click on the tick icon to go straight to the resource.

- Test yourself with multiple-choice and short-answer questions and flashcards.

REFERENCES

Beresford, P. (2002) Thinking about 'mental health': towards a social model. *Journal of Mental Health*, *11*(6), 581–584.

Bracken, P. & Thomas, P. (2001) Postpsychiatry: a new direction for mental health. *British Medical Journal*, *322*(7288), 724.

Brown, G.W. (1959) Experiences of discharged chronic schizophrenic patients in various types of living group. *The Milbank Memorial Fund Quarterly*, *37*(2), 105–131.

Brown, G.W. & Harris, T. (eds) (2012) *The social origins of depression*. London: Tavistock. [Originally published 1978]

Brown, P. (1995) Naming and framing: the social construction of diagnosis and illness. *Journal of Health and Social Behavior*, *36*(Special Issue), 34–52.

Brown, P. & Zavetoski, S. (2005) Social movements in health: an introduction. In P. Brown & S. Zavetoski (eds) *Social movements in health*. Oxford: Blackwell. pp. 1–16.

Burstow, B. (2015) *Psychiatry and the business of madness: An ethical and epistemological accounting*. New York: Palgrave Macmillan.

Burstow, B., LeFrançois, B. & Diamond, S.L. (eds) (2014) *Psychiatry disrupted: Theorizing resistance and crafting the revolution*. Montreal, QC: McGill/Queen's University Press.

Chapman, A. (2016) Re-Coopering anti-psychiatry: David Cooper, revolutionary critic of psychiatry. *Critical and radical social work*, *4*(3), 421–432.

Cooke, B. & Kothari, U. (2002) *Participation: The new tyranny?* London: Zed Books.

Cooper, D. (1968) *Psychiatry and anti-psychiatry*. London: Tavistock.

Coppock, V. & Hopton, J. (2002) *Critical perspectives on mental health*. London: Routledge.

Coulter, J. (1973) *Approaches to insanity: A philosophical and sociological study*. New York: John Wiley & Sons.

Cresswell, M. & Spandler, H. (2009) Psychopolitics: Peter Sedgwick's legacy for the politics of mental health. *Social Theory & Health*, *7*(2), 129–147.

Cresswell, M. & Spandler, H. (2016) Solidarities and tensions in mental health politics: Mad Studies and Psychopolitics. *Critical and Radical Social Work*, *4*(3), 357–373.

Crossley, N. (2006) *Contesting psychiatry: Social movements in mental health*. London: Routledge.

De Swaan, A. (1990) *The management of normality: Critical essays in health and welfare*. London: Routledge.

Foucault, M. (1965) *Madness and civilisation*. New York: Random House.

Foucault, M. (1980) Power/knowledge. In C. Gordon (ed.) *Selected essays and other writings*. Brighton: Harvester Press.

Goffman, E. (1959) *The presentation of self in everyday life*. New York: Anchor Books.

Goffman, E. (1961) *Asylums: Essays on the social situation of mental patients and other inmates*. New York: Anchor Books.

Habermas, J. (1981) New social movements. *Telos*, *48*, 33–37.

Harper, D. & Speed, E. (2012) Uncovering recovery: the resistible rise of recovery and resilience. *Studies in Social Justice*, *6*(1), 9.

Hodge, S. (2005) Participation, discourse and power: a case study in service user involvement. *Critical Social Policy*, *25*(2), 64–179.

Hodge, S. (2009) User involvement in the construction of a mental health charter: an exercise in communicative rationality? *Health Expectations*, *12*(3), 251–261.

Ingleby, D. (1983) Mental health and social order. In S. Cohen & A. Scull (eds) *Social control and the state*. Oxford: Blackwell. pp. 141–190.

Layard, R. (2010) Measuring subjective well-being. *Science, 327*(5965), 534–535.

LeFrançois, B., Menzies, R. & Reaume, G. (eds) (2013) *Mad matters: A critical reader in Canadian mad studies.* Toronto, ON: Canadian Scholars' Press. pp. 122–129.

Lupton, D. (ed.) (1999) *Risk and sociocultural theory: New directions and perspectives.* Cambridge University Press.

McEvoy, P. & Richards, D. (2003) Critical realism: a way forward for evaluation research in nursing? *Journal of Advanced Nursing, 43*(4), 411–420.

McKeown, M. & White, J. (2015) The future of mental health nursing: are we barking up the wrong tree? *Journal of Psychiatric and Mental Health Nursing, 22*, 724–730.

McKeown, M., Cresswell, M. & Spandler, H. (2014) Deeply engaged relationships: alliances between mental health workers and psychiatric survivors in the UK. In B. Burstow, B.A. LeFrançois and S.L. Diamond (eds) *Psychiatry disrupted: Theorizing resistance and crafting the revolution.* Montreal, QC: McGill/Queen's University Press.

Pilgrim, D. (1992) Competing histories of madness: some implications for modern psychiatry. In R.P. Bentall (ed.) *Reconstructing schizophrenia.* London: Routledge. pp. 211–233.

Pilgrim, D. (2005) *Key concepts in mental health.* London: Sage.

Pilgrim, D. (2013) The failure of diagnostic psychiatry and some prospects of scientific progress offered by critical realism. *Journal of Critical Realism, 12*(3), 336–358.

Pilgrim, D. (2016) Peter Sedgwick, proto-critical realist? *Critical and Radical Social Work, 4*(3), 327–341.

Pilgrim, D. and McCranie, A. (2013) *Recovery and mental health: A critical sociological account.* Basingstoke: Palgrave Macmillan.

Proctor, H. (2016) Lost Minds: Sedgwick, Laing and the politics of mental illness. *Radical Philosophy.* 197, 36–48.

Read, J. (2005) The bio-bio-bio model of madness. *The Psychologist, 18*(10), 596–597.

Rogers, A. & Pilgrim, D. (1991) 'Pulling down churches': accounting for the British mental health users' movement. *Sociology of Health & Illness, 13*(2), 129–148.

Rogers, A. & Pilgrim, D. (2014) *A sociology of mental health and illness,* 5th edition. Maidenhead: Open University Press/McGraw-Hill Education.

Rose, N. (1990) *Governing the soul: The shaping of the private self.* London: Routledge.

Russo, J. & Sweeney, A. (2016) *Searching for a rose garden: Challenging psychiatry, fostering Mad Studies.* Wyastone Leys: PCCS Books.

Scheff, T.J. (1966) *Being mentally ill: A sociological theory.* Chicago: Aldine.

Sedgwick, P. (1982) *Psychopolitics.* London: Pluto.

Slemon, A., Jenkins, E. & Bungay, V. (2017) Safety in psychiatric inpatient care: the impact of risk management culture on mental health nursing practice. *Nursing Inquiry, 24*(4), e12199.

Spandler, H. (2006) *Asylum to action: Paddington day hospital, therapeutic communities and beyond.* London: Jessica Kingsley.

Spandler, H. (2014) Letting madness breathe? Critical challenges facing mental health social work today. In J. Weinstein (ed.) *Mental health.* Bristol: Policy Press. pp. 29–38.

Spandler, H. & McKeown, M. (2017) Exploring the case for truth and reconciliation in mental health services. *Mental Health Review Journal, 22*(2), 83–94.

Spandler, H., Moth, R., McKeown, M., et al. (2016) Editorial: psychopolitics in the twenty first century. *Critical & Radical Social Work, 4*(3), 307–312.

Thomas, P. (2016) Psycho politics, neoliberal governmentality and austerity. *Self & Society, 44*(4), 382–393.

Vassilev, I. & Pilgrim, D. (2007) Risk, trust and the myth of mental health services. *Journal of Mental Health, 16*(3), 347–357.

CRITICAL PSYCHOLOGICAL IDEAS AND PRACTICES

RICHARD BENTALL AND MICK McKEOWN

THIS CHAPTER COVERS

- The value of psychological ideas and how these might inform care and treatment interventions for mental distress in a context of multi-disciplinary teamwork
- Key features of critical psychological writings and how these pose a challenge to simple bio-psychiatry
- Arguments against categorical psychiatric classification systems and assumptions surrounding the heritability of mental illness
- Connections between critical psychological ideas and the emergence of service-user-inspired alternative forms of help and support.

> **"** I was advised to see a psychologist by a volunteer at the day centre who had studied psychology. This person had helped me with coping strategies and awareness of some of my negative and illogical thinking. At the first meeting with the psychologist, he saw my distress, anger and aggression. Early in my meeting with him he gave me a task which helped me. I had to write down my thoughts in columns. Doing this made me think he cared. At times for me these sessions were emotionally difficult. But I found I could cry openly, something I could not do with anybody else. I trusted him; he listened. His down to earth manner was important to me, which I responded to, sharing thoughts and feelings. Now I am involved in the education of clinical psychologists and I always recall how this psychologist was one of the first people who really helped me by treating me like a person and being there with my feelings.
>
> **Keith Holt, service user** **"**

I am a Clinical Psychologist and have worked in inpatient psychiatric units for the last three decades, in various different cities across England. I can vividly remember the first time I walked onto a ward, filled with excitement and enthusiastic to start working with patients as a fully-fledged Clinical Psychologist (green as they come!). I was also a bit scared, not quite sure what to expect from the patients. My trepidation was well-founded as it turns out, but entirely misplaced. It wasn't the patients that I should have feared but my naivety, and interactions with some of the other professionals around me. I realised quite quickly that my ideas, knowledge and keenness to make a difference came slap bang up against a system that included war-weary staff, who had no intention of filling out my beautifully prepared behavioural checklists. It didn't take long for me to realise that asking busy staff to complete extra paper-work wasn't going to win me any allies. It hit me that my working aspirations were not going to be something straight out of a book of 'how to do psychological therapy'.

In those days (and sometimes still now it feels), psychologists were talking a completely different language and challenging the prevailing biological perspective needed tact and sensitivity. Patients got it, but many staff didn't, and why should they? My understanding of mental distress came up against a completely different emphasis and training regime. Also, the psychological therapy movement is full of jargon and long titles of unfamiliar words, so a clear challenge was to translate the jargon into everyday language. This definitely helped but the de-mystification sometimes can make quite complex ideas and theories seem more mundane and common-sense. This is not necessarily bad, but can lead to misinterpretation and dilution of 'pure' research findings. Hence, some therapies, often developed with research participants that don't really resemble the people I recognise on the wards, are implemented simplistically and uncritically. This can lead to poor outcomes and undermine psychologically informed practices.

Things have changed over the years but the system still revolves around a medical model, with access to services often dependent on a medical diagnosis, rather than an assessment of need. It takes time, patience and allies to change a culture. I still regularly have conversations about the words used to describe ordinary behaviour and human nature amongst patients. For instance, patients are described sometimes as manipulative, lazy, brittle without taking the wider context into consideration – the lack of choice and the imbalance of power, or the side effects of medication all play a part in why people act as they do. Previous traumas that systems can inadvertently mimic are often not known about or not considered important.

Over the years I have worked with many, many patients, all with different experiences, symptoms and outcomes. I have learnt so much from them, and also from the staff I have worked with. Hopefully I have made a positive difference, and I couldn't have wished for a more interesting system to work within. I will never forget those early days though, and the keenness to improve things. Sometimes this risks overshadowing the reality of the individual experiences of staff and patients, and their ability to make changes to a system so left behind in terms of investment and application of new understandings of mental distress.

Sara Finlayson, clinical psychologist

INTRODUCTION

Psychological understandings of mental health and distress and psychologically inspired interventions are valuable in making sense of mental health problems and informing progressive practices within services. Mental health nurses need to be conversant with this body of knowledge and practice to be better placed to fulfil their role within care teams and more effectively support **service users**. Mental health nurses are typically taught basic psychological ideas and certain of them go on to receive additional training in psychotherapeutic techniques, for example to practise cognitive behavioural therapies as part of IAPT teams. Nurses will routinely work in teams that include clinical psychologists and will increasingly find themselves contributing to sophisticated care-planning approaches grounded in formulation rather than simple diagnosis. Psychological understandings of the human condition also permeate organisational processes and strategies for maintaining personal wellbeing and resilience as workers, and for that matter can illuminate other aspects of society such as marketing and public relations, media influence, prejudice and discrimination.

Psychology as a science and clinical psychology as its largest applied sub-discipline have a long history with diverse schools of foundational knowledge leading to different forms of practice. Broadly speaking, psychology concerns itself with the interrelationship between thoughts, feelings and behaviour and psychological treatments based on psychological theory include psychodynamic, behavioural and cognitive-behavioural interventions, and various forms of counselling approaches such as person-centred counselling. It has been noted that therapist attributes that establish therapeutic alliance, such as an ability to express warmth and empathy, are arguably as important for a positive outcome as any particular type of psychological intervention (Wampold & Imel, 2015), even in the treatment of severe mental **illness** (Goldsmith et al., 2015). The historical development and practicalities of different approaches and roles of psychologists are discussed at length in other texts (e.g. Schultz & Schultz, 2015). In this chapter, however, we restrict ourselves to presenting more recent, critically inspired psychological understandings and practices that have emerged at least in part as a reaction to perceived failings within standard psychiatry. As such, we align ourselves with a rational **anti-psychiatry** which acknowledges important humanistic critique but emphasises the scientific shortcomings of psychiatric practices (Bentall, 2009).

Before attempting a critique of the mistakes of psychiatry and psychiatrically dominated services, that, to some extent, more psychologically informed approaches attempt to overcome, it is worth noting that psychological approaches are not beyond criticism. Rogers and Pilgrim (2014) highlight the fact that, although approaches based on talk are immediately less physically invasive and often more appreciated by service users, this does not, in and of itself, mean that they are always benign. In some circumstances, distress can be amplified by therapy and some therapists can be abusive and take advantage of the power imbalance in the **therapeutic relationship**. Similarly, the professionalisation mission of clinical psychology can be read in simplistic terms as merely an effort to usurp the oppression of psychiatric dominance with an equally dominant psychology. Within this, occupational closure strategies that are designed to reinforce the strength of the **profession** may have the negative effect of restricting the availability of skilled psychological support; limited access to psychological therapies has clearly been an issue for many service users dissatisfied with mainstream psychiatry.

The focus on the individual as the subject of both psychiatric and psychological treatment has been criticised by more socially minded commentators. These critics point out that the focus on individual distress may have ideological benefits for neo-liberal market economies by diverting attention away from the social changes that are necessary to create a more mentally healthy society. Hence, it has been argued, psychology takes its place alongside psychiatry and other psy-professions within a psychological complex, serving subjugation and social control rather than emancipation or therapy (Ingleby, 1985). In response, it should be noted that many psychologists have concerned themselves with the **social determinants** of mental health, both from a research perspective and in the development of trauma-focused psychological interventions (Sweeney et al., 2016). These developments have contributed to more radical curricula for the education of psychologists and clinical psychologists (Cromby et al., 2013).

DOCTORING THE MIND

Arguably, the most widely available psychiatric care is predicated on various misconceptions about psychiatric distress, both with respect to their **classification** and their causation (Bentall, 2003, 2009). Specifically, conventional psychiatric approaches assume a categorical model of mental illness, with clear dividing lines between different **disorders** and between disorders and healthy functioning, and also where disorders are largely the product of internal dysfunction (for example, that they are genetically determined brain **diseases**). In fact, there is no logical link between assuming a categorical model and internal dysfunction (e.g. many physical diseases, for example essential hypertension, are thought to be largely the product of internal dysfunction but are recognised to exist on a continuum with health), but cognitive psychologists have suggested that the human mind has a natural tendency towards essentialist thinking (i.e. both adults and young children usually assume that phenomena grouped together under a common name have a common underlying cause) (Gelman, 2004; Haslam, 2000).

The origins of the categorical model

The categorical model of psychiatric classification can be traced back to the work of German-speaking psychiatrists in the middle and late 19th century, particularly the work of Emil Kraepelin, whose book, *Clinical Psychiatry: A Text-book for Students and Physicians* (1912), was constantly revised and became highly influential (Bentall, 2003). Kraepelin attempted to find a principled way of dividing psychiatric disorders into different natural kinds, noting three possible ways of doing this: first, researchers could attempt to identify groups of symptoms that occurred together and that had a common outcome (the patients suffering from the symptoms tended to get better or not); second, they could attempt to identify discrete types of neuropathological processes that give rise to mental illness; and third, they could attempt to define disorders in terms of their aetiology. In his later life, Kraepelin sponsored the work of Alois Alzheimer, who discovered the histological abnormalities associated with the disease that now bears his name (it was Kraepelin's idea to call this specific type of **dementia** 'Alzheimer's disease'), and Kraepelin hoped that his young colleague would achieve the same kinds of results when he examined the brains of dead psychiatric patients; of course, Alzheimer failed. Given the absence of relevant knowledge of causal biological factors, therefore, Kraepelin was forced to group disorders according to symptoms and outcomes. However, he hoped that this kind of classification would eventually lead to, and indeed map on to, classification according to specific disease processes.

CASE STUDY:
SCHIZOPHRENIA

Kraepelin is mostly remembered today for his concept of 'dementia praecox' (senility of the young) which was eventually renamed '**schizophrenia**' by the Swiss psychiatrist Eugene Bleuler (1911). However, he described a wide range of psychiatric conditions, including what are now termed the affective psychoses, which he grouped under the name of 'manic **depression**', and also disorders such as Alzheimer's disease which would now be considered within the province of neurology. Bleuler's reformulation of the dementia praecox concept was more than just a change of name; whereas Kraepelin emphasised cognitive deterioration as the core feature of the disorder, Bleuler (who was influenced by Freud) emphasised subtle emotional aspects. The concept of schizophrenia shifted again following the work of a later German psychiatrist, Kurt Schneider (1950), who, for entirely pragmatic reasons (he was seeking ways of improving diagnostic precision), emphasised the positive symptoms (**hallucinations** and **delusions**) which are thought to be the core symptoms of the disorder today. These changes over time have led some people, for example the British clinical psychologist Mary Boyle (1990), to question whether Kraepelin, Bleuler and Schneider were talking about the same condition.

Whereas the clinical concepts that led to the categorical model were largely inventions of the German-speaking world, their solidification in diagnostic manuals was largely a project conducted in the English-speaking world, especially the USA. Although diagnostic manuals existed before the Second World War, the two manuals in wide use today – the American Psychiatric Association's *Diagnostic and Statistical Manual* (DSM), currently in its 5th edition (APA, 2013), and the World Health Organization's *International Classification of Disease* (ICD), which is currently in its 10th edition (WHO, 1992) – were products of the post-war period. The processes by which these manuals have been developed and revised are beyond the scope of this chapter, but it is worth noting that a watershed development was the APA's publication of the third edition of the DSM in 1980 (DSM-III). The authors of the manual, who styled themselves as neo-Kraepelinians (Blashfield, 1984), were mindful of the poor reputation that psychiatry at the time enjoyed within the wider family of medicine, and hoped to create a diagnostic system which would have the precision they admired in other medical specialties. Hence, the system contained clear 'operational' rules for assigning diagnoses to patients, which have been adopted in all subsequent editions of the DSM and the ICD.

The reliability problem

Robert Spitzer (the editor of DSM-III) was aware of the need to show that any diagnostic system has scientific and clinical validity. Working with a statistician, Joseph Fleiss (1974), he had observed two conditions that needed to be met. Diagnoses had first to be reliable, which is to say that different independent clinicians should be able to agree on the diagnoses assigned to patients. However, Spitzer and Fliess also noted that a reliable system might not necessarily be scientifically valid (a disorder defined in terms of a random collection of symptoms can be assessed reliably in principle) and that it was therefore important to show that diagnoses had utility for the functions intended (grouping together patients with similar aetiologies and predicting the natural course of a disorder and its likely response to treatment). Importantly, a diagnostic system could only achieve validity if it was reliable, and hence most of the work on psychiatric classification carried out in the latter years of the 20th century focused on the reliability problem.

Because the level of chance agreement between different diagnosticians depends on the number of diagnoses (two independent clinicians using a coin to assign two diagnoses at random would agree 50% of the time), Spitzer and Fliess suggested a statistical measure of agreement – kappa – which takes into account the number and frequency of diagnoses, and which has been used ever since. Kappa varies between 0 (chance agreement) and 1 (perfect agreement) with 0.7 considered acceptable. Whereas reanalysis of reliability data collected before the introduction of DSM-III suggested that this criterion was very rarely met, Spitzer later claimed that it was met in the field trials carried out to test the new manual (Hyler et al., 1982).

In fact, this claim has been disputed, and re-examination of the DSM-III field trials has led some commentators to conclude that the DSM revolution in reliability was 'a revolution in rhetoric and not reality' (Kirk & Kutchins, 1992). Nor is there any evidence that reliability has improved in the intervening years; in the field trials for DSM-5, the latest version of the manual, only one diagnosis (major neurocognitive disorder; in effect, brain damage) beat the 0.7 criterion, schizophrenia came in at 0.46, and major depressive disorder at a miserly 0.28 (although, by now, anything above 0.4 had been rebranded as 'good agreement') (Regier et al., 2013).

At the time of writing, the limitations of the categorical system described here are being acknowledged, even within mainstream psychiatry to some extent, with various proposals for the development of alternative approaches that are too complex to be discussed here (e.g. Insel et al., 2010; Kotov et al., 2017). Although it is not clear how these approaches will develop, there is emerging agreement that experiences currently diagnosed under different categories of mental illness exist along a continuum of human experience (see Shevlin et al., 2016).

THE HEREDITY MYTH

The idea that psychiatric disorders are inherited brain diseases has a history that is at least as long as the categorical model of psychiatric classification, and played a dark role in the murder of psychiatric patients during the German Third Reich (Meyer, 1988). This view has been apparently maintained by family, twin and adoption studies that have been used to claim that major psychiatric disorders are highly heritable (Gottesman and Shield's (1973) estimate that schizophrenia is 80% heritable is still widely cited), launching a concerted effort to find specific mental illness genes following the development of molecular genetic approaches over the past two decades.

In fact, heritability estimates are perhaps the most misunderstood statistic in the history of psychology. These estimates, which purport to estimate the amount of variation in a trait or disorder in a particular population that can be attributable to genes, are in fact just complex correlation coefficients, and it is a mistake to assume, for example, that an estimate of 80% means that 80% of the cause of a disorder is genetic (see Bentall, 2009 for a detailed explanation). High heritability estimates can mask major environmental influences if environmental variation is low (for example, the heritability of IQ is much higher in middle-class than in working-class families, probably because middle-class families more consistently promote educational attainment in their children), or if there are gene–environment interactions, which are probably ubiquitous in life (for example, if people with particular genes are more likely to be exposed to different causal environments).

Recent findings from psychiatric genetics undermine rather than support standard genetic models of mental illness. For example, recent family studies have found that psychiatric disorders do not run true in a family, so that a child of a parent with a psychiatric disorder is not only at risk of the same disorder but also at risk of other disorders (e.g. Gureje et al., 2011). At the same time, molecular genetic studies have shown that psychiatric disorders are massively polygenic (a very large number of genes each confer a tiny increase in risk, with many linked to multiple diagnoses) so that, for example, 'The genetic risk of schizophrenia is widely distributed in human populations so that we all carry some degree of risk' (Kendler, 2015: 1).

These developments have been paralleled by findings in psychiatric **epidemiology**, which demonstrate that social factors play an important causal role in mental illness. Whereas it has been known for many years that depression is strongly associated with negative life events, particularly involving loss (Brown & Harris, 2012), the discovery that social factors play an important role in the more severe forms of mental illness has been more recent. Social factors now known to be important include poverty and social deprivation (especially if experienced in childhood), migration and belonging to an ethnic minority (particularly if living in a neighbourhood with a low number of people from the same ethnic minority), living in an urban **environment** (especially in childhood), and personal adversities such as early separation from parents, bullying at school, neglect, and sexual or physical abuse (for a brief review, see Bentall et al., 2015). Recent meta-analyses (studies in which statistical techniques are used to synthesise the findings from all available studies) have shown that childhood trauma markedly increases the risk of later meeting the diagnostic criteria for both schizophrenia (Varese et al., 2012) and bipolar disorder (Palmier-Claus et al., 2016).

These findings have important implications for the care of psychiatric patients in general, and for the practice of mental health nursing in particular. On the most general level, they show that psychiatric services that focus exclusively on diagnosis and medical intervention neglect an important aspect of patients' lives. Traditionally, trained psychiatrists are often uncomfortable when discussing the meaning of patients' symptoms and how they are related to their life experiences, but patients find the failure to do this distressing (McCabe et al., 2004). On a more specific level, there is currently a great deal of interest in the **value** of trauma-focused psychological interventions for people with severe mental illness (Sin et al., 2017).

THE VALUE OF PSYCHOLOGICAL THERAPIES

If psychological factors and **coping** are important, then it would appear that a range of psychological interventions for mental distress ought to be justified, along with the desirability of not interfering in the lives of people who do not express they are distressed, even if their experiences appear strange or unusual to others. So-called 'talking' therapies are often appreciated by service users, especially when contrasted with more physical interventions. The research evidence for effectiveness is somewhat mixed, compounded by issues in evaluating success using standard experimental design studies. There is evidence that psychotherapies work, but it is difficult to state clearly which work best and predict which people or which aspects of their experiences, such as voice hearing, might benefit from different approaches (Smith & Glass, 1977; Thomas et al., 2014). One way out of this uncertainty is to focus on factors that successful therapies have in common, such as the quality of therapeutic alliance, rather than try to disentangle differences in effectiveness across treatment modalities (Martin et al., 2000; Wampold & Imel, 2015). For a long time, mental health nurses have been taught to practise these core skills, and latterly there has been a resurgence of interest in therapeutic alliance and engagement within nursing research (McAndrew et al., 2014).

For the last 7 years I have been working as an IAPT therapist. I always thought that people in contact with mental health services deserved more in the way of talking therapies rather than just being prescribed medication, and IAPT promises to make this happen. The service I work in does really valuable work and offers a range of services at different levels including 1:1 guided self-help, 1:1 high intensity therapy, EMDR, couple's therapy, counselling for depression, computerised CBT and group work. However, these are all short term interventions within primary care and therapists may need to refer on to secondary care services. A number of people I have worked with have experienced complex obsessions and compulsions or trauma, and can be military veterans or survivors of disasters such as Hillsborough. It can be really heartening for me to be able to help someone in enduring distress to get some relief from this pain and move on with their life. Doing this work requires effective and supportive supervision and opportunities for professional development, all of which are provided.

Having worked in the IAPT system I can see the real benefits that have been made possible for many people with recourse to CBT type interventions. That said, it is hard not to have concerns with some aspects of the programme. Cuts and financial pressures have contributed to a stressful work atmosphere, where therapists have to stick to inflexible and short timescales. This can create personal dilemmas and even burnout for staff. I am dispirited to see that elsewhere IAPT workers are being located in job centres and their therapy is tied to benefit entitlements. This is a further sign of how work and employment are politicised, benefits claimants are demonised, and professional roles are corrupted. My own post was previously contracted out from the NHS to the voluntary sector, which for me resulted in a substantial pay cut.

I believe that the interpersonal skills I had before IAPT training are most important for helping people: the ability to listen and express warmth, empathy and positive regard.

Bob McGrae, mental health nurse

An emphasis on essential human relational skills is a central feature of this book. Such skills can underpin effective psychotherapeutic interventions of different sorts which can be delivered by nurses with the appropriate training and supervision. They would also appear to be the necessary skills for supportive and collegiate team-working and leadership. Professional practitioners, however, do not have a monopoly on such skills, and we turn now to discuss some alternatives.

ALTERNATIVE FORMS OF HELP AND SUPPORT

Arguably, there is a substantial crossover between psychologically informed ideas for making sense of mental distress, the autonomous **recovery** that can result from supporting individuals in such distress, user-inspired self-help and alternative forms of help. Both the shift away from categorical diagnostic practices towards continua frameworks of human experience and the increasing acknowledgement of trauma as a major factor in the causation of mental distress are evident in movements for more progressive interventions for persons deemed to be suffering from psychotic experiences and, indeed, not intervening when this is neither warranted nor wanted. In contrast to psychiatry, these perspectives view phenomena such as hearing voices as part of normal human experience necessitating understanding, rather than as symptoms to be got rid of (Corstens et al., 2008).

A number of **peer support** groups have developed over the years by people who struggle with certain mental health-related issues such as **self-harm**, hearing voices or **mood** swings. These developments provide an important alternative to conventional support structures, and can also be encouraged within routine care services. Notable amongst these is the Hearing Voices Network initiated by Marius Romme and Sandra Escher (1993). In 1987, voice hearer Patsy Hague persuaded Romme, her psychiatrist, to accept and take her voices seriously and they appeared together on television to promote this new approach. Thus, the hearing voices movement proceeded to normalise the experience of voice hearing and support people who have these experiences, noting the extensiveness of people living with voices and not wishing for psychiatric intervention. A central tenet is accepting the voices and attempting to make sense of their meaning.

The network has on online presence and supports the establishment of local community-based self-help groups. Increasingly, professional voice-hearing facilitators often organise groups within psychiatric services to support detained service users. The ethos of the network is to raise awareness of sensory experiences that are typically diagnosed as hallucinations and symptoms of **psychosis** within mainstream services. The groups are organised to give people who hear voices, have visions or other sensory experiences the chance to talk openly amongst peers and offer each other mutual support. Alongside supporting each other, members of the network are encouraged to make personal sense of their experiences and learn from them in their own way. It is generally acknowledged that many members will have had traumatic experiences in their life and that this may lie behind their voice-hearing experiences, but no single explanation is forced on people. This movement has spawned lots of valuable off-shoot projects, including the *Compassion for Voices* initiative which provides support and information to enable people to develop self-compassion and greater understanding of the function that voices and other unusual experiences might serve in their lives. Inspired by Romme and Escher, the ***Maastricht Approach*** to supporting people who hear voices has led to the development of a treatment intervention for distressing voices called voice dialogue, that involves talking directly to individual voices (Stone & Stone, 1989).

When hearing voices groups started, there was some concern that talking about voices might collude with people's beliefs that they were 'real'. In fact, for most people, accepting the existence of their voices (but not necessarily believing what the voices say) proved extremely helpful. Similarly, when people who self-harmed started to set up their own support groups, concerns were initially expressed that people might encourage each other to self-harm, but this rarely happened. More commonly, people supported each other to find strategies to minimise the physical harm (**harm-minimisation** strategies); find alternatives; and support cessation, when desired. Similarly, in the USA the Icarus Project (Hall, 2012) is an exciting initiative which supports people who experience mania, 'highs' and other extraordinary states of mind (which would usually be referred to as bipolar or psychosis). Rather than seeing these as necessarily negative states to be prevented at all costs, they provide support and information to find creative ways of accepting and channelling these experiences (see http://theicarusproject.net).

Support groups provide an important space for people to relate to and socialise with others who have had similar experiences. One of the difficulties with self-help groups is that their resources are usually very limited and they are not always able to sufficiently support someone who is in crisis, especially over a long period of time.

The **Open Dialogue** approach is notable for fusing psychologically inspired systemic practices with a focus on supportive family networks and the social nature of dialogic communication between members (Seikkula & Arnkil, 2014). There also appear to be some resonances of Laingian commitments to contain psychic distress by empathically being with people, attending to and seeking meaning in unintelligible speech and behaviour, without feeling the need to superimpose a psychiatric frame. Evaluations of Open Dialogue have been very positive, and to some extent the Finnish implementation of the approach has represented a large natural experiment (e.g. Seikkula et al., 2006, 2011). Despite some methodological criticisms, these studies appear to show that: first episodes of psychosis are less likely to be converted into 'chronic cases'; much larger numbers of individuals obtain meaningful employment or enrol in education (about 85% of service users); relatively low numbers are prescribed ongoing **antipsychotic** medication (around 15%); and services are much more acceptable to service users. These figures are almost completely the reverse of what we usually see in standard western models of psychiatry for service users who would attract a psychosis diagnosis (the target group for Open Dialogue), especially in terms of medication prescribing.

CONCLUSION

We suggest that the implications of the critique presented here and the compatibility of progressive psychological and social ideas with emergent service-user-inspired alternatives make a case for working together in productive alliances to support individuals in mental distress and to value notions of autonomous recovery. Rejecting simplistic models of psychopathology and preferring to see various psychic phenomena on a continuum of human experience also leads to the conclusion that some people who do not want clinical help should legitimately be left alone. For those who do want help to minimise distress or cope with distressing experiences, critical psychological ideas can provide a framework for mental health care teams to organise their support based on multi-factor formulations that attempt to make sense of people's distress, taking account of social factors and previous experiences of trauma and stress. Team-based formulations respectfully bring together the views of all disciplines and service users' own attempts to make sense of their experiences, to collectively plan and evaluate care (Johnstone, 2015).

CRITICAL THINKING STOP POINT 14.1

How might the implications of the Maastricht Approach to hearing voices be implemented in the routine practices of acute inpatient or community mental health teams?

CRITICAL
THINKING
STOP
POINT 14.1
ANSWER

CHAPTER SUMMARY

This chapter has covered:

- The discussion of critical psychological ideas
- A critique of standard approaches to psychiatric classification of mental disorders
- Criticism of psychiatric assumptions regarding the heritability of mental illness
- Connections between the implications of critical psychological ideas and alternative approaches to support and self-help inspired by service users' experiences
- The desirability of multi-disciplinary approaches to organising care, including the value of team formulations.

BUILD YOUR BIBLIOGRAPHY

Books

- A particularly good critical textbook written by psychologists is Cromby, J., Harper, D. & Reavey, P. (2013) *Psychology, mental health and distress*. Basingstoke: Palgrave Macmillan.
- Many of the ideas developed in this chapter are discussed in more depth in Bentall, R.P. (2009) *Doctoring the mind*. London: Allen Lane.
- The importance of therapeutic alliance and therapist characteristics for the success of therapy was most obviously taken up in the work of Carl Rogers: see Rogers, C. (1961) *On becoming a person: A therapist's view of psychotherapy*. London: Constable. Later in life, Rogers came to recognise an implicit politics in his work, using dialogic approaches in pursuit of democratic solutions and reconciliation amidst conflict: see Proctor, G., Cooper, M., Sanders, et al. (eds) (2006) *Politicizing the person-centered approach: An agenda for social change*. Ross on Wye: PCCS Books.

SAGE journal articles

Go to https://study.sagepub.com/essentialmentalhealth for further free online journal articles related to this chapter. If you are using the interactive ebook, simply click on the book icon in the margin to go straight to the resource.

FURTHER
READING:
JOURNAL
ARTICLES

- Kinderman, P., Allsopp, K. & Cooke, A. (2017) Responses to the publication of the American Psychiatric Association's DSM-5. *Journal of Humanistic Psychology*, 57(6), 625–649.
- Pilgrim, D. (2014) Historical resonances of the DSM-5 dispute: American exceptionalism or Eurocentrism? *History of the Human Sciences*, 27(2), 97–117.

Other journal articles

- Harper, D.J. (2010) Clinical psychology in context: a commentary on David Pilgrim's 'British clinical psychology and society'. *Psychology Learning & Teaching, 9*(2), 13-14.

Weblinks

Go to https://study.sagepub.com/essentialmentalhealth for further weblinks related to this chapter. If you are using the interactive ebook, simply click on the book icon in the margin to go straight to the resource.

FURTHER
READING:
WEBLINKS

- Compassion for Voices: http://compassionforvoices.com
- Hearing Voices Network: www.hearing-voices.org
- Intervoice: www.intervoiceonline.org
- Jacqui Dillon, writer, activist, international speaker and trainer concerned with voice hearing, trauma and 'psychosis': www.jacquidillon.org

GREAT FOR
REVISION

ACE YOUR ASSESSMENT

Revise what you have learned by visiting https://study.sagepub.com/essentialmentalhealth. If you are using the interactive ebook, simply click on the tick icon to go straight to the resource.

ONLINE
QUIZZES &
ACTIVITY
ANSWERS

- Test yourself with multiple-choice and short-answer questions and flashcards.

REFERENCES

American Psychiatric Association (APA) (2013) *Diagnostic and statistical manual of mental disorders (DSM–5)*, 5th edition. Arlington, VA: APA.

Bentall, R.P. (2003) *Madness explained*. London: Allen Lane.

Bentall, R.P. (2009) *Doctoring the mind: Is our current treatment of mental illness really any good?* London: Allen Lane.

Bentall, R.P., de Sousa, P., Varese, F., et al. (2015) From adversity to psychosis: pathways and mechanisms from specific adversities to specific symptoms. *Social Psychiatry and Psychiatric Epidemiology, 49*, 1011–1022.

Blashfield, R.K. (1984) *DSM-III. In The Classification of Psychopathology* (pp. 111–137). New York: Springer US.

Bleuler, E. (1911) *Dementia Praecox oder Gruppe der Schizophrenien*. Leipzig, Germany: Deuticke.

Boyle, M. (1990) Is schizophrenia what it was? A re-analysis of Kraepelin's and Bleuler's population. *Journal of the History of the Behavioral Sciences, 26*(4), 323–333.

Brown, G.W. & Harris, T. (eds) (2012) *The social origins of depression*. London: Tavistock. [Originally published 1978]

Corstens, D., Escher, S. & Romme, M. (2008) Accepting and working with voices: the Maastricht approach. In A. Moskowitz (ed.) *Psychosis, trauma and dissociation: Emerging perspectives on severe psychopathology*. Oxford: Wiley & Sons. pp. 319–332.

Cromby, J., Harper, D. & Reavey, P. (2013) *Psychology, mental health and distress*. London: Palgrave Macmillan.

Gelman, S.A. (2004) Psychological essentialism in children. *Trends in cognitive sciences*, 8(9), 404–409.

Goldsmith, L.P., Lewis, S.W., Dunn, G., et al. (2015) Psychological treatments for early psychosis can be beneficial or harmful, depending on the therapeutic alliance: an instrumental variable analysis. *Psychological Medicine*, *45*, 2365–2373.

Gottesman, I.I. & Shields, J. (1973) Genetic theorizing and schizophrenia. *British Journal of Psychiatry*, *122*, 15–30.

Gureje, O., Oladeji, B., Hwang, I., et al. (2011) Parental psychopathology and the risk of suicidal behavior in their offspring: results from the World Mental Health surveys. *Molecular Psychiatry*, *16*(12), 1221–1233.

Hall, W. (2012) Icarus Project & Freedom Centre. Available at: http://theicarusproject.net/resources/publications/harm-reduction-guide-to-coming-off-psychiatric-drugs-and-withdrawal (accessed 3 May 2017).

Haslam, N. (2000) Psychiatric categories as natural kinds: Essentialist thinking about mental disorder. *Social Research*, *67*, 1031–1058.

Hyler, S.E., Williams, J.B. and Spitzer, R.L. (1982) Reliability in the DSM-III field trials: interview v case summary. *Archives of General Psychiatry*, *39*(11), 1275–1278.

Ingleby, D. (1985) Professionals as socialisers: the 'psy-complex'. In A.Scull & S. Spitzer (eds) *Research in law, deviance and social control*. New York: Jai Press. pp. 79–109.

Insel, T., Cuthbert, B., Garvey, M., et al. (2010) Research Domain Criteria (RDoC): toward a new classification framework for research on mental disorders. *American Journal of Psychiatry*, *167*, 748–751.

Johnstone, L. (2015) Editorial. *Clinical Psychology Forum*, Special Issue: Team Formulation, *275*, 1–2.

Kendler, K.S. (2015) A joint history of the nature of genetic variation and the nature of schizophrenia. *Molecular Psychiatry*, *20*(1), 77–83.

Kirk, S.A. and Kutchins, H. (1992) *The selling of DSM: The rhetoric of science in psychiatry*. Piscataway, NJ: Transaction Publishers.

Kotov, R., Krueger, R.F., Watson, D., et al. (2017) The Hierarchical Taxonomy of Psychopathology (HiTOP): a dimensional alternative to traditional nosologies. *Journal of Abnormal Psychology*, *126*, 454–477.

Kraepelin, E. (1912) *Clinical psychiatry: A textbook for students and physicians*. New York: Macmillan.

Martin, D.J., Garske, J.P. & Davis, M.K. (2000) Relation of the therapeutic alliance with outcome and other variables: a meta-analytic review. *Journal of Consulting and Clinical Psychology*, *68*(3), 438–450.

McAndrew, S., Chambers, M., Nolan, F., et al. (2014) Measuring the evidence: reviewing the literature of the measurement of therapeutic engagement in acute mental health inpatient wards. *International Journal of Mental Health Nursing*, *23*(3), 212–220.

McCabe, R., Heath, C., Burns, T., et al. (2004) Engagement of patients with psychosis in the consultation: conversation analytic study. *British Medical Journal*, *325*, 1148–1151.

Meyer, J.E. (1988) The fate of the mentally ill in Germany under the Third Reich. *Psychological Medicine*, *18*, 575–581.

Palmier-Claus, J.E., Berry, K., Bucci, S., et al. (2016) Relationship between childhood adversity and bipolar affective disorder: systematic review and meta-analysis. *British Journal of Psychiatry*, *209*(6): 454–459.

Regier, D.A., Narrow, W.E., Clarke, D.E., et al. (2013) DSM-5 field trials in the United States and Canada, Part II: test-retest reliability of selected categorical diagnoses. *American journal of psychiatry*, 170(1), 59–70.

Rogers, A. & Pilgrim, D. (2014) *A sociology of mental health and illness*, 5th edition. Maidenhead: Open University Press/McGraw-Hill Education.

Romme, M. & Escher, S. (1993) *Accepting voices*. London: MIND Publications.

Schneider, K. (1950) *Klinische Psychopathologie*. Stuttgart: Thieme Verlag.

Schultz, D.P. & Schultz, S.E. (2015) *A history of modern psychology*, 11th edition. Boston, MA: Cengage Learning.

Seikkula, J. & Arnkil, T. (2014) *Open dialogues and anticipations: Respecting otherness in the present moment*. Tampere, FL: National Institute for Health and Welfare.

Shevlin, M., McElroy, E., Bentall, R.P., et al. (2016) The psychosis continuum: testing a bifactor model of psychosis in a general population sample. *Schizophrenia Bulletin, 43*(1), 133–141.

Sin, J., Spain, D., Furuta, M., et al. (2017) Psychological interventions for post-traumatic stress in people with severe mental illness. *Cochrane Database of Systematic Reviews, 1*, CD011464.

Smith, M.L. & Glass, G.V. (1977) Meta-analysis of psychotherapy outcome studies. *American Psychologist, 32*(9), 752–760.

Spitzer, R.L. and Fleiss, J.L. (1974) A re-analysis of the reliability of psychiatric diagnosis. *Br J Psychiatry, 125*(0), 341–347.

Stone, H. & Stone, S. (1989) *Embracing our selves: The voice dialogue training manual*. New York: Nataraj Publishing.

Sweeney, A., Clement, S., Filson, B., et al. (2016) Trauma-informed mental healthcare in the UK: what is it and how can we further its development? *Mental Health Review Journal, 21*(3), 174–192.

Thomas, N., Hayward, M., Peters, E., et al. (2014) Psychological therapies for auditory hallucinations (voices): current status and key directions for future research. *Schizophrenia Bulletin, 40*(Suppl. 4), S202–S212.

Varese, F., Smeets, F., Drukker, M., et al. (2012) Childhood adversities increase the risk of psychosis: a meta-analysis of patient-control, prospective and cross-sectional cohort studies. *Schizophrenia Bulletin, 38*(4), 661–671.

Wampold, B.E. & Imel, Z.E. (2015) *The great psychotherapy debate: The evidence for what makes psychotherapy work*. New York: Routledge.

World Health Organization (WHO) (1992) *International classification of disease (ICD)*, 10th edition. Geneva: WHO.

PHILOSOPHICAL UNDERSTANDING OF MENTAL HEALTH

15

TIM THORNTON

--- **THIS CHAPTER COVERS** ---

- Understanding Thomas Szasz and the 'myth of mental illness'
- Kendell, Boorse and value-free accounts of mental illness
- Fulford and value-laden accounts of mental illness
- The link between the nature of mental illness and other key issues.

> I don't think that I ever really thought about 'the philosophy of nursing' when I was training. It all seems to be about the pragmatics, the down to earth stuff that gets the job done and keeps people alive. That's not to say that we weren't encourage to 'reflect', we certainly were, but it was focused on us developing our competencies in a 'novice to expert', Benner sort of way. The times when we could avoid the deep thinking, introspection was when the dust had settled. I remember going home after a night shift on a thoracic ward. I was newly qualified. During the night I had attempted to resuscitate an elderly man who, in retrospect, would have been on an 'end of life pathway' in today's world. I didn't manage to resuscitate him and the resus team told me not to try too hard. Then they disappeared and I had to break the news to his frail wife, waiting in the side room. That was probably the first time in my nursing career that I challenged my assumptions about what made me do this job and what was important. Had I acted ethically? Had I spared suffering? Had I been absolutely honest when I told his wife that we had tried really hard, but there was nothing we could do? In the end, I concluded that truth is important, and kindness is also important.
>
> **Karen, nurse**

Visit **https://study.sagepub.com/essentialmentalhealth** to access a wealth of online resources for this chapter - watch out for the margin icons throughout the chapter. If you are using the interactive ebook, simply click on the margin icon to go straight to the resource.

INTRODUCTION

The philosophy of mental health care is a branch of philosophy which focuses on a number of deep and difficult issues concerning mental **illness**, health and health care. Philosophy itself has been called 'human thought become self-conscious. Its topics are life, the universe and everything' (Blackburn, 2008: vii). It involves the abstract investigation of the world, including ourselves, prior to the establishment of particular empirical methods. Thus, philosophy predates the invention of science by at least 2000 years and natural science can be seen as a recent offshoot of philosophy dedicated to more specific and particular methods of investigation.

Mental health care calls for philosophical investigation because it raises a number of difficult deep and abstract questions. Here are just a few:

- What is the difference between just being different and having a mental illness?
- What, if anything, is the justification for detaining people merely because they have a particular kind of illness?
- Should someone with a mental illness have less say over the nature of their **recovery** than someone with a physical illness?
- Can a **classification** or taxonomy of mental illness, such as the recently published DSM-5, aspire to be as objective as the Periodic Table in chemistry? Or is it more like the Top 40?

Questions such as these seem to arise not just from quirky or accidental features of health care in this particular country at this particular time but from something deeper and more general: the very idea of mental health and illness. If that is so, they cannot be answered by empirical means – experiments, questionnaires, etc. – because such means presuppose that we already know what we mean by 'mental health' and 'mental illness'. Thus, trying to answer questions like these calls for a method based on investigating our concepts, what we mean by key words. That method is philosophy. So, in thinking about questions such as these, we are doing, or rather *researching*, the philosophy of mental health care.

In this chapter, we will examine some recent attempts to answer the first question, starting with Thomas Szasz' suggestion that the answer is 'nothing' because there is no such thing as mental illness. We will then trace some connections between accounts of mental illness and answers to the other questions set out above. Understanding these issues will help you understand the sometimes contested nature of the field of mental health care.

SZASZ AND THE 'MYTH OF MENTAL ILLNESS'

Thomas Szasz' attack on the very idea of mental illness is often thought of as belonging to a wider movement, called '**anti-psychiatry**', which began in the 1960s, questioning the legitimacy of psychiatry. Other thinkers grouped under the same label include the French philosophical historian Michel Foucault, who argued that mental health care was a form of social control developed to support capitalism, and the radical British psychiatrist R.D. Laing. In fact, Szasz rejected the label 'anti-psychiatry' as firmly as he rejected the idea of mental illness, calling it 'quackery squared' (Szasz, 2009).

The centrepiece of Szasz' critique is an article and then a book called *The Myth of Mental Illness*. A key argument is expressed in this passage:

> The concept of illness, whether bodily or mental, implies deviation from some clearly defined norm. In the case of physical illness, the norm is the structural and functional integrity of the human body. Thus, although the desirability of physical health, as such, is an ethical value, what health is can be

stated in anatomical and physiological terms. What is the norm, deviation from which is regarded as mental illness? This question cannot be easily answered. But whatever this norm may be, we can be certain of only one thing: namely, that it must be stated in terms of psychological, ethical, and legal concepts … [W]hen one speaks of mental illness, the norm from which deviation is measured is a psychosocial and ethical standard. Yet the remedy is sought in terms of medical measures that – it is hoped and assumed – are free from wide differences of ethical value. The definition of the disorder and the terms in which its remedy are sought are therefore at serious odds with one another. (Szasz, 1972: 15)

The argument here starts from the assumption that mental and physical illness involve deviations from different norms. Medical intervention, however, is capable of addressing only one sort of deviation – that corresponding to physical illness – and thus it cannot address the kind of deviation from a norm implicit in mental illness. Since the conception of mental illness involves the idea that it can be so treated, there is something incoherent about the very idea: 'Since medical interventions are designed to remedy only medical problems, it is logically absurd to expect that they will help solve problems whose very existence have been defined and established on non-medical grounds' (Szasz, 1972: 17).

Szasz also develops a shorter argument. If mental illness is a deviation from a psychosocial norm, then this leads by itself to an objection of circularity: 'Clearly, this is faulty reasoning, for it makes the abstraction "mental illness" into a cause of, even though this abstraction was originally created to serve only as a shorthand expression for, certain types of human behaviour' (Szasz, 1972: 15).

CRITICAL THINKING STOP POINT 15.1

Think about both these arguments. Are they successful in implying that mental illness could not exist? It might help to summarise them on the back of an envelope. How might one challenge them?

Neither of Szasz' arguments is compelling. Consider the argument of circularity. We can set it out in logical steps as follows:

- Mental illness is an abstraction from a description of deviant behaviour. It is defined in terms of behaviour.
- Mental illness is supposed to be a cause of deviant behaviour.
- Nothing can cause itself.
- So there is no such thing as mental illness.

The argument is driven by a tension between the claims in the first two steps or 'premises'. But, on reflection, there is a natural view of mental illness that captures what seems right about the first premiss without leading to tension with the second. We can concede that mental illnesses are identi-fied via someone's behaviour (for example, what they say and do) without thinking that the illness *is* the behaviour. It may be that the illness is the *cause* of the deviation such that, even though it is picked out by its characteristic effects, it is not identical to them.

Here is an example of this sort of reasoning from a different and clearer context. Lee Harvey Oswald's action of pulling the trigger on 22 November 1963 may be described as his *murdering president John F. Kennedy*, the action of the moment described by its slightly later effect. The action of pulling the trigger thus both caused the death of the president and is labelled using that later event. As the philosopher of mind, Donald Davidson, argues, we often label actions via their effects

(Davidson, 1980: 3-20). Pulling the trigger is just firing the gun and is just murdering the president. Lee Harvey Oswald did all three in a single action because that single action can be described in all three ways. But it is also true, however, that pulling the trigger *causes* the gun to fire and *causes* the president to die. Putting these two sentences together means that we can call pulling the trigger 'murdering the president' but we can also say it causes the death of the president. According to Szasz, however, it is incoherent to identify something by its effects and to say it causes them. But we do this all the time in other areas. (No Szasz-influenced defence lawyer could have argued that, because nothing can cause itself, there could be no such act.) If the analogy holds, then Szasz' argument also fails. To succeed, he would need some independent reason to rule out the claim that the idea of a mental illness is the idea of something that *causes* characteristic behaviour.

The same objection also applies to the argument from different norms. Just because mental illness is identified via divergence from psychological, ethical and legal norms does not rule out the idea that it comprises some underlying biological cause of such divergence and hence might be subject to medical treatment, thus undermining Szasz' argument. This is not to insist that mental illness is such a cause, or that all so-called mental illnesses really are such causes. But Szasz has not shown that they are not.

Despite these objections, however, it may seem that such a defence of mental illness gives too much in conceding that it is defined in essentially value-laden terms. After all, that alone suggests that the status of mental illness cannot be *objective*. Hence, whether someone is mentally ill is not an *objective fact* about them. It is thus worth briefly examining two responses from Christopher Boorse (1975) and Robert Kendell (1975) which challenged just this point.

KENDELL, BOORSE AND VALUE-FREE ACCOUNTS OF MENTAL ILLNESS

Like Thomas Szasz, R.E. Kendell was a professor of psychiatry but, unlike Szasz, he was an establishment figure, becoming chief medical officer for Scotland *and* president of the Royal College of Psychiatrists in the UK. In his article, 'The concept of **disease** and its implications for psychiatry', he argues in defence of mental illness or disease by suggesting a method for assessing the status of mental illness: 'before we can begin to decide whether mental illnesses are legitimately so called we have first to agree on an adequate definition of illness; to decide if you like what is the defining characteristic or the hallmark of disease' (Kendell, 1975: 306).

Reviewing the history of the debate, he comments:

> By 1960 the 'lesion' concept of disease, and its associated assumptions of a single cause and a qualitative difference between sickness and health had been discredited beyond redemption, but nothing had yet been put in its place. It was clear, though, that its successor would have to be based on a statistical model. (Kendell, 1975: 309)

But, as Kendell goes on to say, whilst a statistical model may address some of the weaknesses of a lesion model, statistical abnormality by itself cannot distinguish between 'deviations from the norm which are harmful, like hypertension, those which are neutral, like great height, and those which are positively beneficial, like superior intelligence' (Kendell, 1975: 309). It cannot distinguish disease from mere difference. Some further criterion is needed to address the fact that illness is a specific *kind* of deviation from the norm.

Kendell's preferred solution is based on the work of the British chest physician, J.G. Scadding:

> Scadding was the first to recognise the need for a criterion distinguishing between disease and other deviations from the norm that were not matters for medical concern, and suggested that the crucial issue was whether or not the abnormality placed the individual at a 'biological disadvantage'... He defines illness not by its antecedents – the aetiological agent or the lesion producing the overt manifestations – but by its consequences. (Kendell, 1975: 309)

Kendell goes on to argue that 'biological disadvantage' must involve increased mortality and reduced fertility; 'whether it should embrace other impairments as well is less obvious' (Kendell, 1975: 310). Thus, he uses this criterion to test the idea of mental illness. Does it produce biological disadvantage by reducing fertility or life expectancy? After some investigation – which turns on empirical facts about the effects of these putative illnesses – he is able to come to a modest, positive conclusion:

> Schizophrenia, manic depressive illness, and also some sexual disorders and some forms of drug dependence, carry with them an intrinsic biological disadvantage, and on these grounds are justifiably regarded as illness; but it is not clear whether the same is true of neurotic illness and the ill-defined territory of personality disorder. (Kendell, 1975: 315)

Two things are worth noting about Kendell's approach:

1. His criterion or test of illness is general. It applies to physical and mental illness. Any condition is an illness if it leads to biological disadvantage of the right sort. That said, it is originally derived from considerations of paradigmatic physical illnesses.
2. The criterion is purely factual and **value**-free. It is a matter simply of empirical fact whether a condition increases mortality and reduces fertility. If it does, then it is an illness. If not, then not.

Kendell's approach faces a dilemma, however. On the one hand, there is ambiguity about what 'biological disadvantage' means. Without some further specification, it will not shed light on the nature of mental illness. But, on the other, attempting to solve that problem by appeal to the idea of increased mortality and reduced fertility produces a theory of illness or disease which is vulnerable to the objection that it does not capture what is *essential* to the idea of all illnesses. Roughly speaking, it seems plausible that one might be genuinely ill without this leading to increased mortality and reduced fertility. Whilst those measures might well address illnesses which, specifically, are life-threatening and undermine reproductive ability, neither risk seems to be an essential feature of everything that we might call 'illness' or 'disease'.

At the same time as Kendell's account, the US philosopher Christopher Boorse (1975) also attempted to set out a value-free, purely descriptive account of disease – which he contrasts with illness, although we will ignore that distinction here – but using a conceptually richer notion: biological function. In his article, 'On the distinction between disease and illness', Boorse (1975) claims that:

> The state of an organism is theoretically healthy, i.e. free of disease, insofar as its mode of functioning conforms to the natural design of that kind of organism ... the single unifying property of all recognized diseases of plants and animals appears to be this: that they interfere with one or more functions typically performed within members of the species. (Boorse, 1975: 57)

More precisely, the theory runs:

> An organism is healthy at any moment in proportion as it is not diseased; and a disease is a type of internal state of the organism which:
>
> (i) interferes with the performance of some natural function - i.e. some species-typical contribution to survival and reproduction - characteristic of the organism's age
> (ii) is not simply in the nature of the species, ie is either atypical of the species, or, if typical, mainly due to environmental causes. (Boorse, 1998: 108)

Like Kendell, Boorse suggests that there is more to being diseased than being different. His is not a merely statistical approach. Instead, the sense that there is something wrong about having a disease is captured by the idea that it threatens natural biological functions. But whilst there is a connection between such functions and the contribution they make to an organism's overall fitness, not every such failure of function need be directly correlated with actual increased mortality and reduced fertility. Biological function is thus a more fine-grained approach to the concept of disease or illness than Kendell's appeal to biological disadvantage.

CRITICAL THINKING STOP POINT 15.2

Think about the idea that illness or disease is a failure of biological function. Is this a good definition? Are there any illnesses that are not such failures and are there any failures that are not illnesses? How well does the idea apply to mental illness?

There are two main difficulties with Boorse's approach. The first is that failure of biological function seems more widespread than disease. In other words, not every failure of function deserves to be called a disease. For example, the main function of sperm is surely to fertilise an egg. That function explains why sperm production continues in populations. But very little sperm actually does this. The benefit is so great that widespread failure can be accommodated without any implication of disease. To cope with this problem, Jerome Wakefield has proposed more recently that disease be restricted to the harmful failures of function. His approach combines biological function and dysfunction with the value: harm (Wakefield, 1999). Although his is perhaps the most famous contemporary account, it faces the second of the objections to Boorse.

The second problem concerns the application of the idea of function and dysfunction to mental phenomena: to thoughts and experiences. It seems relatively straightforward to describe the function of the eye, for example, but rather less clear what the function is of the profound sadness of bereavement or even whether it is functional – since it is widespread – or the dysfunctional consequence of emotional bonds that are elsewhere functional (see Critical thinking stop point 15.2). In such cases, it may be that our assumptions about what is and is not mental illness **drive** our assumptions about mental functions, rather than the other way round. If so, the account does not shed any light on what we mean by 'illness' or 'disease'.

FULFORD AND VALUE-LADEN ACCOUNTS OF MENTAL ILLNESS

So far we have contrasted Szasz' claim that mental illness is value-laden with Kendell's and Boorse's claims that it is value-free. How can we referee their dispute? A useful perspective is provided by the psychiatrist and philosopher Bill Fulford (1999). The significant feature of the debate, he argues, is not so much what they *explicitly* disagree on but what they *implicitly* agree and disagree on. Once this is highlighted, a different conclusion can be drawn. Taking Szasz and Kendell to represent the poles of the debate, Fulford argues that:

> Both authors assume that mental illness is the target problem: Szasz wants to 'raise the question, is there such a thing as mental illness?' Kendell, similarly, seeks to 'decide whether mental illnesses are legitimately so-called'. Both then turn to the concept of physical illness, acknowledging certain difficulties of definition, but suggesting criteria which they take to be self-evidently essential to its meaning: Szasz' criterion is 'deviation from the clearly defined norms of the structural and functional integrity of the body'. Kendell's is 'biological disadvantage, which must embrace both increased mortality and reduced fertility'. Finally, both return to mental illness. Szasz points out that for mental illness, the relevant norms of bodily structure and functioning are not available: on the contrary, he argues, the norms of mental illness are 'ethical, legal and social'. Kendell, on the other hand, draws on epidemiological and statistical data to show that many mental illnesses are biologically disadvantageous in his sense, being associated with reduced life and/or reproductive expectations. Hence by Szasz' criteria of physical illness, mental illness is a myth, whereas by Kendell's it is not. (Fulford, 1999: 169)

According to Fulford, Szasz and Kendell both agree that mental illness is conceptually difficult and, by contrast, that physical illness is straightforward, in part because the latter is value-free. From this they deduce value-free criteria for illness and apply them to mental illness with different results. As described above, Szasz argues that supposed mental illnesses are deviations from value-laden norms and thus do not meet the value-free criteria for illness. Kendell argues that they do fit his preferred criteria of increased mortality and decreased fertility.

Fulford argues, however, that the assumption that Szasz and Kendell, and Boorse for that matter, share is wrong. Physical illness is not value-free. It merely seems that way because we tend to agree on the values that underpin physical health and illness, whilst there is much more variation in the values governing mental health and illness. Further, it is a general feature of value judgements that when we agree on underlying values they can become disguised by value-free criteria.

WHAT'S THE EVIDENCE? 15.1

R.M. Hare on value terms

Fulford's account of value terms draws on the work of philosophers such as R.M. Hare (1919-2002) and J.L. Austin (1911-1960), writing particularly in the middle decades of the 20th century, in the 'Oxford school' of linguistic analytic philosophy. In his *Language of Morals* (1952), Hare discusses the logical properties of value terms.

The value *judgements* expressed by (or implicit in) value *terms* are made on the basis of criteria that, in themselves, are *descriptive* (or purely factual) in nature. The value judgement expressed by 'this is a good strawberry', in one of Hare's examples, is made on the basis that the strawberry in question is, as a matter of fact, 'sweet, grub-free'. Hare points out that where the descriptive criteria for a given value judgement are widely agreed, the *descriptive* criteria may come to dominate the use of the value term as a consequence of repeated association. In the case of strawberries, most people in most contexts prefer or value strawberries that are sweet and grub-free. Hence, the use of 'good strawberry' comes to be associated with descriptions such as 'sweet, grub-free', etc. A complaint to a grocer that a strawberry was sour and filled with grubs would not normally elicit the response: 'And you do not like those things?' This contrasts with, say, pictures where there are no settled descriptive criteria for a good picture because there is no general agreement about pictorial aesthetics.

Hare's general conclusion is this: value terms by which *shared* values are expressed may come, by a process of association, to look like *descriptive* (or factual) terms, whereas value terms expressing values over which there is disagreement, remain obviously value-laden in use.

Fulford argues that the same contrast applies to mental and physical illness. It is because mental health care is concerned with areas of human experience and behaviour, such as emotion, desire, volition and belief, where people's values are highly diverse, that it seems more value-laden than physical illness.

Fulford's positive account of the nature of illness draws on the idea of ordinary doing as the kind of action that one 'gets on and does' without having to try, without having intentions explicitly in mind (Austin, 1957). A failure to be able to do this kind of thing, in the absence of external constraint, captures, Fulford argues, the character of experiences of illness. As a hypothesis, moreover, it helps to explain a number of the key features of medicine. In particular, the idea that illness comprises an internally generated failure of ordinary doing explains its value-ladenness because the ineliminable concept of *failure* of ordinary doing itself suggests an ineliminable negative value judgement.

This is true of physical illness as well as of mental illness but because there is much more agreement about the sorts of things we should be able physically or bodily to do, the underlying values can become hidden behind factual criteria for working muscles, hearts and lungs, etc. This contrast between divergent values in mental health care and shared values in physical medicine explains why there is an anti-psychiatry movement but not an anti-cardiology one.

Having now sketched out some competing views of mental illness, and highlighted the potential connection between illness and values, we can now see what connections there are to the other questions raised at the start of the chapter.

THE LINK BETWEEN THE NATURE OF MENTAL ILLNESS AND OTHER KEY ISSUES

First, is there a connection between mental illness and a justification for compulsory treatment? Fulford argues that his account sheds light on why psychotic illness justifies **coercion**. On his account, illness is an internally caused failure of ordinary doing. In the case of other illnesses, the failures concern difficulties in carrying out actions. But **psychosis** involves a loss of **insight**. It thus involves a defect in the reasons someone has for acting. And because actions are the actions they are on the basis of why someone did them, this leads to a constitutive failure to form, rather than merely to carry out, an action.

CASE STUDY:
BILL
FULFORD

Further, in general, people's actions can be excused when there is a breakdown in intention. If one does something which might normally deserve blame merely by accident, mistake or impaired consciousness, one can be excused because one is not responsible for the act. If on a crowded station platform, one steps on someone else's foot, then that is very different from deliberately doing so in an empty art gallery.

Illness can also act as an excuse. A famous example was the trial of Daniel McNaughton who, in the 1800s, shot and killed the secretary of the UK prime minister, believing that the prime minister was conspiring against him. He was acquitted 'by reason of insanity' though detained in a mental institution for life. As a result of the case, British courts adopted the 'McNaughton rule' which allowed for a defence if, at the time of committing the act, the accused was labouring under such a defect of reason, from disease of the mind, as not to know the nature and quality of the act he was doing or, if he did know it, he did not know that what he was doing was wrong. Fulford attempts to shed light on this intuitive idea and to connect it with coercion in the following way:

> All non-psychotic illnesses ... involve ... instrumental failures of 'ordinary' doing, difficulties in doing what one intends to do. And difficulties of this sort often mitigate and, if very severe, may even excuse. But in the case of psychotic illness, the failure of 'ordinary' doing ... is a failure in the very specification of what is done. The psychotic, therefore ... lacks intent ... [H]e is thus in the same position as others who lack intent in that he is not responsible for what he does, and, hence, excused. (Fulford, 1989: 242-243)

This idea that lack of intent excuses an action can be connected through two links to the problem of justifying compulsory treatment. First, psychotic illness, in which a person lacks insight into his or her condition, undermines the person's capacity to form reasons and thus connects to defective intent. Second, someone whose purported actions can be excused by defective intent, which may undermine their status *as* actions, is also by that fact the kind of subject whose autonomy can justifiably be overridden.

As Fulford spells out, there is of course a sense in which people with psychotic loss of insight clearly do form intentions, just as there is a sense in which they clearly do have reasons for their actions. The point is rather that, to the extent that their actions reflect psychotic loss of insight, those reasons are defective, in whatever (as yet to be determined) way delusional reasoning is defective. Defective reasons for action imply defective intentions, hence excuse and hence also provide a rationale for **compulsion** by others.

This general approach promises to shed light on the key justification for compulsory treatment. There are, however, still some questions remaining. Do all cases that merit compulsory treatment involve defective intent? Why precisely does such a defect justify treatment? What exactly is the connection between the possibility of excusing purported actions because of some failure of intent and overriding the agent's remaining autonomy? And what precisely comprises a relevant defect of intent? Is it right to say that there is a lack of intent, or a failure within the specification of intention, or an impaired intention or what? Nevertheless, it suggests that psychiatry carries with it quite specific medical ethical complexities which flow from the fact that it centres on **disorders** of human agency.

This line of reasoning suggests one factor in an answer to the next question raised at the start, too: should someone with a mental illness have less say over the nature of their recovery than someone with a physical illness? The extent to which mental illness can undermine a capacity to form decisions has to be addressed in decisions about treatment and management. But there is another factor which pulls in the opposite direction. Just as both Fulford and, to a lesser extent, Wakefield argue that the very idea of mental illness is value-laden, so it seems that recovery in mental health care is also value-laden. This is because it is not merely a matter of getting better, or returning to how one was before its onset, or returning to a statistically normal set of mental capacities. Rather, it involves the selection of a way of living which is right for the person concerned.

The Sainsbury Centre for Mental Health policy paper 'Making recovery a reality', begins by summarising some key points of emphasis which, it is suggested, characterise any broadly conceived recovery-based approach. Some of these points are listed below:

- Recovery is about building a meaningful and satisfying life, as defined by the person themselves, whether or not there are ongoing or recurring symptoms or problems.
- Recovery represents a movement away from pathology, illness and symptoms to health, strengths and wellness.
- Hope is central to recovery and can be enhanced by each person seeing how they can have more active control over their lives ('agency') and by seeing how others have found a way forward.
- Self-management is encouraged and facilitated. The processes of self-management are similar, but what works may be very different for each individual – there is no 'one size fits all'.
- Recovery is about discovering – or re-discovering – a sense of personal identity, separate from illness or disability. (Shepherd et al., 2008)

The Scottish Recovery Network summarises its views of recovery in similar terms:

> Recovery is about living a satisfying and fulfilling life. Recovery is about more than the absence of the symptoms of illness. Some people describe themselves as being in recovery whilst still experiencing symptoms … Some people consider recovery as being 'back to the way things were' or back to 'normal' but for others recovery is more about discovering a new life or a new way of being. (Brown and Kandirikirira, 2007: 3)

On this conception, recovery involves a value-rich personal choice. But given, as we have already described, there is a wide divergence of views about the values relevant to mental health and illness, especially to living a good life, this creates a much greater need for those with mental illnesses to be centrally involved in decisions about their care and their hopes for recovery.

Although particularly suited to *mental* health, the recovery model is, however, made more difficult by forms of mental illness. Consider this extract from a first-person narrative of recovering from severe **depression**:

> It took me a long time, for example, to understand, or to re-understand, why people do things. Why, in fact, they do anything at all. What is it that occupies their time? What is the point of doing? During my long morning walks, I watched people hurrying along in suits and trainers. Where was it they were going, and why were they in such haste? I simply couldn't imagine feeling such urgency. I watched others throwing a ball for a dog, picking it up, and throwing it again. Why? Where was the sense in such pointless repetition? (Brampton, 2008: 249)

The complication this raises is this. When she was in the depths of her depression, Sally Brampton ceased to understand why anyone does anything at all. So how could she have set herself goals for her recovery, conceptions of what living well would be, if the very idea of doing things for reasons no longer made sense? On the other hand, imposing ideas of recovery on her risks paternalism. As the medical anthropologist Kim Hopper points out, the experience of mental health and sometimes mental health care may call for 'sensitive work' by nursing staff: 'Deprivation and disgrace can so corrode one's self-worth that aspiration can be distorted, initiative undercut and preferences deformed. Sensitive work will be needed to recover that suppressed sense of injustice and reclaim lost possibility' (Hopper, 2007: 877).

The final question is harder. Can a classification or taxonomy of mental illness, such as the recently published DSM-5, aspire to be as objective as the Periodic Table in chemistry? Or is it more like the Top 40 music charts?

A shameful historical example may illustrate some of the difficulties raised by the value-laden nature of mental illlness. In 1851, the American doctor Samual A. Cartwright delivered a paper to the Medical Association of Louisiana setting out a new mental illness: drapetomania. This was an illness apparently suffered by plantation slaves whose main diagnostic criterion was the disposition to attempt to escape captivity.

Such cases of obviously value-laden diagnoses make a value-free account of illness attractive. As we have seen, according to Kendell and Boorse, mental illness (or, more precisely, disease in Boorse's case) is indeed a value-free, purely factual notion. But, as we have also seen, their accounts face objections. According to Fulford and Wakefield, mental illness is an essentially value-laden notion. For Wakefield, this is a single value: harm. For Fulford, there may be a plethora of values. Indeed, the US psychiatrist John Sadler published a lengthy book on the wide variety of values and even kinds of values in DSM-IV (Sadler, 2004). If this is the case, what kind of values and what kind of classification or taxonomy can underpin mental health care?

First, any value-laden classification will be different from the value-free Periodic Table in chemistry. Even if the criteria for including symptoms or experiences in a particular category are factual and descriptive – like the criteria for a good strawberry – they will reflect original value judgements which cannot be measured by any instrument.

But, second, the issue of the objectivity of a value-laden classification depends on the nature of the values involved. If they are mere expressions of subjective preference, like the Top 40, then they do not answer to anything objective and cannot aspire to being true. On the other hand, they might be thought to be expressions of something independent of any individual's judgement, as moral codes are often thought to be. If so, whilst distinct from the purely descriptive objectivity of the Periodic Table, classifications of mental illnesses would still have a more complex form of objectivity. This raises a key question: what is it to get such judgements right? Recognising the possibility that diagnosis is value-laden at least highlights the potential complexity of clinical decisions and the need to explore differences of views about values as well as the facts involved.

CRITICAL DEBATE 15.1

Grief, depression and the bereavement exclusion criterion

The label 'bereavement exclusion' refers to the way that in the fourth edition (1994) of the *Diagnostic and Statistical Manual* (DSM-IV), individuals could not be diagnosed with major depressive disorder if their symptoms began within two months of the death of a loved one, unless the depressive mood was 'severely' impairing. Given that major depressive disorder could otherwise be diagnosed as early as two weeks after symptoms appeared, bereavement excluded a diagnosis of depression. The rationale was that such symptoms as sadness, loss of interest in activities, difficulty sleeping and concentrating, and decreased appetite can occur in either depression or bereavement. The result, however, was that bereavement, in effect, seemed to immunise people against depression since one could not be depressed and bereaved. Also, no other potentially excluding factors such as job loss were counted. In response to these counter-intuitive features of the diagnosis, the 2013 edition of the *Diagnostic and Statistical Manual* (DSM-5), rather than adding more factors, simply removed the bereavement exclusion. This has led some authors, such as Horwitz and Wakefield (2007), to argue that cases of bereavement will be wrongly regarded as a form of illness when in fact the 'symptoms' of bereavement serve some positive biological function.

CONCLUSION

By its very nature, mental health care raises profound conceptual questions, which call for philosophical rather than empirical research aimed at arriving at a clearer understanding of the underpinning ideas guiding health care. This chapter has illustrated this need by addressing the fundamental question of what, if anything, mental illness is and briefly sketching out some of the key ideas advanced over the last 50 years. One question these rival views differ on is whether mental illness, or disease, is a value-laden or value-free concept and, if the former, what kind of values are involved.

Addressing that question, however, suggests connections to others, such as the justification of coercion, the nature of recovery and decisions made about it, and the objectivity of basic psychiatric taxonomy. A full and proper understanding of the nature of mental illness – the very idea of it – connects to other pressing areas. Philosophical understanding of mental health care is thus not merely an optional extra but a key guide to and resource for good practice.

CHAPTER SUMMARY

This chapter has covered the following ideas:

- Mental health care raises fundamental conceptual issues calling for philosophical reflection.
- The very idea of mental illness is contested and different definitions of what illness is have been debated.
- One key disagreement is whether illness in general is a value-laden or a value-free notion.
- The nature and value-ladenness, or otherwise, of mental illness has connections to the justification of coercion, the role of mental health service users' decision making and the objectivity of classification.

BUILD YOUR BIBLIOGRAPHY

Books

- Fulford, K.W.M., Thornton, T. & Graham, G. (2006) *The Oxford textbook of philosophy and psychiatry.* Oxford: Oxford University Press.
- Fulford, K.W.M., Davies, M., Gipps, R., et al. (eds) (2013) *Oxford handbook of philosophy and psychiatry.* Oxford: Oxford University Press.
- Thornton, T. (2007) *Essential philosophy of psychiatry.* Oxford: Oxford University Press.

SAGE journal articles

Go to https://study.sagepub.com/essentialmentalhealth for further free online journal articles related to this chapter. If you are using the interactive ebook, simply click on the book icon in the margin to go straight to the resource.

FURTHER READING: JOURNAL ARTICLES

- Bas, J.L., Armstrong, D., King, R., Blomfield, J.D. & Phillips, N. (2002) A discussion with D.M. Armstrong about the nexus between philosophy and psychiatry. *Australasian Psychiatry,* *10*(4), 319-324.

- Campbell, A.V. (2005) Mental health practice: can philosophy help? *Australian and New Zealand Journal of Psychiatry, 39*(11-12), 1008-1010.
- Robertson, M. & Walter, G. (2007) Overview of psychiatric ethics I: Professional ethics and psychiatry. *Australasian Psychiatry, 15*(3), 201-206.

Weblinks

FURTHER
READING:
WEBLINKS

Go to https://study.sagepub.com/essentialmentalhealth for further weblinks related to this chapter. If you are using the interactive ebook, simply click on the book icon in the margin to go straight to the resource.

- Association for the Advancement of Philosophy and Psychiatry is an American association promoting cross-disciplinary research in the philosophical aspects of psychiatry and supporting educational initiatives and graduate training programmes: http://philosophyandpsychiatry.org
- International Network for Philosophy and Psychiatry provides a collaborative research and education forum to support organisations and individuals involved in conceptual and ethical work in psychiatry and related disciplines: http://innponline.com
- Metapsychology Online reviews books about mental health and other psychological and philosophical issues: http://metapsychology.mentalhelp.net
- PPP: *Philosophy, Psychiatry & Psychology*, the main journal in the field, is published by Johns Hopkins University Press: www.press.jhu.edu/journals/philosophy_psychiatry_and_psychology

Video

- An overview of the field of philosophy of mental health by Bill Fulford: www.youtube.com/watch?v=g76tETaqfLc

VIDEO LINK
15: BILL
FULFORD

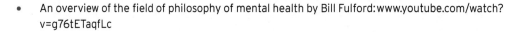

ACE YOUR ASSESSMENT

Revise what you have learned by visiting https://study.sagepub.com/essentialmentalhealth. If you are using the interactive ebook, simply click on the tick icon to go straight to the resource.

ONLINE
QUIZZES &
ACTIVITY
ANSWERS

- Test yourself with multiple-choice and short-answer questions and flashcards.

REFERENCES

American Psychiatric Association (APA) (1994) *Diagnostic and statistical manual of mental disorders,* 4th edition *(DSM-IV)*. Arlington, VA: APA.

American Psychiatric Association (APA) (2013) *Diagnostic and statistical manual of mental disorders,* 5th edition *(DSM-5)*. Arlington, VA: APA.

Austin, J.L. (1957) A plea for excuses. *Proceedings of the Aristotelian Society, 57,* 1–30.

Blackburn, S. (2008) *The Oxford dictionary of philosophy.* Oxford: Oxford University Press.

Boorse, C. (1975) On the distinction between disease and illness. *Philosophy and Public Affairs, 5,* 49–68.

Boorse, C. (1998) What a theory of mental health should be. In S.A. Green & S. Bloch (eds) *An anthology of psychiatric ethics.* Oxford: Oxford University Press. pp. 108–115.

Brampton, S. (2008) *Shoot the Damn Dog: A Memoir of Depression*. London: Bloomsbury.

Brown, W. & Kandirikirira, N. (2007) *Recovering mental health in Scotland: Report on narrative investigation of mental health recovery*. Glasgow: Scottish Recovery Network.

Davidson, D. (1980) *Essays on actions and events*. Oxford: Oxford University Press.

Fulford, K.W.M. (1989) *Moral theory and medical practice*. Cambridge: Cambridge University Press.

Fulford, K.W.M. (1999) Analytic philosophy, brain science and the concept of disorder. In S. Bloch, P. Chodoff & S.A. Green (eds) *Psychiatric ethics*, 3rd edition. Oxford: Oxford University Press. pp. 161–192.

Hare, R.M. (1952) *The language of morals*. Oxford: Oxford University Press.

Hopper, K. (2007) Rethinking social recovery in schizophrenia: what a capabilities approach might offer. *Social Science & Medicine, 65*, 868–879.

Horwitz, A.V. & Wakefield, J.C. (2007) *The loss of sadness*. Oxford: Oxford University Press.

Kendell, R.E. (1975) The concept of disease and its implications for psychiatry. *British Journal of Psychiatry, 127*, 305–315.

Sadler, J.Z. (2004) *Values and psychiatric diagnosis*. Oxford: Oxford University Press.

Shepherd, G., Boardman, J. & Slade, M. (2008) *Making recovery a reality*. London: Sainsbury Centre for Mental Health.

Szasz, T. (1972) *The myth of mental illness*. London: Paladin.

Szasz, T. (2009) *Antipsychiatry: Quackery squared*. New York: Syracuse University Press.

Wakefield, J.C. (1999) Mental disorder as a black box essentialist concept. *Journal of Abnormal Psychology, 108*, 465–472.

SPIRITUAL CARE: UNDERSTANDING SERVICE USERS, UNDERSTANDING OURSELVES

16

JULIAN RAFFAY AND DON BRYANT

THIS CHAPTER COVERS

- Spiritual care and its relevance to nursing
- Spiritual care in practice
- Understanding spiritual strengths
- Spiritual care and diversity
- Issues in spiritual care.

> The account below is factual (though anonymised). It shows the multi-disciplinary approach used by chaplains:
>
> Tom, a community psychiatric nurse, approaches the chaplain for advice on Jane who has a diagnosis of schizophrenia, believes her house is haunted and she reports seeing ghosts. The chaplain meets Tom who outlines Jane's history and reports her hearing crackling sounds around the house and getting electric shocks. He also describes Jane experiencing unpleasant smells coming from under the stairs and hearing voices. The chaplain considers Tom's report, considers various explanations, and they visit Jane. After a reasoned conversation with Jane, the chaplain seeks to rule out alternatives to the diagnosis. An electrician is brought in and condemns the electrical installation. The smells under the stairs vanish after removing a load of damp, unwashed clothes. Much encouraged and a couple of visits later, Jane tells the chaplain her parents threatened her with ghosts when she misbehaved. To reassure Jane, the chaplain sprinkles holy water around the house, praying that Jane may find peace in every room. The chaplain and Tom decide that Jane's root problem is social isolation and arrange for her to join a church sports group. Jane is eased off her medication and discharged within three months.
>
> Lisa, chaplain

> Mental illness can be an extremely frightening place to be. The feeling of inadequacy, worthlessness, lack of interest and emotion can be all-consuming and self-defeating in terms of recovery. Often stimuli are required to address these issues. These may take the form of medicines, psychological therapies, love and support from family and friends, together with spiritual care. If we believe that recovery is the objective then we need a strong core belief that it is possible. Medicines can help treat the immediacy of the illness and to an extent control it but alone will not enable recovery. The will to recover comes from within and is aided by many external factors including, very importantly, spiritual care in all its aspects. Giving service users a belief and reason for things to get better is vital to recovery. By understanding and expounding on service users' beliefs, faith and fears, chaplains have a vital role to play in both inpatient and community settings.

Don Bryant, service user

INTRODUCTION

This chapter locates an important aspect of nursing care – attending to spirituality – as crucial to a broader holistic approach. Participatory practices are emphasised within a context of meaning-making and self-reflection:

> Terms such as 'participation' and 'self-determination' are so broad [...] they can mean different things to different people. [...] The result, as research studies of user involvement have shown, is that there is often a huge gap between what professionals claim [sic] to be doing in this respect and the reality, despite the 'good intentions' of the professionals involved. (Ferguson, 1997: 27)

Just for a moment, recall the last time you went to a supermarket. What did you experience at the checkout? Respect, care, good humour, or disrespect, disinterest, resentment? Suppose for a moment that, everywhere you went, day after day, people appeared to have no time for you or interest in you. That, sadly, is how **service users** often describe their experience of ward staff. By contrast, Forrest et al. (2000: 52) observe:

> A 'good' nurse was frequently described by users as someone with the lay qualities of: 'common sense'; 'warmth and sensitivity'; 'being nice'; and 'someone who can be a friend'. These findings are consistent with other research which suggests that service users appear to value professionals' interpersonal and 'human' qualities rather than specific therapeutic approaches.

Whenever I (JR) have asked nurses what they would hope for if admitted, similar 'human' qualities top the list. Perhaps they recognise Forrest et al.'s (2000: 53) further point that: 'If a nurse cannot function at the "human" end of the [professional–human] continuum there cannot be progress towards professional help'. So, why the mismatch between what nurses would personally **value** and what they deliver?

CRITICAL THINKING STOP POINT 16.1

What do you think is the meaning of 'someone who can be a friend'? We can easily devalue service users by imagining such remarks to be naïve and unrealistic. However, they may reflect a depth of insight we struggle to engage with.

In this chapter, we argue that spiritual care lies at the heart of effective and compassionate care. It is something we ignore at our own peril, rather than an optional bolt-on for the religiously minded. However we see it, hope is pivotal, central to our wellbeing (Loehr & Schwartz, 2003; Frankl, 1962). Its presence makes a 'good' nurse and its absence will powerfully **affect** the presentation of self and the quality of relationships. The film *Patch Adams* (Shadyac, 1998) illustrates the point well.

I (JR) remember when I started out as a support worker, realising one day that I was drinking to excess. What shocked me was discovering it had crept up on me. Inevitably, there will be times when, as a registered nurse, you will find yourself under pressure at work and potentially in your personal life. In the face of the 'perfect storm' (Raffay, 2012), what will serve as your compass? Where will you find resilience? What resources will equip you to recover? You may not experience the perfect storm, but relentless shifts, lack of clarity, staff shortages and excessive targets can do just as much damage (Anthony & Crawford, 2000; Francis, 2013).

Balancing the technical and human aspects of nursing demands careful attention to each. It demands proper attention to continuing professional development and to ourselves as spiritual beings. We need to be honest with ourselves and take responsibility for our own and our team's wellbeing day in, day out, building resilience for the hard times. Kara, from her perspective as a **carer**, remarks that service users, carers and staff are altogether more alike than is often acknowledged (Francis, 2013: 131). What works for one works for all.

SPIRITUAL CARE AND ITS RELEVANCE TO NURSING PRACTICE

In an online survey of 4054 nurses, 43% strongly agreed and 40% agreed that 'spirituality and spiritual care are fundamental aspects of nursing' (McSherry & Jamieson, 2011: 1764). The authors inferred: 'many nurses [...] feel inadequately prepared to deal with spiritual issues and this aspect of nursing care is not sufficiently addressed within the programmes of nurse education' (p. 1765). McSherry (undated: 10) suggests that perseverance will more than pay off:

> Spirituality is a difficult concept to define but this should not diminish its significance or credibility. It is no more complex than other commonly used terms within health care. Think how difficult it is to define everyday terms such as care, community, love, attention, affection and so forth. The fact that spirituality is difficult to define and that people tend to define it in different ways is not unusual in terms of the language we use as health care professionals.

NHS Education for Scotland (2009) defines spiritual care as:

> that care which recognises and responds to the needs of the human spirit when faced with trauma, ill health or sadness and can include the need for meaning, for self worth, to express oneself, for faith support, perhaps for rites or prayer or sacrament, or simply for a sensitive listener. Spiritual care begins with encouraging human contact in compassionate relationship, and *moves in whatever direction need requires.* [our italics]

The last six words put the patient rather than the nurse in control of the conversation (an approach consistent with client-centred therapy and its derivatives).

CRITICAL THINKING STOP POINT 16.2

Do you consider spiritual care relevant to nursing practice? If not, why not?

The importance of the human dimension becomes clear when we 'imagine the case of a fast food outlet that prioritizes keeping queue length to a minimum, but is avoided by customers who find the staff uncommunicative. Any further emphasis on minimizing queue length would only exacerbate the problem' (Raffay, 2014: 942).

Jay (2013: 55) suggests why Forrest's (2000) observations might hold:

I have sought to define spiritual care not as a particular activity or intervention, but as a quality of relationship that is a professional relationship, [...] one focused on the person rather than the illness, and that allows for a degree of reciprocity in order to be a real rather than a wholly one-sided relationship. It is concerned with discernment rather than diagnosis, it refrains from imposing solutions – indeed it has at its heart the ability to stay with a person when there are no solutions, no answers, and because of this is not afraid, indeed is obliged sometimes to stand without apology on the edge of mystery.

CRITICAL THINKING STOP POINT 16.3

Spend some time considering your work this week. What might you have done differently? How might you include Jay's approach in your work over the coming months?

Jay (2013: 46) cites Mitchell and Roberts who suggest that spiritual care:

is not something extra that we do, but the application of insight and understanding to all that we do. It is as much a way of being as a way of doing ... Spirituality is not a special form of treatment; there are no technical routines that are inherently spiritual. It is the way in which the work is carried out that imparts the spiritual quality. (2009: 50)

Their definition explains why spiritual care cannot be left to chaplains alone.

CRITICAL THINKING STOP POINT 16.4

Spend a moment thinking about the characteristics of a good nurse. You may find it helpful to reflect on individual colleagues, especially those you admire. Think about asking patients, friends or relatives who they consider to be the best nurses and why.

SPIRITUAL CARE, RECOVERY AND CO-PRODUCTION

Spiritual care, like **recovery**, is a rallying point as well as a concept. People turn to (or from) spirituality to express their wish for a different service or different emphasis. As a movement, spiritual care has political power within the organisation. It may, in time, become more influential or may, amidst the shifting sands of policy, jargon and concepts, find itself absorbed by recovery approaches. Some new idea such as **co-production** may eventually absorb both. What matters is service improvement and recovery, however framed (Raffay, 2011). Concepts like spiritual care can enlarge the human spirit and deepen our understanding and respect for one another. We need to be wary of any tendency to over-reach ourselves and encompass all human experience (Jay, 2013).

CRITICAL THINKING STOP POINT 16.5

Describing spiritual care and recovery as rallying points recognises these approaches as movements rather than purely as ideas.

SPIRITUAL CARE IN PRACTICE

CASE STUDY:
SPIRITUAL
CARE

About 15 years ago, the NHS focused on so-called 'spiritual needs'. This ensured staff provided special diets, prayer mats, Bibles and similar. The approach had two disadvantages. First, it cast religious people as needing an emotional crutch. Second, it failed to recognise that a person's spirituality could be their most important source of resilience, a protective factor, reducing the likelihood of **self-harm** and suicide.

SPIRITUAL STRENGTHS

Gilbert et al. (2011) and Parkes and Barber (2011) advocated redefining spirituality to recognise strengths as well as needs. A wise nurse will recognise that time spent affirming a person's spirituality will, usually, speed recovery. Parkes and Barber (2011) offer invaluable 'how to' tips. You may wish to consider your own spiritual strengths/resilience and how you will preserve (or find) hope during your work (and home life). How might you help service users, carers or colleagues to do similar?

CASE STUDY 16.1

Ahmed, a service user on an acute ward, won't take his morning medication. He becomes hostile and is put on 1:1 observation. During that time, a support worker gets to know Ahmed and asks what's bothering him. He explains that it is Ramadan and the medication makes him drowsy for midday prayers.

The support worker mentions this to the qualified staff who immediately arrange for Ahmed's medication to be rescheduled. Ahmed is delighted. His relationship with the staff improves dramatically. He makes a speedy recovery and continues to volunteer on the ward as a gardener after his discharge.

Questions

- If you were (or have been) admitted to a psychiatric unit, what resources would you (or did you) draw on for resilience?
- How can you build your readiness to cope with pressure and distress?
- How can you become more aware of how people find resilience (e.g. Ahmed and prayer)?
- Do you think the ward staff could have avoided the stand-off with Ahmed?

WORKING ALONGSIDE A SERVICE USER AND USING ASSESSMENT TOOLS AND CARE PLANS

Steele (2012) remarked: 'As a service user, it frightens me silly that my spirituality might be overlooked. If that was overlooked, I don't see any point in even looking at recovery because that is what my recovery would be about.' We agree with Steele and consider the problem largely one of formation. Nurses can easily imagine that spiritual care is another discipline like pharmacology that they can learn. But this approach disappoints when their typically limited knowledge fails to elicit the anticipated response from the service user. Spiritual care is essentially different from technical skill and is chiefly about human encounter. It is naïve to imagine a 25-year-old nurse could, after reading a textbook, know more about the faith experience of a 50-year-old Sikh than the person themselves. They are likely to gain little by reading about the 5 Ks of Sikhism. They could more usefully learn from the service user what their faith means to them and how they frame their **illness**. Nurses and other staff will almost certainly receive a welcome response and confer dignity by listening with interest, by supporting that person's experience of life. In doing this, they will be undertaking assessment (Raffay, 2012; see also Edwards & Gilbert, 2007 – 'assessment' comes from the Latin, to sit alongside).

SPIRITUAL CARE AND DIVERSITY

Keeping diversity in mind is essential when we consider broad comments about spirituality in different clinical settings. For instance, older people are often considered more religious. This could simply be because older people have time to reflect. Middle-aged people may be assuming the role and values of their elders. What matters is whether an individual service user considers themselves spiritual and/or religious and how that shapes their understanding of their context and expectations of care.

This, too, is shallow thinking. It is wrong to imagine two groups: the religious and others. Most people are religious and/or spiritual in differing degrees, in differing ways, at different times of their lives and in different circumstances. There is no substitute for spending time with a service user and learning what makes them tick. It takes time to understand, for instance, the mind of a Christian who considers they have a problem with pornography. You need trust before you hear the account of a Muslim who fasts in Ramadan and goes for a pint with his colleagues after sunset. When it comes to diversity, we often do best with those most like ourselves!

CRITICAL THINKING STOP POINT 16.6

Saying there can be no substitute for spending time with a service user raises the question of who defines success in mental health. Co-production implies that it has to be both the service user and the staff, each making their 'vital' contribution (Slay & Stephens, 2013). Staff experience enormous pressure from the 'perfect storm' to be in the office rather than on the ward with service users. How will you respond?

In forensic settings, we need to recognise the emotional significance of 'born again' or redemptive experiences; indeed, authors writing from a clinical perspective have used redemption metaphors in this context (Adshead, 2011; Adshead et al., 2015; Dorkins & Adshead, 2011; Ferrito et al., 2012; McKeown et al., 2016). Teachings about the possibility of a new start are highly relevant as people reflect on crimes they have been charged with. Transformation may be deep and genuine. Others may 'fake it', hoping to reduce their minimum term. Many aspire to a better life but also experience temptation to return to 'old ways' (as we do ourselves). Conversions can bring advantages, including extra visits and better food. Being practical, chaplains usually look for evidence over time before acknowledging change. Positively, the closeness of forensic life can bring influence to bear when fellow patients share what 'works' for them. Reflection on our own personal resolutions and failures may make us more compassionate.

In the case of Islam, a nurse's apprehension around radicalisation can make conversation more difficult yet also more important. Muslim chaplains are greatly valued for their expertise. In the face of apprehensions around national security, members of other faiths, not least Christians, can find their religious concerns and values pushed to one side. Although 'religion or belief' is a protected characteristic under the Equality Act 2010 (HM Government, 2010), we should give equitable attention to all, including those of no faith. The term 'spiritual but not religious' (SBNR) is a slowly growing research field in its own right and Ammerman's (2013) work provides a good introduction.

Substance misuse services have an interesting relationship with spirituality (Cook et al., 2011). The word 'recovery' originates in Alcoholics Anonymous (AA). AA in turn traces its roots to the York Retreat founded in 1796, a Quaker foundation established to deliver more humane care. The third of AA's Twelve Steps refers directly to God or a Higher Power (defined by the member). As in forensics, we may recognise the need for something akin to a 'born again' experience to find the will to overcome substance misuse. Interestingly, such matters offer pause for thought about the balance between self-reliance and belief in greater power and reflection on the fact that twelve-step programmes also emphasise **peer support**, perhaps connecting to co-production values.

In **dementia** services, spirituality offers ritual. Familiar words provide powerful resources for wellbeing. Chaplains and nurses may be familiar with service users who, having lost the ability to communicate, 'come to life' when reciting the Lord's Prayer or a familiar hymn, completing them without help. Enabling a person with dementia to attend church (or equivalent) can reinforce these reminiscences and may reassure and settle them beyond the immediate experience.

People with learning disabilities are often assumed incapable of spirituality (Harshaw, 2016) but such passive discrimination reveals deep prejudice. People with learning disabilities have equal rights to a rich and interesting life, including opportunities to explore or reject a religious faith. Indeed, Harshaw (2016) suggests their spirituality may run deeper than other people's. Co-production with people with learning disabilities can be hugely valuable in developing suitable services and provision.

THE ROLE OF SPIRITUAL AND PASTORAL CARE DEPARTMENTS (CHAPLAINCIES)

Marie Curie Cancer Care's (2010) *Spiritual and Religious Care Competencies* offers a helpful approach. The charity considers that spiritual care is everyone's responsibility, with some staff exercising leadership as specialists at different levels. Chaplains are responsible for advising on policy and supporting practice. They may liaise with a ward or unit through a member of staff (e.g. a spirituality champion).

Chaplains support staff as well as service users and carers. They often act as shock absorbers within the organisation, easing conflict, improving communication and offering advocacy. They can be especially helpful if there is a death or an injury on the ward and offer valuable support to ward managers, senior staff, frontline staff and service users alike. In such circumstances it is important to involve a chaplain swiftly rather than as an afterthought a few days later. Chaplains typically spend at least as much time with people of no faith as with people of faith. They are comfortable working with people of other faiths to themselves. Contrary to popular opinion, most people of faith welcome a leader of another faith.

Referrals to spiritual and pastoral care teams are easy to make, though, depending on the type of hospital, it may be realistic to allow for a few days' delay in getting a response. Seek guidance from the teams' publicity, spirituality pages of your Trust's website, or contact the switchboard. It is helpful to advise on urgency, risk issues and whether the service user would like to see a chaplain from any particular faith. Email may be as good as phone, depending on the hardware available locally. When referring, we suggest using service user initials for confidentiality, except where these are unusual.

WORKING WITH FAITH COMMUNITIES AND OTHER ORGANISATIONS

It would obviously be offensive to suggest people from a particular **culture** invariably like music with a certain beat. However, nurses often stereotype people around religious faith. We may instinctively call a Buddhist for a Buddhist service user, but from what Buddhist tradition? Why assume all Buddhists hold the same beliefs and worship in a similar manner? Buddhism has existed some 2500 years. Long before modern communications, it spanned the entire south-Asian continent.

Inevitably, there are different schools of Buddhism and a conversation with the service user may identify which they belong to. They may prefer one temple or leadership style to another (for reasons perhaps not wholly different to why someone might prefer a particular Zumba class). Uninformed public broadcasting has regrettably given the impression Muslims all hold the same opinion. In reality, there are Sunnis and Shi'as. Adherents within either may adopt a Sufi approach. Similar issues reflect the richness of most, if not all, faith groups.

CASE STUDY 16.2

Ken enjoys the church he attends and Sunday morning is the highlight of his week. He values the friendship of the small groups and contributing to his faith community. He loves working the sound mixing desk and the projection system. The church members recognise his valuable contribution. He considers that his faith helps him cope with his bipolar condition. The ward staff have asked him to draw up a wellness recovery action plan/Recovery Star but he hasn't said anything about his faith

(Continued)

as he feels they wouldn't be interested and his discharge might be delayed. This lack of communication stands in the way of the possibility that church leaders might, with Ken's consent, work with the mental health team. Cooperation would enable the team to be alerted when Ken's condition began to deteriorate. It could also enable exploration of how Ken's strengths could contribute to fuller and potentially paid occupation.

Questions

- How does your own stance on faith influence your reaction to Ken's belief that his faith helps him cope with his mental health problems?
- Why do you think Ken might not feel able to talk about his faith and fear discrimination if he did?
- How do we balance the opportunities faith communities provide with concerns for vulnerable adults?

Safeguarding presents an interesting issue when it comes to inviting non-NHS staff in to support service users, often at short notice. Centrally organised religious groups (such as Church of England and Roman Catholic) have robust policies, whose standards may be better than those within the NHS. Less regulated faith groups may pose greater risk. In assessing risk, it is worth considering the frequency and intensity of visits. We are not suggesting that faith leaders necessarily pose any greater risk than other visitors or professionals. However, except for chaplains and volunteers recruited through NHS procedures, nursing staff need to be aware that spiritual care (chaplaincy) teams cannot monitor the credentials of people on lists of religious leaders.

Possible anxieties around safeguarding should not cause us to overlook the significant support service users can get from faith communities. Some service users may not want their illness known about, but others would welcome a thoughtful offer to contact their faith community leader. Sadly, many do not raise the matter, expecting staff prejudice, whereas it is simple to consult the service user. Visits, fetching personal items and overseeing accommodation are just some of the obvious advantages for inpatients (though it may be advisable, as a precaution, to document such arrangements). Other advantages include comradeship and support and follow-up (or collaborative working with the service user's agreement) after discharge.

SPIRITUAL CARE AND THE MENTAL HEALTH ACT CODE OF PRACTICE

The Mental Health Act Code of Practice (2015) in England and Wales considers 'religion or belief' (p.24 § 1.14). This is clearly framed within the Equality Act 2010 and that should encourage the compassionate nurse to give due and fair consideration to all nine Protected Characteristics without partiality. Section 23.9 specifically states that **medical treatment** can only be appropriate if 'particular circumstances, including cultural, ethnic and religious or belief considerations' (p. 247) are fully taken into account. It is hard to see how this might be assured without a proper spiritual assessment (Raffay, 2012) and we may lament staff disregard, given its importance to service users (Walsh et al., 2013). Strangely, the Code of Practice only mentions spirituality explicitly when considering aftercare (p. 357, § 33.4) and care planning (p. 366, § 34.19). However, its second Guiding Principle, 'Empowerment and Involvement' (p. 23, §1.7), clearly implies that whatever is important to the service user (or carer) should be important to the nurse. It may alert us to beware of the commonly used phrase 'patient needs', which often actually means 'nursing needs' and may have limited bearing on what actually concerns the service user. Though our brief analysis identifies the Code of Practice as favourable to spiritual care, we need to recognise issues staff should consider if they are to have a rounded understanding.

ISSUES IN SPIRITUAL CARE

WHAT'S THE EVIDENCE? 16.1

Much of the research is US-based and has been conducted by Koenig (2015). Overall, Koenig reports a positive impact between belonging to a faith community, practising a faith, and mental wellbeing. UK-based research on spiritual care is limited. Indeed, there are no robust studies on the impact of spiritual care in mental health (Jankowski et al., 2011; Mowat, 2008; Pesut et al., 2016; Snowden et al., 2013). The main reasons for this are the barriers small chaplaincy teams experience in becoming research active and the diffuse nature of spirituality. This lack of evidence should not lead us to conclude that spiritual care is irrelevant as it is greatly valued by service users (Raffay et al., 2016). It may suggest that arguments for evidence-based practice are more complex than they first appear (Kendall et al., 2011).

EXPLORATION OF THE INDIVIDUAL NURSE'S CONTRIBUTION, VALUES AND ATTITUDE

Our values interact with those of our colleagues. Whether support worker, nurse or ward manager, we exercise leadership by example, even if we are unaware of this. Edwards and Gilbert (2007) have diagrammatically represented how staff shape the culture of their services and either foster or deny the spiritual. Few appreciate how their personal preferences may either advantage or compromise the recovery of service users. Koslander and Arvidsson (2006: 597), in their grounded theory study, reported that service users 'actively sought the assistance of nurses to meet their spiritual needs. [When they met disinterest,] they turned their thoughts inwards and found community with other patients, while nurses often avoided addressing the spiritual dimension'. Burkhart and Hogan (2008) offer a theoretical framework with nurses awaiting cues from patients. They suggest that some nurses will seek to convey openness in their manner but imply they will be reluctant to take the initiative. While this approach appears laudable, the account of Ken (Case study 16.2) explains why standoff is the most likely outcome. Service users are often fearful of raising spiritual matters and the opportunity for doing so safely needs to be communicated explicitly within an atmosphere of trust and mutual respect.

HEALTHY AND UNHEALTHY INDIVIDUAL SPIRITUALITY

Anyone who has worked in mental health will have faced claims of demonic possession. Collusion with such thinking may be harmful when abused people blame themselves for crimes perpetrated against them (Faith and Order Commission, 2016). Supervision is essential in this area, especially when newly appointed, but also throughout one's career. I (JR) have found it helpful to open the conversation (and build relationship) by asking the service user what makes them think they might be demon-possessed. In one instance, I offered much reassurance to someone who believed they were the 'whore' described in Revelation 17.1:16. I pointed out that theologians commonly understood the whore to refer to a city or state rather than to an individual. What was interesting was how spiritual expertise brought about lasting change. Ideas around possession are commonplace in Islam (jinn) and traditional African religion, and cultural sensitivity is invaluable. Absence of cultural competence can cause confusion as when an African-Caribbean service user told me Satan had entered his foot. Thankfully, I realised that this was an expression meaning he had pain rather than anything more sinister. We gain perspective through repeated attentive listening and genuine care. Stuckenbruck (2013) offers interesting **insights** into this world.

Religious **psychosis** is often cited as evidence that religion is harmful in mental health. A nurse colleague pointed out that ward staff inevitably encounter failures of pastoral care in faith communities. Those who benefit from the protective factors and remain in the community (Koenig, 2015) are invisible to secondary care services. Even where an individual imagines they are Jesus or Mohammed, telling them they are deluded and fixated or avoiding facing the situation does little good. Far better to help the person to make sense of their experience, remaining calm and seeking to understand what may be fuelling particular beliefs. It could be powerlessness, self-hatred, childhood abuse, or any manner of things that may become evident over time and with genuine trust and respect.

Crowley and Jenkinson (2009: 255) explore harmful spirituality and suggest that:

> Rather than attempting to classify groups into 'good or bad', 'harmful and not harmful', and their beliefs into 'true' and 'false', it can be helpful to consider a continuum with a critical point after which a group can progress to become harmful, if it takes its beliefs and/or practices to the extreme.

From my (JR) experiences as a vicar, I have found the Johari window very useful (Ingham & Luft, 1955). Either person in a conversation brings aspects of themselves of which they are unaware, whether vicar, nurse, psychiatrist or chaplain. At times, the interaction will be positive but sometimes harmful. A church may invite people to donate to charity and a person who is manic may give more than they can afford. A gurdwara may seek volunteers to help with its hospitality and someone whose marriage is failing may use the opportunity to avoid addressing their domestic life. This recognises the complexity that can be lost when we pathologise spirituality. It goes without saying that there are predatory and dangerous religious groups, though assuming all are dangerous makes no more sense than to assume the same of nurses.

CASE STUDY 16.3

A few years ago, Precious used to describe herself as a new ager. She continues to be interested in crystals and their impact on her health. She is concerned the ward she is on is dirty and that this affects her mind. She says that God has told her she must get pregnant and give birth to his second son. She claims that being on an all-female ward is a Deprivation of Liberties. She wants to involve advocacy and her solicitor.

Questions

- What models or approaches might you use to frame your understanding of Precious?
- What assumptions underlie each of these?
- What do you think would be the relative advantages (and potentially disadvantages) of involving a chaplain or nurse?
- How might listening to Precious pre-empt conflict?

People identifying themselves as LGBTQIA (**lesbian**, gay, **bisexual**, **transgender** queer/questioning, intersex or asexual) often struggle with orthodox religious teaching, especially with Christianity, Islam and Judaism. Though some churches, mosques and synagogues are harsh in singling out sexual difference, many are inclusive. A service user may benefit by moving to the latter. Suggesting LGBT people give up their faith altogether may be dangerous as it may also provide them with resilience. A willingness on nurses' part to discuss (appropriately and sensitively) matters of sexuality is likely to prove invaluable. A referral to (or working with) a chaplain may be suitable (though, occasionally, the chaplain may be the last person they would wish to see).

In the face of a mental health crisis, it is small wonder many service users reach towards sources of identity, purpose and hope. This reaching typically has concurrent positive and negative elements. Service users may explore taking up a faith, giving up their faith, trying another faith, occasionally doing this several times a day. At such times, it is important to offer support but also to allow questioning and exploration. Service users do not need you to have answers but look for reassurance and (implicitly) the core conditions of counselling (Forrest et al., 2000). If they ask for a faith community leader, it may sometimes be worth exploring with them whether the timing is right. It is usually wise to discourage people from making major life changes until they have achieved at least some measure of recovery.

CRITICAL THINKING STOP POINT 16.7

NHS staff generally score best on diversity with those most like themselves. To what extent are we genuinely interested in those whose perspectives, values and upbringing are quite different from our own? Do we experience interest and curiosity or threat and challenge?

HEALTHY AND UNHEALTHY ORGANISATIONAL SPIRITUALITY

It is not only individuals (or indeed faith communities) that are vulnerable to unhealthy spirituality. The same is true of any institution. For instance, staff and students are more fraught towards the end of term. Institutions that once had an excellent reputation nose-dive and up-and-coming ones take their place. On a ward, there is misgiving when a manager takes early retirement. On shifts, some staff mixes work well and everything is hunky-dory – the next day, you find yourself on the shift from hell. Keyes (2002) proposes that we understand mental wellbeing as a continuum rather than as the absence of illnesses we may either have or not have. His approach alerts us to our own vulnerability and helps us better understand our own 'good' days and 'bad' days. It reminds us that we should not interpret every failure of *a* faith community (or nursing team) as evidence *all* are failing.

CASE STUDY 16.4

Sarah attends a mental health support group at her local day centre. She has found this very helpful in the past. More recently, things have not been so good and she would like to leave. She feels that the staff have become distant and formal. Because of fears around rejection, she feels anxious in the days leading up to the group. She has not felt able to share this. Last time she wanted to leave, her care coordinator coldly told her that attendance was a condition of her community treatment order.

(Continued)

Questions

- How might the understanding of spirituality that you have developed in reading this chapter shed light on how you would deal with this situation if you were the team leader?
- What can we do to foster flourishing healthy teams where we work?
- When might it be appropriate to consider raising an issue with senior management or whistle-blowing?

HEALTHY AND UNHEALTHY PERSPECTIVES

May, a clinical psychologist and service user, offers us some invaluable insights. He warns specifically against the way health care professionals can dominate service users by insisting that their frame of reference is the correct one:

> I do not have one formulation of my own experiences of being treated for psychosis, I have several which lend themselves to different paradigms. The psycho-social, the spiritual and the pathological explanations I consider, at various times, all have strengths and weaknesses. (May, 2001: 16)

He challenges the professional model, implying that it is unhealthy and exclusive:

> Recently, at a workshop about challenging 'them and us' prejudices in mental health services, a psychology assistant described to me how, when she mentioned she had experienced a panic attack in a psychology department, everyone went quiet and looked very uncomfortable. If we really want to improve people's mental health then we need to challenge processes of social exclusion that are within the mental health profession's own practices. This includes valuing the diversity of personal experiences and the process of reflection. (May, 2001: 16)

May warns how the odds can be stacked against service users voicing their opinion.

DEVELOPMENTS IN SPIRITUAL CARE

Our own Liverpool-based research is attempting to break through the plateau in conceptualising spiritual care. Our insight lies in seeing co-production (Slay & Stephens, 2013) as opening up new horizons, not simply in spiritual care but potentially across all disciplines. Rather than guessing what matters to service users and carers, we can potentially deliver more effective services by working alongside them in the research, design and delivery of services. To this end, we are conducting an action research cycle. In the first part, we explored service user and carer aspirations for spiritual care (Raffay et al., 2016); and in the second part, we conducted a service evaluation of current practice (alluded to in Wood et al., 2016).

CRITICAL DEBATE 16.1

The National Secular Society (Paley, 2009) has repeatedly argued that religious care should be paid for by faith communities and that it is a misappropriation of NHS funds. Such an approach however flies in the face of NHS obligations under the Equality Act 2010. Yet issues around spiritual care raise the wider issue of what is care, what constitutes evidence and who decides. Co-production suggests service users and carers should have a voice alongside professional bodies and NHS managers. It may resolve the difference between what staff think their job is about and user aspirations. What's more, the example of Ahmed (in Case study 16.1) suggests that spiritual care may save money:

- Do you consider spiritual care to be: (a) the compassionate heart of the NHS and a vital part of safe humane services, (b) something best left to chaplains, or (c) a waste of money?

CONCLUSION

Swinton (2000: 20) gives us insight into the social processes associated with **stigma**:

It is through the myriad of unnoticed social gestures and negative assumptions that people with mental health problems find their sense of self-worth and personhood constantly being eroded. It is through that same process that they come to be perceived, consciously or subconsciously, as 'nonpersons' and consequently excluded from meaningful participation in society.

Effective spiritual care, set within a broader holism, can be protective against these exclusionary forces. We have made a case here that such care is worthy of support within **multi-disciplinary teams**, though this is not necessarily systematically taken up, and such deficiencies contribute to a negative impact for many service users. Such a state of affairs requires attention, and mental health nurses may be the most capable and relevant staff to take up this challenge.

CHAPTER SUMMARY

This chapter has covered:

- The relevance of spiritual care to nursing
- What spiritual care looks like in practice
- Spiritual strengths
- Spiritual care and diversity
- Issues in spiritual care.

BUILD YOUR BIBLIOGRAPHY

Books

- Coyte, M.E., Gilbert, P. & Nicholls, V. (2007) *Spirituality, values and mental health: Jewels for the journey.* London: Jessica Kingsley.
- Morgan, G. (2017) *Independent advocacy and spiritual care: Insights from service users, advocates, health care professionals and chaplains.* London: Palgrave Macmillan.
- Watts, F. (ed.) (2011) *Spiritual healing: Scientific and religious perspectives.* Cambridge: Cambridge University Press.

SAGE journal articles

Go to https://study.sagepub.com/essentialmentalhealth for further free online journal articles related to this chapter. If you are using the interactive ebook, simply click on the book icon in the margin to go straight to the resource.

- Koslander, T., da Silva, A.B. & Roxberg, Å. (2009) Existential and spiritual needs in mental health care: an ethical and holistic perspective. *Journal of Holistic Nursing, 27*(1), 34-42.
- Walton, M.N. (2012) Assessing the construction of spirituality: conceptualizing spirituality in health care settings. *Journal of Pastoral Care & Counseling, 66*(3), 1-16.
- White, M.L., Peters, R. & Schim, S.M. (2011) Spirituality and spiritual self-care: expanding self-care deficit nursing theory. *Nursing Science Quarterly, 24*(1), 48-56.

Weblinks

Go to https://study.sagepub.com/essentialmentalhealth for further weblinks related to this chapter. If you are using the interactive ebook, simply click on the book icon in the margin to go straight to the resource.

- Church of England – Promoting mental health: a resource for spiritual and pastoral care: www.catholicmentalhealthproject.org.uk/new/wp-content/uploads/2016/09/Promoting-Mental-Health-Anglican-resource.pdf
- Compassionate Mind Foundation: https://compassionatemind.co.uk
- NHS England Chaplaincy Programme: www.england.nhs.uk/ourwork/pe/chaplaincy

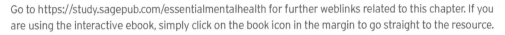

ACE YOUR ASSESSMENT

Revise what you have learned by visiting https://study.sagepub.com/essentialmentalhealth. If you are using the interactive ebook, simply click on the tick icon to go straight to the resource.

- Test yourself with multiple-choice and short-answer questions and flashcards.

REFERENCES

Adshead, G. (2011) The life sentence: narrative group therapy with men who have killed. *Group Analysis, 44*, 1–21.

Adshead, G., Ferrito, M. & Bose, S. (2015) Recovery after homicide: narrative shifts in therapy with homicide perpetrators. *Criminal Justice and Behavior, 42*(1), 70–81.

Ammerman, N. (2013) Spiritual but not religious? Beyond binary choices in the study of religion. *Journal for the Scientific Study of Religion, 52*(2), 258–278.

Anthony, P. & Crawford, P. (2000) Service user involvement in care planning: the mental health nurse's perspective. *Journal of Psychiatric and Mental Health Nursing, 7*, 425–434.

Burkhart, L. & Hogan, N. (2008) An experiential theory of spiritual care in nursing practice. *Qualitative Health Research, 18*, 928–938.

Cook, C., Powell, R. & Sims, A. (2011) Spirituality, mental health, substance misuse. In D.B. Cooper (ed.) *Developing services in mental health: Substance use*. Abingdon: Radcliffe Publishing.

Crowley, N. & Jenkinson, G. (2009) Pathological spirituality. In C. Cook, A. Powell & A. Sims (eds) *Spirituality and psychiatry*. London: RCPsych Publications.

Dorkins, E. & Adshead, G. (2011) Working with offenders: challenges to the recovery agenda. *Advances in Psychiatric Treatment, 17*, 178–187.

Edwards, W. & Gilbert, P. (2007) Spiritual assessment: narratives and responses. In M.E. Coyte, P. Gilbert & V. Nicholls (eds) *Spirituality, values and mental health: Jewels for the journey*. London: Jessica Kingsley.

Faith and Order Commission (2016) *Sexual abuse and the church: A theological resource for the local church*. London: Church House Publishing. pp. 20–21.

Ferguson, I. (1997) The impact of mental health user involvement. *Research Policy and Planning, 15*, 26–30.

Ferrito, M., Vetere, A., Adshead, G., et al. (2012) Life after homicide: accounts of recovery and redemption of offender patients in a high secure hospital. *Journal of Forensic Psychiatry & Psychology, 23*, 322–344.

Forrest, S., Risk, I., Masters, H., et al. (2000) Mental health service user involvement in nurse education: exploring the issues. *Journal of Psychiatric and Mental Health Nursing, 7*, 51–58.

Francis, R. (2013) *Report of the Mid Staffordshire NHS Foundation Trust public inquiry: Executive summary*. London: The Stationery Office.

Frankl, V.E. (1962) *Man's search for meaning: An introduction to logotherapy*. London: Hodder & Stoughton.

Gilbert, P., Barber, J. & Parkes, M. (2011) The service user view. In P. Gilbert (ed.) *Spirituality and mental health*. Brighton: Pavilion.

Harshaw, J. (2016) *God beyond words: Christian theology and the spiritual experiences of people with profound intellectual disabilities*. London: Jessica Kingsley.

HM Goverment (2010) *Equality Act 2010*. London: The Stationery Office.

Ingham, H. & Luft, J. (1955) The Johari Window: a graphic model of interpersonal awareness. *Proceedings of the Western Training Laboratory in Group Development*. Los Angeles: UCLA.

Jankowski, K., Handzo, G. & Flannelly, K. (2011) Testing the efficacy of chaplaincy care. *Journal of Health Care Chaplaincy, 17*(3–4), 100–125.

Jay, C. (2013) What is spiritual care? In C. Cook (ed.) *Spirituality, theology and mental health: Multidisciplinary perspectives*. Norwich: SCM Press.

Kendall, T., Glover, N., Taylor, C., et al. (2011) Quality, bias and service user experience in healthcare: 10 years of mental health guidelines at the UK National Collaborating Centre for Mental Health. *International Review of Psychiatry, 23*(4), 342–351.

Keyes, C. (2002) The mental health continuum: from languishing to flourishing in life. *Journal of Health and Social Behaviour, 43*, 207–222.

Koenig, H.G. (2015) Religion, spirituality, and health: a review and update. *Advances in Mind–Body Medicine, 29*, 19–26.

Koslander, T. & Arvidsson, B. (2006) Patients' conceptions of how the spiritual dimension is addressed in mental health care: a qualitative study. *Journal of Advanced Nursing, 57*, 597–604.

Loehr, J.E. & Schwartz, T. (2003) *On form*. London: Nicholas Brealey.

Marie Curie Cancer Care (2010) *Spiritual and religious care competencies for specialist palliative care*. London: Marie Curie Cancer Care.

May, R. (2001) Crossing the 'them and us' barriers: an inside perspective on user involvement in clinical psychology. *Clinical Psychology Forum, 150*, 14–17.

McKeown, M., Jones, F., Foy, P., et al. (2016) Looking back, looking forward: recovery journeys in a high secure hospital. *International Journal of Mental Health Nursing, 25*, 234–242.

McSherry, W. (Undated) *Spirituality in nursing care*. Available at: www2.rcn.org.uk/__data/assets/pdf_file/0008/395864/Sprituality_online_resource_Final.pdf (accessed 30/10/16).

McSherry, W. & Jamieson, S. (2011) An online survey of nurses' perceptions of spirituality and spiritual care. *Journal of Clinical Nursing, 20,* 1757–1767.

Mitchell, S. & Roberts, G. (2009) Spirituality and psychiatry. In C. Cook, A. Powell & A. Sims (eds) *Psychosis.* London: RCPsych Publications.

Mowat, H. (2008) *The potential for efficacy of healthcare chaplaincy and spiritual care provision in the NHS (UK): A scoping review of recent research.* Commissioned by NHS Yorkshire and Aberdeen: Mowat Research Aberdeen, Scotland.

NHS Education for Scotland (2009) *Spiritual care matters: An introductory resource for all NHS Scotland staff.* Edinburgh: NHS Education for Scotland.

Paley, J. (2009) Keep the NHS secular: John Paley calls for a debate on whether the NHS should be advocating spirituality in health care. *Nursing Standard, 23*(43), 26.

Parkes, M. & Barber, J. (2011) Professional attitudes. In P. Gilbert (ed.) *Spirituality and mental health.* Brighton: Pavilion.

Pesut, B., Sinclair, S., Fitchett, G., et al. (2016) Health care chaplaincy: a scoping review of the evidence 2009–2014. *Journal of Health Care Chaplaincy, 22*(2), 67–84.

Raffay, J. (2011) Assessing spiritual strengths and needs. *The Journal of Health Care Chaplaincy, 11,* 50–64.

Raffay, J. (2012) Are our mental health practices beyond HOPE? *Journal of Healthcare Chaplaincy, 12,* 68–80.

Raffay, J. (2014) How staff and patient experience shapes our perception of spiritual care in a psychiatric setting. *Journal of Nursing Management, 22,* 940–950.

Raffay, J., Wood, E. & Todd, A. (2016) Service user views of spiritual and pastoral care (chaplaincy) in NHS mental health services: a co-produced constructivist grounded theory investigation. *BMC Psychiatry,* 16, 200.

Shadyac, T. (1998) *Patch Adams.* London: Universal Pictures.

Slay, J. & Stephens, L. (2013) *Co-production in mental health: A literature review.* London: New Economics Foundation.

Snowden, A., Telfer, I., Kelly, E., et al. (2013) The construction of the Lothian PROM. *The Scottish Journal of Healthcare Chaplaincy, 16,* 3–32.

Steele, K. (2012) Personal conversation (with permission to publish), 14 May.

Stuckenbruck, L. (2013) The human being and demonic invasion: therapeutic models in ancient Jewish and Christian texts. In C. Cook (ed.) *Spirituality, theology and mental health: Multidisciplinary perspectives.* Norwich: SCM Press.

Swinton, J. (2000) *Resurrecting the person: Friendship and the care of people with mental health problems.* Nashville, TN: Abingdon Press.

Walsh, J., McSherry, W. & Kevern, P. (2013) The representation of service users' religious and spiritual concerns in care plans. *Journal of Public Mental Health, 12*(3), 153–164.

Wood, E., Raffay, J. & Todd, A. (2016) How could co-production principles improve mental health spiritual and pastoral care (chaplaincy) services? *Health and Social Care Chaplaincy, 4*(1), 51–56.

WELLBEING IN MENTAL HEALTH CARE

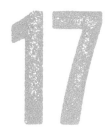

KEVIN ACOTT, EMILY GRIFFIN AND HARVEY WELLS

THIS CHAPTER COVERS

- Aspects of life that enhance or hinder wellbeing
- Contemporary understandings of wellbeing within its historical, social and political contexts
- Wellbeing from key theoretical perspectives, focusing on a dialectical understanding
- Concepts of wellbeing from a service user and carer perspective
- Treatment and care approaches to enhancing wellbeing
- The importance of wellbeing in mental health care and mental health nursing
- Contribution of wellbeing to our own lives, learning and clinical practice.

Visit **https://study.sagepub.com/essentialmentalhealth** to access a wealth of online resources for this chapter - watch out for the margin icons throughout the chapter. If you are using the interactive ebook, simply click on the margin icon to go straight to the resource.

INTRODUCTION

'Wellbeing' is a core part of understanding ourselves and our learning, of understanding people's experiences of mental health and **mental disorder** and of understanding how we can work, live and learn effectively and compassionately. The aim of this chapter is to help the reader consider this much-discussed but often slippery concept, to begin to understand it from a 'dialectical' point of view and to apply its ideas and practices both to your own experiences and to those of **service users**. We will explore some of the evidence and controversies in the area and encourage you to understand the limits and possibilities of examining wellbeing in the contexts of mental health and mental ill health. We will draw heavily on the experiences of Emily, who was a student nurse, and Hannah, who has previously used mental health services. We hope the chapter will help you grow as a student, as a nurse and as a person – and enhance your own wellbeing.

Table 17.1 The Warwick-Edinburgh Mental Well-being Scale (WEMWBS)

Below are some statements about feelings and thoughts.

Please tick (✓) the box that best describes your experience of each over the **last 2 weeks**

STATEMENTS	None of the time	Rarely	Some of the time	Often	All of the time
I've been feeling optimistic about the future	1	2	3	4	5
I've been feeling useful	1	2	3	4	5
I've been feeling relaxed	1	2	3	4	5
I've been feeling interested in other people	1	2	3	4	5
I've had energy to spare	1	2	3	4	5
I've been dealing with problems well	1	2	3	4	5
I've been thinking clearly	1	2	3	4	5
I've been feeling good about myself	1	2	3	4	5
I've been feeling close to other people	1	2	3	4	5
I've been feeling confident	1	2	3	4	5
I've been able to make up my own mind about things	1	2	3	4	5
I've been feeling loved	1	2	3	4	5
I've been interested in new things	1	2	3	4	5
I've been feeling cheerful	1	2	3	4	5

From Tennant, et al. (2007) ©NHS Health Scotland, University of Warwick and University of Edinburgh, 2006, all rights reserved.

Now ask yourself a few questions:

How might you have responded to this scale a year ago?

Five years ago?

How would you like to answer it in a year's time?

How might your best friend answer it?

How much did work **affect** your answers?

How much did your relationships affect your answers?

How much did your physical health affect them?

How much did your mental health affect them?

Source: The Warwick-Edinburgh Mental Well-being Scale (WEMWBS) from Tennant et al. (2007) ©NHS Health Scotland, University of Warwick and University of Edinburgh, 2006, all rights reserved.

SCORING THE WEMWBS

To get a total wellbeing score, add all of the numbers from the boxes you have ticked. If you have experienced each of those statements, more often than not you will be scoring 4 or 5 for each. If they apply rarely or not at all, then you would score 1 or 2. The total score should be between 14 and 70. Figure 17.1 shows the statistical breakdown of the WEMWBS.

Interpreting the scores

Someone's wellbeing is poor, or '**languishing**', if the score is between 14 and 41; a person has moderate wellbeing if they score between 42 and 59; and they have an excellent, or '**flourishing**', wellbeing if they score above 60.

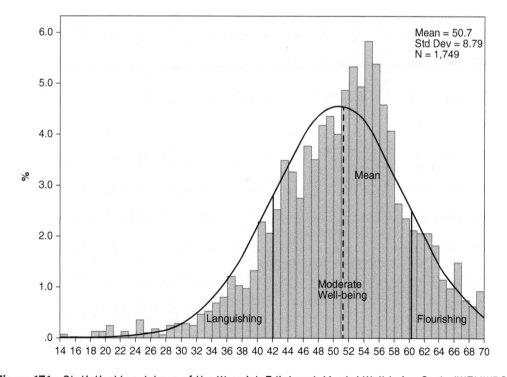

Figure 17.1 Statistical breakdown of the Warwick-Edinburgh Mental Well-being Scale (WEMWBS)

Adults with flourishing wellbeing report the lowest level of helplessness, the highest perception of control over their life choices, the highest level of functional goals, the highest self-reported resilience and the highest level of social interaction (Keyes, 2007). Overall, adults with flourishing wellbeing function better than those with moderate or languishing wellbeing, whereas adults with languishing wellbeing report high numbers of work days missed and high levels of mental and physical ill health (Keyes, 2007).

History and context

The emphasis on wellbeing as a concept and as something worth pursuing and developing is both an ancient and a modern thing. Philosophers, spiritual leaders and ordinary men and women have always sought happiness, balance, health and a sense of connectedness with other people and the **environment**. Yet the term 'wellbeing', as it's now used and as a concept seen as worth studying and enhancing, is relatively recent. In the UK, LSE Professor of Economics Richard Layard founded the Wellbeing Programme at the LSE Centre for Economic Performance (CEP) in 2001. The programme's main aims were to 'promote subjective happiness and wellbeing as the criterion for public policy, and to conduct research that would contribute to the formulation of the most effective policies'. The programme was soon seen as valuable by government agencies and quite quickly became part of the way in which legislators, clinicians and academics talked about health, happiness and **illness**.

Meanings and definitions

Thinking about the questions in the WEMWBS, we can begin to see some of the ideas that can help shape our understanding of 'wellbeing'. The developers of the scale talk about both '*hedonic* perspectives' of wellbeing (those that focus 'on the subjective, *feeling* experience of happiness') and '*eudaemonic* perspectives' of wellbeing, i.e. 'those that focus on psychological functioning, good relationships with others and self-realisation', in other words are '*cognitive*'. The WEMWBS 'derives from a model of mental wellbeing that is more than the absence of mental illness, and involves both feeling good and functioning well'. What does this mean? We will soon see these two elements of wellbeing overlap and interweave; and they interweave in the one area that was deliberately left out of the scale: '(The scale) *does not include spirituality or purpose in life*. These were deemed to extend beyond the general population's current understanding of mental wellbeing and their inclusion was thought likely to increase non-response.' Yet that – we would contend – is what wellbeing is all about: feeling good, functioning effectively *but with a sense of purpose*.

According to the Department of Health (2014):

> There is a two way relationship between wellbeing and health: health influences wellbeing and wellbeing itself influences health … Health is one of the top things people say matters for wellbeing … Both physical and mental health influence wellbeing, however mental health and wellbeing are independent dimensions [and] mental health is not simply the opposite of mental illness.

The World Health Organization (WHO) states that 'wellbeing exists in two dimensions, subjective and objective. It comprises an individual's experience of their life as well as a comparison of life circumstances with social norms and **values**' (WHO, 2012). 'Subjective' experiences can include a person's overall sense of wellbeing, psychological functioning and emotional states.

The Office for National Statistics (2015) suggests that key 'objective' measures are:

- where we live
- personal finance
- the economy
- education and skills
- governance (for example, trust in politicians/voting)
- the natural environment
- our relationships
- health.

We can see that to understand wellbeing, we need to consider subjective and objective elements – and how they interact. It may also be becoming clear that in order to understand mental health and mental disorder, we need to understand wellbeing – and vice versa. Is this not complicating things? Aren't mental health and wellbeing the same thing?

The short answer is no. A person can have a diagnosis of a mental health problem yet experience flourishing wellbeing; in the same way that someone can have a chronic physical illness and still experience a high level of functioning, satisfaction with life and a high degree of social integration. One way to conceptualise the relationship between mental illness and emotional wellbeing is to consider them on separate but related continua.

Figure 17.2 shows the dual axis model of mental illness and emotional wellbeing. It provides simple examples of a person who may fall within each of those quadrants; for example, someone who would score highly on the mental illness axis *and* highly on the wellbeing axis (top-left quadrant) might have a diagnosed severe mental illness and be flourishing: functioning very well, have a sense of purpose

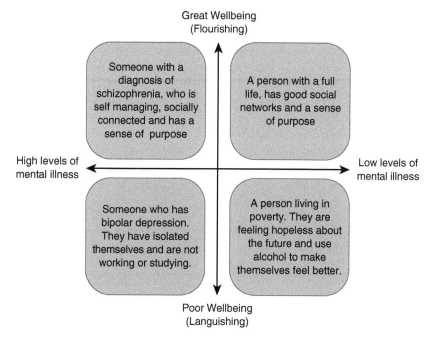

Figure 17.2 Dual Axis Model of Mental Health. Keyes (2007), American Psychological Association, adapted with permission.

and a good social network. However, someone who scores low on both the mental illness axis and the wellbeing axis (bottom-right quadrant) might be someone who is unemployed, struggling to make ends meet, lacking social contact, without a sense of purpose, yet does not have a diagnosable mental health problem. Clearly, the person in the first example is doing much better in terms of overall wellbeing than the person in the second example. Despite the importance of wellbeing to a person's overall functioning, in mental health services we tend to focus on the mental illness rather than the person's wellbeing. We will pick this discussion up again under the section, 'Implications for mental health nursing'.

A DIALECTICAL VIEW OF WELLBEING

We would suggest that one way to understand wellbeing – for ourselves and for the people we are trying to help – is by looking at things in a 'dialectical' way.

The term 'dialectical' means there are opposites, two ends of a pole, two extremes, that can mask our understanding of an aspect of our lives. In order to find a new, helpful truth about these aspects, we need a 'synthesis', or an integration of these opposites: we need to move from 'x' versus 'y' to 'x + y'. We need to find a way to accept the partial truth in both extremes, while rejecting the absolute truth we can be tempted to see in either, and find a new, more accurate and powerful truth emerge. Some of the key dialectics in wellbeing, we would suggest, are:

- hope v hopelessness (we may say to ourselves, 'I must be hopeful at all times to be an effective nurse')
- being well v being ill (we may say to ourselves, 'someone is either well or ill')
- optimism v pessimism (we may say to ourselves, 'everything is going to be alright' or 'everything is going to turn out badly')
- being useful v being useless (we may say to ourselves, 'If I'm not helpful 100% of the time, then I'm a useless nurse')
- being relaxed all the time v being anxious all the time (we may say to ourselves, 'If I'm not cool, calm and collected every minute of every shift, then I'll be anxious and out of control')
- being 100% interested in other people v having absolutely no interest in anyone else (we may say to ourselves, 'I must be 100% interested in everyone I work with, 100% of the time')
- being full of energy all the time v being lazy (we may say to ourselves, 'If I'm not really energetic and full of life all the time, then I'm lazy')
- dealing with problems brilliantly v being rubbish at dealing with problems (we may say to ourselves, 'If I'm not able to solve everyone's problems, then I'm a terrible person')
- being a good person or being a bad person (we may say to ourselves, 'If I'm not functioning all the time at my very best, I must be a really bad person').

All of us may cling to one or other of these extreme positions at times. Our childhood, our upbringing, our genetic make-up, the environment, people around us, our physical health, the use of drugs or alcohol to excess: all of these things may push us to believe in the existence of these extremes. And, at their very worst, these beliefs can be part of us sliding from a poor state of objective and subjective wellbeing into a mental health problem like **depression**, an **anxiety** disorder, or (in very rare cases) **psychosis**.

The answer lies partly in trying to see the truth in both positions at the same time, to notice the extremes, to try and resolve the tensions and to find a middle way. For example, our 'wellness' or 'illness' generally lies on a continuum: our functioning in one or more areas of our lives may be limited, but that doesn't mean there aren't aspects of ourselves that aren't 'well', that aren't exceptions to the problem. Similarly, no one is simply a 'good' or 'bad' person or a 'good' or 'bad' nurse.

CASE STUDY 17.1

Emily was a 29-year-old student nurse who found her wellbeing increasingly compromised by the stresses of her course, her experiences on placement and her personal life. At one point, she became depressed. She was prescribed antidepressants, undertook counselling and studied mindfulness and meditation. Today, she's really enjoying life again, but looks back here at some of the key wellbeing dialectics she feels contributed to her problems.

Being a good nurse v pleasing people

I sometimes felt pressure to conform with the status quo in order to be accepted by the team I was working in, and sometimes that included a tacit acceptance or tolerance of bad nursing practice. This caused me a great deal of stress, because I wasn't sure how to balance pleasing the people who would be signing us off (mentors) with being the best nurse I could be. I wanted very much to be a good, caring nurse, but I didn't want to be that difficult person either.

I think this all contributed to a sense of two mental versions of what a nurse could be - savvy, common sense, real-world nurse who is well-liked but probably breaking every NMC rule in the book (and therefore 'bad' nurse in university's eyes), and by contrast, rule-following, theoretically immaculate 'good' nurse who might win awards for university but whom few will like in practice (and therefore 'difficult' as a team member). I found treading this line, and essentially trying to be the best of both, very stressful at times.

Reflecting too much v reflecting too little

I was told that if things were difficult in practice it's possible I wasn't analysing myself enough, and so when things were difficult I kept trying to reflect my way out of it, and criticise myself more accurately, and work out how I could be closer to perfection. I wasted time reflecting on ways I could further protect patients from my inevitably terrible interactions with them and crashing lack of compassion.

In fact I now think my time would have been better spent learning how to protect myself, from my own harshest judgements. I was convinced that I should be able to find a solution to my own dread and suffering, just by thinking. I wilfully ignored the physical signs that I was becoming unwell (I wasn't sleeping, lost my appetite, became constantly tearful) because I didn't want anyone to think I was a failure.

Being helpful v losing oneself

I am a classic 'people pleaser'. I wanted to please my mentors, the people I worked with, fellow students, teaching staff, family and friends so much that I put my own health and happiness totally on hold. I would always accept the extra shift if no one else could stay, even when I was exhausted. I would go the extra in being friendly and helpful to those around me in the hope that everyone would be satisfied and I would feel right with the world. The more I felt I was losing control of my mental state, the harder I tried to be nice and good and giving, in a sadly paradoxical attempt to earn some kind of mental peace. I believe now that I would have been no less helpful for stopping and taking care of myself first - and probably could have stayed 'helping' for longer. We can assume compassion and niceness are enough - they're not.

(Continued)

Realistic hope v outrageous optimism

It's crucial to stay hopeful. But you need to be gentle to yourself and realistic too. Feeling you are losing hope, or have nearly lost all of it, is the most profoundly terrifying thing. When I needed to I held on to the things I really valued - family, friends, moments of humour, reading something that made me feel heard and not lost, remembering (and actually, asking people who know me best to remind me when I didn't believe myself) that I had suffered these terrible feelings before and that they passed.

What not to do

Looking back, Emily can see that she did things that contributed to the breakdown of her wellbeing, and contributed to her slipping into mental health problems:

When I was trying to convince everyone, including myself that I was fine, I did a few disastrous things that certainly made a difference. One, I used alcohol to numb my emotions - a glass of wine always seemed to 'take the edge off' really bad days. I inevitably felt more anxious the next day. Two, I stopped doing many of the positive things I usually did (calling friends, exercise, eating properly, taking time to relax or do things just for myself), specifically to reserve my energy to solve the problem of my feelings. Throughout my first year I went running regularly and loved the positive impact it had on me physically and mentally. When I started feeling bad in the second year I stopped and of course lost all of those benefits.

Three, I didn't tell a single person how I was feeling and persuaded myself that I could keep my feelings private and simply think my way out of feeling bad.

Finding ways to maintain and develop wellbeing

Like Emily, we need to focus on both hedonic and eudaenomic aspects of our wellbeing; we need to encourage the people we work with - colleagues, service users and carers - and support them in maintaining or regaining their wellbeing in both these areas, and in both subjective and objective realms.

I talked, a lot, to a few people I trusted, made myself eat and take regular exercise. The things I should have been doing more of (rather than stopping) all along, frankly! If I'm honest I think another protective tool in my internal make up is a sense of humour.

In a similar way, writing down what I'm feeling has always proved to be a useful means for me of working through stuff I'm finding difficult. I often keep a diary and have actually since come to consider this a really important part of managing my own mental health and wellbeing. I find it immensely helpful to be able to review the things that helped and the things that were going on which might have contributed to feeling bad.

Books and literature have always offered me a feeling of connection to other people when I feel most alone, too. Sometimes someone you will never have to talk to, or get out of bed and put a smile on for, writes something that for a minute in time makes you feel understood, and I find that endlessly comforting. I find something very healing and calming about that process; when I write I find it easier to follow a solid, single thread without intrusion or distraction, and to achieve stillness around an idea, than I ever can when I talk or think.

I spent time learning mindfulness and meditation. Through mindfulness and meditation, I came to see how much I resisted uncertainty in any area of my life. For the first time I realised that the very thing I had been doing to try and save myself from feeling bad had been making me feel worse. Mentally picking away at the problem of a thought or feeling is not only pointless and harmful, it misses the point by assuming that thoughts and feelings are problems in the first place. Mindfulness has helped me to see that they are not problems. They just are what they are. They are not me, they are them. What's more, they pass. I have learnt that when you stop fighting your own mind so hard, and turn round to face the feelings you dread so much, you often find that they are not as horrifying as all that.

Resilience, strength and mental health

I needed a stronger internal buffer against the emotional demands of the course - something to create a barrier between myself as a nurse and myself as a person. I thought if I gave more, worried more, reflected more, gave more of myself, then I could overcome any imperfections in my nursing, and therefore stamp out the stress I was causing myself! That putting down of defences left me totally vulnerable.

A lot of it is about understanding the importance of boundaries, I think. I never mastered the therapeutic boundary - or rather, looking back, I think I was often letting patients determine the boundaries. I suppose my logic was that it was somehow unkind or selfish to jealously defend an emotional/mental territory for myself, particularly when faced with someone openly welcoming me into theirs. But of course this meant that naturally I often felt invaded, vulnerable or lacking control in a situation.

I guess I needed someone to step in and tell me that we're all just human, that even the best nurses aren't perfect, and that part of being a good nurse is actually about being resilient. The best nurses I knew had a blend of compassion and sturdiness; they genuinely cared about the patients but also seemed to keep something of themselves back, a core bit of them that was safely defended and simply not available to patients or mentors or lecturers. I wonder now if they seemed to cope so effortlessly because it came completely naturally to them that they must care for that part of themselves just as carefully as they cared for patients.

I think we each come to nursing with our own private stash of personal strength: in fact I think of it as a cleared space, like a crop circle, characterised by peace and calm. In my mind everyone's different size - from what I can tell some were just born with an inherently strong sense of themselves, and unshakeable self-esteem, and their circles span imaginary acres. Others have widened the boundaries of their circles by investing in themselves and their wellbeing - doing stuff they enjoy, having relationships which promote rather than destroy their self-esteem, fitness and healthy eating, making time for themselves. And some are always giving away bits of their already small circle to the outside world, until they find they barely have enough room to stand up in. As one of the latter, I think some of us just probably need to do more than others to clear themselves a bigger circle. You have, each of the people you work with has, that cleared space.

Resilience

As we've seen in Case study 17.1, 'resilience' can be seen as a quality we have, built on complex combinations of genetics, experience and the environment around us, that enables us to be 'elastic', to 'bounce back' from stressful events or prolonged periods of pressure. Angie Hart of Boing Boing downplays the importance of genetics, favouring Roisman and colleagues' (2002: 1216) definition:

'Resilience is an emergent property of a hierarchically organized set of protective systems that cumulatively buffer the effects of adversity and can therefore rarely, if ever, be regarded as an intrinsic property of individuals.' How we view ourselves, the world and other people can all influence our resilience. At the same time, we need to be careful that 'having resilience' doesn't become a way in which we judge others or ourselves: 'Overcoming adversity, whilst also potentially changing, or even dramatically transforming, (aspects of) that adversity' (Hart et al. 2016: 3). The Boing Boing organisation offers this definition of 'resilience': 'Beating the odds whilst also changing the odds' (www. boingboing.org.uk/)

CRITICAL THINKING STOP POINT 17.1

Find a quiet place to sit for 5 minutes:

- Think about times in your life when you have needed to call on your capacity to be resilient.
- Try and allow yourself to observe what goes through your mind.
- What did you feel?
- What did you tell yourself?
- What did you do?
- How effective was your strategy?
- What did you discover about yourself?
- How can you apply this to developing your professional capacity for resilience as a nurse?

(Reproduced with the kind permission of Armin Luthi, Senior Lecturer, London Southbank University)

WELLBEING AND EDUCATION: HOW DOES YOUR WELLBEING COMPARE WITH THAT OF OTHER STUDENTS?

In order for students to learn and develop effectively, it is imperative that universities provide an environment that promotes student wellbeing. Several studies have shown that there is a strong correlation between student wellbeing and academic outcome (Abouserie, 1994; Morris, 2011); a high level of personal wellbeing is essential for educational achievement. The demands of higher education, combined with perceptions of low control, can lead to high levels of distress, low levels of satisfaction and poor academic outcomes (Cotton et al., 2002).

We completed a small pilot study at a London university to explore the level of wellbeing in university students. We used an electronic version of the Warwick-Edinburgh Mental Well-being Scale (WEMWBS; Tennant et al., 2007) to gain a measure of student wellbeing. In addition to the WEMWBS, each participant was asked three open-response questions to find out what could be done to help improve their wellbeing: what the student can do and what the university can do to improve student wellbeing.

Thirty participants completed the wellbeing survey. The mean wellbeing score for the participants was 50, indicating that, overall, students experience moderate wellbeing. However, 29% of participants indicated that they experience languishing wellbeing, whilst only 14% indicated that they experience flourishing wellbeing (see Figure 17.3).

Overall wellbeing score

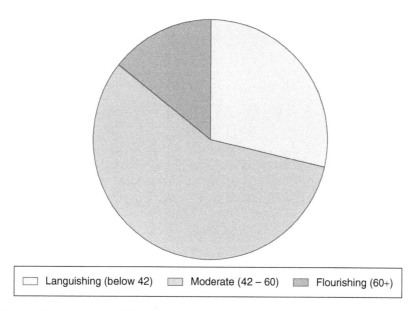

Languishing (below 42)   Moderate (42 – 60)   Flourishing (60+)

Figure 17.3   Breakdown of participants' wellbeing scores by category

Whilst the results show that the majority of students have moderate wellbeing and some students are positively flourishing, there are a significant number of students who are struggling with poor wellbeing. This suggests that universities need to consider ways of supporting these students better in order to maximise their time at university.

The open questions exploring what could be done to improve wellbeing produced some interesting suggestions. In response to '*What can you do to improve your wellbeing?*', the main responses were around getting regular exercise, eating healthier, taking time for oneself and talking to people. These suggestions show that students understand the importance of taking care of themselves and have clear ideas on how to manage their wellbeing.

In response to the question '*What can the university do to improve your wellbeing?*', the two recurrent suggestions were around improved organisation of courses, and for the university to provide better places to eat, socialise and relax. These suggestions imply that students find that facilities on the university sites provide insufficient resources to cater for their wellbeing. These results support the notion that wellbeing, at its basic level, is comprised of some fundamental but simple components: eating healthily, sleeping well, taking time to relax and socialise with others, and having a sense of purpose.

Treatment and care approaches

So how does what we now know about wellbeing affect the treatment and care of people with mental health problems? If we return to think about the dual axis model of mental health, we can consider that many of the treatments offered by mental health services would be aiming to reduce the impact of someone's mental 'illness', yet may fail to attend to their wellbeing. It is certainly true that an episode of mental ill health will impact negatively on someone's wellbeing, as would an episode of physical illness, but should the focus on mental *health* services be on mental *illness*?

Consider for a moment what a service would look like if it were to offer interventions for improving someone's wellbeing rather than focusing on mental illness/disorder? What would it offer? Think about what you would need if you were struggling; take a few minutes to write down your ideas. When you have finished, consider one service user's perspective on her experience of mental illness and wellbeing (Case study 17.2).

CASE STUDY 17.2

Hannah (whose name has been changed to protect her identity) is a 25-year-old, former service user of mental health and substance misuse services. She has received a range of different diagnoses over the period of her treatment; her current diagnoses are bipolar affective disorder and opiate dependency. She has received various treatments, including medication (quetiapine and methadone), various periods of counselling and psychosocial interventions, input from a range of mental health services and from her GP, and she has worked hard in her own life to develop the coping strategies she needs to ensure she remains well.

When did you start to experience problems?

As a child I was really insecure as I was a little bit overweight. I lost all that weight when I got into my teens because I was constantly on the go and I didn't eat. I didn't really sleep a lot either. I just had this inhuman amount of energy all the time. It was really good because I could go to a group of people and I could instantly get along with them. I was the life and soul of anywhere I went.

I wasn't a good friend to people; I'd be horrible to people. I'd pick people up and I'd drop them. You know, people that I cared about and people that cared about me. I remember if I went out for a social occasion I'd be going around and have no control over what I said to people. I'd be quite charismatic and funny but I'd go around insulting people all night.

One day it hit me like a ton of bricks when I woke up; I swear I felt like I was in a hole that I couldn't get out of, like a depressing hole. I didn't feel like myself. Everything I thought I knew about myself just vanished overnight and I felt so lost and suicidal. I pictured the things that I was doing and I'd be so humiliated about it that I just wanted to die.

I got really depressed and I started self-harming. I'd drink when I felt overly depressed. I'd drink and then I'd self-harm or I'd take pills and I'd sleep the whole day and the whole night and the whole day again to the point where I couldn't sleep anymore. I was really awake but really tired and I couldn't turn my mind off. I started trying heroin. Now that for me was the beginning of the end because when I tried heroin it was like the answer to all my problems. It made me just feel like I was wrapped up in this warm bubble and nothing mattered and my mind wasn't racing and I just felt brilliant.

What sort of treatment did you get?

My Dad took me to a drugs service where we met this woman. She took a list of all my problems and of the drugs that I'd used and the activities that I'd been involved in. She said they'd get me some counselling and I've got to stop using. I went away and I thought 'how am I going to do this?' but I couldn't stop and I used all weekend. So when I went back she said, 'okay well that didn't work'. She was quite aggressive about it, 'oh if you can't stop using you should get on the methadone programme and see how you like that!'

So I went to the appointment with the doctor at the drugs service. He asked how much heroin I'm using and said, 'we'll start you on 10mls of methadone'. I wanted to ask some questions and he said 'people who ask questions don't stop using drugs'. I was so desperate I agreed.

At first, when I started treatment, I had the attitude of, 'I'm going to solve my drug problem and then I'm going to put it in a box and that's that'. Now I feel that actually it's a continuous thing; I need to come to terms with it, revisit and make sense of it and accept it. That is part of the journey of becoming a whole person.

What are the things important to you now to ensure you remain well?

For me sleep's the most important thing. I know if I can't sleep properly then I'm in trouble. I'd like to see myself being able to go back to how I was when I was younger; I didn't have to take anything. I liked it when my sleep was real as mine is a medicated sleep but I'm scared what'd happen if I do stop taking the medication. It's a thing I've got to accept but I do wonder what it does to my health.

It's important to give people the skills to handle their mental health problems. It's not a 'I'm telling you' thing and it's not something that can be done to someone; they have to be in control and they have to have the skills to know when they're becoming unwell and how to deal with it. It's the best thing that I've gained.

Reflecting on Hannah's treatment

Hannah's treatment largely consisted of prescriptive interventions and approaches: medication, advice and instruction. It was only when Hannah was referred to a worker who listened to her and worked with her to address her concerns that she gained some control over her difficulties and her wellbeing began to increase. With her growing confidence and support, she found that she had the resources to deal with her problems. Hannah has learned that if she can take care of relatively basic things, like sleeping, social support and having a purpose in life, the other, more problematic aspects of life can be managed.

IMPLICATIONS FOR MENTAL HEALTH NURSING

Having come to the end of this chapter, spend a few minutes thinking about the following questions:

- What do you think is important about wellbeing?
- How does wellbeing apply to the practices of mental health nursing?
- How much does your current practice involve ideas about your patients' wellbeing?
- How can you integrate this into your practice as a mental health nurse?

One could argue that the concept of wellbeing adds an additional layer to the practices of mental health nursing; it is not the same as mental illness and therefore it must require additional work for the professional. However, what would it feel like to have just your 'illness' addressed and not the rest of you? Giving attention to a patient's wellbeing is an acknowledgement that they are more than 'just a patient with a mental health problem'; they are human, triumphs, warts and all. We would suggest that if greater consideration was paid to wellbeing by treatment services, then **recovery** from illness would be more likely to occur quicker and more fully (Keyes, 2007). Addressing the 'whole person' was rightly highlighted as a key message in the King's Fund report (2016), 'Bringing Together Physical and Mental Health', and should be considered the way to approach integrated health care.

CONTROVERSIES IN WELLBEING

CRITICAL DEBATE 17.1

'The language of "well-being" is used to mask an unhelpful medical approach to working compassionately and effectively with people.'

Have another look at the list of 'objective' measures. How many of those affect your wellbeing? How many affect service users you've met? Is there a danger that 'wellbeing' can end up blaming people for their problems, or making something 'medical', when it's actually social and political?

CRITICAL
DEBATE
17.1 ANSWER

So far, we have presented a largely positive and unproblematic view of wellbeing, but wellbeing hasn't been embraced by all. Critics of the current focus on wellbeing argue that it is simply a way of loading blame for society's problems onto the individual. Stating that a person lacks the resilience to manage suggests they are somehow inadequate, rather than that there is a lack of support given or the aims were too high (Christopher, 1999). Blaming the individual for failing to have sufficient wellbeing can end up meaning that the systems or the standards don't have to be reviewed.

It is likely that as a student mental health nurse you will have received a lecture or seminar on self-care; you will have been told that mental health nursing is a demanding professional training and you have to look after your wellbeing or you won't be able to care for your patients, or succeed in your education. Looking after yourself involves eating healthily, getting adequate exercise and sufficient sleep, socialising with family and friends, and enjoying leisure activities. However, all of this is done whilst attending lectures, doing background reading, writing essays, revising for exams, completing placement hours, writing reflective accounts, and all of the other things that are required of your nursing education. Many of these tasks have hard deadlines that cannot be missed (without incurring some penalty). So you have a choice: get eight hours sleep or spend a few more hours work-ing on that essay that is due next week; spend time after a long shift on placement cooking a healthy meal and then going for a run, or grab some fast food and sit in front of the TV for the evening as you are exhausted. Maintaining wellbeing takes effort and that can be a challenge when your efforts are being used to study as a nurse. Take another look at Emily's story (Case study 17.1): when things became difficult, which is inevitable on a programme like nursing, she stopped doing all the things that maintained her wellbeing. Was this a fault with Emily, for not taking care of her wellbeing, or a fault with a system that places high demands on people without offering them sufficient support?

What you should have learned

Now that you have finished reading this chapter, you should be able to:

- identify aspects of your life that enhance or hinder your wellbeing
- describe contemporary understandings of wellbeing within a wider social context

- provide an understanding of wellbeing from various key theoretical perspectives
- understand concepts of wellbeing that include service user and student perspectives
- identify treatment and care approaches to enhancing wellbeing
- recognise the importance of wellbeing in mental health care and mental health nursing
- apply concepts of wellbeing to your own lives, learning and clinical practice.

CHAPTER SUMMARY

In this chapter, you have learned:

- The concept of wellbeing and how it relates both to the demands of being a student mental health nurse and the practices of being a qualified mental health nurse.
- You need to find balance between the demands of your education and what you need to maintain your wellbeing. This balance will be constantly challenged, but by remaining mindful and utilising the support of others around you this is a balance that can be found.
- For success as a *qualified* mental health nurse, the balancing act that you have learned as a student in maintaining your own wellbeing will be tested in different ways. However, you are now responsible for helping your patients build their wellbeing after it has been eroded.
- To keep in mind the things that helped you when you have struggled in the past.
- To take some time with the person to find out what they need.

BUILD YOUR BIBLIOGRAPHY

Sage journal articles

Go to https://study.sagepub.com/essentialmentalhealth for further free online journal articles related to this chapter. If you are using the interactive ebook, simply click on the book icon in the margin to go straight to the resource.

FURTHER
READING:
JOURNAL
ARTICLES

- Campion, J. & Nurse, J. (2007) A dynamic model for wellbeing. *Australasian Psychiatry*, 15(1 suppl.), S24-S28.
- Haramati, A. & Weissinger, P.A. (2015) Resilience, empathy, and wellbeing in the health professions: an educational imperative. *Global Advances in Health and Medicine*, 4(5), 5-6.
- Manning, C. (2016) Resilience: a personal story. *InnovAiT: Education and Inspiration for General Practice*, 9(6), 328-332.

Weblinks

Go to https://study.sagepub.com/essentialmentalhealth for further weblinks related to this chapter. If you are using the interactive ebook, simply click on the book icon in the margin to go straight to the resource.

FURTHER
READING:
WEBLINKS

- Action for Happiness: www.actionforhappiness.org/why-happiness
- Department of Health (2014) The relationship between wellbeing and health: www.gov.uk/government/uploads/system/uploads/attachment_data/file/295474/The_relationship_between_wellbeing_and_health.pdf
- Measuring Wellbeing: www.ons.gov.uk/ons/guide-method/user-guidance/well-being/index.html
- The Resilience Framework: www.boingboing.org.uk/index.php/resources/category/9-resilience-frameworks?download=79:rf-adults

ACE YOUR ASSESSMENT

Revise what you have learned by visiting https://study.sagepub.com/essentialmentalhealth. If you are using the interactive ebook, simply click on the tick icon to go straight to the resource.

• Test yourself with multiple-choice and short-answer questions and flashcards.

REFERENCES

Abouserie, R. (1994) Sources and levels of stress in relation to locus of control and self esteem in university students. *Educational Psychology, 14*(3), 323–330.

Christopher, J.C. (1999) Situating psychological well-being: exploring the cultural roots of its theory and research. *Journal of Counseling & Development, 77*(2), 141–152.

Cotton, S.J., Dollard, M.F. & de Jonge, J. (2002) Stress and student job design: satisfaction, well-being, and performance in university students. *International Journal of Stress Management, 9*(3), 147–162.

Department of Health (2014) The relationship between wellbeing and health. Available at: www.gov.uk/government/uploads/system/uploads/attachment_data/file/295474/The_relationship_between_wellbeing_and_health.pdf (accessed 12.12.17)

Hart, A., Gagnon, E., Eryigit-Madzwamuse, S., et al. (2016) Uniting resilience research and practice with an inequalities approach. *SAGE Open, 6*(4), 1–13.

Keyes, C.L. (2007) Promoting and protecting mental health as flourishing: a complementary strategy for improving national mental health. *American Psychologist, 62*(2), 95.

King's Fund (2016) *Bringing together physical and mental health: A new frontier for integrated care.* London: King's Fund. Available at: www.kingsfund.org.uk/publications/physical-and-mental-health (accessed 09.08.17).

Morris, C. (2011) Open minds: towards a 'mentally well' university. In L. Marshall & C. Morris (eds) *Taking wellbeing forward in higher education: Reflections on theory and practice.* Brighton: University of Brighton Press. pp. 10–20.

Office for National Statistics (ONS) (2015) *Measuring national well-being: Personal well-being in the UK, 2014 to 2015.* Available at: www.ons.gov.uk/peoplepopulationandcommunity/wellbeing/bulletins/measuringnationalwellbeing/2015-09-23 (accessed 09.08.17).

Roisman, G.I., Padrón, E., Sroufe, L.A., et al. (2002) Earned–secure attachment status in retrospect and prospect. *Child development, 73*(4), 1204–1219.

Tennant, R., Hiller, L., Fishwick, R., et al. (2007) The Warwick-Edinburgh Mental Well-being Scale (WEMWBS): development and UK validation. *Health and Quality of Life Outcomes, 5*(1), 63.

World Health Organization (WHO) (2012) *Measurement of and Target-setting for Well-being: An Initiative by the WHO Regional Office for Europe.* Geneva: WHO. Available at: www.euro.who.int/_data/assets/pdf-file/0009/181449/e96732.pdf (accessed 30.11.17).

RECOVERY-ORIENTATED PRACTICE

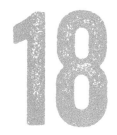

KAREN MACHIN AND EMMA WATSON

THIS CHAPTER COVERS

- History: the transformation of 'recovery'
- Recovery in diverse settings
- Approaches to use for recovery-focused working
- Implementing recovery-focused services
- Measuring recovery.

> " I have found recovery to be something of an abstract concept. I've come across individuals who do not understand or use the word recovery, and given the numerous definitions and uses, this is hardly unexpected. The word implies a return to a previous state of health, where this does not always occur. Understandably, people with mental health problems often feel changed by their experiences. Through the process and adjustment to a new reality, people seldom return to the person they once were, which only highlights the discord between the medical model which psychiatry is built upon and the humanistic philosophy of recovery. Regardless whether a person has experienced mental health problems, change is something which undoubtedly occurs in every person's life. One of the most memorable insights I've had in practice was a person likening recovery to a caterpillar breaking away from its protective cocoon, to the freedom to live as its reformed self as a butterfly.
>
> With recovery at the forefront of policy agenda, in practice I have sometimes found recovery used more as a buzzword, and therefore generated a culture that recovery is something a professional can 'do' to a person. People suggest recovery is more about a personal journey, and as such I think we as future nurses need to distance ourselves from this attitude. Instead, work towards embracing the role of the facilitator, to re-empower the independence and capacity of people who can often feel marginalised in society.
>
> **Jessica Beaty, nursing student** "

As someone who has used mental health services and is now employed by them, I have seen the 'lightbulb' moment of recovery focused practice from both sides. As a service user and student on the Peer Support Worker course, that moment was learning of a holistic approach to recovery that resonated with me in a way that the traditional biomedical model never had. As a practitioner, there have been numerous examples of this too: from something as simple as role-modelling recovery through my job role, to advocating for a person, ensuring their opinions are valued and the subsequent benefits this has on their overall sense of wellbeing.

The values of hope, autonomy and empowerment are intrinsic to the recovery ethos, and therefore, should be fundamental within mental health care as a whole. A person-centred approach consisting of techniques such as active listening, strength spotting and the use of recovery focused language, combined with innate qualities such as compassion, patience, respect and a desire to understand a person's experiences without judgement, are vital to supporting and facilitating recovery.

The role of the Peer Support Worker is the embodiment of this humanistic approach: the practice of mutuality and reciprocity to develop respectful and trusting therapeutic relationships that aid another person in their own journey to reignite hope and regain a sense of control at a distressing, and sometimes catastrophic, stage of their life.

I have experienced both personally and as a practitioner the loss associated with periods of illness, whether that takes the form of relationships, employment, finance, homes, or perhaps most notably, loss of hope and our sense of self. Rebuilding self-identity through the investigation of who we are and what we enjoy, the recognition of our strengths and what can motivate us to stay well is a fundamental part of recovery. As a practitioner, facilitating this process has often been challenging, but the knowledge that I have empowered someone on their personal journey is the greatest reward.

Virginia Mathieson, peer support worker

INTRODUCTION

Within this chapter, **recovery** will be presented as an important feature of recent mental health policy, leading to various interesting service developments (Perkins & Slade, 2012). Examples of these will be used to illustrate the complexity of working in a recovery-focused way and how this may seem at odds with traditional ways of working. The concept of recovery is open to interpretation and critique, not least from elements of the user/**survivor** movement which has good claim to having initiated it in the first place. This debate will be aired in this chapter.

HISTORY: THE TRANSFORMATION OF 'RECOVERY'

For as long as there has been pain, there has been recovery. Within the context of mental health, recovery has traditionally been considered synonymous with cure or restoration of the brain's chemical balance through treatments, most popularly medication. In recent decades, this view has been consistently challenged, and, as a result, the meaning of the term 'recovery' has undergone a process of transformation.

Challenges to biochemical theories came initially from former and current patients who began to share their experiences of the treatment they received. United by a shared sense of anger, the **service user** movement began, in the 1970s, to challenge the assertion that recovery is something that professionals effect, and argued that recovery is something that individuals must do for themselves (Chamberlin, 1988). This passionate message was communicated within emerging narratives of recovery. The understanding of recovery which they have communicated has a radically different focus from clinical recovery. The centrality of hope, identity and personal responsibility has replaced a focus on functioning, symptoms and interventions (Ralph, 2000).

Recovery, in this modern definition, is described as a process of making sense of what has happened, reconstructing a positive identity, accepting, living and growing beyond the limits of mental health problems (e.g. Anthony, 1993; Deegan, 1993; Leete, 1988). Themes of emotional overload and healing from trauma are commonly described. It has also been widely acknowledged that recovery, in its new meaning, has expanded to recognise the need to recover not only from mental **illness**, but also from societal **stigma** and the sometimes devastating effects of medication (Anthony, 1993).

In 2001, the Department of Health issued a policy statement in relation to recovery:

> We need to create an optimistic, positive approach to all people who use mental health services. The vast majority have real prospects of recovery – if they are supported by appropriate services, driven by the right values and attitudes. The mental health system must support people in settings of their own choosing, enable access to community resources including housing, education, work, friendships or whatever they think is critical to their own recovery. (DH, 2001a: 24)

This sentiment has been reinforced by a series of policy initiatives in relation to the 'expert patient' (DH, 2001b), self-management (DH, 2006a), social inclusion (Cabinet Office, 2006) and choice (DH, 2005). A recovery-promoting approach has also received strong support from all the major mental health professions (see the Royal College of Psychiatrists' *Fair Deal Manifesto* (2008) and the Chief Nursing Officer quinquennial review: *From Values to Action* (DH, 2006b)).

As recovery has become more widely recognised within mainstream mental health services as an important concept, debates surrounding the use of the term, the practical implementation and the philosophy of the concept have erupted. Many feel that the initial grassroots ideas encompassed by recovery have taken on a new and more sinister meaning as recovery is adopted by mainstream services. Common critiques of recovery include that:

- It has been 'hijacked' and subverted within policy to serve the purposes of those in power and remove ownership from survivors themselves. In this way, the personally meaningful has been transformed into a corporate exercise (Mair Edwards, 2015).
- Increasing co-option of recovery by bio-psychiatry is suited to wider forms of socio-economic oppression defined by neo-liberal political ideology concerned with fitness to work under capitalism. Resistance is voiced by groups such as Recovery in the Bin who assert the right to be 'un-recovered' (Thomas, 2016).
- The vagueness of the concept means it is widely accepted as a 'good thing' without consideration of the underlying politics which may be at play (Rose, 2014).
- The term 'recovery' continues to imply illness and deficit and so reinforces the medical model despite arguing otherwise (Beresford, 2015).

- 'Recovery' is difficult to apply to certain contexts such as older people or intellectual and developmental disability (Slade et al., 2014).
- It is an idea that is difficult to apply to non-western, collectivist cultures (Lapsley et al., 2002).
- Its focus on the individual and the **values** of hope, control and opportunity undermine the current and historical abuse that people experience, downplaying the importance of context beyond an individual's ability to influence or change (Arenella, 2015).
- The welcomed emphasis on personal recovery is lost when faced with the reality of assessment and outcome measurement, which default back to a focus on psychosocial rehabilitation (Davidson et al., 2006).
- Staff within mental health services are reluctant to adopt new ways of working and fear that these may be implemented as part of a cost-cutting agenda and will leave people open to neglect and poor care (Thornicroft et al., 2008).
- Recovery is nothing new; we are 'doing it already' (Roberts & Boardman, 2013).

The challenge is now for mental health service providers to create services that nurture the original principles of recovery. However, as the recovery message has begun to demand a higher priority and the debate has grown more complex, the struggle that NHS services face in providing recovery-focused practice has intensified. Indeed, although the 'why?' has grown abundantly clear through policy and personal narrative, the 'how?' of recovery-focused change has remained vague and difficult to articulate.

CRITICAL THINKING STOP POINT 18.1

Is 'recovery' meaningful to you? Do you see the need for services to be 'recovery focused' or is this a vague and meaningless concept?

WHAT'S THE EVIDENCE? 18.1

First-hand accounts of recovery have contributed to the development of a recovery orientation in the literature (Jacobsen, 2001; Jacobsen & Greenley, 2001; Ralph, 2000; Young & Ensing, 1999). Several different domains have been suggested as defining features of recovery orientation, such as the development of spirituality, a sense of identity (Liberman, 2002; Noordsy et al., 2002), hope, choice, social relationships, the availability of peer support, feelings of independence and autonomy, and involvement in meaningful activity (Onken et al., 2002, 2007). The values contained within the recovery orientation have been at the core of a grassroots social movement that envisions and advocates for major reform of the mental health service system (Resnick et al., 2005).

Many advocates of recovery have rejected the overreliance on evidence-based practice in favour of values-based ways of working. Criticisms of evidence-based approaches have been levelled from people with lived experience whose views are often missing from the literature. Service-user-run groups highlight the importance of flexible solutions, which do not match with the need for standards, criteria and practice guidelines for evidence-based practice (Mead & MacNeil, 2002). Because of this, people who use services have emphasised values-based practice as feeling more inclusive to their opinions (Perry et al., 2013).

Values-based practice has been developed as an equal, and essential, counterpart to evidence-based practice, offering theory and skills for making decisions where there are potentially conflicting values. The National Institute for Mental Health in England (NIMHE) includes recovery within the national framework of values for mental health, which underpins the Ten Essential Shared Capabilities (Hope, 2004), identifying it as part of a respect for diversity (Woodbridge & Fulford, 2004: 25). Farkas (2007) suggests that there are four core recovery values: person orientation, person involvement, self-determination or choice, and growth potential, while Repper and Perkins (2003) emphasise hope, control and opportunity.

CRITICAL THINKING STOP POINT 18.2

What would you suggest as the core values of recovery-based practice and how can you evidence these in your own practice?

RECOVERY IN DIVERSE SETTINGS

Recovery in its modern sense has originated among an adult mental health population. Because of this, many of the ideas and approaches contained within a recovery-focused approach appear to be more difficult to translate into other settings. Slade et al. (2014) identify this belief as one of the common 'abuses' of recovery and argue that while the ideology has roots in adult mental health, it is relevant to a wide range of populations. Here we would include family, friends and **carers** (Machin & Repper, 2013).

Within this section, we will consider some of the settings in which recovery is considered to be more challenging to apply.

Across the life span

For older and younger people, identification with the word recovery is less common. For older people, the term recovery may continue to hold connotations of 'getting better' or recovering from illness. In contrast, children and younger people are in the process of establishing their sense of self and are consequently unclear about what they might be recovering from. Daley et al. (2013) found that, for older people, the important components of recovery include finding **coping** strategies, taking personal responsibility and the impact of their mental health on their identity. Unlike younger adults, older people did not strive toward a new sense of self, nor did they seek support from their peers. In **dementia** services, the term recovery has been replaced with a 'living well' approach due to the degenerative nature of dementia being incongruent with the word recovery (DH, 2009). For younger people, many of the components of a recovery-focused approach may apply more naturally. For example, holding hope and facilitating opportunities may be easier in a population where youth and opportunities to develop are abundant. Despite this, it may also be more natural to adopt a paternalistic or directive approach due to the age dynamic between staff and young people.

Multiply-disadvantaged groups

There is very little evidence about the experience of recovery as it applies to groups who face multiple discrimination because of factors such as racism, sexism and homophobia in addition to the challenges around their mental health. It is known that people from these groups are likely to experience a higher incidence of mental health challenges, including suicide and use of mental health legislation (Fitzpatrick et al., 2014). Many people attribute their distress to their negative experiences of society. However, the processes used within organisations and the assumptions made within the literature can serve to reinforce social processes of exclusion. For recovery to be meaningful to people, it needs to take account not only of their personal journey, but also the social and political context within which their recovery occurs. In order to be meaningful, the recovery agenda must consider people's real lives, including their 'pre-story' and underlying causes of distress, which may be rooted in social oppression (Kalathil, 2011).

Forensic health settings

Forensic health settings are one of the most difficult for implementing recovery. Given the confines of the judicial system, it can be difficult to understand how hope can be promoted, control can be offered and meaningful opportunities can be provided. In addition, the stigma experienced by people in forensic services and their families may be increased significantly due to the application of mental health diagnoses and criminal records. Drennan et al. (2014) have set out an approach for implementing recovery within forensic settings which centres on five important components: maintaining safety and security for everyone; participation of people in all aspects of their own care; open and transparent decision making in partnership with people; informed choice; and nurturing enabling relationships with staff, peers, family and friends. Despite the obvious constraints, staff and service users within secure settings have begun to develop recovery initiatives, and accounts of personal journeys include poignant references to redemptive experiences (McKeown et al., 2016; Mezey et al., 2010). Rethink Mental Illness, a mental health charity, convenes a recovery and outcomes network that brings together service users, staff and commissioners from secure services across England to strategically influence care and treatment practices (McKeown et al., 2017).

Following two suicides in 2013, Ranby's mental health team felt a strong need to promote their service and try and reach those who may be hidden due to fear or stigma. One idea generated from a life sentenced prisoner was that the best people to help prisoners were prisoners themselves. He believed that he could reach more individuals than we could as professionals as he had 'walked the walk'. He felt it would be beneficial for prisoners to have basic mental health training to enable them to help and offer support to fellow prisoners who might be struggling. The idea of the Mental Health Awareness Peer Support was born and we are now recruiting for our 5th cohort of Navigators.

We hope that this project will help normalise mental health issues and allow patients to access mental health services without stigma. For the peer support workers, we hope this project provides a framework to support their recovery. To provide a sense of being believed in, being listened to and understood. We hope it promotes a feeling of self-worth which they will be able to take with them when they leave prison. We hope that it provides a belief in their own abilities and that although they may not always have full control over their experiences, they have control over their lives.

Having prisoners work as peer support workers is an innovative idea and one that we think will bring about huge benefits to the prison population. Having been in similar situations themselves, prisoners can relate to the sorts of problems others may be facing, enabling them to offer shared understanding, support and advice in a down to earth way.

Heidi Asplin, occupational therapist

APPROACHES TO USE FOR RECOVERY-FOCUSED WORKING

Certain approaches have become an essential part of recovery-focused working and we consider these in the following sections.

Co-production

Co-production can be challenging to define, but key features include building on people's existing capabilities to see them as assets and working together to achieve a mutual goal in an equal partnership (SCIE, 2013). Boyle and Harris (2009: 11), in a report for the New Economics Foundation, state that:

> Co-production promotes equal partnership between service workers and those intended to benefit from their services – pooling different kinds of knowledge and skill, and working together ... designing and delivering public services in an equal and reciprocal relationship between professionals, people using services, their families and their neighbours.

Co-production can support initiatives such as personal budgeting, and is core to specific projects such as delivering training in **recovery colleges** (Perkins et al., 2012). But it can also be a fundamental value of everyday relationships where staff co-produce with the person they are supporting to achieve their goals.

Strengths focus

Strengths are what make recovery possible and, by drawing these out, it is possible to use them to support the recovery of others. A strengths focus can be adopted by using hobbies and interests both to build social relationships and enable people to (re)discover their sense of capability. In addition, a strengths focus can be expressed in a communication style which consistently acknowledges achievements and 're-frames' experiences of failure into opportunities for learning and growth. This does not mean that important and difficult issues can't be discussed, merely that they are discussed in the context of a person's abilities and whole identity rather than in the context of illness or diagnosis. Positive psychology neatly sums this up as a move from 'what's wrong to what's strong'.

Non-directive approach

A recovery-focused approach is founded on the belief that each person knows what is best for them and is able to reach their own solutions. Instead of offering advice, open questions and active listening skills may help a person gain a better understanding of their situation and find their own direction as a result.

Mental health professionals have the knowledge to suggest available options without directing choices: for example, they might suggest that a recovery college course might be of interest, but they would not make referrals. However, there may be times when they feel they need to act in the person's 'best interests'. Where this produces conflict, they can encourage the person to seek additional support from an advocacy service; indeed, in some circumstances, professionals have a duty to ensure the person has access to independent mental health advocacy (IMHA) (Newbigging et al., 2015).

CASE STUDY:
SUPPORTING
JANE

Mutuality

A recovery-focused approach acknowledges that the personal goals of the person being supported should also be the goal of anyone who supports them. A mutual way of working is one that strives to reduce the power imbalance between supporter and supportee. Mutuality is not a natural process within mental health services; Shery Mead, the creator of the Intentional **Peer Support** model, states that 'everything we have learned about help in the mental health system pushes us to think of it as a one-way process' (Mead & MacNeil, 2006: 32). The development of new roles of 'peer workers' within health care services is one means by which an immediate sense of mutuality can be negotiated (Repper, 2013), as is the co-learning that takes place on recovery college courses where all parties are learning together. The development of mutual relationships requires skilled work and ongoing reflection to review where the power lies and whether this is helpful.

Safety

Given the subjective nature of the concept, it is important to build relationships based on an agreed understanding of what feels 'safe' in terms of personal boundaries, trust and communication. Language can form an important part of a safe relationship, and adopting language which feels comfortable to the person, while gently reframing any highly negative language, is important. Feelings of being 'unsafe' can be triggered by a number of factors which are specific to individuals. These include feeling rejected, dehumanised, embarrassed or judged. These factors are sometimes difficult to identify but are important to attune to. This concept of safety relates closely to the ideas of 'containment' (Bion, 1962) and 'holding' (Winnicott, 1945) in psychology.

Numerous important policies, including a duty of care, health and safety and **safeguarding**, emphasise the central position which risk occupies within modern mental health services. As a result, mental health practice has moved from a therapeutic focus to a risk focus which, according to some, has caused a narrowing of the options provided to people (Sawyer, 2005). People who use services value practitioners who can support them to feel in control of their own lives by taking positive risks that help them to regain a sense of personhood: '(The) biggest risk in life is not to risk at all. We may avoid suffering, but we won't learn or grow' (Young et al., 2008: 1430).

Wellness planning

A popular approach for supporting people's recovery is the use of a '**wellness plan**'. This is sometimes also referred to as a recovery plan or wellbeing plan and may take different forms. The most widely known tool for wellness planning is the Wellness Recovery Action Plan (WRAP; Copeland, 1997). Generally, wellness plans focus on similar themes which include helping people to identify their personal **triggers** (external events which **affect** wellbeing) and **early warning signs** (behaviours, feelings or thoughts which indicate things aren't quite right). Some plans also include a section for what support is helpful in a crisis and how to move on following this. The use of a WRAP has been linked to statistically significant changes in the awareness of early warning signs, the awareness of personal triggers and the ability to use positive coping strategies and take responsibility for personal wellness (e.g. Cook et al., 2012).

In addition to written tools, creative formats such as collage or film may be helpful in supporting people. The use of peer support has also been found to be particularly powerful as a peer support worker can share their own wellness plan and support people to develop theirs. It is important, however, that using a wellness plan is the choice of the individual and is not imposed on them.

CRITICAL THINKING STOP POINT 18.3

How would you use these skills in practice? Do they complement your way of working? Do you recognise these skills as a core part of your role? How might a recovery orientation be supported by thinking about concepts such as therapeutic alliance?

CASE STUDY 18.1

Working with family members

Ann is a carer for her son, Tom, who has recently been admitted to a ward under a Section of the Mental Health Act (England and Wales). This is the first time this has happened in her family and Ann is distressed about what this means and what people from her church will think. But she is also relieved as, for the last few months, she has been unable to make sense of what is happening for him. She has been given a letter that tells her she is the nearest relative. She has also been told all about visiting hours and the ward rounds, but is wondering how to look after the rest of the family, and keep her job, as well as support Tom. She has also asked you how long Tom will be in hospital for. You know that Tom blames his parents for everything.

- What can you do to support Ann?
- How can you support recovery where families have opposing views?

IMPLEMENTING RECOVERY-FOCUSED MENTAL HEALTH SERVICES

The redefinition of recovery demands that services begin to examine their **culture**, structures and practices. Their goal is no longer to eradicate symptoms, but to build the capacity to feel in control of one's life; impart knowledge about recovery and available options; improve satisfaction with quality of life; and inspire hope and optimism for the future (Resnick et al., 2005). An understanding of how this transformation of services can occur is now emerging. International guidance suggests that there needs to be consideration of four levels of practice: what interventions are offered, and how, as well as their place within the organisation and in wider society (Le Boutillier et al., 2011).

The ImROC programme in England has developed a framework by which organisations might become more recovery orientated (Shepherd et al., 2008), including self-assessment centred around four transformational themes:

- a change in the role of mental health professionals and professional expertise
- a redefinition of the purpose of services from reducing symptoms to rebuilding lives
- recognition of the equal importance of both 'professional expertise' and 'lived experience'
- a different relationship between services and the communities that they serve.

However, any change and the creation of new services produce uncertainty for staff and raise anxieties, including fear of redundancy, low morale and concerns about loss of status and power (Thornicroft et al., 2008). In addition, the call to work in a new way can feel like an indirect criticism of traditional ways of working. Ramon (2011) suggests that while these losses need to be acknowledged, attention should remain on the potential gains involved in recovery-focused ways of working so that the process is viewed as a win-win situation (where both staff and people using services stand to benefit).

The pressing need for organisations to adopt recovery-focused ways of working has contributed to the advent of an additional, institutionally defined meaning of the concept. On this definition, recovery is conceptualised as a bureaucratic and economically guided vision which has led people to become suspicious of initiatives labelled as recovery-focused, such as employment targets and reduced inpatient stays (Le Boutillier et al., 2015). As a result, some have argued that statutory mental health services are the wrong place to house attempts to implement recovery-focused ways of working. However, this does not detract from the need for people's experiences of these services to improve.

While it is clear that implementing recovery-focused approaches requires organisational commitment, individuals and staff teams have the potential to transform their ways of working within an organisation to adopt new approaches. Small changes such as using strengths-based language within notes, being led by the person rather than leading them, and using the existing strengths and interests within the team may go a long way to changing cultures. Innovative teams across the country have implemented 'no force first' and collaborative note-writing procedures to great effect.

CASE STUDY 18.2

Supporting Jane

I've been using services now for over 20 years. They sectioned me three times but that was a long while back now. I go to the Clinic to get my depot injection every three weeks and I still see the psychiatrist every few months. I used to go to the drop in centre, but they closed it down three years ago. Now they say we have to be socially included. They told me I should go to the college for creative writing, but I liked the teacher and my friends at the drop in. I don't want to go to the college: it's the other side of town and I don't know anyone else who goes. I liked the drop in. We had a good group. Everyone keeps talking about recovery now: they even have a recovery college. But that makes me panic more. It's just an excuse to stop my benefits. If I recover, they'll make me go to work, won't they?

What support could you offer?

MEASURING RECOVERY

Given that recovery was initially transformed by the voices of people using services, narrative accounts present the most powerful means of communicating recovery-focused change. Qualitative methods allow individuals to self-define recovery and offer a less reductive approach to measuring this. Such methods have been integral to the development of the understanding of peer support, the personal meaning of recovery and people's experiences of crisis. Despite this, the prestige of qualitative approaches remains comparatively low, and quantitative measures, in particular randomised controlled trials, remain the gold standard of clinical research.

The Royal College of Psychiatrists (2013) has described the need to 'value the importance of outcomes and accurate data', one of five key imperatives in improving the quality of mental health services. Initiatives such as 'payment by results' further increase the need to create reliable measures relating to recovery-focused practices. Newman-Taylor et al. (2015) argue that it is feasible to co-produce service evaluations with the equal involvement of people using and working within services. Any research into recovery-focused practice ideally endeavours to model the values of recovery in the process of carrying it out. Therefore, methods which are less directive, more inclusive and, at all times, co-produced are worthy forms of evaluation.

CRITICAL THINKING STOP POINT 18.4

How would you measure recovery within your role? Is measuring 'recovery' important? Is it truly possible?

> If you were to ask me what supporting people towards recovery means to me, I would say fundamentally, it is about forming a partnership with an individual to help support them in managing the mental health problems they may be experiencing. It is not about 'curing' a person or getting them back to where they were necessarily. Instead, I believe it is about working together to find ways of helping them to live with their experiences, with the intent of moving forward.
>
> As students, I feel we have a lot to offer in enabling recovery with the people we work with during placements. For one, I have found that our position as supernumerary learners allows us greater freedom to spend face-to-face time with individuals. I have been able to be there for those who have needed somebody to listen to how they are thinking and feeling. Simply having that time to sit and listen has proved immensely healing for individuals I have worked with, and I think this is a fundamental principle that should never be forgotten.
>
> Of course, it is a common fear among students that once they qualify and enter the profession as staff nurses, this 'luxury' of having time to spend with individuals will be lost. What I have learned is that we have to work with the obstacles that are presented to us and continue learning ways of working in a recovery-oriented manner that makes every interaction, no matter how small, one that encourages understanding and choice between both nurse and individual.
>
> **Sabrina Carter, student nurse**

MAKING A DIFFERENCE 18.1

Picture the scene. Here I am on an acute psychiatric inpatient ward, sat telling the psychiatrist that I have no hope. Nothing to live for. Imagine then, being given a gentle nudge, and I look at him through my tears and he says 'Clare, I think you would make a very good peer support worker.'

Fast forward to now, five months later. I've completed the Peer Support Training Course and submitted my assignment. I'm tempted to write that sentence out again as I can't quite believe it myself! So why am I so amazed? Well there are a few reasons; one is that I had truly lost all hope. I felt that nobody could help me. Several sections and inpatient stays, numerous medications and some talking therapies, yet still I felt worthless and lost. I forgot who I was, and became somebody I didn't know or like.

Then along came Peer Support. How strange it felt, to sit in a room of people, many with shared experiences similar to my own. Then as I talked to others and shared some of my story, peer support became my new **addiction**.

My view of recovery has totally changed. I know that for me, it's not a linear journey.

I hadn't heard about Peer Support until that life changing day on the ward. I hope that Peer Support grows and grows and lifts more people out of their darkness. I hope that more people like me can find their passion and purpose again. I hope that Peer Support becomes available to all that want and need it. Did I just say hope? What a wonderful word...

Clare Knighton, *peer support worker*

CONCLUSION

Arguably, a turn to recovery as an organising theme for policy and practice has been the major development in UK mental health care in recent years. Grounded in user movement politics and demands, concerted efforts at implementation simultaneously offer transformative hope and risk incorporation into the narrower confines of bureaucratised care. Nurses will have a key role in supporting individuals on their chosen recovery journeys and collaborating with new peer worker colleagues. The skills and values necessary to adequately perform this role to become a positive agent in realising recovery are arguably essential to mental health nursing, and compatible with broader thinking about therapeutic alliance and collaborative, person-centred **care planning** (Leese et al., 2014). Mental health nurses have nothing to fear from recovery notions and a great deal to gain. They must, however, be alert to the possibilities of dilution or co-option of core ideals.

───── CHAPTER SUMMARY ─────

This chapter has covered the following ideas:

- The concept of 'recovery' has been transformed by the voices of people using services, united out of a shared passion for change.
- As opposed to clinical recovery, its new meaning is self-defined by individuals. Recovery has now become a dominant theme in mental health policy and practice, which represents both a success and a challenge as there is a risk that it will become co-opted or diluted.
- Values of recovery can be applied to any service setting or group of people, including primary care, forensic settings, carers, older people or BME groups, and staff themselves.
- The use of specific approaches and language facilitates a recovery-focused approach.
- Other markers of recovery-focused services are the use of peer support or recovery education or minimal restraint 'no force first' initiatives.
- Measuring recovery outcomes is essential for the approaches to continue to be commissioned. However, this can be difficult as self-defined individual recovery is not well suited to broad outcome measurements.

───── BUILD YOUR BIBLIOGRAPHY ─────

Books

- Campbell, P. & Davidson, B. (1999) *From the ashes of experience: Reflections on madness, survival and growth.* Chichester: Wiley.
- Pilgrim, D. & McCranie, A. (2013) *Recovery and mental health: A critical sociological account.* London: Palgrave Macmillan.
- Repper, J. & Perkins, R. (2003) *Social inclusion and recovery: A model for mental health practice.* Sidcup: Bailliere Tindall.
- Slade, M. (2009) *Personal recovery and mental illness: A guide for mental health professionals.* Cambridge: Cambridge University Press.

SAGE journal articles

Go to https://study.sagepub.com/essentialmentalhealth for further free online journal articles related to this chapter. If you are using the interactive ebook, simply click on the book icon in the margin to go straight to the resource.

- Brooks, H.L., Rogers, A., Sanders, C., et al. (2015) Perceptions of recovery and prognosis from long-term conditions: the relevance of hope and imagined futures. *Chronic Illness*, 11(1), 3-20.
- Pilgrim, D. (2008) 'Recovery' and current mental health policy. *Chronic illness*, 4(4), 295-304.
- Topor, A., Borg, M., Di Girolamo, S., et al. (2011) Not just an individual journey: social aspects of recovery. *International Journal of Social Psychiatry*, 57(1), 90-99.

Weblinks

Go to https://study.sagepub.com/essentialmentalhealth for further weblinks related to this chapter. If you are using the interactive ebook, simply click on the book icon in the margin to go straight to the resource.

FURTHER
READING:
WEBLINKS

- Implementing Recovery through Organisational Change (ImROC): www.imroc.org – a collective of consultants who support recovery through changing mental health organisations
- Recovery in the Bin: https://recoveryinthebin.org – website for a radical group committed to challenging the co-option of recovery which also has an active Facebook and Twitter presence
- Research into Recovery: www.researchintorecovery.com/home – led by Mike Slade, this international group was previously situated at King's College London and is now hosted in Nottingham
- Scottish Recovery: www.scottishrecovery.net – established in 2004 to raise awareness about recovery.

ACE YOUR ASSESSMENT

Revise what you have learned by visiting https://study.sagepub.com/essentialmentalhealth. If you are using the interactive ebook, simply click on the tick icon to go straight to the resource.

ONLINE
QUIZZES &
ACTIVITY
ANSWERS

- Test yourself with multiple-choice and short-answer questions and flashcards.

REFERENCES

Anthony, W.A. (1993) Recovery from mental illness: the guiding vision of the mental health service system in the 1990s. *Psychosocial Rehabilitation Journal*, *12*, 55–81.

Arenella, J. (2015) Challenges for the recovery movement in the US: will its light reach the darkest corners? *Clinical Psychology Forum*, *268*, 7–9.

Beresford, P. (2015) From 'recovery' to reclaiming madness. *Clinical Psychology Forum, 268*, 16–20.

Bion, W.R. (1962) *Learning from experience*. London: Heinemann.

Boyle, D. & Harris, M. (2009) *The Challenge of Corruption*. NEF/NESTA. Available at: www.nesta.org.uk/sites/default/files/the-challenge-of-co-production.pdf (accessed 26.11.17).

Cabinet Office (2006) *Reaching out: An action plan on social inclusion*. London: Cabinet Office.

Chamberlin, J. (1988) *On our own*. London: Mind.

Cook, J.A., Copeland, M.E., Jonikas, J., et al. (2012) Results of a randomized controlled trial of mental illness self-management using wellness recovery action planning. *Schizophrenia Bulletin*, *38*, 881–891.

Copeland, M.E. (1997) *Wellness recovery action plan*. Dummerston, VT: Peach Press.

Daley, S., Newton, D., Slade, M., et al. (2013) Development of a framework for recovery in older people with mental disorder. *International Journal of Geriatric Psychiatry*, *28*, 522–529.

Davidson, L., O'Connell, M., Tondora, J., et al. (2006) The top ten concerns about recovery encountered in mental health system transformation. *Psychiatric Services*, *57*, 640–645.

Deegan, P. (1993) Recovering our sense of value after being labeled mentally ill. *Journal of Psychosocial Nursing and Mental Health Services, 31*(4), 7–11.

Department of Health (2001a) *Making it happen: A guide to delivering mental health promotion*. London: DH.

Department of Health (2001b) *The expert patient: A new approach to chronic disease management for the 21st century*. London: DH.

Department of Health (2005) *Creating a patient-led NHS*. London: DH.

Department of Health (2006a) *Supporting people with long-term conditions to self-care: A guide to developing local strategies and good practice*. London: DH.

Department of Health (2006b) *From values to action: The Chief Nursing Officer's review of mental health nursing*. London: DH.

Department of Health (2009) *Living well with dementia: A national dementia strategy*. London: DH.

Drennan, G., Wooldridge, J., Aiyegbusi, A., et al. (2014). *Making Recovery a Reality in Forensic Settings*. [ImROC briefing paper 10]. London: Centre for Mental Health/Mental Health Network/NHS Confederation.

Farkas, M. (2007) The vision of recovery today: what it is and what it means for services. *World Psychiatry, 6*, 68.

Fitzpatrick, R., Kumar, S., Nkansa-Dwamena, O., et al. (2014) *Ethnic inequalities in mental health: Promoting lasting positive change*. London: Lankelly Chase Foundation.

Hope, R. (2004) *The ten essential shared capabilities*. London: NIMHE & Sainsbury Centre for Mental Health.

Jacobsen, N. (2001) Experiencing recovery: a dimensional analysis of recovery narratives. *Psychiatric Rehabilitation Journal, 24*, 248–256.

Jacobsen, N. & Greenley, D. (2001) What is recovery? A conceptual model and explication. *Psychiatric Services, 52*, 482–485.

Kalathil, J. (2011) *Recovery and resilience: African, African-Caribbean and South Asian women's narratives of recovering from mental distress*. London: Mental Health Foundation.

Lapsley, H., Nikora, L.W. & Black, R.M. (2002) *'Kia Mauri Tau!': Narratives of recovery from disabling mental health problems*. Wellington, NZ: Mental Health Commission.

Le Boutillier, C., Chevalier, A., Lawrence, V., et al. (2015) Staff understanding of recovery-orientated mental health practice: a systematic review and narrative synthesis. *Implementation Science, 10*, 445–458.

Le Boutillier, C., Leamy, M., Bird, V.J., et al. (2011) What does recovery mean in practice? A qualitative analysis of international recovery-oriented practice guidance. *Psychiatric Services, 62*, 1470–1476.

Leese, D., Smithies, L. & Green, J. (2014) Recovery focused practice in mental health. *Nursing Times, 110*, 20–22.

Leete, E. (1988) A consumer perspective on psychosocial treatment. *Psychosocial Rehabilitation Journal, 12*, 45–52.

Liberman, R. (2002) Future directions for research studies and clinical work on recovery from schizophrenia: questions with some answers. *International Review of Psychiatry, 14*, 337–342.

Machin, K. & Repper, J. (2013) *Recovery: A carers' perspective*. London: Centre for Mental Health & Mental Health Network, NHS Confederation.

Mair Edwards, B. (2015) Recovery: accepting the unacceptable? *Clinical Psychology Forum, 268*, 26–27.

McKeown, M., Jones, F. & Callaghan, I. (2017) Services for people requiring secure forms of care. In M. Chambers (ed.) *Psychiatric and mental health nursing: The craft of caring*, 3rd edition. Boca Raton, FL: CRC Press.

McKeown, M., Jones, F., Foy, P., et al. (2016) Looking back, looking forward: recovery journeys in a high secure hospital. *International Journal of Mental Health Nursing, 25*, 234–242.

Mead, S. & MacNeil, C. (2002) *Peer support: a systemic approach*. Independent report. Available at: www.semanticscholar.org/paper/peer-support-a-systemic-approach-mead-macneil/5985cf53401a5 3bb4506c67945c38385fc5d3418 (accessed 09.08.17).

Mead, S. & MacNeil, C. (2006) Peer support: what makes it unique? *International Journal of Psychosocial Rehabilitation, 10,* 29–37.

Mezey, G.C., Kavuma, M., Turton, P., et al. (2010) Perceptions, experiences and meanings of recovery in forensic psychiatric patients. *The Journal of Forensic Psychiatry & Psychology, 21*(5), 683–696.

Newbigging, K., Ridley, J., McKeown, M., et al. (2015) *Independent mental health advocacy: The right to be heard.* London: Jessica Kingsley.

Newman-Taylor, K., Herbert, L., Woodfine, C., et al. (2015) Are we delivering recovery-based mental health care? An example of 'co-produced' service evaluation. *Clinical Psychology Forum, 268,* 50–57.

Noordsy, D., Torrey, W., Mueser, K.T., et al. (2002) Recovery from severe mental illness: an intrapersonal and functional outcome definition. *Nursing and Mental Health Services, 31,* 7–11.

Onken, S.J., Craig, C.M., Ridgeway, P., et al. (2007) An analysis of the definitions and elements of recovery: a review of the literature. *Psychiatric Rehabilitation Journal, 31,* 9–22.

Onken, S.J., Dumont, J.M., Ridgway, P., et al. (2002) *Mental health recovery: What helps and what hinders?* A national research project for the development of recovery-facilitating system performance indicators. Alexandria, VA: National Association of State Mental Health Program Directors (NASMHPD) & National Technical Assistance Center (NTAC) for State Mental Health Planning.

Perkins, R. & Slade, M. (2012) Recovery in England: transforming statutory services? *International Review of Psychiatry, 24,* 29–39.

Perkins, R., Repper, J., Rinaldi, M. & Brown, H. (2012) *Recovery colleges briefing.* London: Centre for Mental Health & Mental Health Network, NHS Confederation.

Perry, E., Barber, J. & England, E. (2013) *A review of values-based commissioning.* London: NSUN.

Ralph, R.O. (2000) Recovery. *Psychiatric Rehabilitation Skills, 4,* 480–517.

Ramon, S. (2011) Organisational change in the context of recovery-oriented services. *The Journal of Mental Health Training, Education and Practice, 6,* 38–46.

Repper, J. (2013) *Peer support workers: A practical guide to implementation.* London: Centre for Mental Health & Mental Health Network, NHS Confederation.

Repper, J. & Perkins, R. (2003) *Social inclusion and recovery: A model for mental health practice.* Sidcup: Bailliere Tindall.

Resnick, S., Fontana, A., Lehman, A.F., et al. (2005) An empirical conceptualization of the recovery orientation. *Schizophrenia Research, 75,* 119–128.

Roberts, G. & Boardman, J. (2013) Understanding recovery. *Advances in Psychiatric Treatment, 19,* 400–409.

Rose, D. (2014) Editorial: the mainstreaming of recovery. *Journal of Mental Health, 23*(5), 217–218.

Royal College of Psychiatrists (RCP) (2008) *Fair deal manifesto.* London: RCP.

Royal College of Psychiatrists (RCP) (2013) *Driving quality implementation in the context of the Francis report.* Occasional Paper OP92. London: RCP.

Sawyer, A.M. (2005) From therapy to administration: deinstitutionalisation and the ascendency of psychiatric 'risk thinking'. *Health Sociology Review, 14,* 283–296.

Shepherd, G., Boardman, J. & Slade, M. (2008) *Implementing recovery: A new framework for organisational change.* Briefing Paper. London: Sainsbury Centre for Mental Health.

Slade, M., Amering, A., Farkas, M., et al. (2014) Implementing recovery-orientated practices in mental health systems. *World Psychiatry, 13,* 12–20.

Social Care Institute for Excellence (2013) *Co-production in social care: What it is and how to do it.* SCIE Guide No. 51. London: SCIE.

Thomas, P. (2016) Psycho politics, neoliberal governmentality and austerity. *Self & Society*, *44*(4), 382–393.

Thornicroft, G., Tansella, M. & Law, A. (2008) Steps, challenges and lessons in developing community mental health care. *World Psychiatry*, *7*, 87–92.

Winnicott, D.W. (1945) *Primitive emotional development.* London: Tavistock.

Woodbridge, K. & Fulford, K.W.M. (2004) *Whose values? A workbook for values-based practice in mental health care.* London: Sainsbury Centre for Mental Health.

Young, A., Green, C. & Estroff, S. (2008) New endeavours, risk taking, and personal growth in the recovery process: findings from the STARS study. *Psychiatric Services*, *59*, 1430–1436.

Young, S.L. & Ensing, D.S. (1999) Exploring recovery from the perspective of people with psychiatric disabilities. *Psychiatric Rehabilitation Journal*, *22*, 219–231.

EMPLOYMENT AND RECOVERY IN MENTAL HEALTH CARE

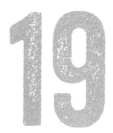

CHRIS ESSEN AND JANE CAHILL

THIS CHAPTER COVERS

- Work, vocation and employment within mental health services and society
- Social inclusion and how labour markets affect mental health service users seeking employment
- Evidence-based practice in the area of vocational rehabilitation
- The work experiences and aspirations of service users
- Principles for practice in vocational rehabilitation.

> "I've seen it myself when we've gone onto wards and we've looked at people's stress and anxiety levels, and people input and say what all their problems are – social housing; they might want to go back to work; they might have a problem with the employer that hasn't been dealt with; you know, families ... And ward staff are really busy, and it's not their fault, but they don't see it as their remit.
>
> **Ann, recovery worker**

> "Is it okay to stick someone with mental health problems, within a month, into a fast food joint? Or is best to wait 6 to 9 months and get them into a job that they're capable of doing, that they want to do, and is actually going to promote and maintain their health? That's the difference between what we do, and what other people do. If we don't do that, if we don't support people into a good job which is going to support their mental health, then we might as well go home.
>
> **Jenny, vocational support worker**

Visit **https://study.sagepub.com/essentialmentalhealth** to access a wealth of online resources for this chapter – watch out for the margin icons throughout the chapter. If you are using the interactive ebook, simply click on the margin icon to go straight to the resource.

Make your work to be in keeping with your purpose. (Leonardo da Vinci)

INTRODUCTION

Consideration of the **value** of employment for mental health **service users**, and the best means to ensure meaningful and rewarding opportunities for work, arguably rest at a significant juncture. In many ways, gainful employment identifies who people are, and may indeed represent the defining characteristic of full **citizenship** (Patrick, 2012). The degradation of services and tightening of welfare entitlements, predicated on a politics of austerity, have presented a recent two-fold squeeze upon mental health service users and this has had particular consequences in the field of employment support. Notably, work capability and personal independence payments (PIP) assessments have quite unashamedly started from an assumption that disability benefits are inappropriately supporting individuals capable of competitive employment, resulting in substantial stress and distress for mental health service users caught up in the system. Forms of therapy have even been deployed entangled in coaching the unemployed, described latterly as 'psycho-**compulsion**' (Friedli & Stearn, 2015; Thomas, 2016). This situation is exacerbated by government-inspired media rhetoric that contrasts 'skivers' (the unemployed) with 'strivers' (the employed), whilst also constructing deserving and undeserving distinctions that depict mental health problems as less deserving forms of disability (Patrick, 2016; Tyler, 2013).

Our experience and knowledge in the area of employment and **recovery** come from having applied collaborative action research to assist a group of stakeholders with attempting to implement an evidence-based approach to vocational support provision within secondary mental health services (Bamford et al., 2012). The above two quotations are from participants in our research, and encapsulate two of the main dilemmas that practising nurses are likely to face when attempting to address vocational issues.

First, as discussed in previous chapters, the established assessment and treatment priorities of mental health nurses have tended to follow those of traditional psychiatry and, as such, have been informed by its frequently reductive biomedical approaches to extremes in human distress, unusual personal perceptions and behaviours which mean some individuals struggle with living according to society's expectations. Despite recent developments in mental health practice, including within psychiatry, evidence suggests that there remain significant tensions between newer, humanistic, recovery-oriented approaches to helping people and the intertwined biomedical and coercive legacies that persist within mental health services (Stickley & Wright, 2011a, 2011b). As our first practitioner voice above suggests, these tensions are worse when there is only limited time available for nurses and other professionals to engage with patients as complex people, with complex lives, rather than as possessors of one or more clinical diagnoses requiring behavioural management and/or pharmacological treatment.

Second, despite vocational issues having received much more attention in recent years, a new form of dogma may be emerging out of some otherwise positive findings – that with intensive in-work support many more mental health service users can take up paid work who might previously have been written off as being unable to. Our second practitioner voice poses some rhetorical questions, which reflect broader concerns in our research group that previous paternalistic projections of incapacity may be being replaced, through the way recovery services are increasingly designed and implemented, by a similarly limited agenda for supporting people into *any paid work at all*. These concerns are in part rooted in growing sensitivity about this political situation in which all sick or disabled welfare benefit claimants are under intense pressure to justify not working. Indeed, uncritical collusion with the most punitive characteristics of recent welfare reforms could undermine the prospect of a more deeply therapeutic approach developing between professionals and service users.

We will go on to look at some of the background to this situation, by exploring a few key constructions of work, employment and vocation that have appeared within mental health services. This grounding is important for maintaining critical distance when examining how work has come to be conceptualised in the present day. The associated rationale, policy and aims behind contemporary practice, intended to be socially inclusive, will briefly be examined, and acknowledgement made of the extent to which people with a mental illness diagnosis are likely to find themselves both impoverished and disproportionately excluded from the paid workforce. The links between poverty, labour markets and how the welfare benefits system operates will be discussed, such that readers can begin to assess for themselves the research evidence behind a current overarching emphasis on assisting unemployed service users with rapid entry into paid employment. Qualitative research literature will illustrate a number of pertinent observations about the motivation and capacity for work among service users themselves. We will then conclude by offering some 'principles for practice' in vocational rehabilitation, derived from our own research, and suggestions for other, progressive, recovery-focused nursing practice to support nurses, occupational therapists and vocational support specialists with working in partnership.

WORK, VOCATION AND EMPLOYMENT IN MENTAL HEALTH SERVICES AND SOCIETY

Despite important differences in their formal definitions, the words 'work', 'employment' and 'vocation' have tended to be used interchangeably across both academic literature and everyday practice talk. A more nuanced appreciation of such language recognises that a career in nursing, for example, constitutes a 'vocation'. Often described by the religiously inclined as a 'calling', having a vocation is, by definition, a career that offers meaning and fulfilment over and above simply earning money, and is on occasion based around an altruistic form of social contract. So, the altruistic commitment associated with a career in nursing is reflected in the fact that, up until fairly recently, the NMC Code explicitly stated that it was the duty of a registered nurse to help out in the event of crisis, when and wherever they encountered it. Although this requirement has since been relaxed, it is still the case that if a suitably qualified nurse were not to offer assistance at the scene of an accident, for instance, when it was safe and appropriate to do so, this would be frowned upon by the NMC. Therefore, at least in principle, registration as a nurse might lead to instances of unpaid work.

Employment, on the other hand, is nothing more than the contractual relationship between an employer and an employee, where an employee carries out a predefined range of work tasks (a job) for an agreed amount of financial reward (pay). Employment need not offer anything deeper, in terms of life meaning, and may indeed precipitate the stress and distress that define alienated work. Thus, we might ask to what degree recovery-oriented support for mental health service users should be concerned with achieving employment, addressing vocational needs, or both. In answering this question, it is additionally relevant to define the limits of what we mean by work. Within most everyday contexts, 'work' refers simply to expending effort to achieve a tangible outcome (albeit that the same word is nominal shorthand for either paid employment or a place of employment). Therefore, a further distinction can be drawn between a person's vocational aspirations, paid employment and a broader understanding of work that encompasses other socially imposed requirements for the completion of tasks (Royal College of Psychiatrists, 2002). Some of these do not attract financial reward, such as putting the bins out or caring for sick relatives, but may be, in some sense, occupationally meaningful to the individual.

The types of work that mental health service users have been expected to engage in has varied over time. Indeed, their inability or unwillingness to meet the basic work expectations society imposes may have contributed to someone coming to the attention of services, and consequently receiving a mental **illness** diagnosis. Current developments in the creation of **peer support** roles ironically subvert such normative expectations, making a virtue of lived experience as the key characteristic of role expectation (Repper & Carter, 2011).

Laws (2011) provides us with a useful historical overview of these issues and highlights how work in itself came to be viewed as therapeutic, within the burgeoning asylum system. She traces attitudes towards work as these appeared alongside dominant social mores, between 1813 and 1979. Readers are encouraged to digest the full extent of her study for themselves, since we can only cover it briefly here, but her analysis appears motivated at the outset by a significant critical observation that: 'beliefs in the healthful properties of work have become a politically virulent (although comparatively under-theorized) concept in justifying the return of individuals on sickness-related benefits to the free labour market' (Laws, 2011: 184).

Laws is referring here to an influential claim that has emerged this century regarding employment, which we shall return to – that supporting people with rapid entry into competitive employment actually improves mental health (Perkins et al., 2009).

The earliest phase in the development of therapeutic work identified by Laws consisted of religious attempts at moral rehabilitation. Cooperation with the everyday practical tasks essential for both patients and staff to fulfil, in order to sustain the asylum community itself, meant that interventions typically centred on the self-control required for someone to engage in repetitive physical tasks such as farm work, with engagement in these activities seen as an indicator of moral progress. As the 20th century approached, Laws notes, institutions lost sight of this process for directly making a living and were instead preoccupied with reaping the economic benefits of alienated industrialised forms of labour that were becoming characteristic of wider society. It was not then until after the turn of the century that there was a resurgence of interest in simple, pastoral work activity being a source of occupational therapy:

> Through a return to traditional crafts such as basket-weaving and pottery-making, the early occupational therapists thus sought to rescue a restorative work ethic both from the degrading practices of factory work and from the quiet despotism of bed-rest and, in doing so, to rescue the soul of the patient. (2011: 188)

A key point to take from Laws' analysis is that these periodic changes in the role of work within the asylum system were highly influenced by external social factors (in the above case, the arts and crafts movement). This was perhaps most evident with the outbreak of the Second World War, when institutional labour was absorbed into supporting the general war effort, leading to diminished regard for occupational therapy. Resettlement back into a rehabilitative agenda during the post-war period saw two distinct strands of thinking emerge, Laws notes. First, an ascendant biomedical field began to propose restorative potential in the repetitive physical movements characteristic of certain types of work; while, second, Freudian thinking influenced a parallel view that the physical products of work themselves, such as pottery, were a location for patients to express their unconscious psychic world. Notwithstanding the continuation of these strands within specific clinical arenas, by the mid to latter part of the 20th century institutional manufacturing facilities had sprung up as an attempt to replicate modern industrial settings, with the express purpose of preparing patients to enter the general workforce (what is now known as pre-vocational training).

Perhaps the most salient thing to say about Laws' final analysis is that she articulates important and enduring 'tensions' in how work has been conceptualised over the period she covers, centring on an underlying distinction between therapeutic work and work being the goal of therapeutic interventions. Linked to this is recognition of a further difference, that between a patient preparing for the outside world of work, by doing work in a protective **environment** (work as therapy), and them experiencing the conventional rewards of working (work because of therapy). Central to the first of these is a notion that certain forms of work or work environment are inherently therapeutic. We are now experiencing a period during which supported employment is thought therapeutic, for which we might similarly identify significant societal influences.

CRITICAL THINKING STOP POINT 19.1

- What are the distinct moral and political features of how work is thought about in our time?
- How has wider society possibly influenced the way employment support services are delivered?

SOCIAL INCLUSION AND INFLUENCE FROM THE LABOUR MARKET

It can be difficult to disentangle the idea of social inclusion from that of recovery-oriented practice. However, working towards social inclusion principally relies on policymakers and others helping to set the specific social conditions necessary for ensuring that all people in society are valued and able to share in its material and cultural benefits. Whereas, by engaging in recovery-oriented practice, a practitioner works with specific individuals to maximise their social inclusion. In theory, it would seem then that if we can create socially inclusive conditions, and appropriately support the capacity of individuals to engage with these, policy and practice should meet in the middle (Boardman, 2011). However, the individualistic normative thrust of social inclusion attempts may mean that we start to neglect the deeper structural ways that society discriminates against some people, through its dominant socio-economic paradigm. In other words, social inclusion may simply be about providing increased opportunities for people to try harder to fit into mainstream society:

> Rather than being seen as a necessary and unquestionable 'human right' or a top-down form of social engineering, social inclusion can be viewed as a paradoxical claim which both expresses a genuine demand to tackle the consequences of social inequality and yet at the same time could become another way people with mental health problems are subject to moral and social regulation. (Spandler, 2007: 3)

We can say with some certainty that many mental health service users currently experience a high degree of social exclusion, because they are disproportionately impoverished. This exclusion presents a complex causative picture, with people already in poverty much more likely than the general population to start to experience mental health problems, while the emergence of mental health problems also often leads to an individual descending into poverty. A recent report by the Mental Health Foundation (Elliott, 2016) provides a holistic view of poverty in mental health that highlights, among other things, its links to stigmatisation within the context of a normative social environment characterised by unhelpful political and media narratives about both the unemployed and mental health.

One of the main challenges that unemployed mental health service users face, because of problems in the economy since 2008, is the disproportionately negative effect this has had on their prospects (Beatty & Fothergill, 2011; Beatty et al., 2011). For example, a study found nearly one third of the working-age population unemployed in the 100 areas of highest unemployment in the UK outside of London, with those without a strong work record finding it very difficult to compete for jobs (Beatty et al., 2011). Yet targeted job creation schemes are incompatible with the neo-liberal competitive philosophy preferred by governing politicians. Despite evidence for their effectiveness, condition management programmes for the unemployed were wound up and replaced by a work programme in which providers receive payment by results (Beatty et al., 2013). Providers were effectively incentivised to concentrate on the 'low hanging fruit' of those closest to the jobs market, and to neglect those whose support needs were more complex or intensive, such as those who have been residing within forensic mental health services.

Similarly, compelled 'social inclusion' into unrewarding work, or entry into workplaces that are not properly socialised into inclusionary practices, can lead service users into stressful alienating experiences inimical to their wellbeing. While older forms of 'sheltered' employment have been justly criticised as outdated, and associated with disabling institutionalisation, there may still be a case for thinking about some form of protected workspace or transitional spaces as a precursor to mainstream competitive employment. A-Way Couriers, a long established user-led social enterprise in Toronto, Canada, is a competitive business that only employs mental health service users. People can work anything from two hours a week to full-time, in the booking office or as a courier, and the pace of the work and management practices suit people who have suffered quite disabling experiences. Crucially, shared experiences amongst workmates ensure a lack of **stigma** and positive, comradely relationships. Many people have used employment in this somewhat protected environment to launch subsequent careers in the mainstream labour market.

CRITICAL THINKING STOP POINT 19.2

The economic climate is one factor that can under-write the approach taken to supporting people. Can you think of any other salient contextual factors? What would their likely impact be on how service users are treated?

INDIVIDUAL PLACEMENT AND SUPPORT (IPS) AS EVIDENCE-BASED PRACTICE

Multiple randomised controlled trials have revealed that Individual Placement and Support (IPS) is the most successful approach for achieving entry into competitive employment, its main desirable outcome measurement (Bond et al., 2008; Burns et al., 2008; Crowther et al., 2001; Drake et al., 2003; Twamley et al., 2003). Effective implementation of IPS occurs according to seven fundamental principles, as listed by Rinaldi et al. (2010: 163):

competitive employment is the goal, the job search occurs rapidly, eligibility is based on client choice, job choice follows client preference, support is ongoing and is based on client need, employment and mental health services are integrated, and personalised welfare benefits advice and guidance is provided.

IPS contrasts with sheltered work or pre-vocational training, the main forms that vocational services took prior to IPS gaining popularity, in that it imposes a strict 'place then train' requirement, and is accepted as being the only evidence-based practice in this specific area of service provision.

However, our own analysis of the IPS research data (Essen, 2012) discovered significant problems with how IPS research evidence had been constructed and presented in relation to policymaking. We found that some of the statistical claims made in support of IPS, which implied most unemployed service users wanted to work in competitive employment, were quite misleading. Scratching below the surface of the evidence cited by proponents, we found, for instance, that only a minority of people surveyed actually said that they wanted this kind of work (Secker et al., 2001). Further, there continues to be a lack of research evidence about the range of aspirations people have and are likely to express when asked within a non-stigmatising context.

A further, confusing claim found in an important review of vocational support provision, called Realising Ambitions, asserted that: 'There is strong evidence that appropriate work actively improves mental health and protects against relapse' (Perkins et al., 2009: 19).

The formulation of 'recovery' used within the document was linked to a dual model of mental illness and health, where mental 'wellness' is considered to be a lack of diagnosable mental illness, and is treated separately from mental 'wellbeing', which is presented as shorthand for good mental health (Westerhof & Keyes, 2009). So, it may be said that an individual can experience the symptoms of a diagnosable mental illness, while simultaneously being in either good or bad mental health, according to whether or not they have a 'meaningful, valued and satisfying life – including gainful employment' (Perkins et al., 2009: 22). This is certainly an interesting distinction, that may have its merits, but we found no evidence that working does anything to ameliorate mental illness symptoms in the sense that most people would probably interpret the statement (Essen, 2012).

On top of our critical analysis of previous research, our own research group provided useful insights that led us to emphasise the importance of a pragmatic, needs-led (rather than model-led) approach to recovery-focused support, that we will come onto.

WHAT IS THE EVIDENCE? 19.1

Randomised controlled trials rely on the willing engagement of research participants who have already identified themselves as amenable to the main proposed outcomes of the approach tested, by virtue of having volunteered to join a study with those aims. In the case of IPS, which aims solely for sustained employment in the competitive jobs market, there appears to be a lack of rich foundational evidence about what it is service users actually want from vocational support services. Therefore, we have to wonder to what extent the participants in IPS trials actually represent the true range of vocational aspirations found in the service user population.

CRITICAL THINKING STOP POINT 19.3

What, in your view, are the benefits of rapid entry into paid employment for service users?

THE EXPERIENCES AND ASPIRATIONS OF SERVICE USERS

Service users have reported that participation in a job provides an opportunity to reflect on their performance alongside that of others, in a way that may eventually lead to the establishment of a more mainstream identity (Borg & Kristiansen, 2008; Boyce et al., 2008; Leufstadius et al., 2009; Nithsdale et al., 2008; Provencher et al., 2002; van Niekerk, 2009). Engaging with a 'normal' community and participating in 'normal' activities, with the 'right' people (Broer et al., 2011), may offer the improved status of being considered a 'normal' person (Marwaha & Johnson, 2005).

The stability of a structured everyday routine provides people with controlled exposure to social situations, and opportunities that test their practical abilities (Borg & Kristiansen, 2008; Boyce et al., 2008; Dunn et al., 2008; Hillborg et al., 2010; Leufstadius et al., 2009). A balanced set of appropriately challenging work demands, if successfully engaged with, may, for some, lead to positive feelings of esteem, energy and wellbeing (Boyce et al., 2008; Leufstadius et al., 2009) and distraction from distress (Dunn et al., 2008; Hillborg et al., 2010):

> activities seen as meaningful to the individual (whether paid work or something else), plus a sense of responsibility for problems, personal control and understanding of mental health issues would appear to be important qualities fostered by those reporting a good quality of life. (Nithsdale et al., 2008: 181)

However, these positive attributes are sensitive to variations in **mood** and capacity (van Niekerk, 2009), and issues of **coping** with the other social and practical aspects of working are prominent in many accounts (e.g. Marwaha & Johnson, 2005; Nithsdale et al., 2008). Service users may even give public accounts of wanting a job, without then actually doing anything to seek one (Alverson et al., 2006; Marwaha & Johnson, 2005). There are various reasons for this, including feelings of social stigma (Boyce et al., 2008), along with familial and cultural factors (Alverson et al., 2006; Nithsdale et al., 2008). Individual acceptance and positive adaptation to receiving a mental illness diagnosis are also significant (Borg & Kristiansen, 2008; Nithsdale et al., 2008).

PRINCIPLES FOR PRACTICE IN VOCATIONAL REHABILITATION

> We get this big obsession that the clinical side is the important thing. I think that's only a small part, when I look at my recovery ... you've got this clinical bit, which is important, but you've got the bigger picture which is the outside world of coping with that.
>
> **Clive, service user**

Our research occurred within a special research and development partnership, with Leeds Partnership NHS Trust and Leeds Mind, which sought to find out which aspects, features and processes of professional practice and service design would work best in assisting people who used adult mental health services to retain, or find and sustain, meaningful employment (Bamford et al., 2012). Identifying local good practice and reviewing international research evidence assisted us in making a range of practical changes to service provision. Achieving these changes necessitated a participative approach to engaging with NHS staff, service users and voluntary sector support providers. In very simple terms, we provided a collaborative research process through which stakeholders could harness their personal experiences of delivering or receiving vocational support, in order to develop a consensus on what was best practice, before co-producing a suitable range of provision. We expressed our best practice consensus through a collection of statements, linked to the notion of recovery, described as principles for practice:

- Recovery for someone diagnosed with a mental illness often means simply reclaiming their everyday life with other people in society.
- Vocational rehabilitation assists recovery by working with a person to develop their hopes, confidence and abilities in engaging with a structured routine of everyday life activity that is both personally meaningful and rewarding.
- Vocational rehabilitation is a developmental learning process that should occur at the service user's own pace and be broken down into realistic steps, while recognising that there will be fluctuations in their attitude, opinion and ability over time.
- The most important first step in vocational rehabilitation is starting the journey towards personally meaningful activity, which may or may not include attempting to access paid employment straightaway.
- Recovery can be significantly enhanced if activity is financially rewarding.
- Employment support is specifically about helping someone to retain, gain or maintain paid employment. It can be both a major vehicle for and an end goal of vocational rehabilitation.
- Many service users feel able to take up paid employment, or can be encouraged to do so, when specialist employment support and benefits advice is available to them.
- Some service users might not want to talk about paid work at all, but could still want to explore their vocational options.
- While it is important to be honest with a service user about the steps involved in achieving a particular goal, it is also important not to be over-protective, and to recognise that paid employment is a real possibility for many people diagnosed with a mental illness.
- Inspiring hope is fundamentally important, with service users relying on multiple sources of information in deciding what is possible for someone in their position. People involved in their care should be giving a consistent message of positively supporting vocational goals, including employment.
- Sometimes foundational steps are required to help someone with confidently managing structure and routine, before they are prepared to consider accessing paid employment.
- Some people find that volunteering is useful for building their confidence, gaining work experience and eliciting work references. As such, volunteering is not the final destination for most service users.
- Clinicians may need to focus on helping someone to develop basic life skills, such as using public transport, before progressing to a vocational support specialist. However, vocational goals, particularly job retention-related ones, ought to be identified right from the beginning of somebody's care and reviewed on a regular basis within the context of positive risk taking.

- Support can be strengthened if provided alongside engagement with other activity such as physical exercise, developing a social life or achieving a qualification.
- Clinical support and specialist vocational support should mesh where possible, although some service users do particularly value the normalisation of relationships involved in working with a non-clinician.

We encourage readers to think practically about how they might go about applying these recovery-orientated principles with someone they know.

CASE STUDY 19.1

Gavin spent 10 years living in a secure mental health setting. Prior to receiving a diagnosis of schizo-affective disorder, he spent two years in prison. Three years on, Gavin is 47 years old, married, living in the community, and, with the help of his team, is managing his condition well. He says he is keen to move on with his life and to give something back to society. One day, he would like to be in a position to earn some of his own money. Because Gavin had a difficult upbringing, he struggles with his reading and writing, although he is quite physically fit and enjoys exercise. On several occasions recently, he has been asked to talk to audiences about his experiences of mental health, and he finds this voluntary work very rewarding:

- How would you go about supporting Gavin to meet his vocational aims?
- What barriers and opportunities might there be for you in doing so?

For some time, policy has emphasised recovery-oriented or person-centred care principles and practice (DH, 2001, 2011; NHS England et al., 2014; NIMHE, 2005; Scottish Executive, 2006). Notwithstanding various criticisms regarding the authenticity of policy aspirations and translating these into impact (Davies & Gray, 2015; Pilgrim, 2008; Slade et al., 2014), this position has also been supported by the Nursing and Midwifery Council (NMC, 2010). Nurses are encouraged to reflect on and use their personal qualities, experiences and interpersonal skills to develop therapeutic, recovery-focused relationships with patients, which capitalise on an awareness of their own mental health and an ability to share aspects of their own life to inspire hope.

As much as institutionalising care settings can be disabling, novel approaches to organising care can transform ward environments into places promoting recovery and independence (Kidd et al., 2014). We conclude this chapter by offering a specific example of practice within nursing which we believe is highly appropriate in casting the role of mental health nurses in a way that will assist them to work in partnership with occupational therapists and vocational support specialists to implement the principles for practice we have outlined.

The Tidal Model

The Tidal Model originally emerged out of mental health nursing in the late 1990s, from the work of Phil and Poppy Buchanan-Barker in Newcastle. It exemplifies a robust recovery approach towards person-centered collaborative care, and draws its core philosophical metaphor from chaos theory; comparing the unpredictable – yet bounded – nature of human behaviour and experience to the dynamic flow and power of water and the tides of the sea. **Therapeutic relationships** are a key to the model, with proponents believing these may be more influential in healing potential than any other purely psychological therapy, chemical or psychological intervention. It has been used in a number of settings, from outpatient addictions, through to **acute** care, forensic services and the care of older people with **dementia** (Buchanan-Barker & Barker, 2008).

CRITICAL DEBATE 19.1

Is it the role of nurses to become social activists when advocating on behalf of their service users?

CHAPTER SUMMARY

This chapter has covered the following ideas:

- Work of any kind can be challenging for someone diagnosed with a mental illness.
- Nurses should give consideration for the life that someone has beyond their diagnosis and use of services, including their vocational aims.
- The specific emphasis that services have placed on work, occupational therapy and mental health have varied over time and tended to reflect the dominant priorities of society.
- Recovery can be influenced by labour markets, implementation of the Work Capability Assessment, changes to unemployment benefits and the common features of a workplace.
- The frequently low aspirations of service users are influenced by the beliefs and attitudes displayed by family, carers and clinical staff.
- Service users primarily want to be considered 'normal' and valued members of society.

BUILD YOUR BIBLIOGRAPHY

Books

- Freshwater, D. & Rolfe, G. (2004) *Deconstructing evidence-based practice*. London: Routledge. An insightful book providing a fresh look at evidence based practice. Readers' are assisted to understand using a series of case studies drawing on clinical settings where evidence-based practice has been taken up.
- Johnson, M. (2007) *Wasted*. London: Sphere. This autobiography traces the life of a young man who, after childhood abuse, fell into criminality and addiction. It highlights issues of mental health within the prison system and prefigures him eventually managing to run a successful business.
- Mawson, A. (2008) *The social entrepreneur: Making communities work*. London: Atlantic. Another autobiographical work, but this time from the perspective of a church minister working in a run-down community to support a co-productive approach to building inclusive social enterprises.

SAGE journal articles

Go to https://study.sagepub.com/essentialmentalhealth for further free online journal articles related to this chapter. If you are using the interactive ebook, simply click on the book icon in the margin to go straight to the resource.

FURTHER
READING:
JOURNAL
ARTICLES

- Fossey, E.M. & Harvey, C.A. (2010) Finding and sustaining employment: a qualitative meta-synthesis of mental health consumer views. *The Canadian Journal of Occupational Therapy*, 77(5), 303-314.
- Pacheco, G., Page, D. & Webber, D.J. (2014) Mental and physical health: re-assessing the relationship with employment propensity. *Work, Employment & Society*, 28(3), 407-429.
- Waghorn, G., Stephenson, A. & Browne, D. (2011) The importance of service integration in developing effective employment services for people with severe mental health conditions. *The British Journal of Occupational Therapy*, 74(7), 339-347.

Weblinks

FURTHER READING: WEBLINKS

Go to https://study.sagepub.com/essentialmentalhealth for further weblinks related to this chapter. If you are using the interactive ebook, simply click on the book icon in the margin to go straight to the resource.

- A-Way Couriers: www.awayexpress.ca/a-way-history - history of the A-Way Couriers user-led initiative in Toronto, Canada.
- Centre for Mental Health: www.centreformentalhealth.org.uk/Pages/Category/employment - resources to support the supported employment practice of Individual Placement and Support.
- Tidal Model: www.tidal-model.com - resources to support the Tidal Model of mental health nursing.

ACE YOUR ASSESSMENT

ONLINE QUIZZES & ACTIVITY ANSWERS

Revise what you have learned by visiting https://study.sagepub.com/essentialmentalhealth. If you are using the interactive ebook, simply click on the tick icon to go straight to the resource.

- Test yourself with multiple-choice and short-answer questions and flashcards.

REFERENCES

Alverson, H., Carpenter, E. & Drake, R.E. (2006) An ethnographic study of job seeking among people with severe mental illness. *Psychiatric Rehabilitation Journal*, 30, 15–22.

Bamford, C., Betton, V., Cahill, J., et al. (2012) *Improving the vocational outcomes of mental health service users: A knowledge transfer*. Leeds: University of Leeds & Leeds Partnerships NHS Trust.

Beatty, C. & Fothergill, S. (2011) *Incapacity benefit reform: The local, regional and national impact*. Sheffield: CRESR.

Beatty, C., Duncan, K., Fothergill, S., et al. (2013) *The role of health interventions in reducing incapacity claimant numbers*. Sheffield: Sheffield Hallam University.

Beatty, C., Fothergill, S., Gore, T., et al. (2011) *Tackling worklessness in Britain's weaker local economies*. Sheffield: CRESR/Sheffield Hallam University.

Boardman, J. (2011) Social exclusion and mental health: how people with mental health problems are disadvantaged – an overview. *Mental Health and Social Inclusion*, 15(3), 112–121.

Bond, G.R., Drake, R.E. & Becker, D.R. (2008) An update on randomized controlled trials of evidence-based supported employment. *Psychiatric Rehabilitation Journal*, 31, 280–290.

Borg, M. & Kristiansen, K. (2008) Working on the edge: the meaning of work for people recovering from severe mental distress in Norway. *Disability & Society*, 23, 511–523.

Boyce, M., Secker, J., Johnson, R., et al. (2008). Mental health service users' experiences of returning to paid employment. *Disability & Society*, *23*(1), 77–88.

Broer, T., Nieboer, A.P., Strating, M.M.H., et al. (2011) Constructing the social: an evaluation study of the outcomes and processes of a 'social participation' involvement project. *Journal of Psychiatric and Mental Health Nursing*, *18*, 323–332.

Buchanan-Barker, P. & Barker, P.J. (2008) The Tidal commitments: extending the value base of mental health recovery. *Journal of Psychiatric and Mental Health Nursing*, *15*, 93–100.

Burns, T., White, S.J., Catty, J., et al. (2008) Individual placement and support in Europe: the EQOLISE trial. *International Review of Psychiatry*, *20*, 498–502.

Crowther, R.E., Marshall, M., Bond, G.R., et al. (2001) Helping people with severe mental illness to obtain work: systematic review. *British Medical Journal*, *322*, 204–208.

Davies, K. and Gray, M. (2015) Mental health service users' aspirations for recovery: examining the gaps between what policy promises and practice delivers. *British Journal of Social Work*, *45* (suppl. 1), i45–i61.

Department of Health (2001) *The journey to recovery: The government's vision for mental health care*. London: DH.

Department of Health (2011) *No health without mental health: A cross-government mental health outcomes strategy for people of all ages*. London: DH.

Drake, R.E., Becker, D.R. & Bond, G.R. (2003) Recent research on vocational rehabilitation for persons with severe mental illness. *Current Opinion in Psychiatry*, *16*, 451–455.

Dunn, E.C., Wewiorski, N.J. & Rogers, E.S. (2008) The meaning and importance of employment to people in recovery from serious mental illness: results of a qualitative study. *Psychiatric Rehabilitation Journal*, *32*, 59–62.

Elliott, I. (2016) *Poverty and mental health: a review to inform the Joseph Rowntree Foundation's Anti-Poverty Strategy*. London: Mental Health Foundation.

Essen, C. (2012) Does Individual Placement and Support really 'reflect client goals'? *Journal of psychiatric and mental health nursing*, *19*(3), 231–240.

Friedli, L. & Stearn, R. (2015) Positive affect as coercive strategy: conditionality, activation and the role of psychology in UK government workfare programmes. *Medical Humanities*, *41*(1), 40–7.

Hillborg, H., Svensson, T. & Danermark, B. (2010) Towards a working life? Experiences in a rehabilitation process for people with psychiatric disabilities. *Scandinavian Journal of Occupational Therapy*, *17*, 149–161.

Kidd, S.A., McKenzie, K.J. & Virdee, G. (2014) Mental health reform at a systems level: widening the lens on recovery-oriented care. *The Canadian Journal of Psychiatry*, *59*(5), 243–249.

Laws, J. (2011) Crackpots and basket-cases: a history of therapeutic work and occupation. *History of the Human Sciences*, *24*(2), 183–199.

Leufstadius, C., Eklund, M. & Erlandsson, L.K. (2009) Meaningfulness in work: experiences among employed individuals with persistent mental illness. *Work: A Journal of Prevention Assessment & Rehabilitation*, *34*, 21–32.

Marwaha, S. & Johnson, S. (2005) Views and experiences of employment among people with psychosis: a qualitative descriptive study. *International Journal of Social Psychiatry*, *51*, 302–316.

National Institute for Mental Health Excellence (NIMHE) (2005) *Guiding statement on recovery*. London: DH.

NHS England, Public Health England, Health Education England, Monitor, Care Quality Commission & NHS Trust Development Authority (2014) *Five year forward view*. Available at: www.england.nhs.uk/wp-content/uploads/2014/10/5yfv-web.pdf (accessed 10.08.17).

Nithsdale, V., Davies, J. & Croucher, P. (2008) Psychosis and the experience of employment. *Journal of Occupational Rehabilitation, 18*, 175–182.

Nursing and Midwifery Council (2010) *Standards for pre-registration nurse education.* London: NMC.

Patrick, R. (2012) Work as the primary 'duty' of the responsible citizen: a critique of this work-centric approach. *People, Place and Policy Online, 6*(1), 5–15.

Patrick, R. (2016) Living with and responding to the 'scrounger' narrative in the UK: exploring everyday strategies of acceptance, resistance and deflection. *Journal of Poverty and Social Justice, 24*(3), 245–259.

Perkins, R., Farmer, P. & Litchfield, P. (2009) *Realising ambitions: Better employment support for people with a mental health condition.* London: The Stationery Office.

Pilgrim, D. (2008) Recovery and current mental health policy. *Chronic Illness, 4*(4), 295–304.

Provencher, H.L., Gregg, R., Mead, S., et al. (2002) The role of work in the recovery of persons with psychiatric disabilities. *Psychiatric Rehabilitation Journal, 26*, 132–144.

Repper, J. & Carter, T. (2011) A review of the literature on peer support in mental health services. *Journal of Mental Health, 20*(4), 392–411.

Rinaldi, M., Miller, L. & Perkins, R. (2010) Implementing the individual placement and support (IPS) approach for people with mental health conditions in England. *International Review of Psychiatry, 22*, 163–172.

Royal College of Psychiatrists (2002) *Employment opportunities and psychiatric disability.* Council Report 111. London: RCP.

Scottish Executive (2006) *Rights, relationships and recovery: The report of the National Review of Mental Health Nursing in Scotland.* Edinburgh: SE.

Secker, J., Grove, B. & Seebohom, P. (2001) Challenging barriers to employment, training and education for mental health service users: the service user perspective. *Journal of Mental Health, 10*, 395–404.

Slade, M., Amering, M., Farkas, M., et al. (2014) Uses and abuses of recovery: implementing recovery-oriented practices in mental health systems. *World Psychiatry, 13*(1), 12–20.

Spandler, H. (2007) From social exclusion to inclusion? A critique of the inclusion imperative in mental health. *Medical Sociology, 2*, 3–16.

Stickley, T. & Wright, N. (2011a) The British research evidence for recovery: papers published between 2006 and 2009 (inclusive). Part One: A review of the peer-reviewed literature using a systematic approach. *Journal of Psychiatric and Mental Health Nursing, 18*: 247–256.

Stickley, T. & Wright, N. (2011b) The British research evidence for recovery: papers published between 2006 and 2009 (inclusive). Part Two: A review of the grey literature including book chapters and policy documents. *Journal of Psychiatric and Mental Health Nursing, 18*, 297–307.

Thomas, P. (2016) Psycho politics, neoliberal governmentality and austerity. *Self & Society, 44*(4), 382–393.

Twamley, E.W., Jeste, D.V. & Lehman, A.F. (2003) Vocational rehabilitation in schizophrenia and other psychotic disorders: a literature review and meta-analysis of randomized controlled trials. *Journal of Nervous and Mental Disease, 191*, 515–523.

Tyler, I. (2013) *Revolting subjects: Social abjection and resistance in neoliberal Britain.* London: Zed Books.

van Niekerk, L. (2009) Participation in work: a source of wellness for people with psychiatric disability. *Work, 32*, 455–465.

Westerhof, G. & Keyes, C. (2009) Mental illness and mental health: the two continua model across the lifespan. *Journal of Adult Development, 17*, 110–119.

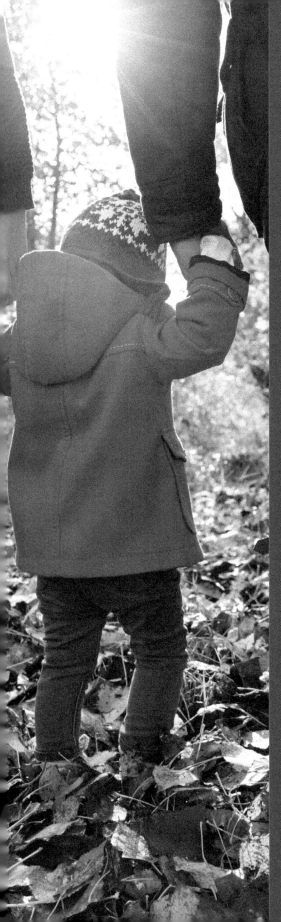

PART C   SKILLS FOR CARE AND THERAPEUTIC APPROACHES

COMPASSIONATE COMMUNICATION IN MENTAL HEALTH CARE

20

SUE BARKER AND SOPHIE WILLIAMS

THIS CHAPTER COVERS

- The development of compassionate care
- The importance of compassionate care
- Communication to provide compassionate care
- Barriers to compassionate communication
- Compassionate communication to facilitate hope and recovery.

"

A husband of one of the women on the unit had been complaining that his wife did not look like herself. The staff mostly assumed that this was due to her health status and made reassuring comments. I was unsure what he meant by 'not looking like herself' so I invited the couple to talk to me in a quiet area. He appeared pleased to be listened to and taken seriously and thanked me for my time. He explained his wife had always taken good care of herself and now her hair was untidy, her clothes lacking coordination and she had no make-up on. She appeared to agree with him but resigned to the situation. He offered to bring some photographs in to show me. The following day we sat down together and looked at the photographs and he pointed out how happy and beautiful she was. She appeared to remember and smiled; when she smiled at her husband he said to her 'you are so beautiful when you smile'. I put the photographs in her room and the next day when she was being assisted with washing and dressing the staff helped her to look more like the photograph. She appeared to be pleased about this and when her husband visited she greeted him with a smile. At this point he cried and said it felt like he was seeing her for the first time in ages.

Rachel, mental health nurse

"

> I feel like I just 'do it' [compassionate communication]. I don't feel that it is a skill I have learnt. I am a compassionate person and my communication demonstrates this. Learning compassionate communication is almost a contradiction, since it could be seen as inauthentic and almost contrived ... patients can see the difference. I care, and the way that I talk to my patients shows that.
>
> **Sara Aspinall, mental health nurse**

> One of the most challenging things is to remember that whenever the service user is communicating with you, even if it's difficult to understand or if they are repeating themselves, the question they are asking or what they are saying is really important to them and whatever they are saying should be acknowledged kindly, respectfully and sensitively. Compassionate care is listening to and appreciating everything communicated to you.
>
> **Sophie Williams, mental health nursing student**

INTRODUCTION

Compassionate care is high on the agenda for all areas of health care (Care Quality Commission, 2011; Royal College of Nursing, 2012; Crawford et al., 2013; NHS England, 2014) and communication is the most important vehicle for delivering this. Sadly, over recent years there have been many occasions where compassionate care and effective communication have been lacking, for example the Francis report on Mid Staffordshire (2013) and the Andrews and Butler report in South Wales (2014). As can be seen in Rachel's story later in the chapter, taking a little extra time can enhance the wellbeing of both the **service user** and their family. This chapter aims to foster an understanding of compassionate communication and how it can be developed.

DEVELOPMENT OF CONTEMPORARY COMPASSIONATE CARE

The NMC (2009) informs us that compassion is about recognising how the person feels, to be empathetic but also to have the desire to care for them to improve their experience. It is 'how care is given through relationships based on empathy, respect and dignity' (Cummings, 2012: 13). For Goetz et al. (2010: 351), compassion is 'a distinct affective experience whose primary function is to facilitate cooperation and protection of the weak and those who suffer'. These all highlight the experience of emotion, a personal feeling response to others' suffering (perhaps empathy), and the motivation to help others.

Stickley and Spandler (2014) encourage us to recognise the link between compassion and empathy and go on to identify compassion in action as human kindness. This shows us that by understanding others' experiences we are able to provide them with comfort. This provision of comfort to a person who is in some way suffering can be identified as compassionate care. Likewise, Buddhists, who believe that to live is to suffer, identify compassion as the motivation to relieve suffering in others, but they do not suggest it involves an emotional experience. In this sense, the person has the interpersonal intention and motivation to relieve distress but this can be undertaken without a personal emotional experience.

Gilbert (2010) recognises compassion in an evolutionary sense, identifying the role of threat, motivation and soothing systems. His model provides an explanation of the use of compassion through an appraisal process. As with Buddhists, Gilbert understands compassion as a concept of motivation. He provides a personal intention and a personal reward, whereas Buddhists focus on the interpersonal intention and not on personal benefit.

We can therefore see that compassion is about the motivation to alleviate another's suffering, whether that is due to personal emotional engagement with them (empathy), personal reward or spiritual beliefs.

CRITICAL THINKING STOP POINT 20.1

Do you think compassion involves empathy, personal reward and/or spiritual beliefs?

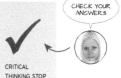

CHECK YOUR ANSWERS

CRITICAL
THINKING STOP
POINT 20.1
ANSWER

Despite compassion being found in all cultures and the implicit understanding that health care is founded on compassion, the **culture** of compassionate approaches to care is more clearly seen in psychological theory development within humanistic psychology. The early humanistic psychologist, Carl Ransom Rogers, focused on the need for skilled helpers or counsellors to be empathetic, offer non-judgemental positive regard and be congruent or 'real' to themselves. This was to influence many nurse care theorists such as Peplau, Leininger, Watson, Roach and Eriksson. Roach, in the 1980s, identified the five 'C's of care which were: compassion, competence, confidence, conscience and commitment.

Alongside the psychological and nurse theory movement towards a focus on compassionate care, there have also been cultural, political and policy developments in this direction. Compassion has been at the heart of the UK government and NHS philosophy of care for a number of years. Compassion is one of the six core **values** of the NHS and the third principle which states that the NHS aspires to the highest standards of excellence and professionalism, which will be achieved through dignity, respect and compassion (NHS, 2015).

As part of this cultural movement through political and professional pressure, the Chief Nursing Officer for England set in motion a new vision for nursing and midwifery labelled the '6 Cs' (Cummings, 2012). The six 'Cs' she identified were care, compassion, competence, courage, communication and commitment. This can be seen to have many similarities to previous nursing theory but it also includes courage and communication, which link to more recent health issues of poor communication and the need for nurses to take a lead in developing high quality practice and to 'whistle blow' when they find poor practice.

WHAT'S THE EVIDENCE? 20.1

A focus on compassion is warranted from reading reports into shocking service failings:

* Francis' report on Mid Staffordshire (2013)
* Andrews and Butler report in South Wales (2014)
* Death by indifference (Mencap, 2007)

(Continued)

- Serious Case Review of Winterbourne (Flynn, 2012)
- The Parliamentary and Health Service Ombudsman (2011)
- Maternity Unit of Furness General Hospital official investigation (Kirkup, 2015)
- Patients First and Foremost (DH, 2013).

Within mental health policy, there is little direct mention of compassionate care despite the plethora of generic guidance such as the competencies established by the NMC for undergraduate nurses (NMC, 2010). There are, though, a number of policy documents that guide mental health nurses towards recovery-focused care and the generation of hope, such as 'No Health without Mental Health' (DH, 2011). Spandler and Stickley (2011) recognise this dearth and suggest that compassionate care allows the mental health nurse a method for creating hope, and posit that mental health nurses who provide compassionate care generate optimism.

CRITICAL THINKING STOP POINT 20.2

- Do you think compassionate care generates optimism?

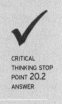

CRITICAL
THINKING STOP
POINT 20.2
ANSWER

There are a number of more recent models of compassion from psychology and nursing. Baughan and Smith (2008) developed one based on nursing research and Gilbert's model (2005) was developed from psychological research and theory. Todres and colleagues' (2009) model developed as a **collaboration** of nursing, psychology and social science research and is called 'the humanising values framework'; it can be considered to be both person-centred and compassionate.

BOND FRAMEWORK OF COMPASSIONATE CARE

CASE STUDY:
JILLY

Baughan and Smith (2013) constructed a framework that unpacks the contemporary nature of compassionate caring. Developed from their analysis of the stories of care gained from nursing students, registered practitioners and service users, it offers a useful tool to explore care. This framework comprises 18 caring indicators; these were categorised into four interrelated or 'bonded' themes which 'clarify and encapsulate what a caring nurse is and does' (2013: 147). The first letter of each theme forms the acronym or composite word BOND, hence the label the BOND framework. BOND is an acronym for:

B = being and becoming

O = overcoming obstacles

N = noticing

D = doing

Being and becoming

Baughan and Smith's research established that being and becoming is an important theme for compassionate care and within this they offer some key features. They state the need for nurses to be adaptable, flexible, creative, conscientious and ready to learn, which are common expectations of professionals. They also identify that nurses need to be a caring empathetic presence for those with whom they work; this is an extra dimension to other professions and can create emotional work for them. In essence, they need to become more emotionally intelligent.

A caring empathetic presence can be seen in Nan's experience with a woman who was experiencing a mental health crisis:

> I do not think I did anything much really. I was called to Angela's house through a neighbour who had called the police. The police asked me to attend to undertake an assessment of her mental state as she was already known to the CMHT. I arrived and Angela invited me in. Once inside the house I sat down next to Angela but then she stood up, started pacing and shouting. She then started throwing objects around. She frequently looked at me, apparently to check how I was responding. I continued to sit quietly in a relaxed and calm manner. I could see that Angela was distressed but she was unable to articulately express this. After some time Angela sat beside me and cried. I touched her forearm and she thanked me for my kindness. I felt I had done very little except try to show her I cared and was there for her.
>
> **Nan, mental health nurse**

Overcoming obstacles

Baughan and Smith's (2013) research also recognises that to provide compassionate care, obstacles will need to be overcome which will require skilful problem management, decision making and collaborative working. Features such as reframing problems and preventative and restorative skills will be useful tools along with non-discriminatory and non-judgemental practice. Effective partnership working will assist in the overcoming of obstacles but nurses will need to foster their **coping** strategies and resilience. Emotional resilience has been explained as 'flexible optimism', where people redirect their thoughts and energy away from fault finding to positive and creative problem solving (Abraham, 2004).

Noticing

Nurses need to notice their own experiences, their interactions with others and the experiences of others. This can be achieved through systematic and holistic assessments, recognising the effects of cues and interactions and the professional and ethical demands of caring. Nurses can struggle to identify indicators of compassion fatigue in themselves and others, but if they do so they can engage with their coping strategies and enhance their resilience. This is necessary if they are to maintain compassionate care.

Noticing is crucial in mental health nursing and has previously been identified as observing oneself and others, but noticing in compassionate care is something deeper. For example, Nan's daughter-in-law had recently had a miscarriage which had been distressing for the whole family and today she visited a newly delivered mother in her home. The house was quiet, clean and tidy, the mother appeared smartly dressed and offered Nan a coffee. Nan accepted the coffee despite feeling uncomfortable and having a desire to leave. The mother was polite and answered all the assessment questions indicating everything was fine. Nan felt something was wrong and so checked her body to ensure she appeared relaxed and managed her breathing. She was unsure whether it was her own feeling related to the death of her potential grandchild that was causing her concern or whether there was something in the mother. Nan stayed in the situation talking to the mother about her plans for the day and whether she intended to go back to work, to give her the opportunity to ascertain the root of her concern.

Doing

Baughan and Smith's (2013) theme of doing includes features such as establishing **therapeutic relationships**, understanding and supporting informal **carers**, engaging in critical analysis and evaluation of practice, and influencing the working **environment**. All of which, they indicate, are important in a proactive approach to compassionate care.

Student tip: Some patients may find it difficult to express their needs clearly but using the 'getting to know you' form from the RCN or speaking to the patient's friends or family may open up forms of communication.

COMPASSION-FOCUSED THERAPY

Gilbert (2005, 2009, 2010) created a theory of human compassion which he developed into a therapy called 'compassion-focused therapy'. His theory originated from a psychological understanding of evolution and neurophysiology. Gilbert (2005) explained compassion through systems of and the interplay between threat, motivation and soothing. The threat system provokes negative emotions such as fear, leading to **aggression** or withdrawal, whereas the motivational and soothing systems are considered positive. The motivational system leads to rewards such as food and shelter, whereas the soothing system is linked to the comfort of attachment and the social nature of mammals. This soothing system provides the recognition and desire to reduce others' distress. Compassion in this sense can be considered an evolutionary adaptive motivational system which reduces negative feelings by engaging with others to share safety, comfort and warmth (MacBeth & Gumley, 2012).

Gilbert's model offers a circular model of compassion with compassion in the central circle, and the next ring containing the attributes of sensitivity, empathy, distress tolerance, care for wellbeing and being non-judgemental. The outer ring contains the required skills he identified as imagery, sensory, reasoning, behaviour, feeling and attention. The whole compassion circle is surrounded by warmth (Gilbert, 2009).

Whilst Rachel was unaware of Gilbert's theory and therapy, her compassionate care can be understood using it. Rachel explained that she was passing the day room of the older person's assessment ward on which she was working. Rachel saw the husband of one of the women patients leaving the room in a hurry; he appeared distressed and she immediately had a *feeling* of concern for him. She looked around the room to see what the problem was and saw his wife with her arms around a male patient. Rachel then followed the husband and invited him to a quiet room. The husband tearfully described how his wife had called him a liar when he said he was her husband, and stated the other patient was her boyfriend. Rachel listened carefully, occasionally touching him gently on his shoulder (*warmth*) and offering him tissues and a drink. Rachel's motivational system was triggered initially as a fear reaction which changed to a soothing reaction when using her *senses* and *reasoning* she *imagined* what was happening. She behaved (*behaviour*) in a manner she believed would soothe the husband's distress by listening (*attention*) and demonstrating *warmth* and *compassion*.

IMPORTANCE OF COMPASSIONATE CARE

Compassionate care is not an optional extra; it is needed according to policy, as seen earlier, but also to enhance the wellbeing of those receiving it.

WHAT IS THE EVIDENCE? 20.2

There is a wealth of literature to support the importance of compassionate, person-centred care within health services. This literature includes increased performance in the activities of daily living as an outcome (Sjögren et al., 2013; Teitelman et al., 2010), an increased sense of wellbeing (McKeown et al., 2010; Sloane et al., 2004; Teitelman et al., 2010) and lowered agitation (Chenoweth et al., 2009; Sloane et al., 2004; Teitelman et al., 2010).

Compassionate care can be conceptualised as a style of communication, given that all behaviour is communicating something.

COMMUNICATION TO PROVIDE COMPASSIONATE CARE

Psychosocial wellbeing can be improved by effective communication where patients feel known, validated, gain hope and feel worthy, reassured and comforted (Hack et al., 2005; Thorne et al., 2005). Street et al. (2009) also found that 44% of people gained physical health improvements in their review of the available studies. They concluded that communication can have both a direct and an indirect impact on health (Street et al., 2009). Crawford et al. (2006) and Brown et al. (2006) indicate that within pressurised modern health care services the use of brief, ordinary effective (BOE) communication is a pragmatic way in which to achieve warm, compassionate, therapeutic relationships with service users. This was also highlighted by Barker (2011) but referred to as the therapeutic use of phatic communication. Regardless of the model of communication used, all communication and compassionate care literature guides the reader towards developing self-awareness to improve their compassionate communication skills. Indeed, self-awareness or 'knowing oneself' was acknowledged as a useful tool as far back as Socrates. Effective therapeutic communication involves the therapeutic use of self which includes self-awareness, self-concept, self-esteem, self-efficacy, self-confidence and the individual's **personality** (Morrissey & Callaghan, 2011).

Self-awareness

In relation to dignity, there are three key messages from the Royal College of Nursing (2015) about self-awareness:

1. We need to know and respect ourselves before we can respect the dignity of others.
2. We need to be aware of the impact of ourselves on others – and vice versa.
3. We need to be able to provide care that takes account of the beliefs and values of others that are very different from our own.

'Self-awareness means being in touch with one's thoughts, feelings and actions ... being consciously aware of one's own existence' (Rungapadiachy, 1999: 282). Morrissey and Callaghan (2011) assert that the mental health nurse who uses themselves therapeutically is likely to be self-aware. For them, self-awareness means to be able to reflect on one's self, to pay attention to one's self and to identify what is within themselves that they can use therapeutically.

There are numerous elements that influence a mental health nurse's behaviour and it may be useful for them to reflect on these to develop self-awareness (Barker, 2007). These include:

- thoughts
- feelings
- behaviour
- beliefs
- attitudes
- values
- hopes and fears
- likes and dislikes
- past experiences.

Self-awareness is one of the five domains of emotional intelligence, the other four being managing emotions, motivating oneself, recognising emotions in others and handling relationships. Emotional intelligence is regarded as an essential skill within modern society for political leaders and business-people through to nurses and patients (Goleman, 2004).

What *is* communication?

The core characteristics of a person-centred approach to communication in mental health nursing are appreciating the individuality, the uniqueness of the person, believing they are doing their best, respecting their worth, behaving genuinely, enabling control to remain with the person, recognising the person's needs and their motivation to achieve these, and realising that all their behaviour is communicating something (Morrisey & Callaghan, 2011).

Communication is about attending, listening and responding (Barker, 2007), but Burnard (2002) states that the most important of these is listening. Listening is important to facilitate a feeling of being valued (Williams & Irurita, 2004) and a feeling of comfort (Morse, 2000). Morrissey and Callaghan (2011: 3) go on to state that listening helps service users to:

- feel cared about and accepted
- feel significant and respected
- feel heard and understood
- connect to other people
- establish a sense of trust
- feel less isolated and alone
- make sense of their current situation and/or past experiences
- ask for help
- give feedback on their care
- express emotions and release tension
- participate in their **care planning**.

The skills of listening, attending and responding are sometimes called the micro skills of communication. These micro skills can be verbal and non-verbal. Listening is seen as a non-verbal skill but can be demonstrated through verbal responding.

NON-VERBAL MICRO SKILLS

Non-verbal communication skills are usually divided into haptics, proxemics and kinesics. Haptics refers to when people respond or communicate through touch or proprioception (awareness of the location of one's own body). Proxemics (from proximity) is the use of distance or space. People tend to sit close together to share intimacy but maintain a distance if they are in a formal situation. Kinesics is communication through the use of gestures such as facial expressions; this can be where the nurse uses their body to project a message or where they interpret the kinesics of the other person. Haptics, proxemics and kinesics are all culturally influenced so nurses need to consider this when interpreting another or managing one's own body to share a message.

Egan (1977) offered those trying to help others a format for one's body in therapeutic interactions and is usually remembered by using the acronym SOLER. SOLER stands for: sit squarely, open posture, lean forward, eye contact and relax. More recently, this model was revisited by Stickley (2011), who offered an alternative model to support nurses in their use of their body in communication. He provided the acronym SURETY which stands for:

- **S**it at an angle
- **U**ncross arms and legs
- **R**elax
- **E**ye contact
- **T**ouch
- **Y**our intuition.

CRITICAL THINKING STOP POINT 20.3

Do you think SOLER or SURETY is most useful to you in your clinical practice?

CRITICAL
THINKING STOP
POINT 20.3
ANSWER

There can be seen to be many similarities between the Egan and Stickley models, the most obvious difference being Stickley's inclusion of touch and use of intuition. Campbell (1984: 110) states, 'The need to be touched, held, nurtured is with us from the very beginning to the end of our life'. Touch can be an important component of therapeutic relationships, along with other non-verbal responses, which could include: postural echo, nodding, smiling and the use of silence. Touch can be a valuable tool when demonstrating compassionate care but mental health nurses need to be sensitive, using their intuition to assess when touch is appropriate. The physical and psychological condition of the person, as well as cultural components, should be taken into consideration.

Alongside the wider culture or hegemony in the USA or the UK, there are a number of other ideologies or belief systems that dictate when touch is and is not appropriate. Some religions give clear rules about who is allowed to touch whom and when – for example, Muslim men and women only shake hands with people of the same sex if they have a close relationship. In health and social care in the UK, touch is seen as something of a minefield, with some professionals fearful of accusation and litigation, believing that they should avoid it (Pemberton, 2010). Professional touch is, though, acknowledged as important within these services. There are no specific laid-down rules for touch but professional bodies offer guidance for their registrants. The guidance relates to ensuring that the patient, client or other person is treated with respect and dignity, facilitating informed decision making and trust (NMC, 2015).

Intuition has also become an area to explore in communication and compassionate care, and as seen above in Stickley's model. He recognises every interaction between people as unique, so, whilst there are some rules and guidance for compassionate communication, mental health nurses need to use their intuitive understanding of people to guide them, which is recognised as the art of mental health nursing. In 1978, Carper offered nurses four ways of knowing, identifying empirical knowledge, or what we know as evidence-based practice (the science of nursing), as only one way. The others were: ethical knowing, aesthetical knowing and personal knowing (the art of nursing). Personal ways of knowing are based on intuition and empathy, whereas ethical knowing is a way of understanding using rules, ethical frameworks, professional guidance and morals. Aesthetic knowing can also be linked to intuition as it is the awareness of the 'here and now'; it is how the nurse perceives, senses or feels what is happening.

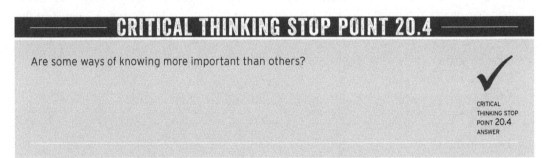

CRITICAL THINKING STOP POINT 20.4

Are some ways of knowing more important than others?

CRITICAL
THINKING STOP
POINT 20.4
ANSWER

Benner (1984) has been recognised as developing an acceptance of intuitive knowing in nursing in her novice-to-expert model. She identified that expert nurses used an implicit intuition as part of their practice. Whilst this is accepted, there is still a problem of definition of the concept. It has been defined as 'individual opinion' supported by 'experience', to an emotional and physical awareness through connection at a physical and spiritual level (Rew & Barrow, 2007).

Three types of intuitive knowing have been identified: intuition based on practice experience, intuition based on spiritual awareness and intuition based on connectiveness, though these are recognised as overlapping and interrelated (Ólafsdóttir, 2008). Inner knowing, based on practice experience, is where the mental health nurse has internalised knowledge derived from clinical experience and then uses this at a subconscious level. This type of intuitive knowing has been accepted for some time in experienced or expert nurses (Traynor et al., 2010), but Stickley (2011) and Smith (2009) recognise that intuition may be useful in practice for novices too. This type of intuition may be more closely linked to spiritual awareness and connection with the other person, which could be considered self-awareness and empathy.

Whilst the use of non-verbal skills may help the mental health nurse to demonstrate their interest and presence, and intuition supports their understanding and guides their actions, mental health nurses also need to communicate verbally.

VERBAL MICRO SKILLS

Verbal micro skills involve all that is said – not only the words but also the tone of voice, the speed and volume. All of these can influence how a message is perceived. Para-linguistics, such as saying 'ahh', 'umm' and 'uh huh', can be useful to demonstrate attention and encourage the person to continue to talk. Techniques such as focusing, reflecting, echoing and probing (asking questions) can also demonstrate attention and encourage further exploration of the problem.

Focusing can involve a technique labelled 'funnelling' where the nurse encourages the person to move from broad statements such as 'I'm useless', through questioning, to help the person to identify the problem more specifically to enable it to become a problem to be solved. An example might be:

Service user: I'm useless.

Nurse: What has happened to make you feel this?

Service user: Everything I do goes wrong, I've never been able to do anything right.

Nurse: I find that hard to believe. Could you explain how you have come to that conclusion?

Service user: My mother didn't love me and threw me out of my home when I was 16. I started a college course but didn't finish it and yesterday I was told that my tenancy agreement for my flat would not be renewed.

Nurse: That must be very worrying for you. What do you think worries you most?

Service user: All of it worries me but I won't be able to prove my mother wrong or get a job if I don't have somewhere to live.

Reflecting and echoing, unlike focusing and funneling, are not directive; they are used in a facilitative way to help the person develop self-understanding. There are two types of reflecting – paraphrasing and mirroring – but both are a type of summarising what has been said. Paraphrasing is where the key message is given back to the service user in the nurse's own words, while mirroring is where the person's words are used to give a summary of the key message. Echoing is very similar to mirroring but is usually briefly repeating what the person has said so that they can hear it and develop their story.

Probing involves asking questions: these can be open or closed and the type of question used will depend on the circumstances. Open questions are useful for encouraging the person to continue to give detail and explore their circumstances or options, whereas closed questions are useful if the nurse needs specific information or the person is struggling with communication due, for example, to cognitive deficits. The most useful type of probing questions start with 'what', 'where', 'when', 'how' and 'who'; generally, 'why' questions are unhelpful as they can lead to the person shutting down and becoming defensive.

As identified above, listening is probably the most important communication skill and, as part of this, silence can be used as a therapeutic tool in mental health nursing. Stickley and Stacey (2009) identified that mental health nurses, as with others, feel the need to immediately respond when the other person stops speaking, but found the use of a 2-second silence before responding facilitated the person understanding they were important, the nurse had time for them, the interaction was more than normal conversation, the response had been considered and it was acceptable to sit and just 'be' with them.

There are numerous communication skills that mental health nurses can use to develop compassionate therapeutic relationships with service users. These relationships, though, are not without a cost to the nurse. They can cause additional stress due to organisational cultures, routine and the emotional labour involved.

BARRIERS TO COMPASSIONATE CARE

The focus within the reports on the lack of compassionate care has been on individuals showing a lack of compassion, but there is a gaining recognition that some organisations do not provide an environment that supports compassionate care and communication. The organisational culture of health services appears to be focused on reductionism and super specialism, with little room for compassionate holistic care, despite the call for health services to be more compassionate. There is a primary **drive** for cost-efficiency by increased throughput of service users, which is acknowledged as tick-box, technically competent care (Cole-King & Gilbert, 2011). Within this culture, young professionals feel traumatised and bullied. A culture that focuses on tasks achieved rather than on the humanity of those requiring the service has been seen over a number of decades to be problematic through the work of Kitwood (1997) and his successors.

CRITICAL THINKING STOP POINT 20.5

Is the culture within the NHS toxic (DH, 2013), as has been suggested, or does it facilitate compassion?

CRITICAL
THINKING STOP
POINT 20.5
ANSWER

The nature of the service users in mental health services may also be a barrier, as a number of service users do not wish to accept health service provision. Some suggest it is impossible to develop trusting compassionate relationships in this situation. People who are acutely mentally ill or have a severe cognitive impairment may not see the benefits of treatments that have significant side-effects and may find it difficult to trust those people, including mental health nurses, who have coerced them into accepting the treatment.

There are also those who indicate that mental health nurses and other health care professionals need education to develop their compassionate care. Alongside this need for initial and continuing education, there is a risk of 'compassion fatigue' in those who do not receive adequate support and do not experience self-compassion. The need for resilience has been identified for continued work in areas that require high emotional labour to reduce burnout, but Gilbert's theory of compassion-focused therapy and model of compassion highlights the need for self-compassion. When a person has self-compassion, they show themselves understanding (self-empathy) and have sensitivity, distress tolerance and a non-judgemental regard for themselves, the need to provide compassionate care can be enhancing for wellbeing rather than draining.

COMPASSIONATE COMMUNICATION TO FACILITATE HOPE AND RECOVERY

As indicated earlier in this chapter, mental health policies do not offer specific guidance on how to provide compassionate care to mental health nurses but they guide us towards a **recovery** approach. The recovery approach encourages mental health nurses to recognise the person as an individual with their own unique story, to provide them with hope for the future and to support them in their recovery, whatever the service user would like that to be. Spandler and Stickley (2011) suggest that the skills identified within compassionate care and communication can provide mental health nurses with tools to generate hope and optimism for those with whom they work.

Student tip: Sometimes if a service user is distressed, refocusing their attention on something positive can help. Doing an activity like playing music, painting nails, doing a jigsaw or even cleaning can refocus their energy. This gives them a meaningful activity which makes them feel valued and can also leave them feeling calmer and happier and reconnect them with how they were before they came into care.

CRITICAL DEBATE 20.1

There is a tension between the science and art of mental health nursing. Scientific understanding and knowledge are derived from a specific approach to developing knowledge. This is accepted by government and academic organisations as the most valid form of evidence on which to base practice.

As demonstrated above in the brief description of intuition, this has also been highlighted as a valuable tool in compassionate mental health care. The tension between science and art within nursing and health care has been an enduring one. Do we accept an individual's intuition, wherever that may come from, or do we accept evidence that has been developed and honed over hundreds of years? Most health care providers and government would guide the mental health nurse to follow the rigorously developed scientific evidence. With contemporary concern over compassionate care, there has been renewed interest in exploring the use of self and intuition. Authors such as Fisher and Freshwater (2014) offer us a way forward called aesthetic rationality that incorporates the appreciation of the art of care in a scientific method. Lapum et al. (2012) also offer a new way of conceptualising the bringing together of intuition and evidence-based practice in their cyborg ontology. It would appear that to provide compassionate care, mental health nurses need to work with both these ways of knowing people with mental health problems, in order to facilitate their recovery journey.

CONCLUSION

Mental health nurses are steeped in the history, knowledge and skills necessary for providing compassionate care. To do so is in line with broader exhortations to support recovery, and ought to underpin commitments to effective therapeutic alliances. At a time when nursing in general stands accused of a lack of compassion, mental health nurses are well placed to renew the public image of nursing through a concerted and self-critical appreciation of the value of compassion within their work, and actually communicating this to service users and colleagues alike.

—————— **CHAPTER SUMMARY** ——————

This chapter has covered:

- The development of compassionate care
- Contemporary models of compassion
- Exploration of the some of the evidence to support the need for compassionate care
- Examination of communication skills that underpin the mental health nurse's ability to show compassion
- How the science and art of mental health nursing can support all the ways in which mental health nurses can generate hope and recovery through compassionate care.

—————— **BUILD YOUR BIBLIOGRAPHY** ——————

Books

- Gault, I., Shapcott, J., Luthi, A. et al. (2016) *Communication in nursing and healthcare: A guide for compassionate practice*. London: SAGE.
- Gilbert, P. (2013) *Mindful compassion: Using the power of mindfulness and compassion to transform our lives*. London: Robinson.
- Watkins, P. (2008) *Mental health practice: A guide to compassionate care*, 2nd edition. Oxford: Elsevier Health Sciences.

SAGE journal articles

FURTHER
READING:
JOURNAL
ARTICLES

Go to https://study.sagepub.com/essentialmentalhealth for further free online journal articles related to this chapter. If you are using the interactive ebook, simply click on the book icon in the margin to go straight to the resource.

- Crawford, P., Gilbert, P., Gilbert, J., et al. (2013) The language of compassion in acute mental health care. *Qualitative Health Research*, 23(6), 719-727.
- Curtis, K., Gallagher, A., Ramage, C., et al. (2016) Using appreciative inquiry to develop, implement and evaluate a multi-organisation 'cultivating compassion' programme for health professionals and support staff. *Journal of Research in Nursing*, 22(1-2), 150-165.
- Zulueta, P.D. (2013) Compassion in 21st century medicine: is it sustainable? *Clinical Ethics*, 8(4), 119-128.

Weblinks

FURTHER
READING:
WEBLINKS

Go to https://study.sagepub.com/essentialmentalhealth for further weblinks related to this chapter. If you are using the interactive ebook, simply click on the book icon in the margin to go straight to the resource.

- Compassionate Mental Health website: http://compassionatementalhealth.co.uk
- Frameworks for Change: www.frameworks4change.co.uk – this website offers some free resources to support self-compassion and a link to a talk on closing the compassion gap by Andy Bradley, the founder
- NHS: www.gov.uk/government/policies/compassionate-care-in-the-nhs – provides information and updates on compassionate care in the NHS with links to policies and facilities to subscribe for updates
- Royal College of Psychiatrists: www.rcpsych.ac.uk/pdf/FR-GAP-02_Compassionate-care.pdf – this suggests ten things to do to improve compassion

ACE YOUR ASSESSMENT

ONLINE
QUIZZES &
ACTIVITY
ANSWERS

Revise what you have learned by visiting https://study.sagepub.com/essentialmentalhealth. If you are using the interactive ebook, simply click on the tick icon to go straight to the resource.

- Test yourself with multiple-choice and short-answer questions and flashcards.

REFERENCES

Abraham, R. (2004) Emotional competence as antecedent to performance: a contingency framework. *Genetic, Social and General Psychology Monographs, 130,* 117–143.

Andrews, J. & Butler, M. (2014) *Trusted to care: An independent review of the Princess of Wales Hospital and Neath Port Talbot Hospital at Abertawe Bro Morgannwg University Health Board.* Available at: http://gov.wales/docs/dhss/publications/140512trustedtocareen.pdf (accessed 10.08.17).

Barker, S. (2007) *Vital notes for nurses: Psychology.* Oxford: Blackwell.

Barker, S. (2011) *Midwives' emotional support of women becoming mothers.* Newcastle upon Tyne: CPS.

Baughan, J. & Smith, A. (2008) *Caring in nursing practice*. London: Pearson Education.

Baughan, J. & Smith, A. (2013) *Compassion, caring and communication: Skills for nursing practice*, 2nd edition. London: Routledge.

Benner, P. (1984) *From novice to expert: Excellence and power in the clinical nursing process*. Menlo Park, CA: Addison-Wiley.

Brown, B., Crawford, P. & Carter, R. (2006) *Evidence-based health communication*. Buckingham: Open University Press.

Burnard, P. (2002) *Learning human skills: An experiential and reflective guide for nurses and health care professionals*, 4th edition. Oxford: Butterworth Heinemann.

Campbell, A.V. (1984) *Moderated Love: A Theology of Professional Care*. London: SPCK.

Care Quality Commission (CQC) (2011) *Dignity and nutrition*. Inspection programme: national overview. Newcastle upon Tyne: CQC.

Carper, B. (1978) Fundamental Patterns of Knowing in Nursing. *Advances in Nursing Science, 1*(1), 13–24.

Chenoweth, L., King, M.T., Jeon, Y.-H., et al. (2009) Caring for Aged Dementia Care Resident Study (CADRES) of person-centred care, dementia-care mapping, and usual care in dementia: a cluster-randomised trial. *The Lancet Neurology, 8*(4), 317–325.

Cole-King, A. & Gilbert, P. (2011) Compassionate care: the theory and the reality. *Journal of Holistic Healthcare, 8*(3), 29–37.

Crawford, P., Brown, B. & Bonham, P. (2006) *Communication in clinical settings*. Cheltenham: Nelson Thornes.

Cummings, J. (2012) *Compassion in practice, nursing, midwifery and care staff: Our vision and strategy*. London: Department of Health and NHS Commissioning Board. Available at: www.england.nhs.uk/wp-content/uploads/2012/12/compassion-in-practice.pdf (accessed 10.08.17).

Department of Health (2011) *No health without mental health*. London: DH.

Department of Health (2013) *Hard Truths: The Journey to putting patients first: volume one of the government response to the Mid Staffordshire NHS foundation trust public inquiry*. London: The Stationery Office.

Department of Health (2013) *Patients First and Foremost: the Initial Government Response to the Report of the Mid Staffordshire NHS Foundation Trust Public Inquiry*. London: DH.

Egan, G. (1977) *The skilled helper*. Monterey, CA: Brooks/Cole.

Fisher, P. and Freshwater, D. (2014) Towards compassionate care through aesthetic rationality. *Scandinavian journal of caring sciences, 28*(4), 767–774.

Flynn, M. (2012) *Winterbourne View Hospital: a serious case review*. South Gloucestershire Safeguarding Adults Board.

Francis, R. (2013) *Report on the Mid Staffordshire NHS Foundation Trust public enquiry*. Available at: www.gov.uk/government/uploads/system/uploads/attachment_data/file/279124/0947.pdf (accessed 10.08.17).

Gilbert, P. (ed.) (2005) *Compassion: Conceptualisations, research and use in psychotherapy*. Abingdon: Routledge.

Gilbert, P. (2009) Introducing compassion-focused therapy. *Advances in Psychiatric Treatment, 15*, 199–208.

Gilbert, P. (2010) An introduction to compassion focused therapy in cognitive behavior therapy. *International Journal of Cognitive Therapy, 3*(2), 97–112.

Goetz, J.L., Keltner, D. & Simon-Thomas, E. (2010) Compassion: an evolutionary analysis and empirical review. *Psychological Review, 136*, 351–374.

Goleman, D. (2004) *Emotional intelligence and working with emotional intelligence*. London: Bloomsbury.

Hack, T., Degner, L. & Parker, P. (2005) The communication goals and needs of cancer patients: a review. *Psychooncology*, *14*, 831–845.

Kirkup B. (2015) *The report of the Morecambe Bay investigation*. March. Available at: www.gov.uk/government/publications/morecambe-bay-investigation-report.(accessed 04.10.2017).

Kitwood, T. (1997) *Dementia reconsidered: The person comes first*. Maidenhead: Open University Press.

Lapum, J., Fredericks, S., Beanlands, H., et al., 2012. A cyborg ontology in health care: traversing into the liminal space between technology and person-centred practice. *Nursing Philosophy*, 13(4), 276–288.

MacBeth, A. & Gumley, A. (2012) Exploring compassion: a meta-analysis of the association between self-compassion and psychopathology. *Clinical Psychology Review*, *32*, 545–552.

McKeown, J., Clarke, A., Ingleton, C., et al. (2010) The use of life story work with people with dementia to enhance person centered care. *International Journal of Older People Nursing*, 5(2), 148–158.

Mencap (2007) *Death by indifference*. London, Mencap.

Morrissey, J. and Callaghan, P. (2011) *Communication skills for mental health nurses*. London: McGraw-Hill Education.

Morse, J.M. (2000) Responding to the cues of suffering. *Health Care for Women International*, *21*, 1–9.

NHS England (2014) *Compassion in practice: two years on*. Available at: www.england.nhs.uk/wp-content/uploads/2014/12/nhs-cip-2yo.pdf (accessed 10.08.17).

NHS (2015) *The handbook to the NHS Constitution*. Available at: www.gov.uk/government/publications/the-nhs-constitution-for-england (accessed 10.08.17).

Nursing and Midwifery Council (2009) *Record keeping guidance*. London: NMC.

Nursing and Midwifery Council (2010) *Standards for Pre-registration nursing education*. London: NMC.

Nursing and Midwifery Council (2015) *The Code: Professional Standards of Practice and Behaviour for Nurses and Midwives*. London: NMC.

Ólafsdóttir, Ó.Á. (2008) Inner knowing and emotions in the midwife–woman relationship. In B. Hunter & R. Deery (eds) *Emotions in midwifery and reproduction*. Basingstoke: Palgrave Macmillan, pp.192–209.

Parliamentary and Health Service Ombudsman (2011) *Care and Compassion?: Report of the Health Service Ombudsman on Ten Investigations Into NHS Care of Older People* (Vol. 778). London: The Stationery Office.

Pemberton, C. (2010) Should children's social work be a touch free zone?' *Community Care*, 20. Available at: www.communitycare.co.uk/2010/08/20/should-childrens-social-work-be-a-touch-free-zone/ (accessed 01.10.17).

Rew, L. & Barrow Jr, E.M. (2007) State of the science: intuition in nursing, a generation of studying the phenomenon. *Advances in Nursing Science*, 30(1), E15–E25.

Royal College of Nursing (RCN) (2012) *Quality with compassion: The future of nursing education*. Report of the Willis Commission on Nursing Education. London: Royal College of Nursing on behalf of the independent Willis Commission on Nursing Education.

Royal College of Nursing (2015) *Dignity and me*. Available at: www.nursingtimes.net/download?ac=1255026 (accessed 01.10.17).

Rungapadiachy, D.M. (1999) *Interpersonal communication and psychology for health care professionals: Theory and practice*. Oxford: Butterworth Heinemann.

Sjögren, K., Lindkvist, M., Sandman, P., et al. (2013) Person-centredness and its association with resident well-being in dementia care units. *Journal of Advanced Nursing*, 69(10), 2196–2206.

Sloane, P.D., Hoeffer, B., Mitchell, C.M., et al. (2004) Effect of person-centered showering and the towel bath on bathing-associated aggression, agitation, and discomfort in nursing home residents with dementia: a randomized, controlled trial. *Journal of the American Geriatrics Society*, *52*(11), 1795–1804.

Smith, A. (2009) Exploring the legitimacy of intuition as a form of nursing knowledge. *Nursing Standard*, *23*(40), 35–40.

Spandler, H. & Stickley, T. (2011) No hope without compassion: the importance of compassion in recovery focused mental health services. *Journal of Mental Health*, *20*(6), 555–566.

Stickley, T. (2011) From SOLER to SURETY for effective non-verbal communication. *Nurse Education in Practice*, 11(6), 395–398.

Stickley, T. & Stacey, G. (2009) Caring: the essence of mental health nursing: In P. Callaghan, J. Playle & L. Cooper (eds) *Mental health nursing skills*. Oxford: Oxford University Press. pp. 44–54.

Stickley, T. & Spandler, H. (2014) Compassion and mental health nursing. In T. Stickley & N. Wright (eds) *Theories for mental health nursing: A guide for practice*. London: Sage.

Street, R., Makoul, G., Neeraj, A., et al. (2009) How does communication heal? Pathways linking clinician–patient communication to health outcomes. *Patient Education and Counseling*, *74*, 295–301.

Teitelman, J., Raber, C. & Watts, J. (2010) The power of the social environment in motivating persons with dementia to engage in occupation: qualitative findings. *Physical and Occupational Therapy Geriatrics*, *28*(4), 321–333.

Thorne, S., Armstrong, E., McPherson, G., et al. (2005) 'Being known': patients' perspectives of the dynamics of human connection in cancer care. *Psychooncology*, *14*, 887–898.

Todres, L., Galvin, K.T. and Holloway, I. (2009) The humanization of healthcare: a value framework for qualitative research. *International Journal of Qualitative Studies on Health and Well-being*, *4*(2), 68–77.

Traynor, M., Boland, M. and Buus, N. (2010) Autonomy, evidence and intuition: nurses and decision-making. *Journal of advanced nursing*, *66*(7), 1584–1591.

Williams, A.M. & Irurita, V.F. (2004) Therapeutic and non-therapeutic interpersonal interactions: the patient's perspective. *Journal of Clinical Nursing*, *13*, 806–815.

21

THERAPEUTIC ENGAGEMENT FOR MENTAL HEALTH CARE

MANDY REED AND SIMON HALL

THIS CHAPTER COVERS

- An exploration of the factors that can affect our reactions to people and situations
- What the evidence tells us about 'good' and 'poor' engagement
- Some examples from practice that demonstrate really good engagement
- Top tips to help you start and end relationships when on placements.

> As nurses, I think we are in a very privileged position as we can establish a therapeutic relationship where, given the right ingredients, the people we work with let us be close and open up. Perhaps the qualities of a nurse convey to those we are working with that we do genuinely care and are worth talking to. Essentially it's about being useful to the individuals we work with and the key for me in engagement is the ability to build a trusting therapeutic relationship. Being able to come alongside someone and understand their experiences from their perspective and to think together about what might be useful.
>
> **Lou, practitioner**

> I have an example of a nurse demonstrating care when I was on the PICU. It is an environment where the turnover of nursing staff seemed to be constantly in flux, with new faces appearing each day. One of the nurses called Michael, was kind enough to give me a tooth brush one day, and I instinctively felt that here was a person I could trust, and looked forward to seeing again. Michael never returned. Nursing care, and forming trust and empathy can be as simple and powerful as giving someone a toothbrush, not just to clean teeth, but also as an emblematic symbol of care and hope.
>
> **Mark, service user**

Visit **https://study.sagepub.com/essentialmentalhealth** to access a wealth of online resources for this chapter - watch out for the margin icons throughout the chapter. If you are using the interactive ebook, simply click on the margin icon to go straight to the resource.

INTRODUCTION

All nursing care starts with the establishment of a relationship which is both therapeutic and based on an 'unconditional positive regard' (Rogers, 1961; Rogers et al., 1967).

This chapter discusses therapeutic *engagement*, which can only occur within a relationship that is considered to be 'therapeutic'. Hence, the **therapeutic relationship** will be considered first, before moving on to strategies and skills for therapeutic engagement.

Clarkson (2003) suggested that there are five types of relationship: the 'working alliance'; the 'transference/counter transference relationship'; the 'developmentally needed/reparative relationship'; the 'person-to-person relationship'; and the 'transpersonal relationship'. In Clarkson's five-relationship framework, there is an implicit assumption that the responsibility for the therapy lies predominantly with the therapist (Clarkson, 2003).

In nursing, the person most renowned for work in this area is Hildegard Peplau (1952, 1988). One of the early pioneers of mental health nursing, Peplau developed the concept of the 'nurse–patient relationship' in her 1952 book *Interpersonal Relations in Nursing*, which is regarded as the first systematic theoretical framework of the therapeutic relationship in psychiatric nursing.

Peplau (1952) identified that as human beings are unique, so are their experiences. With this in mind, Peplau developed a nursing model for practice based on the therapeutic interpersonal process (known as 'Peplau's theory of interpersonal relations model'), which is made up of four 'phases'. The four phases are, first, **orientation**, followed by identification, exploitation and then, finally, resolution (Peplau, 1988). Peplau suggests that the patient engages with the therapeutic relationship by passing through the identified phases. For example, Peplau's orientation phase is the 'getting to know you' stage when the nurse and patient first meet and roles and expectations are laid out (Peplau, 1952: 19). The tasks of this phase are largely to establish trust and to explore ways of interacting that will connect both nurse and patient at the start of their engagement. The skills and knowledge required during this phase fundamentally underpin the qualities of what is termed a therapeutic relationship.

As a student nurse on your placements, you are ideally placed to develop relationships from a perspective of curiosity; being interested in the people in your care is central to the start of a co-produced therapeutic relationship. Engagement is not a 'one-off' intervention but an ongoing process between the person and their workers (Ryan & Morgan, 2004). It is also one that requires conscious, active consideration and effort. Throughout your training, you will observe experienced nurses who seem to effortlessly engage with the people in their care; this may appear so on the surface but is most likely based on empathic skills development built up over time. That is not to say that you will be unable to make these kinds of relationships as students, more so to emphasise how conscious and aware you need to be in all of your interactions with people.

Like **recovery**, there are many definitions of what is meant by the word engagement. Considering the personal recovery philosophy underpinning this book, the following by Ryan and Morgan (2004: 141) is probably most helpful:

> Engagement is a separate and distinct function, the foundation for all aspects of the helping process. It is an attempt to build an ongoing constructive partnership, and will most usually be facilitated by a series of unstructured, informal and shared encounters, that take place at the beginning of the process of relationship-building. It is a therapeutic activity within its own right, needing to be positively monitored and sustained throughout the duration of the helping process.

As can be seen in this definition, there is a symbiotic interchange between the function of engagement and the qualities of a therapeutic relationship. As you develop during your training, you will no doubt be noticing that there are many different ways of considering what/how you approach an individual to begin that process of therapeutic engagement. This will depend partly on your knowledge and experience (are you a first-, second- or third-year student?), partly on the **environment** of the interaction (are you on placement in an **acute** inpatient environment where everyone is compulsorily detained, or are you in a community team working with people to develop their **wellness plans**?), and more specifically on what we can think of as the degree of **collaboration**. If we consider the work of John Heron (2001), we can think of this from two broad perspectives; those interactions based on facilitating the person to work on their own goals (cathartic, catalytic and supportive), and those based on a more authoritative stance (prescriptive, informative and confronting) when the person is unable to work collaboratively with you. Mike Firn (2008) developed this further with his **classification** by degree of collaboration, clarifying three broad types of engagement based on either a collaborative or person-led agenda, an informative one and a restrictive one likely to involve the use of mental health legislation.

CRITICAL THINKING STOP POINT 21.1

Think of two or three occasions when you have connected well with those in your care and, then, using Peplau's model consider which 'role/s' you adopted within those relationships:

The 'mother-surrogate', The 'technician', The 'manager', The 'socialising agent', The 'health teacher' or The 'counsellor or psychotherapist'.

WHAT'S THE EVIDENCE? 21.1

'Good' engagement

Research has consistently shown that the personal qualities of the professional (in this case the mental health nurse) have the biggest influence on the development or otherwise of a positive therapeutic relationship (for example, Clarkson, 2003; DH, 2008; Gunasekara et al., 2014). The personal qualities and skills which help to make up a good mental health nurse have been debated for over half a century, ever since the seminal work of Peplau and colleagues in the 1950s (Peplau, 1952). As a result, interpersonal skills and techniques are taught as an integral part of all mental health nurse training; these are increasingly informed by the lived experience of the people and their families. A number of studies have examined key aspects of therapeutic engagement inherent in best quality mental health nursing care (e.g. Bowers et al., 2009; Dziopa & Ahern, 2009; Gunasekara et al., 2014). These can be summarised as:

- demonstrating understanding and empathy
- offering individualised care
- providing support

- being there/being available
- being genuine
- promoting equality
- demonstrating respect
- demonstrating clear boundaries
- demonstrating self-awareness.

CRITICAL DEBATE 21.1

Ideally, our role as mental health nurses is to help people when they are distressed or need help, but how do you know if you are helping? What can we do if people don't want our help?

'POOR' ENGAGEMENT?

The research and literature contributing to the development of both assertive outreach (AO) and early intervention (EI) service models focus on engagement as a fundamental issue (e.g. French et al., 2010; Ryan & Morgan, 2004). Although at different ends of service provision, one of the hoped-for outcomes from being in contact with EI services is a positive experience of engagement and care to minimise the impact of the **illness** and reduce the likely need for AO services in the longer term.

CASE STUDY: SUPPORT PACKAGE

The factors that can **affect** engagement have been well documented in the literature (e.g. Kreyenbuhl et al., 2009; O'Brien et al., 2009). As with much of life, they are complex; some are related to the design of mental health services on offer, some to the environment and trauma surrounding the individual, and some relate to the person themselves. Although there may not be much you can do as a student to redesign better services, an understanding of these issues will help you to be authentic with the people you work with as a mental health nurse. The importance of empathy and the ability to imagine what you might feel like if in that person's shoes cannot be underestimated.

Some of the practical factors which can affect engagement include the person having difficulty getting to, forgetting or missing appointments. Although services may be designed to suit workers and/or clinic opening hours, they are often not convenient for the people in our care or for their loved ones. Despite recommendations to enhance the availability of services after 5pm on weekdays and at the weekend across the whole of the NHS, most types of team (at the time of writing) only offer limited extensions to their normal 9–5 hours. The cost of getting to meetings with workers may be prohibitive or transport services may be very limited; this especially applies in rural areas and/or for people on very low incomes. Other factors to consider are from a psychological perspective. A person may feel they are either better or that they want to be independent and resolve the issues themselves. Equally, they may be unhappy with the service they have already received; for example, feeling a loss of control when taking prescribed medication. There are clear links between traumatic experiences (of the illness and/or service provision) and future non-concordance and poor engagement (Kreyenbuhl et al., 2009; O'Brien et al., 2009).

CRITICAL THINKING STOP POINT 21.2

- How have you observed appointments being made with service users and/or their families from your clinical experience so far? Are they consulted as to a convenient time and place; if not, why do they say this is the case?
- What have you observed happen when a person does not keep that appointment? Were they offered another automatically, or did the team wonder if they 'really wanted' help at that point in time? What did you think about the team's response?

CASE STUDY 21.1

David

There is no relationship that is close to being automatic other than that of a newborn and their mother. Not even love at first sight is as sacred or as profound, but there are special ones and those meant to be over the course and span of life.

A month after discharge from my first internment, it was another slow day in rural Wiltshire, the doorbell went off and I invited two blokes into my sister's home, but in essence or, as fate would dictate, I was inviting them into my life and we were on the precipice of kick starting my recovery and without me knowing, on that very day and that early, some therapies were being employed. And with some reassurances and a laid out prescription plan by both parties plus understanding, foundations were laid. What started out a mundane and uneventful dead end day, after the visit, ended pervaded by renewed hope, a change of pace, more understanding and at the very basic a glimmer of optimism looking up from the belly of the abyss.

Beforehand, I did what was asked of me, i.e. take my medicine religiously, open our home to my care coordinator and partaking in planned activities but none of it provided me with sense or a way out and I was living my days like a robot not that intellectually or creatively programmed, devoid of emotion and all around numbness of the world around and not being aware of what was happening and finding the point in all that was going on.

Fast forward a bit...

Comes the day of what we agreed to do together, in this case a chance to kick a football after a hiatus of 7-8 years. As good as I was in a previous life, time does a number on you and I have to say I missed my window of opportunity to effect a sporting life for a career. I digress, still I felt like a drone programmed to be lifeless. At the end of that session, I, for the first time in a long time, actually took away something and maybe, just maybe, these Simon and Phil characters were onto something. This therapy by way of (what I now know as) social inclusion would be built on, all the while coaxing me out of the depressed shell I was cocooned in and had accepted as life.

What for me started out as a kick about, became something to look forward to every week although when we used to finish, I would go into a depressive state for having to wait a whole week before we got to do it again and to also see the fellas.

As I became less inhibited about going out, not just for footy but for other groups we fostered and ran, I was having therapy sessions at least twice a week not including the football. We happened upon a little farm shop in our quest to find the best hot chocolate in the county; to this day the farm shop hasn't been beaten. Finally, I had found someone I could vent to and unreservedly talk to about my fears, my illness, my hopes, my life, my family, and at that time not realising how therapeutic this had become.

With my mother, sister, brother, nephew and niece as the only family I've ever known, I was introduced to a group of gentlemen, with whom I only played football for which they ordained me their captain and a leadership role, then later on a liaison, for I helped set precedence for peer support and interaction outside of sanctioned periods, be it taking in a movie, going out for meals, bowling, birthday and milestone celebrations to gaming nights and sleepovers. Such is the strength of our bond, that I regard these men, my brothers and it doesn't end there, I have, outside of my own household gained parents and family.

I say, while many see this as a curse, for me it's in its own way a gift for I wouldn't have had met the extraordinary people I have met on this transcendental journey of mine.

David, service user

- There are many potential barriers that can affect engagement. Can you think of the potential barriers at the societal, organisational and personal levels that could have an impact on service users like David?
- The importance of getting to know somebody and understanding their situation beyond a diagnosis could be aligned to Phil Barker and Poppy Buchanan-Barker's 'Tidal Model'. What key elements from this scenario can be linked to the Tidal Model's 10 key commitments?
- Social engagement is a complex intervention as it is hard to measure and, as a practitioner, how much value do we put on friendship? How is friendship different from peer support?

CASE STUDY 21.2

Mark

My last stay in hospital was on a PICU ward where I was very unwell, not to say challenging to many of the nursing staff whom at the time I perceived as neglectful and disinterested in my psychosis or in the remnants of my personality, which was fragmented. At the time, and occasionally still on reflection, I feel that in a location where nurses outnumbered patients, there should have been more care and curiosity about me and how I was presenting, and attempts to make my stay more comfortable and endurable; even to establish a rationale which I could understand for why I was detained under the Mental Health Act.

(Continued)

This perception was largely filtered and inferred through the fractured lens of paranoid psychosis, and with the benefit of hindsight and credible information I know that broad disinterest might not have been the entire case or explanation. My fear was manifest and real; for a number of weeks subsequent to my admission I laboured under the belief that I might be detained there indefinitely, and this combined with being 'Sectioned' only fed my sense of anger and injustice. Nevertheless one of the nurses, Lou, through her own endeavour and compassion formed a strong therapeutic alliance with me. I think her care and curiosity, her ability to communicate through my psychosis, anger and mistrust clearly demonstrate an example of a person centred and compassionate approach to nursing care. I think it must have been a challenging, brave and difficult thing to do, to approach and create the key and locate that narrow access, no wider than a blade of grass, beyond my illness and into my 'better self', by which I mean that component of my core being which remained somehow intact and reachable. The physical tool and metaphor for this was through my acoustic guitar, which I asked my parents to bring to me on the ward. It was as if some prescient part of me knew that music could genuinely be a lifesaver.

Lou located another acoustic guitar on the ward, which I attempted to tune and which stubbornly wouldn't remain in tune (another metaphor?), and she asked me to teach her a few chords with which we could strum along together. We didn't write a hit song, but through the medium of a few rudimentary chords she communicated to me that she was interested, curious and cared. Although the guitar is not my first instrument, teaching Lou a few simple chords, and indeed whilst on the ward writing a song which I felt quite proud of, reaffirmed my humanity, my worthiness, and my heart.

This activity went beyond the use of medication, which I was refusing to take on occasions, and is a good example that the bio-medical approach isn't everything. Lou's ability to reflect critically on her training and practice, to identify the use of a psychosocial, even artistic, intervention is an outstanding example of transformative practice.

Mark, service user

For me part of being a nurse is being aware of the possible impact on somebody of being admitted to hospital at an already very difficult, stressful and bewildering time in their life. It's about being aware of what is appropriate, at what time, and of understanding there is always a way in. To do this, it is crucial to get to know someone. As nurses, I think we are in a very privileged position as we can establish a therapeutic relationship where, given the right ingredients, the people we work with let us be close and open up. Perhaps the qualities of a nurse convey to those we are working with that we do genuinely care and are worth talking to. As nurses I think we are provided with a number of opportunities to care; for example, in a PICU environment compared to an acute ward you have a higher number of nurses and less people which provide opportunities to spend a lot of time with someone. Essentially it's about being useful to the individuals we work with and the key for me in engagement is the ability to build a trusting therapeutic relationship. Being able to come alongside someone and understand their experiences from their perspective and to think together about what might be useful.

Lou, practitioner

One evening I came close to complete fragmentation, but managed to hold it together. Somewhere, within all that existential malaise and malign illness Mark was still present with the will to live; having a nurse sit with me helped me hang on to that. Being there, however unobtrusively, is surely one of the most powerful and potent things a nurse, or any human being can do for another who is very unwell. All it took was a toothbrush and two guitars to create a sustained tension at the core of my being enabling me to survive the very worse. On discharge from hospital, it would take another three to four years for recovery, including CBT and family therapy, education, art, and then work to rebuild my personality, and fully discover who I was, but it is my belief that Lou helped to prevent me from falling irretrievably into the bloodless maw of schizophrenia. By seizing the opportunity to work 'on the ground', and to think creatively and instinctively about how to work with an individual in a way which reassures their idiosyncratic human validity and identity, however distorted it might be, is the paradigm of mental health nursing.

Mark, service user

Questions

- What were the specific things that Lou did to reach out to Mark during this period?
- Why might these have been such a contrast to the other experiences of care Mark was receiving at that time on a PICU?

BEST PRACTICE DURING FIRST CONTACT WITH SERVICES

As already discussed, having a positive experience when first in contact with mental health services can have a crucially significant impact both on the person themselves and their loved ones. Being met openly and warmly by individuals who listen and offer help can be unbelievingly reassuring at such a distressing time. Often, it is the small things that are particularly noticed and commented on: kindness, ensuring the person knows what is going to happen next, interpersonal warmth, offering practical help (Reed et al., 2010). Other key factors include being seen promptly, in a friendly environment, by knowledgeable and calm professionals (Lebowitz et al., 2015).

CRITICAL THINKING STOP POINT 21.3

Try to imagine how you would feel if your GP said they were concerned about you and wanted to refer you to a mental health team for assessment. What might your hopes and fears be at this time?

ENGAGING WITH PEOPLE WHO HAVE LONG-TERM CONTACT WITH SERVICES

Something very important to be aware of when working with people who have long-term contact with services is how they may manage ending relationships and loss by protecting themselves from further trauma. When people have been in contact with services over a number of years, they will inevitably have had changes in the care team working with them which can be distressing and take time to deal with. It can be easier to not be interested in building a relationship with a person (as in, say, a student nurse) as they will only have to get used again to them not being around. However, the 'gift of time'

(Barker & Buchanan-Barker, 2005) you bring as a student can be very welcome, especially when you are able to focus on working alongside the individual to help them achieve small goals.

CRITICAL THINKING STOP POINT 21.4

Think of an example from your experience so far that has helped you to start or end a relationship on placement. What words or phrases did you use? What might you do differently now in a similar situation?

CASE STUDY 21.3

Martha, service user

I was initially disappointed when I found out my fifth placement was on a 10-bed rehabilitation unit within an inner city specialist hospital. I had an image of a locked art cupboard, service users with no place to go and tired nurses who wanted an easy life. I couldn't have got it more wrong. It was nurse-led with a strong ward manager and deputy, a lack of hierarchy, and a positive, 'can do' team philosophy.

Whilst there, I had my first experience as a named nurse with a 24-year-old woman, 'Sarah', who had a diagnosis of bipolar disorder and had been in and out of hospital numerous times. In the past, staff had not managed to engage Sarah in a meaningful way. Both Sarah and her family later told me this was because she had been treated as a 'mad young girl who didn't understand anything', which had fed into her feelings of powerlessness. I used my student status to address the power imbalance, as the relationship was mutually beneficial; I was supporting her recovery and she was helping me to develop my skills and confidence. We embarked on a number of sessions together aimed at building up our shopping and cooking skills and subsequently spent many hours singing along to the radio whilst trying out recipes in the ward kitchen.

Questions

- What strikes you about the environment and team that helped Martha to both think differently about her placement and engage with Sarah?
- What do you think it was about Martha that helped Sarah to embark on her co-produced journey with her?

Martha's perspective on being a newly qualified mental health nurse

I'm a newly qualified mental health nurse embarking on a preceptorship programme, and constantly reflecting on my journey to becoming a fully-fledged super nurse. I'm a big fan of the 6C's (DH, 2012a) which I've found useful as a framework for reflecting on my practice. However, when it comes to mental health, I think there needs to be a 7th C - collaboration. Collaboration is my favourite word in nursing. The following list is how this makes sense to me personally:

1. Care – be respectful and always explain the rationale for anything you are doing/planning to do with the person. This applies to something you may have done with that person many times before (for example, helping a person with **dementia** to have a wash).

2. Compassion – imagine how you might feel if you had had the life and experiences of the person you are working with. Alternatively, try imagining they are a relative or close friend; some of you will be doing your training partly because you have a friend or relative who has mental health issues. This can be particularly challenging when working with people in the criminal justice or forensic services.

3. Competence – your time as a student allows you to build up your knowledge, skills and your evolving competence. However, not knowing something is a great leveller and it is always better to explain what you do or do not know, rather than trying to pretend otherwise. The people you work with and their loved ones will appreciate your honesty and genuineness far more than if you try to pretend you do know 'the answers'; they will either see through your façade at the time or feel very let down when they do realise you were not being open with them subsequently.

4. Communication (+ Curiosity) – remember to always be interested in the person's story rather than the label of any diagnosis they have been given. Ask what is important to them and how you can help; ask how they are making sense of their current situation; or how they think they have got to where you are meeting and working with them.

5. Courage – sometimes that initial engagement can take place by 'being with' a person. It can take courage to be with a person who is either very distressed or is having difficulty getting their needs met (see Mark's example about being given a toothbrush at the start of this chapter).

6. Commitment – don't ever promise to do something you know is unrealistic. If you make a plan to meet, be SMART and if anything changes make sure you let the person know as soon as possible with an explanation as to why that has happened (for example, if there is an urgent admission when you are on a ward shift and had planned an activity with a person you are working with).

7. Collaboration – we need to be confident about admitting what we don't know. Building the skills, knowledge and confidence of our **service users** is our real priority and a spirit of learning and working collaboratively together can help.

CRITICAL THINKING STOP POINT 21.5

- From your placements and experiences so far, which of the above points do you recognise?
- If you could only choose one that demonstrates how you work as an individual, which one would it be and why?

CRITICAL DEBATE 21.2

National policy (e.g. DH, 2001) often refers to some people with mental health problems being 'hard to engage' or 'non-concordant'. This was the premise behind the setting up of Assertive Outreach teams at the end of the last century, their remit being to work with some of the most complex individuals in

(Continued)

receipt of care. Rather than a reluctance to engage, it quickly emerged that the majority of these individuals were traumatised not only by aspects of their life leading up to becoming unwell, but also by their coercive experiences of care when detained under mental health legislation. Additionally, there was historically a view that individuals had to want to get help to benefit, and things like not keeping an outpatient appointment meant they did not want or need a service. In theory, this view has largely evaporated now with the advent of services built around asking the person how/where and by whom they would wish to be seen, and developing care plans around the person's personal recovery goals (e.g. DH, 2012b; Leamy et al., 2011; Shepherd et al., 2008). When you are on your placements, you are encouraged to reflect on how much contemporary mental health practice, in reality, adopts this recovery philosophy

CONCLUSION

Our relationship and attitudes around engagement with service users have an enormous bearing on engagement. We have a unique job as mental health nurses, often having to try to support people who feel that they don't want or need our services and support. The added complication for others is the potential **stigma** associated with our role which can determine that we may see individuals who have no other options left to them and are feeling vulnerable. Whatever the form of engagement and all our efforts to engage, our success as mental health nurses is measured, ultimately, by making ourselves redundant and supporting the next person needing our help.

———————— CHAPTER SUMMARY ————————

This chapter has covered:

- The importance of engagement in developing collaborative therapeutic relationships
- How to be professional, but also warm in your interactions with the people in your care
- Examples of working with people at different stages of their recovery from first contact to longer term
- A number of the barriers to successful engagement from either a service, personal or service user/carer perspective and what you might do to avoid these
- How to consider a number of useful phrases, practical tips and strategies you can develop throughout the rest of your training and on qualifying as a mental health nurse.

———————— BUILD YOUR BIBLIOGRAPHY ————————

Book chapters

- Kirby, S.D. (2013) Relationships and recovery. In A. Hall, M. Wren & S.D. Kirby (eds) *Care planning in mental health: Promoting recovery*, 2nd edition. Chichester: Wiley-Blackwell. This chapter discusses the therapeutic alliance between the person in our care and ourselves as practitioners, proposing a model linked to personal recovery literature.
- Mutsatsa, S. (2013) The therapeutic alliance and the promotion of adherence to medication. Chapter 3 in *Medicines management in mental health nursing*. London: SAGE. Although not

covered explicitly within this chapter, the importance of good engagement to promote informed adherence to medication is another essential mental health nursing skill.

- Rapp, C.A. & Goscha, R.J. (2012) Engagement and relationship: a new partnership. Chapter 4 in *The strengths model: A recovery oriented approach to mental health services,* 3rd edition. New York: Oxford University Press. This chapter, in a revised edition of the seminal work developing the Strengths Model, expands on some of the concepts covered in this chapter and the ongoing and purposeful nature of engagement with the people in our care.

Book

- Walker, S. (ed.) (2014) *Engagement and therapeutic communication in mental health nursing.* London: SAGE.

SAGE journal articles

Go to https://study.sagepub.com/essentialmentalhealth for further free online journal articles related to this chapter. If you are using the interactive ebook, simply click on the book icon in the margin to go straight to the resource.

FURTHER READING: JOURNAL ARTICLES

- Antoniou, A.S. & Blom, T.G. (2006) The five therapeutic relationships. *Clinical Case Studies,* 5(5), 437–451. This article uses a case study to apply and bring to life Clarkson's seminal theory, documenting the different relationships and transference issues throughout.
- Livingston, J.D., Nijdam-Jones, A., Lapsley, S., et al. (2013) Supporting recovery by improving patient engagement in a forensic mental health hospital results from a demonstration project. *Journal of the American Psychiatric Nurses Association,* 19(3), 132–145 .
- Roy, H. & Gillett, T. (2008) E-mail: a new technique for forming a therapeutic alliance with high-risk young people failing to engage with mental health services? A case study. *Clinical Child Psychology and Psychiatry,* 13(1), 95–103.

Weblinks

Go to https://study.sagepub.com/essentialmentalhealth for further weblinks related to this chapter. If you are using the interactive ebook, simply click on the book icon in the margin to go straight to the resource.

FURTHER READING: WEBLINKS

- Blog article on issues of power in therapeutic relationships: http://blogs.brighton.ac.uk/bjrhs/2016/02/09/the-therapeutic-relationship-and-issues-of-power-in-mental-health-nursing
- Defining a therapeutic relationship and how to recognise the lack of it: www.goodtherapy.org/blog/psychpedia/definition-of-therapeutic-relationship
- Nursing theory of Hildegard Peplau: http://nursingtheories.weebly.com/hildegard-e-peplau.html

---

ACE YOUR ASSESSMENT

Revise what you have learned by visiting https://study.sagepub.com/essentialmentalhealth. If you are using the interactive ebook, simply click on the tick icon to go straight to the resource.

ONLINE QUIZZES & ACTIVITY ANSWERS

- Test yourself with multiple-choice and short-answer questions and flashcards.

REFERENCES

Barker, P. & Buchanan-Barker, P. (2005) *The Tidal Model: A guide for mental health professionals.* London: Routledge.

Bowers, L., Brennan, G., Winship, G., et al. (2009) *Talking with acutely psychotic people: Communication skills for nurses and others spending time with people who are very mentally ill.* London: City University.

Clarkson, P. (2003) *The therapeutic relationship,* 2nd edition. London: Whurr.

Department of Health (2001) *The mental health policy implementation guide.* Available at: http://webarchive.nationalarchives.gov.uk/20081023023730/http://www.dh.gov.uk/en/Publicationsandstatistics/Publications/PublicationsPolicyAndGuidance/DH_4009350 (accessed 29.11.17).

Department of Health (2008) *Refocusing the care programme approach.* Available at: http://webarchive.nationalarchives.gov.uk/20130124042407/http://www.dh.gov.uk/prod_consum_dh/groups/dh_digitalassets/@dh/@en/documents/digitalasset/dh_083649.pdf (accessed 29.11.17).

Department of Health (2012a) *Compassion in practice: Nursing, midwifery and care staff – our vision, our strategy.* Available at: www.england.nhs.uk/wp-content/uploads/2012/12/compassion-in-practice.pdf (accessed 16.11.17).

Department of Health (2012b) *No health without mental health: Implementation framework report.* London: DH.

Dziopa, F. & Ahern, K. (2009) What makes a quality therapeutic relationship in psychiatric/mental health nursing? A review of the research literature. *The Internet Journal of Advanced Nursing Practice,* 10(1), 1–19.

Firn, M. (2008) Engagement within the care planning process. In A. Hall, M. Wren & S. Kirby (eds) *Care planning in mental health: Promoting recovery.* Oxford: Blackwell.

French, P., Smith, J., Shiers, D., et al. (2010) *Promoting recovery in early psychosis: A practice manual.* Oxford: Wiley-Blackwell.

Gunasekara, I., Pentland, T., Rodgers, T., et al. (2014) What makes an excellent mental health nurse? A pragmatic inquiry conducted by people with lived experience of service use. *International Journal of Mental Health Nursing,* 23, 101–109.

Heron, J. (2001) *Helping the client: A creative practical guide,* 5th edition. London: Sage.

Kreyenbuhl, J., Nossel, H. & Dixon, L.B. (2009) Disengagement from mental health treatment among individuals with schizophrenia and strategies for facilitating connections to care: a review of the literature. *Schizophrenia Bulletin,* 35(4), 696–703.

Leamy, M., Bird, V., Le Boutillier, C., et al. (2011) Conceptual framework for personal recovery in mental health: systematic review and narrative synthesis. *The British Journal of Psychiatry,* 199, 445–452.

Lebowitz, S., Ahn, W.-K. & Oltman, K. (2015) Sometimes more competent, but always less warm: perceptions of biologically oriented mental health clinicians. *International Journal of Social Psychiatry,* 61(7), 668–676.

O'Brien, A., Fahmy, R. & Singh, S. (2009) Disengagement from mental health services: a literature review. *Social Psychiatry and Psychiatric Epidemiology,* 44, 558–568.

Peplau, H. (1952) *Interpersonal relations in nursing: A conceptual frame of reference for psychodynamic nursing.* New York: Springer.

Peplau, H. (1988) The art and science of nursing: similarities, differences, and relations. *Nursing Science Quarterly,* 11(1), 8–15.

Peplau, H. (1997) Peplau's theory of interpersonal relations. *Nursing Science Quarterly,* 10(4), 162–167.

Reed, M., Peters, S. & Banks, L. (2010) Sharing care with families. In P. French, J. Smith, D. Shiers, M. Reed & M. Rayne (eds) *Promoting recovery in early psychosis: A practice manual*. Oxford: Wiley-Blackwell.

Rogers, C. (1961) *On becoming a person*. Boston: Houghton Mifflin.

Rogers, C., Gendlin, E., Kiesler, D., et al. (1967) *The therapeutic relationship and its impact*. Madison, WI: Madison University of Wisconsin Press.

Ryan, P. & Morgan, S. (2004) *Assertive outreach: A strengths approach to policy and practice*. Edinburgh: Churchill Livingstone.

Shepherd, G., Boardman, J. & Slade, M. (2008) *Making recovery a reality*. London: Sainsbury Centre for Mental Health.

MENTAL HEALTH ASSESSMENT

22

NICKI MOONE AND STEVE TRENOWETH

THIS CHAPTER COVERS

- An introduction and overview of assessment in mental health
- Comprehensive psychosocial and holistic assessment
- The process of assessment and how this informs clinical decisions
- Examples of the use of assessment tools/rating scales
- Critical debate points, alongside practitioner and service user voices to help develop an understanding of assessment.

> As a practitioner I believe that informal assessment is something that we are all experienced in doing. We develop an art of being able to assess both individuals and situations very quickly and it is this ability that often prevents us from developing a comprehensive approach to assessment of individuals' strengths and needs. In practice we are under increasing demands to measure outcomes and to focus on performance targets and at times this can be at odds with completing robust and comprehensive assessment. However, we can view these challenges as a means to help us develop a shared understanding with a client, identify desirable outcomes and achieve self-management and empowerment. In essence nurses need to have an open mind and focus on client/service user priorities, whilst taking time to ensure that assessment provides accurate and detailed information that helps make sense of service user experiences.
>
> **Asram, clinical nurse specialist**

Visit **https://study.sagepub.com/essentialmentalhealth** to access a wealth of online resources for this chapter – watch out for the margin icons throughout the chapter. If you are using the interactive ebook, simply click on the margin icon to go straight to the resource.

An assessment should be used to have a shared understanding of what is happening and importantly why. The assessment is key and extremely valuable to and for the individual to evaluate/understand their own state of mind/diagnosis – without this how can you make progress? The use of assessment should help the practitioner and the service user get to the heart of the issue. It is most important to remember that doing assessments is not a solitary piece of work and this should not be driven by the practitioner to meet their needs or the organisation. When used well assessments are a shared piece of work that can be added to, used and help determine areas of need. There are inconsistencies in the way that the assessment process is used by practitioners but at the heart the practitioner should: listen, value what is being said, focus on the needs of the service user and not their own priorities. The practitioner needs to be aware that at times service users may be struggling to make sense of their experiences, therefore the assessment may need to be looked at again. Providing an account of how and why you will be doing assessments can help encourage/promote that you are working together to make plans and set goals. Assessment is a vital part of understanding someone and should be part of any working relationship.

Sally Ann, service user

INTRODUCTION AND OVERVIEW OF MENTAL HEALTH ASSESSMENT

This chapter will be written to aid the nurse to develop skills in assessment. It is important to note that we focus here on the nurse role in the **multi-disciplinary team** and in line with local and national guidelines for practice. This chapter offers the reader sufficient detail to help them develop and build their skills and knowledge in conducting assessment of an individual's health and psychosocial functioning. Viewed as the backdrop of quality mental health care, assessment is an essential skill that is well rehearsed and exercised in practice.

Questions asked throughout any **assessment process** should be:

- Why is this information useful?
- What will I do with this information?
- Who should I include in this assessment?
- How will this help the **service user** in their **recovery** journey?

The skill for the nurse lies in being able to manage the expectation of a recovery-focused approach in line with service user expectations and service demands. This is alongside assessment of areas that include: psychological, social, emotional and spiritual needs as well as strengths, needs, physical and mental health. Critical to gaining a comprehensive assessment are **collaboration** with the service user and carers/family, a multi-agency/professional approach, communication and an understanding of how the assessment may be used to inform the decision-making process (National Service Framework, 2012).

NURSE SKILLS NEEDED FOR ASSESSMENT

In contemporary mental health care, there is an assumption that all nurses have personal qualities that enable them to convey compassion, warmth, empathy and commitment (Francis Report, 2010). Assessment is a highly skilled process that requires an ability to gather high quality information that will inform future interventions and provide a baseline against which to measure outcomes. Key skills centre on being able to acknowledge the service user viewpoint, focus on strengths and needs, offer support and facilitate insight and self-management.

The assessment process should include: explaining the process, setting an agenda, listening to and summarising what is said, seeking clarification and using a client-centred approach. The nurse will also need to be able to manage and critically analyse the information to develop a shared understanding between the service user and key individuals involved. It is important to engender hope, optimism and empowerment and a focus on self-management strategies (Slade, 2009). The application of these skills lies in being able to manage expectation of a recovery-focused approach (assessment of strengths and needs) alongside comprehensive assessment of symptoms of mental illness and any distress experienced.

MAKING A DIFFERENCE 22.1

Ensure that the service user remains central to the assessment:

- Convey hope and optimism during the assessment.
- Be culturally sensitive and use assessment to consider potential issues.
- Keep abreast of knowledge and thinking and develop a clear assessment rationale.
- Have regular clinical supervision, discuss findings and what this means in the context of service user experience.
- Communicate assessment findings, ensuring that all key stakeholders are included.
- Be self-aware: are you influencing the assessment process?
- Listen to what is being said and reflect back to convey understanding.
- Be aware that service users are asked many questions, so avoid duplication.

COMPREHENSIVE AND SYSTEMATIC ASSESSMENT IN MENTAL HEALTH

Comprehensive and systematic assessment is complex and dynamic in nature and underpins the work of mental health professionals (Callaghan et al., 2015). Nurses need to be able to understand the process of funnelling down large amounts of assessment information in order to identify issues for further exploration before making any decisions.

There are many different methods and approaches that can be used during the assessment process and this may include: interviews, observations, the use of **rating scales** and specific **assessment tools** related to needs, symptoms, and should include family and carers. It is unlikely that one session with a service user will gather enough information to inform decision making and understand priorities. Key to the interpretation of findings is an ability to understand the interplay and interrelationship between needs and problems and being able to use the information to clarify issues and to understand priorities (Townsend, 2014).

It is important to note that the process of completing this type of broad-based comprehensive assessment is complex. It is essential that nurses have regular clinical supervision, are able to understand findings and interpret them correctly and allow adequate time to complete a thorough assessment (Ross, 2013).

For the nurse, comprehensive and systematic assessment will cover the following broad areas.

Understanding the current situation

CASE STUDY:
BIPOLAR
DISORDER

The starting point of assessment includes an understanding of where and who to get information from in order to gain the fullest picture. To understand the current presentation, the nurse needs to gain a full picture of current mental health and treatment and this includes any forensic or legal issues (Townsend, 2014). This will also include the service user's understanding of their current situation alongside their strengths and needs. Contributing factors such as issues related to current treatment and management plans, existing **coping** strategies, and life situation, including any stressors or **triggers** of relapse, need to be explored (Stuart, 2014).

Psychosocial and holistic assessment

Psychosocial assessment explores psychological and social factors related to the service user experience. This will involve the current family situation and key individuals involved in the service user's life, relationships that are important and social inclusion/functioning. This also includes key areas related to holistic assessment, such as spirituality, work and vocational strengths and needs. General assessment of functioning can be assessed using the General Assessment of Functioning (GAF) tool (First & Pincus, 2002), which is a brief and simple way to assess psychological distress and disturbance.

History

By understanding a client's history, it can help make sense of current experiences and provide context to the current situation. This component covers five key areas:

* history of mental illness
* social and environmental factors
* relationships and employment
* symptoms and diagnosis
* personal understanding on the part of the client/service user. (Nolan, 2000)

Historical assessment enables an in-depth understanding of previous vulnerability factors which may have contributed to the onset of mental health difficulties. It will also encourage an exploration of helpful/unhelpful strategies that have been used and any factors that may have contributed to the onset/relapse of mental health difficulties (Birchwood et al., 2000).

Mental state examination

The mental state examination (MSE) is a clinical assessment using a common format that reflects the service user experience alongside objective observation by the clinician (Simms, 2015; Trzepacz & Baker, 1993). The MSE includes:

* observation of behaviour
* emotional state and **affect**
* **cognition**
* beliefs
* functioning
* impact
* insights.

It also includes: the service user's ability to organise and process information, alongside their current ability to be able to conceptualise their problems, make decisions and make sound judgements.

Risk assessment

Harm minimisation is central to risk assessment and subsequent risk management plans. The assessment should include common themes of risk in mental health care, namely: **self-harm**, self-neglect, suicide and potential violence to self and others. Comprehensive assessment is dynamic and involves a multi-professional/agency approach; it is completed collaboratively with the service user and their **carer**/s at both the outset and throughout the process. Essential elements are: factors that reduce the risk of future risk behaviours, intervention and management strategies, and effective communication (Eales, 2010; Joiner, 2005). The main considerations on the part of the nurse are assessing indicators of: circumstances, intention, history and means, alongside protective factors that the service user has and should include any risks that the service user/client may pose to others. The assessment should be detailed, comprehensive and shared with key individuals, and be sensitively developed with harm minimisation to self and others at the core.

Physical health

In line with a national focus on improving physical health amongst the mental health population, an assessment of physical health needs to be considered (Nash, 2010; Robson et al., 2013). Consideration of comorbid physical health problems and the potential impact on mental health and overall functioning will ensure a baseline of current physical health so that medication regimes reflect any risk issues. Tools that assess attitude to medication, such as the Drug Attitude Inventory (DAI) (Hogan et al., 1983), and those that assess the side-effects of medication, such as the Glasgow **Antipsychotic** Side-effect Scale (GASS) (Waddell & Taylor, 2008), can facilitate discussions on both concordance and service user views on treatment and its impact. Consideration needs to be given to factors that may impact on overall physical health and functioning, which include: motivation on the part of the service user, symptoms, social isolation, lifestyle choices, substance use and non-therapeutic effects of medication. In line with local policy and practice guidelines, areas that are assessed include: medical conditions, lifestyle, diabetes, clinical observations and blood screening. Specifically related to the role of the nurse is the assessment of: smoking, lifestyle, body mass index, blood pressure, glucose and lipids, and weight (Nash, 2014).

Substance use

Exploring the possible use of substances and the possibility of concurrent use existing simultaneously with mental health presentation needs to be considered. Assessment needs to include current use, frequency and amount alongside any risks associated with substance use in terms of behaviour, mental health and overall functioning (Hunt et al., 2013). The aim of the assessment is to determine the nature of current substance use and should consider triggers and any protective factors alongside involving significant others such as family to get more detailed understanding.

Strengths

Assessment of the client/service user's strengths should embrace the principles of the recovery approach. The main aim of assessment is to identify strengths, goals and aspirations alongside building resilience (Shanley & Jubb-Shanley, 2007). An assessment of strengths needs to explore hope, mental wellbeing and satisfaction with life (Ibrahim et al., 2014).

CRITICAL THINKING STOP POINT 22.1

- How do nurses balance a recovery-focused approach (service-user-led priorities) with the needs of mental health services (management of mental health symptoms)?
- Assessment is not just about gaining information; it requires a genuine interest. How can nurses ensure that comprehensive assessment is afforded adequate time and effort?

USING CLARIFYING ASSESSMENTS, TOOLS AND RATING SCALES

Being confronted with large amounts of information, although daunting, provides a broad understanding of current issues and can be used to form the basis of clinical decision making in relation to **care planning** and future interventions. The use of assessment scales and tools can aid understanding of current issues and determine priorities on which to focus.

Clarifying assessments can help make sense of current experiences and understand the interplay between key factors. Most assessment tools and rating scales have guidelines and suggest the time frame that is to be reviewed as part of the assessment. It is imperative that the nurse has familiarised themselves with the tool/rating scale before use to avoid potential error and ensure reliability in the use of the assessment.

The list of clarifying assessment tools and rating scales at the disposal of the nurse is long, but to avoid unnecessary assessment there are several points that nurses need to consider.

CRITICAL THINKING STOP POINT 22.2

- What is the rationale for using this assessment tool/scale?
- How will the tool/scale inform understanding of the current situation?
- Is the tool validated and reliable?
- Am I the most appropriate person to do this assessment?
- What will I do with the findings; how will I share them?

ASSESSING NEED

Assessment of needs includes all areas of an individual's life which enhance quality of life and enable independence. Assessment should focus on aspects that are central to the service user's current mental health, wellbeing and recovery journey. Understanding more about an individual's social functioning, for example, is essential for ongoing growth and development.

Social functioning is a predictor of outcome in mental health and is an outcome valued by service users. The Social Functioning Scale (SFS) developed by Birchwood et al. (1990) focuses on seven main areas:

- social engagement and withdrawal
- interpersonal behaviour
- social activities
- recreation
- independence (competence)
- independence (performance)
- employment/occupation.

As with all assessment tools, an understanding of the limitations of their use is important and the use of SFS is not without consideration. The SFS meets with service-user-valued outcomes of social inclusion; it is comprehensive and will enable an understanding of the impact of **negative symptoms** alongside positive factors of activity and independence. However, some of the questions are outdated and may not be reflective of current social norms. There is a transformational scoring grid that can be hard to use as it can be time-consuming and hard to interpret in light of differing client presentations and demographics. To this end, the SFS has been adapted to ensure the ongoing currency of what is a very useful assessment tool (Mental Health Review Group, 2012).

Using the SFS, the nurse can begin to understand the variables that impact on overall service user presentation and the interplay between symptoms and social functioning. In the scenario provided (see Case Study 22.1), it can be seen that using the SFS has enabled a greater clarity of Mohammad's difficulties. A more in-depth understanding of Ahmed's experiences will ensure that realistic goals and plans can be made, alongside helping the family build on their knowledge and expertise in supporting Ahmed.

FAMILY/CARER ASSESSMENT

Involving a family member or carer in the assessment process is essential to meet the needs of carers and families, hence there is an expectation that all carers will be offered an assessment in their own right and this is stipulated clearly within the Care Act 2014. Nurses are challenged to be increasingly carer aware and to view the carer/family as partners in care (Carers Trust, 2009).

Alongside a statutory responsibility to offer carers assessment, there are other assessment tools/ rating scales that can help to gain a greater understanding of key areas such as: the carer's burden, coping, satisfaction, knowledge of **illness** and the overall experience of caring (Nolan et al., 1995, 2003; Szmukler et al., 1996) To gain more understanding of the **value** of specific family/carer assessment tools, one such tool will be used to highlight how more detailed information can provide insight and clarity into both the service user and family member experience and the background to their difficulties. The Relative Assessment Interview (RAI) (Barrowclough & Tarrier, 1997) and the adapted RAI for use in early intervention **psychosis** (Addington & Burnett, 2004) provide information on and increase understanding of: how the situation has evolved over time, how relationships are managed and the impact on relationships and the impact of stress on family members, and can include the involvement that the family member has in supporting their loved one.

Key factors when using the RAI are to identify and acknowledge experience and expertise, identify strengths and needs and identify any issues relating to stress. It is important when undertaking this type of assessment that the nurse allows adequate time to undertake the assessment and that there is an awareness of the emotional impact that talking through issues may have on the family member/carer.

ASSESSING SYMPTOMS

Further assessment of symptoms or a set of symptoms is warranted, particularly when attributing to the distress experienced. An example of assessment of a broader range of symptoms and commonly used in practice is the Brief Psychiatric Rating Scale (BPRS), developed by Overall and Gorham (1962). With clear guidelines for use, it enables a relatively quick assessment of current presentation. The BPRS is just one example and there are others, all of which allow an assessment of psychopathology. More detailed specific assessment of symptom/s provides a means by which to establish a baseline at the outset and measure outcomes in the future. It is important to note that when evaluating or reviewing progress with an individual, time should be given to selecting the most appropriate tool to measure outcomes, rather than repeating a battery of assessments undertaken at the outset.

Assessment tools/rating scales such as Beck's Depression Inventory (Beck et al., 1996), that look at particular symptoms/diagnosis, are very useful to help begin conversations about what it means in relation to service user experience. Tools that look specifically at **depression** (Beck et al., 1996) and **anxiety** (Beck & Steer, 1990) are commonly used in practice and can help determine links between certain symptoms, such as the link between voice hearing and anxiety.

CRITICAL THINKING STOP POINT 22.3

- Do we really need to use clarifying assessments if we have completed a detailed holistic assessment?
- How do you develop a rationale for undertaking clarifying assessment, and why?
- How can assessment tools and rating scales help establish links between presenting issues and the interplay between different factors such as symptoms and social isolation?

CASE STUDY 22.1

Mohammad is 26 years old and lives with his parents. He has recently been in hospital following a deterioration in his mental health. He smokes cannabis and, prior to admission to hospital, was not going out at all and had refused to leave his bedroom. His mother is very supportive of her son and makes sure that he eats and drinks, as she knows he would not do this for himself. His father feels that Mohammad is lazy and is very frustrated with him. Both parents feel that no one understands what they are going through. Mohammad himself struggles to see a future and says he has no friends and no energy. The challenge is to try and help both Mohammad and his family understand the impact of his illness on his overall functioning. This will include ways in which they can all support

(Continued)

Mohammad on his journey towards recovery and self-management. By using clarifying assessments such as the RAI with the family, they can share their experiences and begin to identify key stressors alongside strengths and needs, thus lessening a sense of isolation. This will also enable a plan to be developed that will build on skills and understanding. By using an adapted SFS with Mohammad, the link between negative symptoms and social isolation can be explored in more depth. This will ensure that realistic and achievable goals can be set with Mohammad and that these meet with his expectations and aspirations for the future.

REFLECTION POINT 22.1

Are there any useful hints that you can share with others about how to ensure the process of comprehensive assessment captures information that will help inform evidence-based interventions or a plan of care, and how you can make best use of the information that is captured?

As a student nurse the importance of a comprehensive systematic assessment is a key topic at university and covered in many modules throughout the course. There are many assessment frameworks as well as assessment tools used within mental health; which can be confusing. It is always worth considering the rationale for each assessment as the framework and tools used may differ from one service user to the next. It is important to seek advice from experienced professionals as well as using up-to-date, relevant evidence-based tools and frameworks. Although assessment frameworks and tools can be great as guidance for a student they can also be a barrier to developing therapeutic relationships. Therefore, it is of paramount importance to ensure that the key skills essential in developing a therapeutic relationship are demonstrated throughout the assessment process. The service user is more likely to know what services and support they will need through their journey of recovery, and which should be at the centre of their care throughout the assessment process.

Kerry White, mental health nursing student

CHALLENGING CONCEPTS 22.1

The challenges faced by undertaking holistic and comprehensive assessment range from the skills that are necessary to undertake assessment through to how to make sense of a wealth of information from many sources. Assessment should underpin any management and intervention plan and help to form a basis for ongoing measurement of valued outcomes. This in itself requires careful negotiation of different priorities alongside confidence and competence in making decisions. The desirability of a co-production approach to care behoves us to consider assessment from the perspective of the recipients of our care. To this end, we should critically reflect on the extent to which formal assessment accurately reflects service users' own subjective views of their needs and wishes for support, care and treatment. Holistic assessments take account of service user priorities and subjective self-assessment as well as perspectives from social networks.

CONCLUSION

This chapter has provided an overview of comprehensive, holistic assessment in mental health. Central to the role of the nurse in the assessment process is working in collaboration with a service user to make sense of the current situation and gain insight into how best to support the recovery journey. The assessment process is not just about asking questions; it is also about wanting to know more and being genuinely interested to find out more. Keeping in mind the management of distress and the promotion of self-management may provide a clear focus for the assessment process.

Assessment includes looking at a broad range of areas. These areas are not assessed in isolation of each other and it is important to understand the interplay and interrelationship between needs and problems and be able to use the information to clarify issues and to understand priorities. Underpinned by collaboration with all relevant individuals, areas to be assessed include: the current situation, psychosocial factors, history, mental and physical health, risk, substance use, alongside client strengths and personal resources.

Understanding a particular distressing experience needs further exploration within the context of overall experience. A service user may be socially isolated; this may be due to anxiety or feeling paranoid, but equally could be due to having no money or social contacts, or be a personal choice. Although a more detailed assessment can provide a clearer picture, consideration needs to be given to ensure there is a clear rationale for the use of the tool, it is fit for purpose and it will provide insight and understanding and add depth to the overall assessment.

CHALLENGING CONCEPTS: TOOLS

- Before beginning the assessment process with a client, it is prudent for the nurse to familiarise themselves with the tools that are available to them, such as:
- Beck's Anxiety Inventory (BAI): a 21-point self-assessment that is completed by the client. The questionnaire helps to discriminate between symptoms of anxiety and those of depression.
- Beck's Depression Inventory (BDI II): a 21-point self-assessment scale that the client can complete. The clinician needs to be mindful of scores that indicate either a denial of depressive symptoms or an over-exaggeration of depressive symptoms, and this needs further exploration.
- Brief Psychiatric Rating Scale (BPRS): quick and easy to use. Once the clinician has familiarised themselves with the tool, it is easy to use in a semi-structured interview format and has guidance and suggestions on the questions to pose to illicit information from the client.
- Drug Attitude Inventory (DAI): a useful tool that helps the clinician to understand the attitude the client has to taking medication. It gives acknowledgement to the client's experiences and attitude to medication and can demonstrate a collaborative approach towards concordance.
- Glasgow Antipsychotic Side-effect Scale (GASS): developed for use to assess the side-effects of atypical antipsychotic medication, it is a very useful tool to begin to explore and understand client experiences of taking medication.
- Global Assessment of Functioning (GAF): simple and easy to use, this brief assessment is a widely acknowledged useful and adaptable tool.
- Relative Assessment Interview (RAI): easily used as a semi-structured interview, the assessment provides family members with the opportunity to talk through their narrative.
- Social Functioning Scale (SFS): although an older tool, the SFS remains a very useful tool to develop critical understanding of the client's level of social functioning and the areas that warrant further attention in the intervention phase.

CHAPTER SUMMARY

In this chapter, you have learned to:

- Understand the principles and processes of comprehensive psychosocial and holistic assessment
- Describe the broad areas which need to be covered in any comprehensive psychosocial and holistic assessment
- Understand critical issues that need consideration from a service user and practitioner perspective when undertaking psychosocial and holistic assessment.

BUILD YOUR BIBLIOGRAPHY

Consider ways to ensure that assessment is developed in line with an understanding of service and service user expectation, to inform and promote self-management and recovery.

Books

- Barker, P.J. (2004) *Assessment in psychiatric and mental health nursing: In search of the whole person.* Cheltenham: Nelson Thornes.
- Norman, I. & Ryrie, I. (2013) *The art and science of mental health nursing: Principles and practice – a textbook of principles and practice.* London: McGraw-Hill Education.
- Trenoweth, S. & Moone, N. (2017) *Psychosocial assessment in mental health.* London: SAGE.
- Walker, S., Carpenter, D. & Middlewick, Y. (2013) *Assessment and decision making in mental health nursing.* Exeter: Learning Matters.

SAGE journal articles

FURTHER READING: JOURNAL ARTICLES

Go to https://study.sagepub.com/essentialmentalhealth for further free online journal articles related to this chapter. If you are using the interactive ebook, simply click on the book icon in the margin to go straight to the resource.

- Littlechild, B. & Hawley, C. (2010) Risk assessments for mental health service users. *Journal of Social Work*, *10*(2), 211–229.
- Stanley, S.H. & Laugharne, J.D. (2011) Clinical guidelines for the physical care of mental health consumers: a comprehensive assessment and monitoring package for mental health and primary care clinicians. *Australian & New Zealand Journal of Psychiatry*, *45*(10), 824–829.
- Woods, S.B., Priest, J.B. & Denton, W.H. (2015) Tell me where it hurts: assessing mental and relational health in primary care using a biopsychosocial assessment intervention. *The Family Journal*, *23*(2), 109–119.

Weblinks

FURTHER READING: WEBLINKS

Go to https://study.sagepub.com/essentialmentalhealth for further weblinks related to this chapter. If you are using the interactive ebook, simply click on the book icon in the margin to go straight to the resource.

- Centre for Mental Health – the value of community mental health needs assessments: www.centreformentalhealth.org.uk/meeting-the-need
- HEARD Alliance – mental health screening and assessment tools for use in primary care: www.heardalliance.org/wp-content/uploads/2011/04/Mental-Health-Assessment.pdf
- NHS Choices –public information about what to expect from mental health assessment: www.nhs.uk/NHSEngland/AboutNHSservices/mental-health-services-explained/Pages/your-mental-health-assessment.aspx

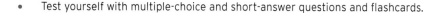

ACE YOUR ASSESSMENT

Revise what you have learned by visiting https://study.sagepub.com/essentialmentalhealth. If you are using the interactive ebook, simply click on the tick icon to go straight to the resource.

- Test yourself with multiple-choice and short-answer questions and flashcards.

ONLINE
QUIZZES &
ACTIVITY
ANSWERS

REFERENCES

Addington, J. & Burnett, P. (2004) Working with families in the early stages of psychosis. In J.F.M. Gleeson & P.D. McGorry (eds) *Psychological interventions in early psychosis: A treatment handbook*. Chichester: Wiley. pp. 99–116.

Barrowclough, C. & Tarrier, N. (1997) *Families of schizophrenic patients: Cognitive behavioural intervention*. London: Chapman & Hall.

Beck, A.T. & Steer, R.A. (1990) *BAI: Beck anxiety inventory*. San Antonio, TX: Psychological Corporation.

Beck, A.T., Steer, R.A. & Brown, G.K. (1996) *Beck depression inventory-II*. San Antonio, TX: Psychological Corporation.

Birchwood, M., Smith, J.O., Cochrane, R., S.O.N.J.A. et al. (1990) The Social Functioning Scale: the development and validation of a new scale of social adjustment for use in family intervention programmes with schizophrenic patients. *The British Journal of Psychiatry*, 157(6), 853–859.

Birchwood, M., Spencer, E. & McGovern, D. (2000) Schizophrenia: early warning signs. *Advances in Psychiatric Treatment*, 6(2), 93–101.

Callaghan, P., O'Carroll, M., Gray, R., et al. (2015) Essential mental health nursing skills. In P. Callaghan & C. Gamble (eds) *Oxford handbook of mental health nursing*. Oxford: Oxford University Press. p. 35.

Carers Trust (2009) Triangle of care for mental health. Available at: https://professionals.carers.org/working-mental-health-carers/triangle-care-mental-health?gclid (accessed 26.07.15).

Eales, S. (2010) Risk assessment and management. In P. Callaghan, J. Playle & L. Cooper (eds) *Mental health nursing skills*. Oxford: Oxford University Press.

First, M.B. & Pincus, H.A. (2002) The DSM-IV text revision: rationale and potential impact on clinical practice. *Psychiatric Services*, 53(3), 288–292.

Francis Report (2010) *Report of the Mid Staffordshire NHS Foundation Trust public inquiry: Executive summary*. London: Crown.

Hogan, T.P., Awad, A.G. & Eastwood, R. (1983) A self-report scale predictive of drug compliance in schizophrenics: reliability and discriminative validity. *Psychological medicine*, 13(1), 177–183.

Hunt, G.E., Siegfried, N., Morley, K., et al. (2013) Psychosocial interventions for people with both severe mental illness and substance misuse. *Schizophrenia Bulletin*, 40(1), 18–20.

Ibrahim, N., Michail, M., & Callaghan, P. (2014) The strengths based approach as a service delivery model for severe mental illness: a meta-analysis of clinical trials. *BMC Psychiatry*, *14*(1), 243.

Joiner, T. (2005*) Why people die by suicide.* Cambridge, MA: Harvard University Press.

Mental Health Review Group (2012) *Mental health assessment tools: The Social Functioning Scale.* Laois, Offaly, Longford, Westmeath Mental Health Services/Janssen.

Nash, M. (2010) Assessing nurses' propositional knowledge of physical health: a training exercise showed that staff need better education to identify clients at risk of experiencing drug reactions and to recognise undiagnosed physical disorders that may affect treatment, says Michael Nash. *Mental Health Practice, 14*(2), 20–23.

Nash, M. (2014) Physical health and well-being in mental health nursing. In *Clinical skills for practice.* London: McGraw-Hill Education.

National Service Framework (NSF) (2012) *No health without mental health.* London: DH.

Nolan, M., Keady, J. & Grant, G. (1995) CAMI: a basis for assessment and support with family carers. *British Journal of Adult/Elderly Care Nursing, 1*, 822–826.

Nolan, M.R., Lundh, U., Grant, G., et al. (eds) (2003) *Partnerships in family care: Understanding the caregiving career.* Maidenhead: Open University Press.

Nolan, P. (2000) *A history of mental health nursing.* Cheltenham: Nelson Thornes.

Overall, J.E. & Gorham, D.R. (1962) The brief psychiatric rating scale. *Psychological reports, 10*(3), 799–812.

Robson, D., Haddad, M., Gray, R., et al. (2013) Mental health nursing and physical health care: a cross-sectional study of nurses' attitudes, practice, and perceived training needs for the physical health care of people with severe mental illness. *International Journal of Mental Health Nursing, 22*(5), 409–417.

Ross, M. (2013) Implementing clinical supervision in mental health practice: the growing number of nurses who use psychological therapies in their work require trained supervisors. Maggie Ross discusses a trial of a cognitive therapy model that aims to support staff in this role. *Mental Health Practice, 17*(2), 34–39.

Shanley, E. & Jubb-Shanley, M. (2007) The recovery alliance theory of mental health nursing. *Journal of Psychiatric and Mental Health Nursing, 14*(8), 734–743.

Simms, A. (2015) *Symptoms of the mind: An introduction at describing psychopathology.* Sidcup: Bailliere Tindall.

Slade, M. (2009) *Personal recovery and mental illness: A guide for mental health professionals.* Cambridge: Cambridge University Press.

Stuart, G.W. (2014) *Principles and practice of psychiatric nursing.* Oxford: Elsevier Health Sciences.

Szmukler, G.I., Burgess, P., Herrman, H., et al. (1996) Caring for relatives with serious mental illness: the development of the experience of caregiving inventory. *Social Psychiatry and Psychiatric Epidemiology, 31*, 137–148.

Townsend, M.C. (2014) *Psychiatric mental health nursing: Concepts of care in evidence-based practice.* Philadelphia, PA: F.A. Davis.

Trzepacz, P. & Baker, R. (1993) *The psychiatric mental status examination.* Oxford: Oxford University Press.

Waddell, L. & Taylor, M. (2008) A new self-rating scale for detecting atypical or second-generation antipsychotic side effects. *Journal of Psychopharmacology, 22*(3), 238–243.

MENTAL HEALTH CARE PLANNING

23

MICHAEL KELLY AND CLAUDETTE KAVIYA

--- **THIS CHAPTER COVERS** ---

- A definition of collaborative and compassionate care planning
- The importance of an holistic approach to care planning
- The role of the nurse in providing person-centred care during the shared care planning process
- How teams can work with service users to promote recovery
- Problems and obstacles that may arise and how they may be overcome.

> **"**
>
> When I first accessed services I viewed care planning as a meeting where I would be told what care would be provided for me and by whom. However, as I accessed services more and more I realised that there were times when what the team felt was best for me, was not the same as what I felt I needed. I began to realise that different teams worked with care planning differently.
>
> For me care planning is about having my views heard, acknowledged and then having people supporting me with the issues that I face and that are priorities for me. It is not about what the team feels is best for me. It is about having a clear plan to enable me to live my life as best I can with the issues I experience.
>
> **Simon, service user**
>
> **"**

Visit **https://study.sagepub.com/essentialmentalhealth** to access a wealth of online resources for this chapter – watch out for the margin icons throughout the chapter. If you are using the interactive ebook, simply click on the margin icon to go straight to the resource.

When I first started as a student I thought care planning was an exercise carried out by nurses to determine the interventions that help service users recover. Although I did appreciate that it had to be person-centered, I viewed this with the professional centered paradigm that the nurse only had to consider the service user's needs and it did not necessarily require the service user's involvement in the planning process. It was an eye opening experience to learn that for care planning to be effective and meaningful the service user must direct and determine their own treatment and recovery. I learnt the concept of professionals working in collaboration with service users to establish effective care plans. I now view care planning as the blueprint that professionals must use to inform service provision; analysing and communicating evidence based information to promote choice for the service user. I believe the most comprehensive care plans are owned and directed by the service user and simultaneously work as a reference point for the professionals. Carrying out recovery-focused and collaborative care plans should be central to the work of nurses and must exemplify their role in the facilitation of care by being in the service user's voice, thereby bridging the gap between the service user and professional goals.

Claudette, mental health nursing student

INTRODUCTION

Shared care planning is one of the central roles undertaken by a nurse in the delivery of personalised care for a **service user**. In 1990, the Department of Health introduced the care programme approach (CPA) to ensure that all mental health service users with complex needs received an individualised plan of care based on their specific needs, and to ensure that relevant professionals, carers and other support networks were identified and actively involved in the delivery of health and social care (Department of Health, 1990). Underlying CPA was the imperative for health and social service teams to work collaboratively to promote the user's recovery through a person-centred holistic approach.

This chapter explores the **value** of developing a shared and collaborative **care plan** and makes connections with some of the benefits and challenges encountered by nurses and users who attempt to work interprofessionally in their delivery.

COLLABORATIVE AND COMPASSIONATE CARE PLANNING

Care planning is the process by which the mental health team and relevant others discuss, agree and review an action plan with the service user so that they can achieve the goals which are the most important to the user. The process of care planning involves:

- teams working in a way which anticipates and works with the needs of the user
- delegating tasks within the team and to the user based on their strengths, knowledge and experience
- negotiating care across all parties involved in the care
- supporting users to manage their own health and wellbeing
- encouraging shared decision making and including carers and family members in this process
- promoting care that is based on evidence and users' preferences. (Burt et al., 2014)

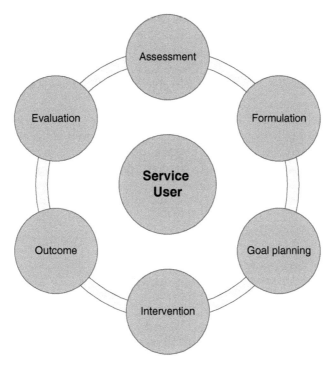

Figure 23.1 The care planning process

The process underlying care planning is continuous and involves a number of ongoing steps: assessing the user's needs, formulating their problem(s), defining an achievable outcome, deciding which interventions are the most appropriate (Hall & Callaghan, 2008) and planning how you will evaluate whether you have been successful at achieving the desired outcome. Based on the work of Hall and Callaghan, Figure 23.1 illustrates how, with the service user at the centre, this is a cyclical process with new goals set as the preceding one has been evaluated.

Engaging users proactively in planning their care is more likely to promote **recovery**, independence and a strong sense of achievement in the long term. Nurses who engage users are more likely to develop better **therapeutic relationships**, foster trust and openness and are more likely to find that users engage better in their treatment (Anthony & Crawford, 2000).

It is important to ask yourself 'who is the care plan for'? Remember they are for the service user to outline their goals and aspirations on their journey to recovery. It must involve the user and mean something to them. Being descriptive and informative in your documentation will allow any professional to provide the necessary service and support to an individual, even in the absence of the primary nurse. Ask yourself: Can a nurse who doesn't know the user pick up the care plan and use it to support the client, especially in times of crisis?

Claudette, mental health nursing student

Having a successful care plan and engaging the user will involve hearing what is said and documenting it in a way that is sensitive and understanding of their problems. Your care plan will show who will do what task, by which dates, and how and when it will be reviewed. It should also be written in the first person so that the user's voice is heard. Pre-written templates should never be used as these are impersonal and do not consider individual need or subtle differences in individual presentations.

Having an agreed, documented and personalised record means that you, the user and the team can have a tool by which progress can be measured, and so all aspects of the plan should be updated and modified as change happens in real time or when the goals of the user, or their outcomes, change (Stacey et al., 2012). Simon's experience below illustrates the distress that a user can experience when care planning is not done in a collaborative and sensitive way.

I first came into contact with services when I was in my late teens. I had real difficulties accepting the fact that I was gay and really struggled to talk to anyone about the feelings that I had. Instead I bottled them inside and eventually tried to hang myself and I was admitted to hospital. It was a horrible experience for me. I was told what was going to happen to me, when it would happen, and that if I didn't like the treatment offered there was the possibility of being sectioned. I was on constant nursing observations but the nurses looking after me sat away from me and would not speak to me. I was terrified and alone.

The staff did not explain to me what the plan of care was and I went to ward rounds where I wasn't even asked my opinion, just sitting there listening to what everyone else thought was wrong with me and what they felt would help. I was just given medication or told to attend occupational and art therapy groups, which I had no real interest in. I had no voice, no say and yet this was my life. I felt so disempowered and useless which made me even more depressed.

Simon, service user

CRITICAL THINKING STOP POINT 23.1

Thinking about Simon's experience, make a list of all the things that you think could have been done differently to provide a less distressing and more person-centred plan of care.

In the example above, it might have been helpful for one of the nurses to meet with Simon and identify some goals he would like to achieve to help him with his recovery. As part of this, they may have worked together to develop SMART goals, which may have helped make his treatment and the care planning process more relevant to him:

- **S**pecific – identify what exactly Simon and you would aim to achieve. Keep it simple and to the point.
- **M**easurable – how would Simon and you know if the goal has been successful or unsuccessful?
- **A**chievable – can Simon achieve the goal, considering his current circumstances?

- **R**ealistic – considering the resources available, is what Simon is hoping to achieve likely?
- **T**ime limited – set a time frame by which you both aim to meet the goal.

Working together to identify immediate and easily attainable SMART goals in the initial stages of care planning can help your therapeutic relationship develop and enable the user to work towards medium- and long-term goals in a more confident way.

THE IMPORTANCE OF AN HOLISTIC APPROACH TO CARE PLANNING

As described in the previous chapter, a holistic assessment identifies the biopsychosocial needs of the service user and covers all potential needs that an individual may have. Once these needs have been identified, the care plan should aim to address each of them in turn. Despite nurses knowing that a biopsychosocial approach is important, service users often do not experience this in practice.

Activity 23.1 has a simple exercise from Slade (2009) which illustrates why this might be the case.

ACTIVITY 23.1

What keeps us well?

- List three things that help keep you well.
- Now list three things that keep your service users well.
- What do you notice?
- Are they the same things that keep you well as keep your service users well?
- If not, why are they different?

Source: Slade (2009)

Activity 23.1 is a very simple exercise and one that can be effective in showing how we sometimes view our needs and those of our service users very differently. For example, you might have mentioned sport or exercise as something that keeps you well, or having supportive friends or stable accommodation. But, in many cases, one of the first things we say that keeps our users well is medication. Why do you think this difference exists? Some reasons given by nurses for this include being too busy to consider the user's needs, not having relevant training, or believing that they know what interventions would best suit (without consulting with the service user) (Mullen, 2009; Ward, 2011).

The exercise also illustrates the importance of taking a wider, more holistic perspective on wellbeing. Identifying all the things that help keep our service users well goes beyond a traditional medical approach. In order to achieve a more holistic recovery and make the plan more meaningful to the user, it might be helpful to ask them to make a list of all the things they enjoy doing and all the things which help keep them well. Meaningful activities do not necessarily mean structured or organised activities undertaken in, for example, a day hospital. It can include joining a local sports or art group, going for a daily walk, having a pet, volunteering, undertaking a course of study or taking a part-time job. All of these have been shown to help improve our mental health and provide a sense of purpose and self-worth (Friedmann & Son, 2009; Teychenne et al., 2008).

One of the best ways that care planning has made a difference to me was when I was allocated a new key nurse. She sat with me every day at the same time for a one-to-one. She listened to my story and really wanted to learn how I had gotten to where I was. She wanted to know what my goals were and she looked at support options for me from local gay support groups, not just from mental health professionals. She saw that I was lonely and the impact that had on me. So we set our first goal for both of us to sit together and call the organizer of a local gay support group. She then encouraged me to attend and explored the things which might prevent me from doing so, helping me think about how to overcome each potential obstacle to meeting my goal of attending the group, including offering to come with me for the first meeting.

Simon, service user

Working together to see how meaningful activities can be incorporated into the care plan, and offering support to help users (re-)engage with activities that perhaps they have struggled with due to being unwell, show that you are putting their needs first and are understanding of the fact that their needs go beyond their **illness**. Focusing on their strengths and aspirations for the future and developing a plan based on these also show that your focus is on recovery and abilities rather than on what cannot be achieved due to illness.

The service user's family and carers can also be very helpful in supporting them, for example by helping create a strengths list or helping to identify what they have observed keeps the user well. They are also in a strong position to help advise, encourage and support users to identify and engage with the action plan, especially at times when their motivation is low or if they struggle to see the point of engaging with the care plan. Don't forget that you may also need to undertake a carer's assessment to see if they too might need support and to make sure they can work with the user in supporting them to meet their needs.

I have found that it is often easier to apply the concepts of service user-led care planning in community settings when the user is often more well and able to engage in the process. However, in inpatient settings where individuals may be very unwell and not able to engage effectively or articulate themselves, the creation of a user-led care plan, although more complex, is not impossible. It is critical to avoid creating generic non-user specific care plans that do not reflect the users' individual needs. You must remember that in these situations the user's mental state may be constantly changing and therefore you must not assume that the person is not able to engage in their care, based on previous experiences. You must persevere and encourage them by tailoring your approach to their preferences and working in collaboration with the individual, their family and other professionals.

Claudette, mental health nursing student

There are times as well when the user relapses and their ability to make decisions about their own care is impaired. At such times, their capacity to make informed choices can impact on the care plan and so it may be helpful to develop an **advance directive** if such an event occurs. When the user has the capacity to consent, both you and the user can identify interventions to be taken in the event of insight being impaired.

Advance directives should be clearly documented, be negotiated with the user and their carers, and be implemented as agreed. This process is much easier if the user has been actively informed and involved throughout the process and the directives and interventions focus on all the things that enable them to get better, rather than taking an approach involving just medication, or extending a hospital admission.

The engagement of family, carers and the use of advance directives can also be helpful when there are risk issues involved. For example, Gus is a 75-year-old gentleman who has impaired mobility and has frequent bouts of **depression**, during which he struggles to take care of himself and there is a risk of self-neglect and falls. In his advance directives, he identified that he wants a particular **carer**, with whom he has a good relationship, to come to his house and support him with his activities of daily living. He has also identified what types of food he likes to eat so that his daughter does not shop for things he has no interest in eating. In his directives, he has chosen to have a small increase in his medication but, if this is not effective, then the team, in the absence of his capacity to consent, may consider ECT which he has found helpful in the past. In this example, the nurse's role is to ensure that these interventions are considered and planned for, identifying all the support mechanisms and people who will assist Gus if required (Hart, 2014).

THE ROLE OF THE NURSE IN PROVIDING PERSON-CENTRED CARE DURING THE PLANNING PROCESS

CASE STUDY: HOLISTIC CARE

Care planning is an essential component in a service user's personal recovery and this can be difficult to achieve when there are so many partners involved. Your role in these situations may be to act as care coordinator, which may involve liaison with people outside of the formal care planning meetings. In some cases, the user may not even need to meet other members of the team as much of the liaison can happen behind the scenes with direct care and support offered by a smaller number of frontline professionals. To manage these numerous partners, you will need to keep a focus on fostering hope with the user (Allott et al., 2002), especially if different team members have differing views on how to support them.

In Simon's case, he found that one of the main things that gave him hope at times of distress was when staff 'just sat and talked with me, allowed me to speak about my difficulties and focused on what we could do together to make things easier for me – not better, easier'.

From this example, you can see that working closely with the user to identify goals that are important to them can help foster hope in someone who struggles to do so themselves (Slade, 2009). Working within this recovery framework, nurses can support users to define their own goals and ambitions and build on their own strengths. Moving away from formulating users' presentations in language that focuses on illness, symptoms and problems is a key step in this process (Shepherd et al., 2008).

It is sometimes the case that the user may look to the nurses' opinion or feel obliged to follow what the nurse advises, due to a view that the nurse is superior or more knowledgeable to them in some way. Sometimes this can lead to issues arising, especially if a user asks for your opinion which you know is in direct opposition to their view or wishes. In this situation I find that honesty that does not disrespect the user and allows them to make an informed decision is critical. You can help achieve this by looking at all the possible outcomes of each decision based on factual verifiable evidence. Another way to do this is to use examples from your own experience and share these with the user. This can be done in a positive and relatable way. However, do not impose these experiences as a fact or the only truth. This can be detrimental to the promotion of choice and personalized care planning.

Claudette, mental health nursing student

Student nurses like Claudette have sometimes come across practice which appears to show that there are many problems with implementing care plans with users collaboratively. Some of the issues identified by students involve witnessing professionals using jargon which the user finds difficult to understand, assessments being undertaken but not informing the care planning process, and care planning not being inclusive of or shared with users (Rylance & Graham, 2014). This would indicate that, in practice, services may not always take a recovery approach to user care, despite the fact that the evidence suggests that users are highly motivated to engage and collaborate in their care in this way (Bee et al., 2015a).

Engaging the user in their recovery plan can happen both informally and formally. Informal care planning might include doing things such as meeting the service user at some point before the formal care plan meeting to discuss likely topics and help them to identify needs and develop an agenda for a care plan meeting.

In the formal care planning process, the nurse may act as a care coordinator overseeing the care planning process, help users identify their needs, identify team members most suited to help meet those needs, and ensure that once a plan has been agreed it is implemented, reviewed and amended as appropriate at regular intervals. Although there is a legal and professional obligation to document the care that you provide, including care plan meetings (Nursing and Midwifery Council, 2009, 2015), informal reviews should also be documented in the user's ongoing care records. Documented information can then be used at more formal reviews when the entire care team is present.

Users can be encouraged to take part in the documentation process through the use of 'My Progress' sheets. These enable you both to catalogue progress since the previous care planning meeting and assist in drawing up an agenda for the formal CPA meeting so that discussions are focused on what the user thinks is important.

HOW TEAMS CAN WORK WITH SERVICE USERS TO PROMOTE RECOVERY IN THE CARE PLANNING PROCESS

When we think of the word 'team' in relation to service users, we often think of the professional care team who works in mental health services. However, 'team' in a recovery-focused approach involves the user, their carers, family and other non-mental-health support networks (e.g. local priest or Imam, housing officer, even neighbours). There is a lot of evidence which shows that teams frequently do not work together with users or with each other (Kelly & Humphrey, 2013), and, as a result, this has led to users disengaging with their care plan and even services, teams showing a lack of understanding of users' needs, and even inappropriate interventions being implemented.

Partnership working aims to overcome these potential pitfalls and is about coming together to plan care and make decisions that positively **affect** the service user and their loved ones. To achieve this, all partners, including the user, must:

- have trust amongst each other
- provide support to each other when decisions cannot be made
- provide advocacy for the user
- take account of the user's wishes and desires. (Minett et al., 2005)

With such a wide network, the service user should consent to the sharing of information and it is important to agree what information may be shared with whom, so as not to breach confidentiality and cause distress. Once confidentiality has been agreed, the team can work together to identify how the user's strengths can be best supported using the skills of the wider team, so that the user is satisfied with their care plan.

Although achieving user satisfaction is the responsibility of all care professionals, the nurse, in particular, is in a unique position to **advocate** on the user's behalf and ensure that their voice is heard in the creation and implementation of the care plan. They also act as a link between the user and the other relevant parties.

WHAT'S THE EVIDENCE? 23.1

Read Grundy et al.'s (2015) work on the 10Cs of care planning and how these are important in the care planning process.

Once you have done this, consider how the 10C's might be applied to a user who is transitioning from child to adult services. How might the nurse work with the user in developing a care plan which considers the 10 C's and supports their transition into adult services?

What can the nurse, team, carers and user do to ensure that such a care plan keeps the user central, especially when the nurse may be ending their professional relationship with them in handing over to new mental health services?

You might find Claudette's experience below helpful in answering these questions:

I have found that when I am creating a transition or a discharge care plan it is helpful to take an IDEAL approach (Nurjannah et al., 2014):

- **I**nclusion - full inclusion of the service user and family in the planning process.
- **D**iscussion - an honest and comprehensive discussion with the user and their family to prevent problems after discharge that may be encountered.
- **E**ducation - provide information to the user and their family about how to manage their mental health problems and what to do to help minimise relapse.
- **A**ssessment - assess how effectively you have explained the user's condition and explained your understanding of the user's issues, based on what they have told you.
- **L**istening - listen to the preferences, goals and concerns of the user and their carers.

Claudette, mental health nursing student

PROBLEMS AND OBSTACLES THAT MAY ARISE IN THE CARE PLANNING PROCESS AND HOW THEY MAY BE OVERCOME

Care planning may seem like a straightforward process. However, a quick scan of the literature shows that care planning is often not done to the satisfaction of users. This section will identify some of the issues that may arise and provide some possible solutions.

Nursing knowledge versus user experience

As a nurse, it can be easy to forget that you have a vast amount of knowledge about mental illness which you have studied from the evidence base. As such, some nurses find it easy to tell users what can work best for them. However, users have a vast amount of knowledge too. This comes from years of experience of having a mental illness. They will often know which medications work best for them, what interventions haven't worked and why, and will frequently be able to help themselves if given the appropriate support. The evidence from the literature suggests that service users are reluctant to engage in discussions which focus on illness and prefer to work with services and staff who take a strengths-based approach underpinned by the principles of recovery and hope (Bee et al., 2015a, 2015b).

When users disagree with the plan of care

There may be times when a user and the team may not agree on particular actions to be taken when the user is unwell. At times such as this, your listening skills are very important and it is essential not to dismiss the user and their views. Listen carefully to what they have to say, acknowledge their point of view and attempt to understand how it is that they have come to that opinion. If your opinions still differ, explain clearly and concisely why your opinion might differ. Document both views in the care plan and try to resolve any differences in your action plan. If this is not effective, being open and honest with the user is important so that they are clear on your role and understand that, at times, although they may not like what you have to do, you are doing so for their own safety and in their best interests.

Care planning is often seen as a tick-box exercise

Fractures in the therapeutic relationship are more likely to occur when the care planning process is viewed as a tick-box exercise, rather than something which is needed by the user to keep them on a recovery pathway. Avoid the use of template care plans and ensure that any plan developed is specific to the user. Using 'My Progress' sheets can help with ensuring care is individualised.

Care plans are created and then filed away until the next CPA meeting

The actions above will help overcome another problem which many nurses experience – having a care plan which is not read and which is not meaningful in any way. Working closely with everyone involved and ensuring that the user's own voice and own words are heard consistently throughout will make the plan more meaningful to everyone involved and therefore more likely to become more than a paper exercise. It can become a working document from which relevant personalised interventions can be planned and implemented. Regular informal care planning reviews which are clearly documented and chart the user's progress also make the formal CPA meetings more meaningful to the user and show how the team remain focused on the user's aspirations and goals.

Nurses are a limited resource and therefore their time is scarce. This is not an excuse to create substandard, or use generic, care plans. The nurse must employ effective self-management and time management skills in order to better manage their workload, and not compromise on either the service provided or the paperwork produced. Where you do feel overloaded and cannot cope I think it is critical to take forward what we as students are encouraged to do: seek help through peer, managerial and non-managerial supervision.

Claudette (reflections on practice)

This list of potential problems is not exhaustive. However, most problems which arise in the care planning process can be resolved when the team works together and equally values the user's perspective and opinions. You, as the nurse, are in an important advocacy position and you must use your role to ensure that any potential problems are resolved together, in a way which is focused on ensuring the user's needs and aspirations remain central to discussions.

CRITICAL DEBATE 23.1

This chapter has highlighted the importance of engaging users in the care planning process to ensure that their needs and wishes are prioritised at all stages of the mental health team's intervention. However, there are times when the user may neither agree that they need your help nor be able to acknowledge that they have a mental health problem which is impacting on themselves and/or others.

There are a number of viewpoints on how to address this. Some might argue that sectioning the user first of all may be best. That way medication can be given to the user with the hope that their mental health improves and they gain insight. Others might argue that the best approach is to engage the user first and try to build a relationship, so that potential barriers to engagement can be explored in the hope that the user engages voluntarily with services.

Based on your reading of this chapter and your experience from practice, it might be helpful here to think about how you and the team may go about supporting users in these circumstances in developing a plan of care, whilst being aware that the user may not be open to engaging with you:

- Where do you stand?
- What clinical, interpersonal and professional skills do you think are necessary for both scenarios?
- How would you work collaboratively with users and sometimes your colleagues who might take a different viewpoint to you?

CHAPTER SUMMARY

Having read this chapter, you should be able to:

- Define what a collaborative and compassionate care planning process is like
- Understand why taking a holistic approach to care planning is important
- Understand your role as a student/nurse in the care planning process
- See the importance of a shared team-working approach to promoting recovery in developing a care plan
- Think critically about potential barriers or problems that may arise and how you, the team and the service user may overcome them.

BUILD YOUR BIBLIOGRAPHY

Books

- Grundy, A.C., Bee, P., Meade, O., et al. (2015) Bringing meaning to user involvement in mental health care planning: a qualitative exploration of service user perspectives. *Journal of Psychiatric and Mental Health Nursing, 23*(1), 12-21. An excellent resource which tells us what it is that users want from care planning. It shows how to make care planning more meaningful for those whom care planning is for.
- Hart, C. (2014) *A pocket guide to risk assessment and management in mental health*. London: Routledge. This handy guide will help you to consider ways to balance person-centred care planning whilst taking positive risks with users.

FIND OUT MORE

FURTHER READING: JOURNAL ARTICLES

SAGE journal articles

Go to https://study.sagepub.com/essentialmentalhealth for further free online journal articles related to this chapter. If you are using the interactive ebook, simply click on the book icon in the margin to go straight to the resource.

- Hall, J. & Callaghan, P. (2011) Focus group study of service user and carer experience of an Integrated Care Pathway. *International Journal of Care Pathways, 15*(2), 44-48.
- Hobbs, P. & Hobbs, P. (2007) The limitations of advance directives and statements in mental health. *Australasian Psychiatry, 15*(1), 22-25.
- Sorrentino, M., Guglielmetti, C., Gilardi, S., et al. (2015) Health care services and the coproduction puzzle filling in the blanks. *Administration & Society, 34*, 32-56.

FURTHER READING: WEBLINKS

Weblinks

Go to https://study.sagepub.com/essentialmentalhealth for further weblinks related to this chapter. If you are using the interactive ebook, simply click on the book icon in the margin to go straight to the resource.

- Integrated care pathways for mental health: www.icptoolkit.org/home.aspx – this resource identifies all the key components of holistic assessment and care planning, with direct links to the evidence base
- Wellness Recovery Action Plan (WRAP): http://mentalhealthrecovery.com/wrap-is – a self-designed prevention and wellness process to help people stay well.

ACE YOUR ASSESSMENT

ONLINE QUIZZES & ACTIVITY ANSWERS

Revise what you have learned by visiting https://study.sagepub.com/essentialmentalhealth. If you are using the interactive ebook, simply click on the tick icon to go straight to the resource.

- Test yourself with multiple-choice and short-answer questions and flashcards.

REFERENCES

Allott, P., Loganathan, L. & Fulford, K.W.M. (2002) Discovering hope for recovery. *Canadian Journal of Community Mental Health, 21*(2), 13–33.

Anthony, P. & Crawford, P. (2000) Service user involvement in care planning: the mental health nurse's perspective. *Journal of Psychiatric and Mental Health Nursing*, 7(5), 425–434.

Bee, P., Brooks, H., Fraser, C., et al. (2015a) Professional perspectives on service user and carer involvement in mental health care planning: a qualitative study. *International Journal of Nursing Studies*, 52, 1834–1845.

Bee, P., Price, O., Baker, J., et al. (2015b) Systematic synthesis barriers and facilitators to service user-led care planning. *The British Journal of Psychiatry*, 207, 104–114.

Burt, J., Rick, J., Blakeman, T., et al. (2014) Care plans and care planning in long-term conditions: a conceptual model. *Primary Health Care Research and Development*, 15, 342–354.

Department of Health (1990) *The care programme approach for people with a mental illness referred to the specialist psychiatric services*. London: DH.

Friedmann, E. & Son, H. (2009) The human–companion animal bond: how humans benefit. *Veterinary Clinics of North America: Small Animal Practice*, 39(2), 293–326.

Grundy, A.C., Bee, P., Meade, O., et al. (2015) Bringing meaning to user involvement in mental health care planning: a qualitative exploration of service user perspectives. *Journal of Psychiatric and Mental Health Nursing*, 23(1), 12–21.

Hall, J. & Callaghan, P. (2008) Developments in managing mental health care: a review of the literature. *Issues in Mental Health Nursing*, 29, 1245–1272.

Hart, C. (2014) *A pocket guide to risk assessment and management in mental health*. London: Routledge.

Kelly, M. & Humphrey, C. (2013) Implementation of the care programme approach across health and social services for dual diagnosis clients. *Journal of Intellectual Disabilities*, 17(4), 314–328.

Minett, R. and members of the North East Warwickshire User Involvement Project (2005) Partnership with the service user. In R. Tummey (ed.) *Planning care in mental health nursing*. Basingstoke: Palgrave Macmillan.

Mullen, A. (2009) Mental health nurses establishing psychosocial interventions within acute inpatient settings. *International Journal of Mental Health Nursing*, 18(2), 83–90.

Nurjannah, I., Mills, J., Usher, K., et al. (2014) Discharge planning in mental health care: an integrated review of the literature. *Journal of Clinical Nursing*, 23(9), 1175–1185.

Nursing and Midwifery Council (NMC) (2009) *Record keeping guidance*. London: NMC.

Nursing and Midwifery Council (2015) *The Code: Professional standards of practice and behavior for nurses and midwives*. London: NMC.

Rylance, R. & Graham, P. (2014) Does the practice of care planning live up to the theory for mental health nursing students? *Mental Health Practice*, 18(2), 30–36.

Shepherd, G., Boardman, J. & Slade, M. (2008) *Making recovery a reality*. London: Sainsbury Centre for Mental Health.

Slade, M. (2009) *Personal recovery and mental illness: A guide for mental health professionals*. Cambridge: Cambridge University Press.

Stacey, G., Felton, A. & Bonham, P. (2012) *Placement learning in mental health nursing: A guide for students in practice*. Edinburgh: Bailliere Tindall.

Teychenne, M., Ball, K. & Salmon, J. (2008) Physical activity and likelihood of depression in adults: a review. *Preventative Medicine*, 46(5), 397–411.

Ward, L. (2011) Mental health nursing and stress: maintaining balance. *International Journal of Mental Health Nursing*, 20(2), 77–85.

MENTAL HEALTH CARE COORDINATION

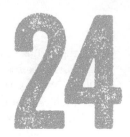

MICHAEL COFFEY, RACHEL COHEN AND BETHAN EDWARDS

THIS CHAPTER COVERS

- Understanding care coordination
- Definitions of care coordination
- Understanding the importance of communicative relationships
- The core tasks of case management
- Distinctions between care coordination and care planning
- The origins of care coordination in the UK
- The care programme approach
- Different approaches to care coordination
- The Strengths Model
- Wellness Recovery Action Plans
- Research findings on care coordination.

Care coordination is one of those things that is 'good on the label' and when it works well, it makes such a difference to the service user, their family and the service. Working in an inpatient service I see the good, the bad and the indifferent. It's as though when the person is admitted to hospital it is such a relief to the care coordinator that they often seem to 'back off' for a while. Most of them are run off their feet and, by the time they find a bed for the person that they are struggling to keep safe at home, they have to get back to all of their other service users who they've not been able to care for during the period of crisis management for another. If we can get a bit of time with the care coordinator on admission to find out what precipitated the crisis, who is important in their lives and previous responses to care, then we can pull a care plan together with them and thus maintain a level of consistency that has a chance of creating seamless care.

Glenda, ward manager

Visit **https://study.sagepub.com/essentialmentalhealth** to access a wealth of online resources for this chapter – watch out for the margin icons throughout the chapter. If you are using the interactive ebook, simply click on the margin icon to go straight to the resource.

INTRODUCTION

In this chapter, we will introduce the role of care coordination in mental health care as structured in contemporary service delivery. You will learn about the historical development of these provisions in relation to the relevant international literature, but we will focus primarily on how this works in the UK. We provide a critical discussion of the development and mobilisation of different models of care coordination, and the implications of this for service configuration. Using evidence from recent studies, the strengths and weaknesses of the care programme approach (CPA) will be evaluated. Emphasising the contemporary **drive** towards **collaboration**, **co-production** and service-user-centred care, recent developments in mental health care services will be critically assessed. Mindful of the focus on recovery-oriented mental health care, examples will be provided from recent case studies, which serve to illustrate some of the inevitable difficulties and complexities that organisations (at both national and local levels) must confront, in order to achieve care coordination that is **recovery** focused and personalised.

UNDERSTANDING CARE COORDINATION

The role of care coordination in maintaining and delivering good quality, person-centred mental health care is widely acknowledged, and has been an area of particular focus in recent years.

Efficient care coordination across all long-term conditions is of concern for policymakers, clinicians, patients and **carers** alike, especially in terms of how inconsistencies and deficiencies **affect** the standard of service provision. For example, governments in the UK, such as in England and Wales, have introduced mechanisms for care coordination in mental health care and recent research funding is now beginning to see evidence published on these developments (Simpson et al., 2016). These systems require there to be an identified worker (called a care coordinator or similar) who takes responsibility for being the main contact with the person, working with them to conclude an assessment of their mental health needs and devising a **care plan** in collaboration with them, which is targeted at meeting identified needs.

Care coordination positions the person as the target of the care to be delivered, with services seeking to engage or involve the person, and gain their participation. Care coordination can be seen largely as a concern of the system and, to some extent, this plays out in the way nursing has approached notions of care planning. In mental health care, the idea of coordinating care for individuals has been around for 40 years and arguably longer if we consider how services have been organised across the last two centuries (Jones, 1960). It is therefore surprising that no 'consensus definition' (Schultz & McDonald, 2014) of care coordination exists. Indeed, the heterogeneity of conceptualisations regarding its political, ideological and practical elements is understood to create significant challenges and difficulties in efforts to establish helpful connections between processes and outcomes, and the absence of a clear definition is felt to have exacerbated matters considerably (Chen et al., 2000; Skrove et al., 2016). In a recent study, Schultz and McDonald (2014: 6) identified 57 different definitions of care coordination. Moreover, existing definitions relate to different aspects of the care coordination model, pertaining, for instance, to various patient populations, or are used to describe different contexts and settings of delivery, including inpatient care, community and social services. It may be argued that since the term is not used exclusively within mental health contexts, this merely adds to the existing ambiguity.

DEFINITIONS OF CARE COORDINATION

By way of illustration, definitions have ranged historically from precise descriptions – for example, the integration of organisational structures (Van de Ven et al., 1976) or the regulation of activity between nurse and case manager (Allred et al., 2005) – to more ambiguous ones, such as 'an activity that is fundamentally about connections among interdependent actors who must transfer information and other resources to achieve outcomes' (Gittell & Weiss, 2004:132). Whilst one of the main objectives of the care coordination role is, arguably, to provide 'real world substance to the abstract concept of continuity of care' (Bachrach, 1993: 465), it would seem that the parameters and attributes of the very role itself are perhaps no less difficult to secure.

Defining and describing care coordination in so many disparate ways creates far more than a mere 'semantic challenge' (Burns, 1997: 394), and has far wider-reaching implications. For example, each definition carries a different expectation of responsibility for practitioners, **service users** and carers alike, and these, arguably, have a significant impact on their understandings of the actions and processes that are necessary to ensure and maintain good quality services.

The extent to which service users might expect to receive active support, as opposed to more indirect guidance, for example, is clearly implied by some definitions:

> getting a person clinically appropriate care in a timely manner without wasting resources ... seek[ing] primarily to help a patient navigate the system, working across care settings and providers and frequently assessing other services. (Sprague, 2003: 3)

or, conversely,

> A way of tailoring help to meet individual need through placing the responsibility for assessment and service coordination with one individual worker or team. (Onyett, 1992: 3)

UNDERSTANDING THE IMPORTANCE OF COMMUNICATIVE RELATIONSHIPS

Many of the definitions of care coordination given here emphasise the importance of communicative relationships. A recent study by Simpson et al. (2016) found that, for mental health service users and their family members, it was the quality of their relationship with workers, rather than the formal mechanisms of care delivery, that were prioritised. However, they also found that the lack of clarity and agreement, regarding where (and from whom) service users and carers might seek out help and support within the care coordination process, produced significant challenges for all involved. This would suggest that, despite clear objectives to the contrary, care coordination as a form of comprehensive case management does not necessarily succeed in its purpose as 'a process or method for ensuring that consumers are provided with whatever services they need in a coordinated, effective and efficient manner' (Intagliata, 1982: 657).

THE 'CORE TASKS' OF CASE MANAGEMENT

Onyett (1992) described what he saw as the 'core tasks' of case management and these can be seen to clearly apply to care coordination in mental health care. They include:

1. Assessment – the care coordinator provides a comprehensive assessment of the person's needs and strengths.
2. Planning – a care plan is devised with the direct involvement of the person on the basis of the assessment and includes specified outcomes.
3. Implementation – the plan is put into action with the involvement of the person, their significant others and all the agencies who will be providing elements of the care.
4. Monitoring – the achievement of the specified outcomes, or lack of it, is regularly monitored and this is recorded.
5. Reviewing – outcomes are evaluated with everyone involved and this leads to a re-assessment, which starts the cycle again.

Care coordination in mental health care is therefore a supportive system which assertively helps the person with the above requirements while recording and monitoring this activity. The key element of care coordination is the direct engagement and involvement of the person in all of these steps so that decisions are shared and based on an understanding of the **values** of the individual and an assessment of the costs versus benefits of any action (Charles et al., 1997).

SOME DISTINCTIONS BETWEEN CARE COORDINATION AND CARE PLANNING

Care coordination is therefore the system or mechanism for ensuring the delivery of care based on research developments introduced by case management studies. It enables care delivery to be monitored and provides the means to achieve information flow between disciplines, the person and their family. One aspect of care coordination is that it requires inputs from various disciplines directed by the care coordinator. In some respects, for nurses who take on the role, this opens up challenges as well as possibilities for more empowered working relations with other disciplines.

Care planning is the shared written agreement between the person and their care coordinator about the goals and intentions of the care to be provided. The care coordination system itself can be oriented around particular approaches, such as recovery, which is then played out in the discussion with the person to agree on a plan for their treatment, recovery and/or care.

I've had many care co-ordinators since using mental health services, but one stood out and helped me through a really difficult time. She was always my point of contact if anything was wrong or I just needed to speak to someone. She just understood me and spent a lot of time getting to know me. She knew for example that my outward appearance doesn't necessarily reflect how I felt inside – something many people don't consider. When I was in hospital and had absconded, she came to see me to check how things were. I really valued this because she remained my point of contact and the person who knew the most about me whether I was in hospital or in the community. When I received my care plan, I couldn't understand why there was no mention of my diagnosis, until my friend pointed out that she had written the entire plan using my words – that meant a lot, I knew she understood me.

Carys, service user

CRITICAL THINKING STOP POINT 24.1

Review the definitions and descriptions provided above and contrast the differences in each defini-tion. You may notice, for instance, similarities between definitions of case management and later developments in care coordination. Some differences are also perhaps due to the fact that case management originated in North America. This means that there are specific cultural and structural elements in the development of these approaches that may limit their transferability.

Consider what this means for definitions of care coordination. Is it possible to achieve the same types of outcomes when we transfer a system of care from a largely market-led, insurance-funded health care economy and apply it to a system such as the NHS in the UK, which is free at the point of delivery for all?

CRITICAL DEBATE 24.1

SEE ALSO
CHAPTER 8

It has been suggested that care coordination via the CPA was largely seen as a policy to leverage change in the system of care rather than purely for the purposes of delivering evidenced-based ser-vices. Does it really matter if it is policy (also see Chapter 8 on policy) or practice?

THE ORIGINS OF CARE COORDINATION IN THE UK

CASE STUDY:
COMMUNITY
MENTAL
HEALTH
TEAM

Care coordination has its origins in the post-Second World War move towards community provision of mental health care. Prior to this, forms of community mental health care existed but these were patchy and largely dependent on the availability of limited numbers of psychiatric social workers (Jones, 1960).

The occupancy of inpatient beds fell from its peak of 350 per 100,000 population in 1954 to 151 per 100,000 population in 1982 (Boardman, 2005). Goodwin (1997) summarised a variety of factors driving forward community care which included:

- the development of new medications
- more enlightened professional attitudes
- imperatives to reduce the cost of expensive hospital services
- increased lobbying from organised groups of carers and service users
- the influence of anti-institutional critiques
- the emergence of **anti-psychiatry** ideas.

These factors combined to raise questions about biomedically-dominated, hospital-centred mental health services (Goodwin, 1997).

These developments led to a greater emphasis on the provision of care and treatment outside of large institutions. As greater numbers of people were discharged from psychiatric hospitals, there was a need for improved community support services.

The first community psychiatric nurse, Lena Peat, was employed at Warlingham Park Hospital, near Croydon in Surrey, in the 1950s, to provide psychological support and medication supervision to service users and their families in their own homes (Nolan, 2003). This was seen as a means to support people to stay well and out of hospital. The large-scale hospital closures of the 1970s and 1980s meant larger numbers of people living outside mental hospitals.

One consequence of growing provision in the community was that this led to a complex and often fragmented system of care which was difficult to negotiate for people with significant problems when securing the help they needed. As a result, people experienced sub-optimal care, poor outcomes and the system itself incurred added costs associated with repeated hospital admissions (Goodwin et al., 2013).

In the USA, Leonard Stein and Mary Ann Test (Stein & Test, 1980) examined the re-provision of care from the hospital to the community. This programme was originally called 'Training in community living' but is commonly seen as the forerunner for what was later titled case management approaches, and further iterations saw the development of assertive community treatment (ACT) approaches. Case management essentially involved the provision of a key individual or team to coordinate care for an individual or group of individuals for the purpose of sustaining community tenure – that is, keeping people well and out of hospital.

It is the case management approach that informed the development of care coordination approaches which we see today in UK mental health services, for example the care programme approach (CPA) in England and Scotland, and care and treatment planning (CTP) in Wales.

THE CARE PROGRAMME APPROACH

The introduction of the care programme approach[1] in England came with little underpinning detail and remained largely patchy for many years (Simpson et al., 2003). Significant criticism of the ways in which care coordination for mental health was becoming overly bureaucratic (Simpson, 2005) and lacked supporting materials, such as training and education of the workforce, forced a number of changes in the care programme approach (Department of Health, 2008) and later changes to provision in Wales (Elias & Singer, 2009). It is the case, too, that over the years subtle changes have occurred in what it was imagined care coordination via the CPA could deliver. The advent of ideas of recovery in mental health care have resulted in newer iterations of care coordination being seen as the means to deliver recovery-focused and personalised mental health care. In the next section, we outline some of the different approaches to care coordination.

FIND OUT MORE

NHS CARE APPROACH

WHAT'S THE EVIDENCE? 24.1

In 2016, Simpson et al. conducted a cross-national comparative mixed-methods study, which involved six NHS sites in England and Wales providing mental health care in the community (Simpson et al., 2016). The study found significant differences for scores on therapeutic relationships related to positive collaboration and clinician input, suggesting that relationships with workers are key to recovery from mental health problems when using care coordination approaches. This suggests that perceptions relating to how recovery-focused care planning works in practice vary across different sites.

By conducting interviews, the study found great variance in experiences of care planning and understandings of recovery and personalisation across sites, with some differences between England

(Continued)

[1]Further reading is available at: www.nhs.uk/Conditions/social-care-and-support-guide/Pages/care-programme-approach.aspx

and Wales. Care plans were seen as largely irrelevant by service users who rarely consulted them. Care coordinators saw care plans as useful records but also as an inflexible administrative burden that restricted time with service users. Service users valued their relationship with care coordinators and saw this as being central to their recovery. Carers reported varying levels of involvement in care planning. Risk was a significant concern for workers but appeared to be rarely discussed with service users, who were often unaware of the content of risk assessments. The study concluded that there are a limited number of shared understandings of recovery, which may limit shared goals. Conversations on risk appeared to be neglected and assessments kept from service users. A reluctance to engage in a dialogue about risk management may therefore work against opportunities for positive risk-taking as part of recovery-focused work (Coffey et al., 2017).

DIFFERENT APPROACHES TO CARE COORDINATION

CARE &
TREATMENT
PLAN WALES

Care coordination in the UK takes on different forms in each individual country, in part as a result of constitutional changes that have devolved responsibilities for health care to regional governments. For example, in England there is the care programme approach (CPA) policy, while in Wales care and treatment plans[2] have been enshrined as law and as such are the legal responsibility of local authorities and local health boards. In Wales, the care plan documentation is standardised and the law mandates who is allowed to be a care coordinator (they must be a qualified health professional), while in England there is likely to be more variation in documentation and a much broader range of staff working as care coordinators, including those without formal professional qualifications. Within these approaches, however, there is scope to adopt strategies that allow people to achieve recovery.

The introduction of case management systems in the USA was in the context of a largely personally funded insurance system that limited lifetime inpatient mental health care and created large gaps in provision between inpatient and community care (Blair & Espinoza, 2015). Case management can then be seen to be a solution to a particular wicked problem (Hannigan & Coffey, 2011). *Wicked problems* are those public policy issues which can only be defined in relation to their possible solutions and for which there is contested and often contrary evidence. Note too that while case management approaches have been developed with particular philosophies and underpinning empirical evidence, the same cannot be said of early iterations of care coordination in the form of the care programme approach.

As contemporary mental health services now seek to move towards enabling people to achieve recovery, there is a need to shift thinking away from overly biomedical approaches, to systems that support clearer social goals (Tew, 2011). One issue with our systems is that they can be overly focused on deficit models of ill health and on supposed pathology models of mental ill health (Beresford, 2002). All types of workers in these systems can become too centred on what the person cannot do and neglect or completely miss what the person can do and could be helped to continue to do.

THE STRENGTHS MODEL

The Strengths Model was developed by Charles Rapp based on the recognition that integration of the person into their community required focusing on the resources and relationships they had available to them. At its core, the Strengths Model is concerned with the quality of life of an individual as

---

[2]For more details on Care and Treatment Plan Wales, see www.mentalhealthwales.net/care-and-treatment-planning

defined by the person themselves. People who experience persistent mental distress prioritise everyday issues just like anyone else. These include adequate income, jobs, opportunities to reciprocate in a range of relationships and independent living in good quality accommodation.

The Strengths Model (Rapp & Goscha, 2006: 54) therefore presents key contrasts with existing deficit-focused models of mental health care. These include:

- assisting a human being versus treating a patient
- valued consumer versus compliant client
- collaboration in community versus office-based brokering
- sustaining activities versus **palliative care**
- focus on daily living circumstances versus focus on intrapsychic factors
- concrete goals versus abstract goals
- interdependence of people versus independence of people
- community options and alternatives versus hospital as a social welfare response.

The governing principles of a strengths model include recognition that people experiencing mental distress can recover, reclaim and transform their lives. The focus of the helping process is on the person's strengths, interests, abilities and competencies, and not on their deficits, weaknesses or problems. The entire community is viewed as an oasis of potential resources for the person, rather than as an obstacle. Naturally occurring resources are considered as a possibility before institutionalised or segregated mental health services. The person is viewed as central to the helping process, leading and directing decisions about their care.

The relationship between the person and those helping is primary and essential – becoming one of collaboration, mutuality and partnership. The helping process takes place in the community, not at the mental health centre or other specialised building. The Strengths Model can be seen to fit well with contemporary notions of recovery for people with enduring mental health problems.

THE WELLNESS RECOVERY ACTION PLAN

The Wellness Recovery Action Plan (WRAP) system was developed in 1997 by Mary Ellen Copeland and is based on the psychological principle of self-determination. The WRAP system strives to achieve and maintain empowerment for people with mental illness, and is linked to the concepts of recovery and personalisation.

A WRAP is a personal plan drawn up by individuals themselves, via a system of **peer support**. Research has shown that WRAPs function as valuable tools for helping people to improve control over their symptoms and to manage their **illness** effectively (Cook et al., 2012). The self-designed plans also help individuals to identify and cope with problematic behaviours and feelings, supporting them in recognising crisis **triggers**, facilitating pre- and post-crisis planning, and enabling them to maintain their own safety.

The WRAP system has several potential benefits, for example it:

- helps participants create a personalised action plan
- encourages learning to develop individual wellness strategies
- enhances their self-awareness
- enhances self-management
- offers families and carers a guide to responding when individuals cannot make decisions for themselves
- helps in acquiring new skills, and broadening knowledge and understanding of the condition to improve quality of life.

It is also important to consider, however, that the emphasis on recovery as a key initiative of the WRAP system confers a considerable degree of responsibility on participants, and may result in under-acknowledgement of structural inequalities such as discrimination, which are also experienced by some as a hindrance to their progress in terms of recovering from mental illness. It might also be noted that for some older or longer-term service users, the shift away from medicalised models of mental health care planning and coordination can prove challenging or worrying, and that such individuals may be less willing to engage with self-management strategies more broadly.

Whilst the WRAP and a strengths based approach towards care co-ordination have challenged the bio-medical emphasis upon the provision of mental health services, they are based upon the notion that the community is a recovery promoting community and that the person themselves has the resources to recover. However, living in the age of austerity, which has condoned successive cuts to social welfare, local government funding and a lack of investment in the NHS, I do not believe that we live in a society where recovery is possible for all. People experiencing a mental health crisis are having to live on £70 a week, and are relying on food banks. Many are living in constant fear of the Work Capability Assessment. Maslow's 'Hierarchy of needs' argues that our basic needs must be met before we have the potential for 'self-actualisation'. We need to start talking in these terms about recovery.

Carys, service user

CRITICAL THINKING STOP POINT 24.2

- Compare the different orientations to care coordination above with the ways in which care is delivered in your clinical placements.
- What elements are similar or different in your placement and how could care be delivered in your practice area to achieve some of the above?
- Are there circumstances in which some parts of the models are difficult to deliver?
- How should these challenges be overcome?

We pose these questions to help you reflect on and challenge the many caveats that are repeatedly used to explain or justify why people are not involved in decisions about their care. For example, we often hear that people don't wish to be involved or are too unwell to participate in decisions about their care.

Paternalism in mental health care can be necessary and justified for people who are highly distressed and needing safety. Mental health nurses must intervene in such circumstances. However, this can be achieved by providing the person with information so that they are fully informed. In the vast majority of cases, people are not so unwell that they cannot be engaged and involved in their care. Many people will have learned, from their long contact with mental health services, that their decisions and wishes are either ignored or not prioritised by staff. In such circumstances, it is not unusual that individuals may give up trying to be involved. Mental health nurses have to be consistent in engaging and involving people and may have significant work to do with people to ensure that new commitments to involvement and recovery are fully realised in their actions.

RESEARCH FINDINGS ON CARE COORDINATION

In this section, we will take a brief look at emergent findings from a number of recent studies which are beginning to lift the lid on care coordination and care planning in contemporary mental health care.

The main duties and responsibilities of the mental health care coordinator's role in the UK are generally understood to involve assembling a care package, central to which is the setting up of a care plan. The care plan is then mobilised by the care coordinator, who acts as the main point of contact for service users, carers, **multi-disciplinary team** (MDT) staff and other organisations involved in the service user's care, and is responsible for overseeing the effective delivery of that care.

Two sets of emerging findings from the Collaborative Care Planning Project (COCAPP) studies provide us with some new evidence on contemporary care coordination in England and Wales, in both community and **acute** inpatient mental health settings (Coffey et al., 2017; Simpson et al., 2016).

As we have noted earlier, there is much emphasis on biomedical elements of mental health care and sometimes a lack of attention to the social aspects of this care. Tew et al.'s (2012) systematic review has shown that control over aspects of one's life and building social connectedness are important factors in recovery. Increased involvement and gaining control in treatment decisions is possible through shared decision making (Charles et al., 1997). In a mixed methods study of people (n = 163) using or providing support via non-statutory services, Coffey et al. (2016) found that greater involvement in decisions about care and improving social contacts were associated with better recovery and quality of life outcomes compared with those who are less involved or have more limited social ties. The area of most conflict in decision making centred on medication and condition-specific decisions, suggesting that much less time and effort were afforded to discussions of social issues.

This study found that there were three central themes of concern for the participants involved:

- connectedness and recovery
- the system of care
- the degree of choice and involvement offered to individuals seeking help via the system of care.

These studies suggest that there is something important about the way in which nurses engage with people to achieve an agreed plan of care, and how care planning does not always operate in ways we might expect. In a series of ongoing studies known as Enhancing the Quality of User Involved Care Planning (EQUIP), a team led by Professor Karina Lovell are training workers in user-involved care planning and then testing the outcomes of this training (Bower et al., 2015). This emerging research is slowly starting to appear from a programme of studies which may help us begin to understand what helps and what we might do differently in mental health care planning and care coordination.

Although care coordination has been around for some time, there has been little research on how it has worked in mental health care over the last 20 years. New research may help us begin to understand how care coordination works today and how it can be developed for the future. Note that these research projects are all asking different questions about care planning and care coordination. To this end, they have approached the topic using different types of methods. All of these methods can tell us something about everyday work.

CRITICAL THINKING STOP POINT 24.3

How might the different approaches to generating new knowledge help us in learning about care coordination?

CONCLUSION

This chapter has introduced the primary importance of care coordination in mental health care settings and has considered contemporary ways of organising and coordinating care in mental health settings, in part derived from earlier research on case management approaches.

In part, these ways of delivering services are the result of policy levers intended to influence and prescribe specific sets of operational criteria for mental health care. There remain many outstanding questions, however, about care coordination. These approaches were initially designed for adult populations within secondary mental health care. We know less about how these approaches play out in specialist tertiary services, such as forensic mental health care or specialist child and adolescent services. Claims of recovery-focused mental health care are also problematic and care coordination is not as person-centred as is often claimed. This may be related to external pressures such as the challenges presented by policies pulling in opposite directions, for example recovery focus versus risk avoidance. Some of this may be related to economic pressures, leading to a reduction in alternatives to mental health care and limited available resources within the system. The challenge for mental health nursing is to remember that in the midst of health technologies such as care coordination, there is still a person to be helped.

CHAPTER SUMMARY

Having read this chapter you should be able to:

- Define care coordination
- Appreciate the importance of communicative relationships
- Identify the core tasks of case management
- Understand distinctions between care coordination and care planning
- Be aware of the origins of care coordination in the UK
- Recognise the value of the care programme approach and the different approaches to care coordination
- See how wellness recovery action plans are congruent with effective care coordination
- Acknowledge the evidence base for care coordination.

BUILD YOUR BIBLIOGRAPHY

Book

- Rapp, C.A. & Goscha, R.J. (2006) *The strengths model: Case management with people with psychiatric disabilities*, 2nd edition. Oxford, Oxford University Press. This is the source material for a discussion on the Strengths Model from the originator of the idea, Charles Rapp.

SAGE journal articles

Go to https://study.sagepub.com/essentialmentalhealth for further free online journal articles related to this chapter. If you are using the interactive ebook, simply click on the book icon in the margin to go straight to the resource.

FURTHER READING: JOURNAL ARTICLES

- El-Ghorr, A., Cameron, R., Fleming, M., et al. (2010) Scotland's national approach to improving mental health services: integrated care pathways as tools for redesign and continuous quality improvement. *International Journal of Care Pathways*, 14(2), 57-64.
- Schultz, E.M. & McDonald, K.M. (2014) What is care coordination? *International Journal of Care Coordination*, 17(1-2), 5-24. This article appears in a SAGE journal which is now focusing specifically on care coordination across a range of health and social care topics.
- Van Hoof, F., Van Weeghel, J. & Kroon, H. (2000) Community care: exploring the priorities of clients, mental health professionals and community providers. *International Journal of Social Psychiatry*, 46(3), 208-219.

Journal article

- Simpson, A., Hannigan, B., Coffey, M., et al. (2016) Cross-national comparative mixed-methods case study of recovery-focused mental health care planning and coordination: Collaborative Care Planning Project (COCAPP). *Health Services and Delivery Research*, 4(5). This is the latest research on care coordination in England and Wales and is open access and free to read direct from the National Institute for Health Research website (www.nihr.ac.uk/about-us/publications).

Weblinks

Go to https://study.sagepub.com/essentialmentalhealth for further weblinks related to this chapter. If you are using the interactive ebook, simply click on the book icon in the margin to go straight to the resource.

FURTHER READING: WEBLINKS

- Scottish Recovery Network: www.scottishrecovery.net - excellent initiatives, useful resources and high quality materials
- University of Kansas Center for Mental Health Research and Innovation: https://mentalhealth.socwel.ku.edu/principles-strengths - a useful resource on the Strengths Model.

ACE YOUR ASSESSMENT

ONLINE
QUIZZES &
ACTIVITY
ANSWERS

Revise what you have learned by visiting https://study.sagepub.com/essentialmentalhealth. If you are using the interactive ebook, simply click on the tick icon to go straight to the resource.

- Test yourself with multiple-choice and short-answer questions and flashcards.

REFERENCES

Allred, C.A., Burns, B.J. & Phillips, S.D. (2005) The assertive community treatment team as a complex dynamic system of care. *Administration and Policy in Mental Health*, *32*(3), 211–220.

Bachrach, L.L. (1993) Continuity of care and approaches to case management for long-term mentally ill patients. *Hospital and Community Psychiatry*, *44*(5), 465–468.

Beresford, P. (2002) Thinking about 'mental health': towards a social model. *Journal of Mental Health*, *11*(6), 581–584.

Blair, T.R. & Espinoza, R.T. (2015) Medicare, medicaid, and mental health care: historical perspectives on reforms before the US congress. JAMA, *314*(21), 2231–2232.

Boardman, J. (2005) New services for old: an overview of mental health policy. In A. Bell & P. Lindley (eds) *Beyond the water towers: The unfinished revolution in mental health services 1985–2005*. London: Sainsbury Centre for Mental Health.

Bower, P., Roberts, C., O'Leary, N., et al. (2015) A cluster randomised controlled trial and process evaluation of a training programme for mental health professionals to enhance user involvement in care planning in service users with severe mental health issues (EQUIP): study protocol for a randomised controlled trial. *Trials*, *16*, 348.

Burns, T. (1997) Case management, care management and care programming. *The British Journal of Psychiatry*, *170*(5), 93–395.

Charles, C., Gafni, A. & Whelan, T. (1997) Shared decision-making in the medical encounter: what does it mean? (or it takes at least two to tango). *Social Science & Medicine*, *44*(5), 681–692.

Chen, A., Brown, R., Archibald, N., et al. (2000) *Best practices in coordinated care*. Available at: www.communitycarenc.org/media/.../best-practices-in-coordinated-care.pdf (accessed 11.08.17).

Coffey, M., Cohen, R., Faulkner, A., et al. (2017) Ordinary risks and accepted fictions: how contrasting and competing priorities work in risk assessment and mental health care planning. *Health Expectations*, *20*(3), 471–483.

Coffey, M., Hannigan, B., Meudell, A., et al. (2016) Study protocol: a mixed methods study to assess mental health recovery, shared decision-making and quality of life (Plan4Recovery). *BMC Health Services Research*, *16*(1), 1–7.

Cook, J.A., Copeland, M.E., Jonikas, J.A., et al. (2012) Results of a randomized controlled trial of mental illness self-management using wellness recovery action planning. *Schizophrenia Bulletin*, *38*(4), 881–891.

Department of Health (2008) *Refocusing the care programme approach: Policy and positive practice guidance*. London: DH.

Elias, E. & Singer, L. (2009) *Review of the care programme approach in Wales*. Llanharan: National Leadership and Innovation Agency for Healthcare.

Gittell, J.H. & Weiss, L. (2004) Coordination networks within and across organizations: a multi-level framework. *Journal of Management Studies*, *41*, 127–153.

Goodwin, N., Sonola, L. & Thiel, V. (2013) *Co-ordinated care for people with complex chronic conditions: Key lessons and markers for success*. London: King's Fund.

Goodwin, S. (1997) *Comparative mental health policy: From institutional to community care*. London: Sage.

Hannigan, B. & Coffey, M. (2011) Where the wicked problems are: the case of mental health. *Health Policy, 101*(3), 220–227.

Intagliata, J. (1982) Improving the quality of life for the chronically mentally disabled: the role of case management. *Schizophrenia Bulletin, 8*(4), 655–674.

Jones, K. (1960) *Mental health and social policy 1845–1959*. London: Routledge & Kegan Paul.

Nolan, P. (2003) The history of community mental health nursing. In B. Hannigan & M. Coffey (eds) *The handbook of community mental health nursing*. London: Routledge. pp. 7–18.

Onyett, S. (1992) *Case management in mental health*. London: Chapman & Hall.

Rapp, C.A. & Goscha, R.J. (2006) *The strengths model: Case management with people with psychiatric disabilities*, 2nd edition. Oxford: Oxford University Press.

Schultz, E.M. & McDonald, K.M. (2014) What is care coordination? *International Journal of Care Coordination, 17*(1–2), 5–24.

Simpson, A. (2005) Community psychiatric nurses and the care co-ordinator role: squeezed to provide 'limited nursing'. *Journal of Advanced Nursing, 52*, 689–99.

Simpson, A., Miller, C. & Bowers, L. (2003) The history of the care programme approach in England: where did it go wrong? *Journal of Mental Health, 12*, 489–504.

Simpson, A., Hannigan, B., Coffey, M., et al. (2016) Cross-national comparative mixed-methods case study of recovery-focused mental health care planning and coordination. *Health Services and Delivery Research, 4*(5).

Skrove, G.K., Bachmann, K. & Aarseth, T. (2016) Integrated care pathways: a strategy towards better care coordination in municipalities? A qualitative study. *International Journal of Care Coordination, 19*(1–2), 20–28.

Sprague, L. (2003) *Disease management to population-based health: steps in the right direction?* NHPF Issue Brief No. 791, 16 May. Washington, DC: National Health Policy Forum.

Stein, L.I. & Test, M.A. (1980) Alternative to mental hospital treatment 1: conceptual model, treatment program, and clinical evaluation. *Archives of General Psychiatry, 37*, 392–397.

Tew, J. (2011) *Social approaches to mental distress*. Basingstoke: Palgrave Macmillan.

Tew, J., Ramon, S., Slade, M., et al. (2012) Social factors and recovery from mental health difficulties: a review of the evidence. *British Journal of Social Work, 42*(3), 443-460.

Van de Ven, A.H., Delbecq, A.L. & Koenig, J.R. (1976) Determinants of coordination modes within organizations. *American Sociological Review, 41*, 322–338.

MENTAL HEALTH RISK ASSESSMENT: A PERSONALISED APPROACH

JOHN BUTLER, ALISON COMMISSIONG AND CHRISTINE CROSSMAN

THIS CHAPTER COVERS

- Ways of thinking of about risk
- Using a practical, formulation-driven approach to working with risk within mental health practice
- Conducting a risk assessment:
    - accessing and gathering information
    - considering the presence of historical and recent risk and protective factors
    - considering the use of structured assessment tools
    - developing the risk formulation

- Working alongside the individual in negotiating a meaningful care and risk (management) plan:
    - negotiating an action plan
    - undertaking frequent and regular review
    - forming a meaningful account

- Issues/factors that may facilitate or hinder meaningful risk assessment and risk management.

Visit **https://study.sagepub.com/essentialmentalhealth** to access a wealth of online resources for this chapter – watch out for the margin icons throughout the chapter. If you are using the interactive ebook, simply click on the margin icon to go straight to the resource.

An accepted yet challenging feature of mental health practice, working with risk necessarily requires an involving and responsive approach. How else would it be possible to make and be confident about important decisions on managing risk – for example, when giving leave or supporting the discharge of a patient who when unwell had stabbed and seriously injured their partner, or when deciding to offer home-based support rather than seeking hospital admission for a service user who has been experiencing suicidal ideas, knowing that they have made three serious suicide attempts in the past, or when considering how best to respond to a family member who is very concerned about the risk behaviour of their son.

Suzanne, mental health nurse

Realising the importance of not making assumptions, I've often found the service user and their family open to discussing and understanding more about risk issues, and witnessed the positive value of agreeing actions that build on strengths, consider and offer opportunities for positive risk taking, and form a 'least restrictive' approach to managing identified risks. This means creating opportunities to actively involve the individual in their own care, and accepting the challenges of working with risk: some may not wish to actively engage; risk is dynamic and often unpredictable; managing differences of opinion about the individual's risk status and most beneficial care responses is difficult; and there's often a tension between wishing to prevent harm and providing opportunities for positive risk taking. What seems most important is shared and supportive decision-making, in which mutual expectations and responsibilities for action are clear and realistic.

Mark, community mental health nurse

INTRODUCTION

In this chapter, we will focus on the specific role of the mental health nurse in conducting meaningful risk assessment and co-producing a care and risk (management) plan. As a central aspect of high quality mental health nursing practice, we will provide an outline of a practical, formulation-driven approach, clarifying key aspects and considerations through the use of case studies, as adapted from our own practice.

WAYS OF THINKING ABOUT RISK

Of course, risk is a feature of our everyday behaviour and life experience. *Stop and think* for a few moments about the scope and nature of things that you do that involve taking risks.

CRITICAL THINKING STOP POINT 25.1

Have you ever driven a car, flown in an aeroplane, or been on a cruise? What about times when you've cooked some food, ironed your clothes, or tried to fix an electrical appliance? Have you ever exceeded the recommended limits for alcohol? Have you ever walked home on your own late at night, through an unfamiliar area? Or perhaps you enjoy more adventurous activities, such as bungee jumping or other high-risk sports.

Though we may consciously think about the risks involved in some, perhaps new and less familiar, activities, we may not stop to think about the more routine activities. Think about some of your examples: What could happen? What's the chance of it happening? How serious would this be? What do you do/could you do to minimise the risk and enhance safety?

Risk may be considered the possibility, chance, probability or likelihood of a beneficial or, more importantly, a harmful or undesirable event/behaviour/outcome within a stated timescale, often in response to changing personal circumstances (Alberg et al., 1996; Morgan, 2000; Wellman, 2006), whilst taking a risk involves taking action when you are uncertain of the actual outcomes.

Having considered examples of the many risks that naturally form part of our lives, it is important to consider the particular risks that are commonly encountered and require specific assessment within mental health practice – for example:

- primary risk to self, e.g. self-neglect, **self-harm**, suicide
- primary risk to others, e.g. **aggression**, violence, offending, neglect of dependents
- primary risk to self or others, e.g. substance misuse, exploitation.

Importantly, particular types of risk may be more evident than others within certain care settings. The experiences of primarily working within a specific care setting is likely to influence the practitioner's threshold for viewing certain behaviours as risks. So, too, the seriousness with which a particular behaviour is viewed as a risk will be influenced by the practitioner's views, beliefs and prejudices.

CONDUCTING A RISK ASSESSMENT

The recognition and assessment of specific risk issues is a first step in the process towards managing risk, and forms an integral part of mental health assessment. A core '*skill* that needs to be learned, practiced and refined' (Wellman, 2006: 146), this involves determining the circumstances, likelihood and severity of specified risk behaviours occurring.

Structured professional judgement

In contrast to unstructured clinical/professional judgement, or the use of a purely actuarial approach in which formal methods and procedures based on statistical predictions are used for assessing risk, the recommended approach to clinical risk assessment has been described as structured professional judgement (DH, 2007a). This aims to combine the evidence base for risk factors with individualised assessment, taking account of the person's particular circumstances, needs and strengths. With the option for complementary use of structured **assessment tools**, this approach involves undertaking a structured assessment and formulation as the basis for developing a care and risk (management) plan.

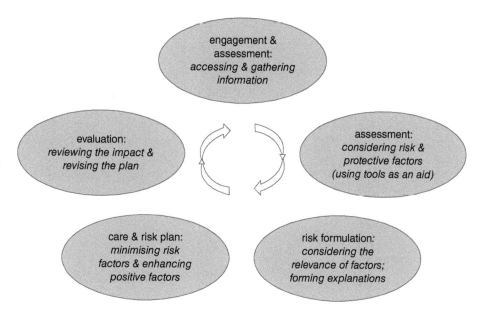

Figure 25.1 A risk formulation cycle

This is a multi-disciplinary and multi-agency activity that actively involves the individual and their **carer** (DH, 2007b, 2008). This process is represented as a cyclical series of key steps in Figure 25.1 (adapted from Duffy, 2008; Doyle & Logan, 2012).

A highly collaborative approach to risk assessment and risk management planning will promote understanding, choice and **recovery**, improve consistency and transparency in decision making, and promote the targeting of resources (DH, 2007b). However, this remains a particular challenge.

Consistent with our own local survey of student mental health nurses, Langan and Lindow (2004) found that few professionals were undertaking systematic risk assessment and that the involvement of **service users** in risk assessment and management was highly variable, with some not even being aware that a formal risk assessment was being undertaken, nor aware of being deemed a risk to others. The reasons given for this lack of involvement included increasing **stigma** and distress, prompting disagreement or disengagement, and fears for personal safety. However, the consequences of such lack of involvement included the over- or underestimation of risk, mislabelling, areas of disagreement, and poorly informed care plans that included overly restrictive interventions and/or a lack of support. Notably, they highlighted some positive examples of a more collaborative and systematic approach, though this often depended on individual professional initiative, being more likely if the practitioner had formed a trusting relationship with the service user, such that s/he was able to influence their **care plan**. A case was made for ensuring that:

- the service user's views are considered
- there is a willingness to take appropriate risks
- effective responses are provided in the event of a crisis/early stages of becoming unwell.

Step 1: Accessing and gathering information

Meaningful risk assessment requires the systematic gathering of information. In practice, the practitioner should always try to gather and *validate information* by consulting informal and professional sources using different methods of enquiry: interviewing; observation; and data-collection from records and significant others (Butler & Lees, 2000). Furthermore, it is almost always helpful to discuss the assessment with a peer or supervisor.

This requires the effective use of interpersonal skills in engaging the individual – for example, developing rapport, using active listening and responding skills, framing questions, and observational skills. One of the challenges reported by student mental health nurses concerns the difficulty in asking direct questions about 'risk', thus highlighting the importance of continued practice, with access to support and supervision. Hart (2014: 59–133) provides a useful practical guide to undertaking a risk assessment.

As information about 'risk behaviour' emerges, it is important to clarify and consider the following (adapted from Alberg et al., 1996; Butler & Lees, 2000), which uses the easy-to-remember acronym HI RISK:

- **H**istory of risk behaviour
- **I**ntent
- **R**ecency and frequency
- **I**deation
- **S**everity/impact
- **K**nowledge of the person and any known patterns of risk behaviour – for example, circumstances, **triggers**, planning and their understanding of their behaviour.

CASE STUDY 25.1

John

John is 42 and was recently released from prison to reside in approved premises (a probation hostel) after serving 5÷ years in custody. He is a MAPPA (Multi-Agency Public Protection Arrangements) Category 1 case, currently managed at Level 2. He attends the probation office weekly and is participating in a group programme in the community. He has been known to mental health services and had a previous admission to a psychiatric hospital in 1996. His probation officer has referred the case for consultation and for a formulation of his needs and risks.

Questions

- What would be your initial view about John's risk status?
- What further information would you wish to gather?
- Who would you consult/involve in gathering information?
- How would gathering information from different sources aid the risk assessment process?
- Recognising the importance of involving John, how would you best do this?

You may have considered:

- whether being managed under MAPPA would suggest that John represents a risk to himself/others
- what category 1 (*a registered sexual offender*) and level 2 (*active multi-agency management*) actually mean (see National Offender Management Service, 2012)

- whether his long prison sentence suggests his committal of a serious offence and/or previous offence patterns
- given that he is residing in approved premises following his release, whether he should be considered a high risk.

You may have considered gathering further information – for example:

- speaking with his probation officer to obtain further information
- clarifying the reasons for his conviction and whether he has any previous convictions
- clarifying the nature, focus and his progress thus far in attending the group programme
- accessing a previous psychiatric report from the Court, which would have been used to assist with sentencing
- reviewing any health care records relating to his previous admission in 1996.

For safety, it would be important to clarify information about his risk behaviour before arranging to meet him – for example, in this case, you would have found out that: John had committed serious sexual violence on women who were strangers to him, involving strangulation with the potential for fatality, thus heightening his level of risk; you would have learned that John was previously charged with an offence of assault against a female member of mental health staff, which involved grabbing her neck.

Step 2: Considering the presence of historical and recent risk and protective factors

Clarifying the presence and relative strength of risk and protective factors assists in the overall evaluation of a person's level of risk in the long term, and in the development of evidence-based risk assessment, better targeting intervention (Witt et al., 2013).

It is helpful to consider the presence of *risk factors* as a series of indicators and warning signs, which may be associated with an increase in the likelihood of risk behaviour.

Different types of *risk factors* have been described (for further information, see Morgan, 2000; Bouch & Marshall, 2005; DH, 2007a; Meaden & Hacker, 2011; Hawton et al., 2013; Witt et al., 2013):

- *Static* – fixed and historical factors that are helpful in predicting future risk behaviour, and are not changed by treatment or over time – for example, age, gender, previous suicide attempts; being based on statistical trends, on their own these factors say little about the person, their background or current intentions
- *Stable dynamic* – long-term and enduring factors that may change over time, although this will take time to happen, and are useful for focusing long-term intervention and care – for example, **depression**, isolation, lack of social supports
- *Acute dynamic* – **acute** factors that are present for an uncertain length of time tend to fluctuate in intensity and duration, and are useful for informing the focus of timely, short-term intervention and care – for example, distress, hopelessness, command **hallucinations**
- *Future* – factors that relate to anticipating potential risks and are useful in informing the focus of immediate and long-term treatment and care – for example, plans to harm self/others, active preparation to harm self/others.

There are a number of helpful sources of information on risk factors, for example: Hawton et al. (2013) provide a helpful systematic review of risk factors for suicide in depression; Witt et al. (2013) provide a helpful systematic review of risk factors for violence in **psychosis**; the National

Confidential Inquiry into Homicide and Suicide (NCIHS) programme summarises statistical trends and patterns (University of Manchester, 2015, 2016); and a summary is provided at http://study.sage pub.com/essentialmentalhealth.

Of course, the most important risk factor is regarded as history, and so particular attention should be given to: previous behaviour/incidents, especially within the past year; the threat of violence or harm; and reports by others of fears for the safety of themselves or others (Butler & Lees, 2000).

Just as it is important to ask direct questions to identify risks and precipitating factors, it is important to remember to ask about *protective (or positive) factors* and **coping** strategies in adopting a balanced approach to clinical risk assessment – for example, what has helped so far/previously? How has this helped? What might help now? This involves identifying personal strengths, skills and supports that will help to influence the reduction of symptoms, increase resilience and contribute to optimism and hope (MacNeil et al., 2012; Dudley & Kuyken, 2014). For examples, see Table 25.1.

Considering the use of structured assessment tools

The assessment of risk can be enhanced through the use of general and specific assessment tools, recommended as a core feature of local procedures (DH, 2007a). The use of structured tools will complement the more common use of a locally developed risk assessment proforma, for which there is more limited evidence and considerable variation in structure, content and quality (Gale et al., 2003; Hawley et al., 2006). The adjunct use of specific risk assessment tools may help to structure the risk assessment approach, though it is clearly important to select such tools carefully, considering their validity, reliability, appropriateness and practical utility, in addition to accessing any related training requirements and abiding by any copyright rules.

Some examples of general and specific tools available to and used by mental health nurses are shown in Table 25.2.

As a good example, Doyle & Logan (2012) recommend the use of START: a brief clinical guide for the dynamic assessment of risks, strengths and treatability. Applicable for use within a variety of mental health settings, use of a manualised guide involves considering 20 dynamic characteristics of the individual (e.g. mental state, social support, coping), each of which may be considered a risk factor or a strength, allowing the practitioner to form a balanced judgement about the role of the individual's characteristics in the context of their living circumstances at the current time. This guide, which

Table 25.1 Examples of positive factors

Hopefulness	Feeling supported/having a confidante[1,2]	Economic security[1,2]
Plans for the future[1]	Strong social and family supports/connectedness[1,2]	Resilient personality[1]
Good problem-solving skills[1,2]	Feeling responsible for dependents/related concerns[1,2]	Cognitive flexibility
Strong faith or spiritual beliefs[1]	Relationship & integration with community[1,2]	Positive coping beliefs[2] & a belief that suicide/violence is wrong
Positive engagement/attitude towards help, care and support[2]	Perception of self-control	Having valued and meaningful roles[2]
	Fear of suicide/pain	
Strong commitment to work/education	Fear of social disapproval	Lack of precipitating life events/losses

For further information, see: [1]Hart, 2014: 30; [2]Meaden & Hacker, 2011: 49, 82

Table 25.2 Some examples of assessment tools

General Assessment Tools	Specific Multiple Risk Tools	Specific Risk Tools
PANSS (Positive & Negative Symptoms Scale)	START (Short Term Assessment of Risk & Treatability)	HCR-20 (Historical & Clinical Risk - 20 items): *for violence & aggression*
KGV(M) (Krawiecka, Goldberg & Vaughan Scale (Modified))		
OQ45.2 (Outcome Questionnaire)	FACE (Functional Analysis of Care Environment)	Beck Hopelessness Scale
		Beck Suicide Intent Scale

involves the identification of signature risk signs, can inform structured professional judgement and link risk assessment, formulation and management, offering a valuable guideline for clinical practice.

As a further well-known example, Woods and Kettles (2009: 91–93) offer an outline of the HCR-20 violence risk assessment: intended for use by all disciplines, who have first completed training, this involves the use of a manualised guide to consider 10 historical, 5 clinical and 5 risk management items in evaluating risk over the medium to long term.

Step 3: Developing the risk formulation – a rationale for action

Forming a personalised explanation of the individual's difficulties, experiences and behaviour, and identifying relevant factors and patterns of circumstances indicative of heightened risk, formulation

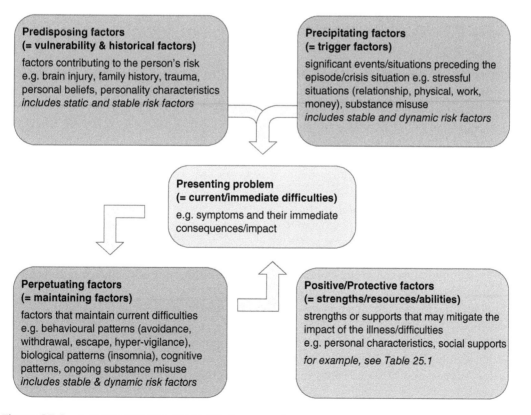

Figure 25.2 A representation of the 5Ps framework

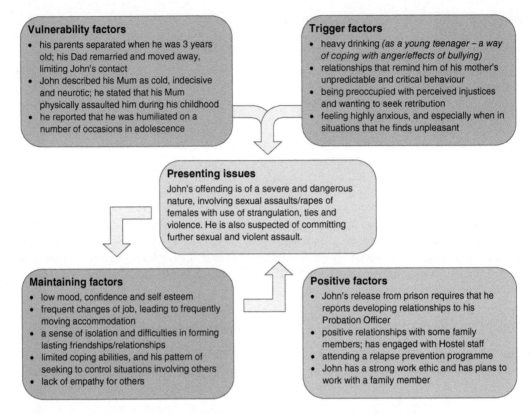

Vulnerability factors
- his parents separated when he was 3 years old; his Dad remarried and moved away, limiting John's contact
- John described his Mum as cold, indecisive and neurotic; he stated that his Mum physically assaulted him during his childhood
- he reported that he was humiliated on a number of occasions in adolescence

Trigger factors
- heavy drinking *(as a young teenager – a way of coping with anger/effects of bullying)*
- relationships that remind him of his mother's unpredictable and critical behaviour
- being preoccupied with perceived injustices and wanting to seek retribution
- feeling highly anxious, and especially when in situations that he finds unpleasant

Presenting issues
John's offending is of a severe and dangerous nature, involving sexual assaults/rapes of females with use of strangulation, ties and violence. He is also suspected of committing further sexual and violent assault.

Maintaining factors
- low mood, confidence and self esteem
- frequent changes of job, leading to frequently moving accommodation
- a sense of isolation and difficulties in forming lasting friendships/relationships
- limited coping abilities, and his pattern of seeking to control situations involving others
- lack of empathy for others

Positive factors
- John's release from prison requires that he reports developing relationships to his Probation Officer
- positive relationships with some family members; has engaged with Hostel staff
- attending a relapse prevention programme
- John has a strong work ethic and has plans to work with a family member

Figure 25.3 Excerpts from the 5Ps formulation for John (Case study 25.1)

acts as a bridge between assessment and intervention. This requires working alongside the individual, and involved others, to identify and understand trigger and mediating factors, their impact and ways of alleviating distress and promoting positive change (Crowe et al., 2008).

This process is aided by using a recognised framework, such as the well-known 5Ps framework (MacNeil et al., 2012; Dudley & Kuyken, 2014). A helpful way of recognising and summarising relevant vulnerability, trigger, maintaining and positive factors, use of the 5Ps framework will provide a focus on identifying and using specific interventions/approaches – an explanatory representation is shown in Figure 25.2.

To ensure that this is meaningful, the formulation will need to be highly personalised and specific to the individual's experience. It is also important to realise that it is an evolving and dynamic statement of understanding, which should be revised as new information emerges and as change occurs (Crowe et al., 2008: 800). However, whilst many experience a sense of hope and understanding, some may find formulation difficult and distressing, especially where not sufficiently considering strengths/protective factors (Chadwick et al., 2003).

In illustrating the use and potential **value** of the 5Ps framework, consider the excerpts from the formulation that was developed with John, in Figure 25.3.

Given the above, the collaborative development of a formulation offers the opportunity to consider the identified risks/concerns and risk and protective factors in the context of the individual's situation, supporting a better informed judgement about their situation/behaviour and leading to evidence-based decision making.

CASE STUDY 25.2

Jenny

Jenny is 35 and lives with her husband and 9-year-old son. Though employed as a welfare officer, she has felt unable to work for over three months. A new manager joined her team six months ago and has criticised her work performance on several occasions. Jenny has felt low since her mother died a year ago, to whom she was very close. She has been finding it difficult to motivate herself, is struggling to sleep properly, has begun to think that everything is pointless and is going wrong, and has again begun to think about taking an overdose. She believes that her husband has had enough of her 'moods' and irritability, and fears he may leave her.

Jenny has had two inpatient admissions in the last four years, each precipitated by her taking a significant overdose of prescribed antidepressant and anxiolytic medication, with alcohol. On each occasion, she had felt highly stressed for a prolonged period: moving accommodation; trying to complete a college course; trying to look after her young son; missing her husband whilst he was away working as a lorry driver.

Jenny has again been feeling very stressed, particularly when trying to respond to the demands of her 77-year-old, proud and independent father, who lives nearby - becoming increasingly infirm, he has had a couple of recent falls. Jenny has always had a difficult relationship with her father, who is often critical of her and always favoured her brother. Though close to her only brother, he lives over 200 miles away.

Questions

- What are some relevant examples of static and dynamic risk factors? Which would merit special attention as 'high' risk indicators?
- What are some relevant protective factors?
- Which structured assessment tools might be helpful in complementing the assessment process? What might be some limitations of these tools?
- Sketch out a formulation using the 5Ps framework. What ideas would this give you about the specific focus for treatment and care?

Providing a summary risk rating: a short discussion

Whilst highly recommended, whether or not a distinct risk formulation is completed, summary ratings of the individual's risk status are a common feature of current practice, often being expressed using categorical terms: low, medium or high risk. The value of such categorical risk ratings has been questioned (Littlechild & Hawley, 2010; Gale et al., 2011; Cahill & Rakow, 2012) as practitioners differ in their understanding of such terms, often hold differing views as to whether risk primarily concerns the likelihood and/or severity of outcomes, and differ in both their assessment of risk status and confidence in their judgement, which is affected by gender, professional background and experience (Gale et al., 2016). If making a summary risk judgement, it is clearly important that the terms to be used are clearly and explicitly defined, to support meaningful and consistent use. Furthermore, reliability in making risk judgements will be enhanced if adopting a teamwork approach (Cahill & Rakow, 2012) and including narrative descriptions that clarify the key issues.

So as an example, it would be reasonable to consider Jenny (Case study 25.2) as presenting a high risk if she was preoccupied with suicidal thoughts, with evidence of intent, planning and preparation, though it would still be important to provide a personalised description of the key issues.

Step 4: Negotiating an action plan using a positive risk-taking approach

Identifying risk carries a responsibility to act, and so risk management will involve considering the relative merits and drawbacks of different options, strategies and plans for minimising the identified risks, by reducing the likelihood or potency of identified risk factors and enhancing the influence of protective factors and strengths (see Wellman, 2006; Morgan, 2007; Doyle & Logan, 2012).

In promoting the individual's recovery, it is highly recommended to adopt a positive risk-taking approach that will involve working alongside the individual, carers and others to decide on the plan of action. Recognising that risk can rarely be eliminated, this requires being willing to take a decision that carries some risk, communicating the rationale, the potential risks and benefits, the plan for promoting safety, and the support available for implementing the agreed actions to all those who are involved (DH, 2007a: 8–10; see also Morgan, 2004; Morgan & Williamson, 2014). Coffey and colleagues (2017) have highlighted how overly risk averse services can put aside uncertainties over the effectiveness of risk assessment and management processes, maintaining a fiction of accuracy and reliability that justifies not taking positive risks.

In John's case (Case study 25.1), risk management actions took the form of (see National Offender Management Service, 2012):

- *restrictive interventions* – for example, residing in the probation hostel, having required contact with his probation officer, complying with regulations and reporting new relationships
- *rehabilitative interventions* – for example, enhancing his ability to manage risk situations through his attendance at a sexual offenders' treatment programme whilst in custody, and his participation within the relapse prevention course in the community
- *protective interventions* – for example, his active engagement in and commitment to change, maintaining stable relationships with those providing support, forming and acting on realistic plans for employment, and not drinking or taking illicit substances.

As a focus for risk management, it is helpful to consider the following (Morgan & Hemming, 1999; Doyle & Logan, 2012):

- the use of specific therapeutic strategies/interventions (psychopharmacological, psychological, psychosocial)
- the use of supervision, which may take the form of applying restrictions or conditions, or supporting the individual to secure and maintain meaningful social and work roles
- identifying, actively monitoring and responding to triggers and **early warning signs** in an efficient and timely way
- implementing emergency/safety plans, with the aim of maintaining the safety of the individual and previous/future victims
- post-incident support, which will involve supporting those affected, learning from the experience and implementing measures to minimise the chance of recurrence.

Step 5: Undertaking frequent and regular review

CASE STUDY:
HIGH RISK
INDICATORS

Risk is dynamic and ever changing: though historical (static) risk factors will remain relevant, stable and acute (dynamic) risk factors will change, and new risks may emerge as a consequence of what's going on for the person at the time.

The assessment and management of risk is therefore an ongoing process that requires regular review. This will involve gathering new information to further inform the (re)assessment, revisiting the formulation and reconsidering the relevance of the care and risk plan. In particular, this will be essential whenever there is any substantial change to the person's circumstances.

FORMING A MEANINGFUL ACCOUNT

It is important to remember that a risk assessment and management plan is only as good as the information that is verbally communicated and provided within written care records, which will be the product of the information gathered, and how well this is perceived, interpreted and written (DH, 2007a; Morgan, 2007). A clear, specific, detailed yet concise description of current and historical risk factors and relevant circumstances that are indicative of risk must be provided. A meaningful care and risk plan will provide specific details of actions to be taken in the event of heightened risk/relapse – what, how, when, where and by whom. Hart (2014) provides further practical guidance on writing a care and risk plan.

Drawing attention to this important yet challenging aspect of the process, in testing the feasibility and reliability of a qualitative evaluation tool, National Confidential Inquiry into Suicide and Homicide by People with Mentall **Illness** (NCISH) (2013) investigated the assessment and management of risk in mental health patients following a suicide/homicide. Conducted by two independent experienced psychiatrists, a retrospective case note audit was undertaken of 42 patients who had completed suicide and 39 patients who had committed homicide: the overall quality of risk assessment and management was considered unsatisfactory in 36% of suicide cases and 41% of homicide cases, most often being related to the quality of risk formulation and management plans. Whilst this pilot study highlighted issues with the quality of record keeping, it was noted that it may also raise questions about the quality of care provided.

If the information provided within the care record leaves you wondering, with many immediate unanswered questions, then further specific information is needed. In determining whether the risk assessment, formulation, and care and risk plan requires further detail, consider:

- Is it comprehensive?
- Is it specific?
- Is it concise, yet providing sufficient detail?
- Are you clear about: what, with/to whom, when, where and for what reasons?
- Is it meaningful and clear as a communication tool?

Student perspective

In a recent local survey of over 50 student mental health nurses, all of whom had undertaken at least four practice placements, a number of challenges and top tips on conducting risk assessment were offered, as summarised in Table 25.3.

As is evident in Table 25.3, whilst variable experiences were highlighted by student mental health nurses, a series of positive principles for practice were identified, which included the importance of undertaking a systematic, formulation-driven approach that actively engages the individual and their family. Indeed, the drawbacks of adopting a practitioner-led, unsystematic approach were highlighted: more subjective assessment; the loss of opportunities for promoting self-disclosure or observing non-verbal communication; and missed opportunities for promoting learning and positive change.

Table 25.3 The student mental health nurse perspective

Key Challenges for Risk Assessment	Top Tips for Meaningful Practice
engaging the individual and/or their family	strive to engage the individual/their family: listen and talk; be non-judgemental; adopt an informal and team approach
insufficient emphasis upon working with the person in managing risk	actively involve the individual, family/carers and professionals
accessing the information	be open and honest about potential risks and explore ways of reducing/managing such
the personal challenge of asking direct questions about risk	though important to recognise and consider historical risk factors, focus upon the present and adopt a structured professional judgement approach
the repetitive nature of some risk proformas/tools	before assessment, carefully select tools and use these in a meaningful way
the lack of specific detail and questionable accuracy of some information	undertake risk formulation as the basis for decision making, focusing upon the person's needs and promoting their recovery
how best to trust your instinct/intuition	plan for positive risk taking with the person, adopting a least restrictive approach in promoting safety and well-being, that follows clinical guidelines
the level of communication with the team	ensure written records have adequate detail, so that others find these useful
some view risk assessment, and the available proformas and tools, as having limited value	regularly review and update
time constraints	undertake training and access supervision

Contributions made by the 2013 cohort of mental health nursing students at UCLan

CRITICAL DEBATE 25.1

Reflect on practice in considering and debating the following questions/statements:

- Generic and specific risk assessment tools are of limited value in meaningfully assessing risk.
- A written assessment of risk is a helpful communication tool that offers both the practitioner and service user a clear focus for talking about how best to manage risk issues.
- Given that different practitioners will often arrive at different judgements/views about an individual's risk status, what are the value and limitations of risk assessment?
- How can we best enable the service user and support their growth and development when undertaking a risk assessment?

CHALLENGING CONCEPTS 25.1

As a key concept within contemporary mental health practice, *positive risk taking* (as a preferred and more meaningful term than 'positive risk management') refers to taking risks to achieve personal 'positive' outcomes (Morgan & Williamson, 2014), which is something that we all do (Morgan, 2004).

As a form of intervention, this involves working with the individual and involved others to think in detail about their situation, considering the merits and drawbacks of different options in making a decision that involves taking a degree of risk, where the identified benefits and positive outcomes clearly outweigh the risk(s) involved. A key feature of this approach, this will involve anticipating difficulties and identifying early warning signs and indicators of heightened risk, that are addressed through a specific contingency plan in minimising harmful outcomes and promoting safety.

Positive risk taking enables involvement in good decision making about risk, offering opportunities to utilise and build on strengths, and for learning and personal development.

CONCLUSION

We have presented a practical, formulation-driven approach to the assessment and management of risk, as a key aspect of the mental health nurse's role. As recommended within both national policy and guidance (DH, 2007a, 2007b, 2012) and through related research, achieving proficiency requires access to initial and follow-up training, supervision and support, good leadership and teamwork.

As outlined, a systematic and structured professional judgement approach that actively engages the individual and those others involved in their care is likely to enhance the meaning and quality of risk decision making.

Following this introduction to the process of working with risk in practice, we would recommend going further by considering the questions posed within Critical debate 25.1, and literature on a number of related initiatives – for example, the use of clinical risk management methods, such as zoning; and the use of anti-absconding and 'safe ward' best practice initiatives. These are just some examples of the many related initiatives to further explore.

CHAPTER SUMMARY

This chapter has covered:

- Ways of thinking about risk and risk assessment as a feature of everyday life experience
- A collaborative and personalised approach to the assessment and formulation of risk, which involves the identification of relevant risk and protective factors, the selection of relevant standardised assessment tools, and use of a structured framework for understanding - *the 5Ps*
- The negotiation of a meaningful care and risk plan that considers and promotes opportunities for positive risk taking and is subject to regular review
- A series of factors that facilitate or hinder meaningful risk assessment and risk management, influencing the quality of mental health practice.

BUILD YOUR BIBLIOGRAPHY

Books

- Hart, C. (2014) *A pocket guide to risk assessment and management in mental health*. London: Routledge. Highly recommended as a very useful and informative practical guide to undertaking a risk assessment and negotiating a risk management plan.
- Woods, P. & Kettles, A.M. (2009) *Risk assessment and management in mental health nursing*. Chichester: Wiley-Blackwell. A highly recommended text providing mental health nurses with a good foundation in issues relating to the assessment and management of risk in practice. A very useful introduction is given to the use of general and specific risk assessment tools in Chapter 4.

SAGE journal articles

FURTHER
READING:
JOURNAL
ARTICLES

Go to https://study.sagepub.com/essentialmentalhealth for further free online journal articles related to this chapter. If you are using the interactive ebook, simply click on the book icon in the margin to go straight to the resource.

- Bouch, J. & Marshall, J.J. (2005) Suicide risk: structured professional judgement. *Advances in Psychiatric Treatment, 11*, 84–91. A useful introduction is given on structured professional judgement and the consideration of different types of risk factors.
- Doyle, M. & Logan, C. (2012) Operationalising the assessment and management of violence risk in the short-term. *Behavioral Sciences & the Law, 30*, 406–419. An excellent discussion is given of the use of a specific multiple risk assessment tool, START, as part of a formulation-driven approach to risk management.

Weblinks

FURTHER
READING:
WEBLINKS

Go to https://study.sagepub.com/essentialmentalhealth for further weblinks related to this chapter. If you are using the interactive ebook, simply click on the book icon in the margin to go straight to the resource.

- For access to national mental health policy and related guidance: www.gov.uk/government/organisations/department-of-health
- For access to national mental health guidance, technology appraisals and related quality standards for practice: www.nice.org.uk
- For access to the National Confidential Inquiry into Suicide and Homicide reports and related resources: www.bbmh.manchester.ac.uk/cmhs/research/centreforsuicideprevention/nci
- For access to learning resources on inpatient suicide prevention: www.youtube.com/channel/UCn7iVOnLS-R5SB7u1I5FCLA

ACE YOUR ASSESSMENT

ONLINE
QUIZZES &
ACTIVITY
ANSWERS

Revise what you have learned by visiting https://study.sagepub.com/essentialmentalhealth. If you are using the interactive ebook, simply click on the tick icon to go straight to the resource.

- Test yourself with multiple-choice and short-answer questions and flashcards.

REFERENCES

Alberg, C., Hatfield, B. & Huxley, P. (eds) (1996) *Learning materials on mental health: Risk assessment.* Manchester: University of Manchester/Department of Health.

Bouch, J. & Marshall, J.J. (2005) Suicide risk: structured professional judgement. *Advances in Psychiatric Treatment, 11,* 84–91.

Butler, J. & Lees, G. (2000) Assessing and managing risk in people with severe mental illness. In L. Cotterill & W. Barr (eds) *Targeting in mental health services: A multi-disciplinary challenge.* Aldershot: Ashgate Publishing. pp. 287–315.

Cahill, S. & Rakow, T. (2012) Assessing risk and prioritizing referral for self-harm: when and why is my judgment different from yours? *Clinical Psychology & Psychotherapy, 19,* 399–410.

Chadwick, P., Williams, C. & Mackenzie, J. (2003) Impact of case formulation in cognitive behaviour therapy for psychosis. *Behaviour Research & Therapy, 41,* 671–680.

Coffey, M., Cohen, R., Faulkner, A., et al. (2017) Ordinary risks and accepted fictions: how contrasting and competing priorities work in risk assessment and mental health care planning. *Health Expectations, 20*(3), 471–483.

Crowe, M., Carlyle, D. & Farmar, R. (2008) Clinical formulation for mental health nursing practice. *Journal of Psychiatric & Mental Health Nursing, 15,* 800–807.

Department of Health (2007a) *Best practice in managing risk: Principles and guidance for best practice in the assessment and managing of risk to self and others in mental health services.* London: DH.

Department of Health (2007b) *Independence, choice and risk: A guide to best practice in supported decision-making.* London: DH.

Department of Health (2008) *Refocusing the care programme approach: Policy and positive practice guidance.* London: DH.

Department of Health (2012) *Preventing suicide in England: A cross-government outcomes strategy to save lives.* London: DH.

Doyle, M. & Logan, C. (2012) Operationalising the assessment and management of violence risk in the short-term. *Behavioral Sciences & the Law, 30,* 406–419.

Dudley, R. & Kuyken, W. (2014) Case formulation in cognitive behaviour therapy: a principle-driven approach. In L. Johnstone & R. Dallos (eds) *Formulation in psychology and psychotherapy: Making sense of people's problems,* 2nd edition. London: Routledge. pp. 18–44.

Duffy, D. (2008) Therapeutic risk and care planning in mental health. In A. Hall, M. Wren & S. Kirby (eds) *Care planning in mental health: Promoting recovery.* Oxford: Blackwell. pp. 37–47.

Gale, T.M., Hawley, C.J., Butler, J., et al. (2016) Perception of suicide risk in mental health professionals. *PLoS ONE, 11*(2): e0149791.

Gale, T.M., Hawley, C.J. & Sivakumaran, T. (2003) Do mental health professionals really understand probability? Implications for risk assessment and evidence-based practice. *Journal of Mental Health, 12*(4), 417–30.

Gale, T.M., Hawley, C. & Sivakumaran, T. (2011) Classification of risk in psychiatry. *Psychiatria Danubina, 23*(Suppl. 1), 198–202.

Hart, C. (2014) *A pocket guide to risk assessment & management in mental health.* London: Routledge.

Hawley, C.J., Littlechild, B., Sivakumaran, T., et al. (2006) Structure and content of risk assessment proformas in mental health care. *Journal of Mental Health, 15*(4), 437–448.

Hawton, K., Casanas, I., Comabella, C., et al. (2013) Risk factors for suicide in individuals with depression: a systematic review. *Journal of Affective Disorders, 147,* 17–28.

Langan, J. & Lindow, V. (2004) *Living with risk: Mental health service user involvement in risk assessment and management*. York: Joseph Rowntree Foundation.

Littlechild, B. & Hawley, C. (2010) Risk assessments for mental health service users: ethical, valid and reliable? *Journal of Social Work, 10*(2), 211–229.

MacNeil, C.A., Hasty, M.K., Conus, P., et al. (2012) Is diagnosis enough to guide interventions in mental health? Using case formulation in clinical practice. *BMC Medicine, 10*, 111.

Meaden, A. & Hacker, D. (2011) *Problematic and risk behaviours in psychosis: A shared formulation approach*. Hove, East Sussex: Routledge.

Morgan, S. (2000) *Clinical risk management: A clinical tool and practitioner's manual*. London: Sainsbury Centre for Mental Health.

Morgan, S. (2004) *Positive risk taking: an idea whose time has come*. Open Mind health care risk report. Available at: http://practicebasedevidence.squarespace.com/blog/2010/9/21/positive-risk-taking-an-idea-whose-time-has-come.html (accessed 30.08.17).

Morgan, S. (2007) *Working with risk: Practitioner's manual*. Brighton: Pavilion Publishing.

Morgan, S. & Hemming, M. (1999) Balancing care and control: risk management and compulsory treatment. *Mental Health Care, 3*(1), 19–21.

Morgan, S. & Williamson, T. (2014) *Viewpoint: How can positive risk taking help build dementia-friendly communities?* Mental Health Foundation/Joseph Rowntree Foundation. Available at: www.jrf.org.uk/report/how-can-positive-risk-taking-help-build-dementia-friendly-communities (accessed 11.08.17).

National Offender Management Service (2012) *MAPPA Guidance 2012, Version 4*. Available at: www.gov.uk/government/uploads/system/uploads/attachment_data/file/406117/MAPPA_guidance_2012_part1_v4_Feb_2015.pdf (accessed 11.08.17).

NCISH (2013) *Quality of risk assessment prior to suicide and homicide: A pilot study*. Manchester: NCISH.

University of Manchester (2015) *The national confidential inquiry into suicide and homicide by people with mental illness: Annual report*. Manchester: Centre for Mental Health & Safety, University of Manchester.

University of Manchester (2016) *Suicide by children and young people in England: The national confidential inquiry into suicide and homicide by people with mental illness*. Manchester: University of Manchester.

Wellman, N. (2006) Assessing risk. In C. Gamble & G. Brennan (eds) *Working with serious mental illness: A manual for clinical practice*, 2nd edition. London: Elsevier. pp. 145–164.

Witt, K., van Dorn, R. & Fazel, S. (2013) Risk factors for violence in psychosis: systematic review and meta-regression analysis of 110 studies. *PLoS ONE, 8*(2): e55942.

Woods, P. & Kettles, A.M. (2009) *Risk assessment and management in mental health nursing*. Chichester: Wiley-Blackwell.

MINIMISING VIOLENCE AND RELATED HARMS

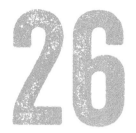

JOY A. DUXBURY AND AMY SCHOLES

THIS CHAPTER COVERS

- Differentiating between the terms aggression and violence
- Identifying predisposing factors to the development and expression of aggression
- Exploring ways of reducing the potential for aggression in health care settings
- Navigating personal and organisational approaches to addressing aggression
- Outlining ways of minimising the use of restrictive interventions.

> "
>
> The thorny issue of aggression management has been a concern for me for many years. In particular, it sits very uncomfortably with me as to how we fail to balance the tension of using coercive practices to manage difficult situations with our nursing roles, recovery orientated focus of care and the need to be therapeutic. This chapter aims to encourage practitioners to be more prevention focused and to consider their roles in minimising conflict and the use of restrictive practices which can be harmful to staff and service users alike. It gives us a lot to think about, particularly the need to change our thinking with regards to trauma informed care. I was fortunate enough to be involved in a training programme called REsTRAIN YOURSELF (RY) (based on the Six Core Strategies) in the North West of England. This has inspired me to make changes in practice and to use strategies that focus on making meaningful changes to the clinical environment, interpersonal, therapeutic relationships and minimising trauma to those we care for using a number of person centred tools such as personal safety plans.
>
> **Tracey, nurse**
>
> "

Visit **https://study.sagepub.com/essentialmentalhealth** to access a wealth of online resources for this chapter – watch out for the margin icons throughout the chapter. If you are using the interactive ebook, simply click on the margin icon to go straight to the resource.

From the same project mentioned above, a number of service users gave their views on their experiences of being 'managed' using restrictive practices such as restraint:

'To me, for me it's like they only use it to show their power. That's what it feels like to me because every time I've self-harmed or anything, it's always been straight to that, never speaking to and showing you things, it's just straight to the restraints. And it just makes me feel like, to me, it's just them showing the power over you.'

'Maybe they've just got out of the wrong side of bed and, you know, or maybe something's playing on their minds outside of the, all this. Maybe something's been going on before they came, stress and worries in the home, like, you know, a cheating wife or a, you know, worrying about the kids, and they just want to make a phone call and they can't.'

'These nurses just appeared in the room and lifted me off the chair physically, pinned me to the floor [...] They had me faced down on the floor, pulled my trousers down and injected me. And that was done in the lady's lounge. And when I got back to my room I just really started to cry because I felt, such a shock and I did feel violated.'

Service users

INTRODUCTION

This chapter explores the prevention and management of **aggression** using multi-model indicators and approaches. With a view to adopting a least restrictive approach, an understanding of the individual who becomes aggressive is explored. Interventions that focus on prevention from an individual and organisational perspective, including **therapeutic relationships**, partnership working, and management, are identified. The importance of employing strategies that are underpinned by 'trauma-informed care' is highlighted with a view to minimising the need for reactive and **restrictive practices**. These can be harmful to both **service users** and staff alike.

In order to highlight the importance of and distinction between the prevention and management of aggression, it is first important to define some key terms:

The terms violence and aggression are often used interchangeably. They are used to describe a range of behaviours or actions that can result in harm, hurt or injury to another person, regardless of whether the violence or aggression is physically or verbally expressed, physical harm is sustained or the intention is clear. (NICE, 2015: 6)

Restrictive practices are:

deliberate acts on the part of other person(s) that restrict an individual's movement, liberty, and/or freedom to act independently in order to:

Take immediate control of a dangerous situation where there is a real possibility of harm to the person or others if no action is undertaken and

End or reduce significantly the danger to the person or others and,

Contain or limit the person's freedom for no longer than is necessary. (DH, 2014: 14)

Violence and aggression are universal phenomena and something that most individuals will encounter to varying degrees at some point. Aggression towards health care professionals is well documented in the literature (Roche et al., 2010). Expressions of aggression can range from verbal abuse through to assault, and whilst aggression cannot be avoided altogether, its incidence can and should be reduced significantly using prevention and proactive strategies.

EXPLANATORY MODELS OF VIOLENCE IN HEALTH CARE SETTINGS

The rise of patient aggression in health and social care settings continues to attract attention both professionally and politically (DH, 2014), so much so that some have coined the term clinical aggression which specifically refers to aggressive behaviour arising out of or during a clinical context (Gerdtz et al., 2013). A number of theories have been developed that endeavour to explain the causes of this, many of which are socially driven. Aspects of that which we refer to as a 'therapeutic triad' include internal, external and contextual factors that can be significantly influential and interlinked. Nijman et al. (1999) first brought our attention to the multifaceted nature of aggression, and this work was later developed by Duxbury (2002).

With regards to internal factors, a number of studies have endeavoured to make an association between mental **illness** and violence (Steinert et al., 2000). This was highlighted some time ago in a report from the Royal College of Psychiatrists (1998) suggesting a number of variables that can be attributed to violence, mental illness being an argued predictor.

The external stance, in contrast, asserts that it is the **environment** that leads to aggression and violence. Factors such as a lack of privacy and space, location, treatment regimes, and rules and rituals, including limit setting, have been identified as contributory (Duxbury & Whittington, 2005). The latter points are more about restrictive regimes as opposed to the physical environment. There is significant evidence suggesting that changes to the physical and psychosocial environment can be beneficial, as indicated in the recent DH guidance (2014).

Using a more social lens, a number of studies have supported the view that non-therapeutic interpersonal styles can **affect** staff and patient relationships and lead to aggression. Conflict with staff is commonly reported to be contributory (Duxbury & Whittington, 2005) and Kamchuchat et al. (2008), for example, suggest that miscommunication is often an underlying cause associated with physical assault. Holmes et al. (2012) questions assumptions that violence is always enacted by patients. Violence can be seen to be intimately bound up with the mental health care system, where bio-technologies squeeze out relational care (Choiniere et al. 2014), and service users are on the receiving end of both subtle and profound violent acts themselves. Indeed, there is a growing view that this violence reflects a dominance of psychiatric knowledge within services, constituting an epistemic injustice (Fricker 2007), thus making the case for seeking systemic approaches to minimise violence in how violence is bred in organisational practices

These explanatory models combined have been identified by a number of authors as helpful in explaining expressions of frustration and dissatisfaction by service users and in challenging a reliance on coercive practices (Duxbury & Whittington, 2005; Huckshorn, 2004). Whilst there is some evidence that training and experience in the management of aggression can help reduce negative outcomes, this remains limited, and the more recent focus has shifted somewhat significantly on preventing aggression by improving the therapeutic environment, both personal and organisational (LeBel, 2011).

Amidst the various theories on the causation of aggression and violence is the need to understand the views of participants, namely patients and health care staff. The experiences and perceptions of both can contribute to the development of aggression, its management and also its consequences.

AVOIDING CONFLICT

When endeavouring to prevent the development of aggression and violence in health care settings and to avoid conflict in the first instance, a solid foundation on which to provide care and foster therapeutic environments and relationships is needed. This requires both primary and secondary prevention strategies, including pre-escalation and de-escalation respectively.

PRIMARY PREVENTION

Cowin et al. (2003) argue that, when endeavouring to prevent the development of conflict, staff must be prepared to recognise environments and relationships that prevent the promotion of therapeutic approaches. This they refer to as pre-escalation. Distasio (1994) and later Paterson et al. (1997) have both suggested a number of strategies that may assist when looking to pre-escalate a situation, some of which include:

approaching the patient with caution

avoiding provocation where possible

using clear, calm and respectful language

using open-ended sentences

avoiding challenges and promises that can't be kept

remaining firm but compassionate.

This has implications for communication styles, understanding the needs of the individual, using good assessment and advance planning tools, and promoting cultures based on person-centredness, as opposed to restriction. These key elements are also reflected more recently in the DH (2014) guidelines on 'Positive and Proactive' and in Bowers' (2014) work on 'Safewards', described in more detail later in the chapter.

The prevention and management of aggression and violence require a multifaceted approach including behavioural and environmental strategies (DH, 2014; NICE, 2015). Bowers et al. (2004) suggest that a focus on containment rather than a therapeutic approach is part of the problem and contributes to the development of aggression and violence in clinical settings. One way of minimising a reliance on **coercion** is the use of **advance directives**.

TARGETED CARE PLANNING FOR THE PREVENTION AND MANAGEMENT OF AGGRESSION: ADVANCE DIRECTIVES (AD)

One approach to promote the principles of person-centred planned care is the advance directive (AD). An advance directive is a document not dissimilar to a targeted **care plan**, used significantly to register advance instructions about future treatment (of aggressive behaviour) in the event of an incapacitating psychiatric crisis. It is intended to support patients' self-determination at a time when they are vulnerable to loss of autonomy, to help them ensure their preferences are known and to minimise unwanted treatments (Papageorgiou, 2002).

ADs encourage respectful dialogue between practitioners and patients to explore their past experiences and preferences, with a view to anticipating conflict and planning for the future. However, some patients find them difficult to understand. For clinicians, barriers are reported, including lack of access to relevant documents, lack of training, lack of communication and lack of time (Amering et al., 2005). Consequently, there is scepticism about their benefit and use, which has yet to be tested (DH, 2014).

There is no doubt that strategies for the prevention and management of disturbed behaviour should be discussed with service users on admission to mental health inpatient services, or as soon as possible to promote positive communication between staff and patients (DH, 2014; Duxbury & Wright, 2011). Whilst research in this area is limited to date, Maitre et al. (2013) reported that patients show a strong interest in creating directives of this sort, have a high level of satisfaction when using them, feel more in control over their mental health care and more respected and valued. Swanson et al. (2013) have also identified their **value** when coupled with dedicated facilitation sessions to help patients complete and use them. System-level policies, however, are required to embed them into practice.

Despite everybody's best efforts, nonetheless, some situations may present where prevention has failed and de-escalation is required as a secondary preventative approach.

SECONDARY PREVENTION

De-escalation, a key secondary intervention in this field, can be beneficial when organisational and personal issues have been addressed or planned for, but have failed to prevent the escalation of aggression.

De-escalation has been defined as: 'The gradual resolution of a potentially violent and/or aggressive situation through the use of verbal and physical expressions of empathy, alliance and non-confrontational limit setting that is based on respect' (Cowin et al., 2003: 65). It is a complex intervention with interacting components operating at individual, team and organisation level. Therefore, de-escalation is not a discrete event, but part of a process of behaviours, actions and staff management strategies which typically characterise life on inpatient wards. Such processes, or sequences, may be short and involve sudden crises, necessitating swift and severe containment interventions (Lavelle et al., 2016).

In order to avoid further confrontation, it is suggested that de-escalation strategies should include basic therapeutic communication skills, most notably active listening, cooperation, compassion, negotiating workable options, the use of open-ended questions, and distraction (Cowin et al., 2003; Price & Baker, 2012).

I have argued for some time now that de-escalation is a reactive approach and that prevention is much more useful than waiting for an incident to occur. In order to explore the value of secondary prevention in more detail, Case study 26.1 is a good example of the use of person-centred strategies and de-escalation.

CASE STUDY 26.1

Ben: An example of the positive management of an aggressive episode

At approximately 9.00am, Ben was rapidly pacing the unit, shouting outside the staff office and making various aggressive demands and accusations towards staff. At this point, the majority of the staff team came out of the staff office and positioned themselves spaciously around communal areas on the ward.

(Continued)

One health care assistant appeared to take the lead in responding to the demands and complaints being voiced by Ben. This staff member's tone was calm and unhesitant. Ben demanded to see the doctor in order to discuss what he believed to be a mismanagement of his medication. The health care assistant was efficient in contacting the doctor, and regularly revisited Ben with updates of every step of progress she was making.

Approximately an hour later, and still very agitated, a meeting was held in a small room on the ward with the health care assistant, doctor and Ben. Ben explained that on previous days his medication was late, due to scheduling difficulties that did not fit in with set medication rounds. Sam had previously complained about this, and staff had produced a document detailing when he was entitled to PRN ('as needed', pro re nata) medication. Ben had asked for PRN early this morning and was repeatedly told by staff, 'I'll be there in 10 minutes'.

Question

- What do you think precipitated this event?

CRITICAL THINKING STOP POINT 26.1

Based on what you have read and considered so far about causation and possible trigger points, can we be sure that primary and secondary prevention, as opposed to tertiary prevention, is prioritised? It may be that services and organisations are risk averse and therefore find it difficult to take therapeutic risks. Indeed, some caring environments and social spaces might have become toxic, precipitating rather than availing conflict. This may be down to a mixture of tensions including limited resources, poor staffing and interpersonal conflicts.

COERCIVE PRACTICES

Coercive practices have been defined as a cluster of interventions used widely around the world to control behaviour which is perceived by staff as indicating that violence by a patient is either already happening or is imminent (Whittington et al., 2006: 146). More recently, the term restrictive interventions/practice has emerged denoting: 'The implementation of a practice or practices that restrict an individual's movement, liberty and/or freedom to act independently' (DH, 2014: 14).

The use of restrictive practices in care settings continues to be controversial. Seclusion and restraint are both restrictive approaches designed as emergency measures to contain and deal with situations on a short-term basis (Mattson & Sachs, 1978; Putkonen et al., 2013; Wale et al., 2011). However, despite the importance of choosing to use a restrictive practice as a last resort only, it continues to be used. Deveau & McDonnell (2009: 175) argue that reliance on the 'last resort' principle has the major drawback that it is an easily voiced rhetorical device and very difficult to observe or challenge.

There is undoubtedly growing evidence indicating that the use of restraint is counter-therapeutic, coercive, punishing, traumatic and unnecessary (Curran, 2007; Soininen et al., 2013). Restraint is also considered to be over-used as a means to manage violence and aggression (Cutcliffe & Santos, 2012).

As mental health nurses are generally those who implement restraint in mental health settings, further research to explore how 'last resort' is enacted within their practice is therefore warranted.

Consider Case study 26.2 and reflect on the key moments when a different course of action might have been more helpful.

CASE STUDY 26.2

Pete: Using overly reactive approaches – what can we learn?

At approx. 2.45pm, a member of staff commented that the ward atmosphere was unsettled and attributed this to the behaviour of one service user (Pete) who was described as a 'ticking time-bomb'. This staff member then finished their shift and left for the day.

At approximately 3.30pm, Pete began pacing the ward and hammering on the ward door, shouting aggressively 'get me out of here, let me out!' This initiated a reactive response from the nurse in charge (NIC) who began frantically calling neighbouring psychiatric intensive care units (PICU) for available beds, attempting to secure an admission for this individual. During this time, different staff members would repeatedly enter the staff office, using it as an area of respite from the threatening atmosphere of the ward.

Whilst the NIC was organising a PICU admission, the intensity of the threats and frequency of shouting increased, exacerbated by other patients reacting to the aggressive behaviour.

With an atmosphere of high expressed emotion and chaos unfolding on the ward, this provoked a demand from the NIC, that the consultant of the ward stand in front of the office door to prevent Pete from entering the office. The NIC, evidently very uncomfortable and afraid of the events unfolding, asked another nurse to ring the police immediately 'before someone gets hurt'. This staff member hesitated, clearly attempting to reflect on whether calling for external force would be necessary. However, the NIC raised her voice and demanded that the call be made. At this point, a lack of communication with the patient who had precipitated this incident was significant, and no options were offered as to what could help ease his current distress.

Eventually, the police arrived and at this point the individual was placed in prone restraint for a short period of time and medication was administered. After returning to the office, the five staff members involved in the incident conducted a 'debrief', which was less than 10 minutes in duration. The primary focus being: 'how did people think it went?' and 'is everyone alright?' There was no discussion as to how the situation escalated to this point or what could be learnt from the incident. There was no formal debrief of patients either.

Question

- How could this situation have been avoided?

REDUCTION MODELS

Reduction models have developed over recent years to reduce the use of restrictive practices. These effectively focus on well-informed systems of therapeutic relationships and cultures, governance, strong leadership, the use of prevention strategies, a focus on users' rights and ensuring that reflective models support learning from incidents where restrictive interventions are used.

There are some small pockets of evidence of implementation in sectors of the UK, although their use remains far from universal. The strongest evidence base to date is the international literature (Huckshorn, 2004).

Approaches based on sophisticated systems to make significant multi-faceted changes across organisations seem to provide the most impressive outcomes. For example, studies using a complex intervention approach with a focus on behavioural leadership, service user-centered care and **culture** shift have reported significantly reduced frequency and duration of restraint and seclusion (McVilly, 2008; Putkonen et al., 2013).

Recent studies have shown that it is possible to reduce the rate of restrictive interventions in organisations where there is an overarching strategy to address their minimisation (McVilly, 2008). Some studies have also linked the importance of clear leadership with targeting a reduction in the use of restrictive interventions (Huckshorn, 2004). Plans should include a mission statement that clearly articulates the organisation's philosophy about seclusion and restraint reduction, for example, and describe the roles and responsibilities of all staff in working towards this.

THE SIX CORE STRATEGIES: THE US APPROACH

The 'six core strategies' (6Cs) were developed in the USA by the National Technical Assistance Center of the National Association of State Mental Health Program Directors (Huckshorn, 2004). They provide an organisational model through which to make significant change in reducing the use of restrictive practices, particularly seclusion and restraint. The strategies focus on six fundamental elements:

- leadership towards organisational change
- the use of data to inform practice
- workforce development
- the use of restraint and seclusion reduction tools
- service users' role in the organisation
- debriefing techniques.

Growing evidence suggesting the value and positive impact of this approach in terms of achieving sustained reductions in seclusion and/or restraint episodes, across a range of service types, has been reported (McVilly, 2008; Putkonen et al., 2013).

UK INITIATIVES

CASE STUDY:
LILY

As part of a rise in work in the UK looking at this area, we have recently completed a project called REsTRAIN YOURSELF (RY). This is an adaptation of the 6CS in a UK setting. Fourteen mental health wards, in the north-west region of England, were included comprising seven implementation wards and seven comparison wards (control) (LeBel et al., 2014).

The primary aim of the project was to reduce the incidence of physical restraint by 40%. This involved four stages: training the trainers; training the staff in participating teams; improving **collaboration** to support the adoption of RY; and evaluation. As part of this project, an overarching multi-method evaluative design was adopted. The principles employed have been tested and positively reported on in non-UK settings (LeBel, 2011; LeBel & Goldstein, 2005; McVilly, 2008). A reduction of 22% in restraint was found across the intervention wards overall.

Focusing on reducing conflict and containment in mental health settings, Bowers has recently developed and launched the Safewards model (Bowers, 2014). Arising from an RCT, selected interventions include using clear mutual expectations, soft words, talk-down approaches, positive words, bad news mitigation, ways to know each other, mutual help meetings, calm-down methods, reassurance, and discharge messages. A control intervention was introduced on 15 wards, and the 10 experimental interventions on the others. The Safewards interventions produced a 15% decrease in the rate of conflict and a 24% decrease in the rate of containment (Bowers, 2014).

Aligned to the need to explore alternatives to and minimise restrictive practices, a plethora of policy activity has emerged in the UK over the last 10 years, dating back from a number of high-profile safety incidents in 2003/4 and resulting in the development of guidelines in this area by the National Institute for Health and Care Excellence (NICE) (2015). Whilst guidance and strategies were instigated prior to this period, the real impetus began back then. This has continued to increase and 2011 onwards has been a particularly significant period, which has included a report of restraint-related deaths in the UK (Aiken et al., 2012; Duxbury et al., 2011), the Francis Report on care deficits (Francis, 2013), Winterbourne (DH, 2012), the 2012 Mind report on crisis in care, which focused on the negative impact of restraint, and, most recently, a report by Agenda (2017) looking at the use of restraint on women. Both the Mind and Agenda reports have highlighted the reported overuse of restraint in a number of trusts across England, with the resultant call for a ban of prone restraint in some circles, however contentious this may be.

WHAT IS THE EVIDENCE FOR THE MINIMISATION OF COERCIVE AND RESTRICTIVE PRACTICES?

There is a plethora of research on the causation of aggression, which I have touched on, however research on the minimisation of approaches to reduce the use of coercive and/or restrictive practices is in its relative infancy.

Recent guidance from NICE has highlighted that restrictive physical interventions (RPIs) such as restraint should be avoided, if at all possible, given the identified risks. But where they are used, staff should communicate with service users in order to attempt to de-escalate the situation and cease the use of an RPI as soon as possible.

Individual risk factors, which suggest a service user is more likely to suffer physical and/or emotional trauma, as a result of restrictive practices must be recognised and taken account of. This might include recording a history of traumatic sexual abuse and related emotional trauma for some patients, or the risk of being held in a restraint position, for patients who are obese or suffering from contraindicated pre-existing conditions (Aiken et al., 2012). Planned interventions should therefore seek to minimise such risks, particularly as patients can associate seclusion with punishment, increased **anxiety** and fears associated with confinement (Mattson & Sachs, 1978; Putkonen et al., 2013).

At the extreme, a number of adverse effects have been reported as a result of the use of physical restraint, ranging from service user and staff discomfort to injuries resulting in death. In 2011, in a *Review of the Medical Theories and Research Relating to Restraint Related Deaths in the UK* (Aiken et al., 2012), an analysis of what is known about the hazardous nature of the use of RPIs, including the use of 'prone restraint', was examined. Duxbury et al. (2011) reported a growing evidence base that suggests that there are individuals who may be more at risk of being restrained than others, whether because of biophysiological, interpersonal, situational or attitudinal factors. These groups are those with serious mental illness or learning disabilities, those from black and minority ethnic communities, those with a high body mass index; men aged 30–40 years; and young people (under the age of 20). It is essential that such evidence be used to inform planning around how best to work with people who present behavioural challenges at both an organisational and an individual level.

In the recent Department of Health (2014) guidance, *Positive and Proactive Care*, based on current literature, six key principles have been identified as fundamental to fostering a safe and positive caring environment for staff and patients: basic human rights and needs such as participation; compassion; dignity; kindness; safety; and freedom of choice.

Empirical evidence from the UK and North America clearly demonstrates that rate variation in restraint and seclusion is largely influenced by environmental, interpersonal or contextual factors such as unclear guidelines, crowded and restrictive environments, staffing problems, poor information sharing and patient acuity (NICE, 2015; Nijman et al., 1999). Unsurprisingly, staff characteristics such as authoritative and confrontational styles have also been linked to patient aggression and violence (Bonner et al., 2002; Duxbury & Whittington, 2005; Tunde-Ayinmode & Little, 2004; Wynaden et al., 2002), as highlighted earlier. It is not surprising therefore that a variation in the use of coercion can occur in different settings and can indeed be avoidable if contributory factors are recognised and addressed (Livingstone, 2007; Stewart et al., 2009).

CRITICAL THINKING STOP POINT 26.2

Consider the implications of restrictive interventions in your practice area. If you do a scan of your environment, you might rebadge some of your practices and those of the organisation as restrictive. If this is the case, consider any potential negative implications of this and what changes can be proposed.

CRITICAL DEBATE 26.1

Contrasting perspectives: staff and patient experiences of aggression

Given the nature of aggression in health care settings, it is not surprising that there are different views on its causation between service users and practitioners.

Patients, for example, commonly express concerns about the aggressive or controlling behaviours of staff. In a study by Duxbury and Whittington (2005), over 25% of patients surveyed felt that staff had significantly contributed to their own aggressive outbursts. Furthermore, coercive practices can have significant negative connotations and outcomes and be perceived by patients as hostile and non-therapeutic actions (Meehan et al., 2006). As a result, patients can be severely traumatised by the use of practices such as seclusion and/or restraint and this can affect both their needs and their road to recovery. This will be discussed in more detail later when examining trauma-informed care. Nurses, in contrast, can perceive and then respond to aggression in a number of different ways. First, given the powerful nature of anger as an emotion, people exposed to anger may feel fearful and intimidated. Nurses, as a result, may avoid patients if they are fearful of them (Smith & Hart, 1994) or they may 'go in strong', as referred to by Whittington and Wykes (1994). Clearly, this is neither helpful nor therapeutic for nurse or patient. A number of studies have suggested that staff behaviour can contribute to the development of patient aggression and, indeed, some staff have expressed concerns about the use and negative impact of restrictive practices. For example, when surveyed, practitioners reported feeling unrest with the techniques taught in relation to restraint, particularly when trying to balance safety with service users' rights and less invasive procedures (Duxbury & Whittington, 2005). Staff have also raised concerns about the impact of coercive practices that can result in personal physical and psychological strain, a lack of confidence, prolonged sickness and dissonance (LeBel, 2011).

Question

Think about the different views that individuals hold about the reasons for conflict and aggression. Reflect on your own views and how they might be different from other members of your team and the service users you care for. What are the implications of different views on the prevention and management of aggression?

CHALLENGING CONCEPTS 26.1

The term restrictive intervention is a relatively new concept that has taken shape since the release of the DH Guidance in 2014, *Positive and Proactive Care*. Prior to this, broader terms such as coercion and individual practices including seclusion, 'control and restraint' and rapid tranquillisation have been commonly used to refer to nursing approaches of this nature. Restrictive interventions now more broadly refer to any intervention that restricts the rights of a service user in health and/or social care settings, and as such can include restrictive environments and organisational practices such as the blanket introduction of set rules and regimes.

CONCLUSION

Caring for individuals who may become upset and violent can be challenging, particularly given the instability of **acute** inpatient settings today. Consequently, staff and patients can experience a sense of powerlessness and frustration. Nurses and their organisations need special personal attributes, skills, education and training to prevent and to intervene when difficult situations arise, safely, therapeutically and in a least restrictive manner. Organisations, however, need to ensure that clear directives are in place to minimise the use of restrictive practices. This includes an understanding of the complex institutional contributory factors that can lead to conflict in the first place (Duxbury & Whittington, 2005).

Effective post-incident debriefing of service users may help, as might supporting service users to record and utilise advance decisions about how staff should use RPIs if necessary. Reduction plans should consider the least restrictive options (NICE, 2015).

Debriefing and post-incident reviews of all incidents of aggression and violence for staff as well as patients is an important component of aggression management. Individuals need opportunities to work through their own feelings and to evaluate the efficacy of nursing interventions, to reduce burnout and enhance personal and professional growth.

This chapter has explored personal, professional and organisational strategies for critically thinking about and preventing aggression. Ongoing reflection and critique of personal and team practices are significant elements in maintaining therapeutic environments for patients under duress.

There is increasing evidence today that restrictive practices cause serious physical and psychological trauma (Aiken et al., 2012). Such outcomes, when they occur, can be among the most controversial because they have occurred as a result of the actions of those charged with the care of vulnerable individuals (Paterson et al., 2003)

Coercion and related restrictive practices should only ever be employed as a last resort. In order to achieve this, however, major environmental, cultural and organisational changes underpinned by a philosophy of trauma-informed care (TIC) are required. Elliot et al. (2005) suggest that best practice is to apply universal trauma precautions that nurses routinely use that are growth promoting and **recovery** focused and that are less likely to re-traumatise those already exposed to interpersonal trauma. Many practices such as the rigid implementation of ward rules and restrictions, locked doors, mixed-sex facilities and coercive practices such as restraint and seclusion are experienced by service users as emotionally unsafe and disempowering and therefore traumatising. Effective TIC services are those where the staff are aware of and sensitive to doing no further harm and make this their priority. Trauma-informed care starts with and goes to the heart of the enabling nature of the nurse–patient relationship and the values services place on person-centred care, with a view to reducing conflict and maintaining the 'caring' status quo at all times. An understanding of factors that can influence the therapeutic triad, both positively and negatively, is essential and practitioners and their organisations need to work together in order to address the challenges outlined in this chapter.

CHAPTER SUMMARY

This chapter has covered:

- How aggression and violence can be defined and the complexities of this
- Various causes and triggers for aggressive behaviour
- How to prevent the development of aggression and violence and the use of de-escalation as a secondary prevention
- The concept of restrictive interventions and the current debate
- Approaches to minimise conflict and restrictive practices and the growing evidence
- Insights into personal triggers and responses to conflict in health and care settings.

BUILD YOUR BIBLIOGRAPHY

Books

- Daley, A., Costa, L. & Beresford, P. (eds) (2017) *Madness, violence and power: A radical anthology*. Toronto: University of Toronto Press.
- Duxbury, J. (2000) *Difficult patients*. London: Butterworth-Heinemann. This book, whilst over a decade old, outlines the principles of therapeutic practice. It introduces the reader to a number of therapeutic universal rules for practitioners to follow in order to be facilitative and supportive when preventing and managing difficult situations.

SAGE journal articles

Go to https://study.sagepub.com/essentialmentalhealth for further free online journal articles related to this chapter. If you are using the interactive ebook, simply click on the book icon in the margin to go straight to the resource.

FURTHER READING: JOURNAL ARTICLES

- Larsen, I.B. & Terkelsen, T.B. (2014) Coercion in a locked psychiatric ward: perspectives of patients and staff. *Nursing Ethics*, 21(4), 426-436.
- Middleby-Clements, J.L. & Grenyer, B.F. (2007) Zero tolerance approach to aggression and its impact upon mental health staff attitudes. *Australian & New Zealand Journal of Psychiatry*, 41(2),187-191.
- Paterson, B. & Duxbury, J. (2007) Restraint and the question of validity. *Nursing Ethics*, 14(4), 535-545.

Weblinks

Go to https://study.sagepub.com/essentialmentalhealth for further weblinks related to this chapter. If you are using the interactive ebook, simply click on the book icon in the margin to go straight to the resource.

FURTHER READING: WEBLINKS

- Agenda: http://weareagenda.org/face-down-restraint-use-widespread-against-women-and-girls – an alliance for women and girls at risk
- Department of Health: www.gov.uk/government/publications/positive-and-proactive-care-reducing-restrictive-interventions – this site has materials to support the policy guidance from Department of Health (2014) *Positive and proactive care: Reducing the need for restrictive interventions*. London: DH. This DH guidance on the DH website has been produced with health and social care settings in mind to address the thorny issue of minimising restrictive interventions that may precipitate violence and conflict
- NICE: www.nice.org.uk/guidance/ng10/resources – this site has a number of resources to support the 2015 NICE guidelines on violence. The NICE guidance is an excellent and robust guide for practitioners to find the best evidence base available to support their practice in prevention and managing violence in clinical and care settings.
- Overall, these websites give a mixture of invaluable information and resources about the presentation of, causes of and responses to aggressive behaviour and conflict within health and social care settings.

Video link

WATCH A VIDEO!

- BBC: www.bbc.co.uk/news/uk-england-bristol-15622930 – Winterbourne View was a milestone in the development of guidelines on minimising restrictive practices following outcries from the public as a result of a BBC panorama exposé in 2012.

VIDEO LINK 26: BBC

ACE YOUR ASSESSMENT

Revise what you have learned by visiting https://study.sagepub.com/essentialmentalhealth. If you are using the interactive ebook, simply click on the tick icon to go straight to the resource.

- Test yourself with multiple-choice and short-answer questions and flashcards.

ONLINE QUIZZES & ACTIVITY ANSWERS

REFERENCES

Agenda (2017) *Face-down restraint use widespread against women and girls*. Available at: http://weareagenda.org/face-down-restraint-use-widespread-against-women-and-girls (accessed 12.08.17).

Aiken, F., Duxbury, J., Dale, C., et al. (2012) *Review of the medical theories and research relating to restraint related deaths*. London: MOJ.

Amering, M., Stastny, P. & Hopper, K. (2005) Psychiatric advance directives: qualitative study of informed deliberations by mental health service users. *British Journal of Psychiatry*, *186*, 247–252.

Bonner, G., Lowe,T., Rawcliffe, D., et al. (2002) Trauma for all: a pilot study of the subjective experience of physical restraint for mental health inpatients and staff in the UK. *Journal of Psychiatric and Mental Health Nursing*, *9*, 465–473.

Bowers, L. (2014) Safewards: a new model of conflict and containment on psychiatric wards. *Journal of Psychiatric and Mental Health Nursing*, *21*(6), 499–508.

Bowers, L., Alexander, J., Simpson, A., et al. (2004) Cultures of psychiatry and the professional socialization process: the case of containment methods for disturbed patients. *Nurse Education Today*, *24*(6), 435–442.

Choiniere, J.A., MacDonnell, J.A., Campbell, A.L., et al. (2014) Conceptualizing structural violence in the context of mental health nursing. *Nursing inquiry*, 21(1), 39–50.

Cowin, L.S., Davies, R., Estall, G., et al. (2003) De-escalating aggression and violence in the mental health setting. *International Journal of Mental Health Nursing*, *12*, 64–67.

Curran, S.S. (2007) Staff resistance to restraint reduction: identifying and overcoming barriers. *Journal of Psychosocial Nursing and Mental Health Services*, *45*, 45–50.

Cutcliffe, J. & Santos, J. (2012) *Suicide and self-harm: An evidence-informed approach*. London: Quay Books.

Department of Health (2012) *Transforming care: A national response to Winterbourne View Hospital*. London: DH.

Department of Health (2014) *Positive and proactive care: Reducing the need for restrictive interventions*. London: DH.

Deveau, R. & McDonnell, A. (2009) As the last resort: reducing the use of restrictive physical interventions using organisational approaches. *British Journal of Learning Disabilities*, *37*, 172–177.

Distasio, C.A. (1994) Violence in health care: institutional strategies to cope with the phenomenon. *The Health Care Supervisor*, *12*(4), 1–27.

Duxbury, J. (2002) An evaluation of staff and patient views of and strategies employed to manage inpatient aggression and violence on one mental health unit: a pluralistic design. *Journal of Psychiatric and Mental Health Nursing*, *9*, 325–337

Duxbury, J. & Whittington, R. (2005) Causes and management of patient aggression and violence: staff and patient perspectives. *Journal of Advanced Nursing*, *50*(5), 469–478.

Duxbury, J. & Wright, K. (2011) Should nurses restrain violent and aggressive patients? *Nursing Times*, *107*, 9.

Duxbury, J., Aiken, F. & Dale, D. (2011) Deaths in custody: the role of restraint. *Journal of Learning Disabilities and Offending Behaviour*, *2*(4), 178–189.

Elliott, D., Bjelajac, P., Fallot, R. et al. (2005) Trauma-informed or trauma-denied: principles and implementation of trauma-informed services for women. *Journal of Community Psychology*, 33(4), 461–477.

Francis, R. (2013) *Report of the Mid Staffordshire NHS Foundation Trust public inquiry: Executive summary*. London: The Stationery Office.

Fricker, M. (2007) *Epistemic injustice: Power and the ethics of knowing.* Oxford: Oxford University Press.

Gerdtz, M., Daniel, C., Dearie, V., et al. (2013) The outcome of a rapid training program on nurses' attitudes regarding the prevention of aggression in emergency departments: a multi-site evaluation. *International Journal of Nursing Studies, 50*(11), 1434–1445.

Holmes, D., Rudge, T. and Perron, A. (eds) (2012) *(Re) thinking violence in health care settings: A critical approach.* Farnham: Ashgate Publishing, Ltd.

Huckshorn, K.A. (2004) Reducing the use of seclusion and restraint in mental health systems: a public health prevention approach with interventions. *Journal of Psychosocial Nursing and Mental Health Services, 42*, 22–33.

Kamchuchat, C., Chongsuvivatwong, V., Oncheunjit, S., et al. (2008) Workplace violence directed at nursing staff at a general hospital in Southern Thailand. *Journal of Occupational Health, 50*, 201–207.

Lavelle, M., Stewart, D., James, K., et al. (2016) Predictors of effective de-escalation in acute inpatient psychiatric settings. *Journal of Clinical Nursing, 25*(15–16), 2180–2188.

LeBel, J. (2011) *The business case for preventing and reducing restraint and seclusion use.* HHS Publication No. (SMA) 11–4632. Rockville, MD: Center for Mental Health Services, Substance Abuse and Mental Health Services Administration.

LeBel, J. & Goldstein, R. (2005) The economic cost of using restraint and the value added by restraint reduction or elimination. *Psychiatric Services, 56*(9), 1109–1114.

LeBel, J., Duxbury, J., Putkonen, A., et al. (2014) Multinational experiences in reducing and preventing the use of restraint and seclusion. *Journal of Psychosocial Nursing and Mental Health Services, 52*(11), 22–29.

Livingstone, A. (2007) *Seclusion practice: A literature review.* Melbourne, VIC, Australia: Victorian Quality Council and Chief Psychiatrist's Quality Assurance Committee.

Maitre, E., Debien, C., Nicaise, P., et al. (2013) Advance directives in psychiatry: a review of the qualitative literature. *Encephale, 39*(4), 244–251.

Mattson, M.R. & Sachs, M.H. (1978) Seclusion: uses and complications. *American Journal of Psychiatry, 135*(10): 1210–1213.

McVilly, K.R. (2008) *Physical restraint in disability services: Current practices, contemporary concerns and future directions.* Melbourne, VIC, Australia: Department of Human Services.

Meehan, T., McIntosh, W. & Bergen, H. (2006) Aggressive behaviour in the high-secure forensic setting: the perceptions of patients. *Journal of Psychiatric and Mental Health Nursing, 13*, 19–25.

Mind (2012) *Mental health crisis care: Physical restraint in crisis.* London: Mind.

National Institute for Health and Care Excellence (2015) *Violence and aggression: Short-term management in mental health, health and community settings.* London: NICE.

Nijman, H.L.I., Muris, P., Merckelbach, H.L.G.J., et al. (1999) The Staff Observation Aggression Scale- Revised (SOAS-R). *Aggressive Behavior, 25*, 197–209.

Papageorgiou, A. (2002) Advance directives for patients' compulsorily admitted to hospital with serious mental illness: randomised controlled trial. *British Journal of Psychiatry, 181*, 513–519.

Paterson, B., Bradley, P., Stark, C., et al. (2003) Deaths associated with restraint use in health and social care in the UK: the results of a preliminary survey. *Journal of Psychiatric and Mental Health Nursing, 10*, 3–15.

Paterson, B., Leadbetter, D. & McComish, A. (1997) Deescalation in the management of aggression and violence. *Nursing Times, 93*(36), 58–61.

Price, O. & Baker, J. (2012) Key components of de-escalation techniques: a thematic synthesis. *International Journal of Mental Health Nursing, 21*(4), 310–319.

Putkonen, A., Kuivalainen, S. & Louheranta, O. (2013) Cluster randomized control trial of reducing seclusion and restraint in secured care of men with schizophrenia. *Psychiatric Services, 64*(9), 850–855

Roche, M.A., Diers, D., Duffield, C., et al. (2010) Violence toward nurses, the work environment, and patient outcomes. *Journal of Nursing Scholarship*, *42*(1), 13–22.

Royal College of Psychiatrists (1998) *Violence in psychiatry*. London: RCP.

Smith, M.E. & Hart, G. (1994) Nurse's responses to patient anger: from disconnecting to connecting. *Journal of Advanced Nursing*, *20*, 634–651.

Soininen, P., Valimaki, M., Noda, T., et al. (2013) Secluded and restrained patients' perceptions of their treatment. *International Journal of Mental Health Nursing*, *22*, 47–55.

Steinert, T., Wölfle, M. & Gebhardt, R.P. (2000) Measurement of violence during inpatient treatment and association with psychopathy. *Acta Psychiatrica Scandinavica*, *102*(2), 107–112.

Stewart, D., Bowers, L., Simpson, A., et al. (2009) Manual restraint of adult psychiatric inpatients: a literature review. *Journal of Psychiatric and Mental Health Nursing*, *16*, 749–757.

Swanson, J.W., Swartz, M.S., Elbogen, E.B., et al. (2013) Facilitated psychiatric advance directives: a randomised control trial of an intervention to foster advance treatment planning among persons with severe mental illness. *American Journal of Psychiatry*, *163*(11), 1943–1951.

Tunde-Ayinmode, M. & Little, J. (2004) Use of seclusion in a psychiatric acute inpatient unit. *Australasian Psychiatry*, *12*(4): 347–351.

Wale, J.B., Belkin, G.S. & Moon, R. (2011) Reducing the use of seclusion and restraint in psychiatric emergency and adult inpatient services: improving patient-centered care. *The Permanente Journal*, *15*(2), 57–62.

Whittington, R. & Wykes, T. (1994) Going in strong: confrontative coping by staff. *Journal of Forensic Psychiatry*, *5*(3), 609–614.

Whittington, R., Baskind, E. & Paterson, B. (2006) Coercive measures in the management of imminent violence: restraint, seclusion and enhanced observation. In D. Richter & R. Whittington (eds) *Violence in Mental Heath Settings*. London: Springer.

Wynaden, D., Chapman, R., McGowan, S., et al. (2002) Through the eye of the beholder: to seclude or not to seclude. *International Journal of Mental Health Nursing*, *11*(4), 260–268.

COGNITIVE BEHAVIOURAL THERAPIES

27

SARAH TRAILL AND ADAM TRAILL

THIS CHAPTER COVERS

- The origins and development of CBT
- An overview of the principles of CBT
- CBT assessment and basic formulation
- Cognitive behavioural interventions.

> **"**
>
> I first became interested in CBT as a student nurse in my final year of training. The idea that thoughts, moods and behaviours could maintain problems was a new concept for me. I remember feeling happy that I was able to help someone overcome a debilitating anxiety problem via discussion and action. The approach is accessible and democratic with collaboration being an essential element, and over the last 20 years I have seen first-hand what a difference it can make to people's lives.
>
> **Katherine, community mental health nurse**
>
> **"**

Visit **https://study.sagepub.com/essentialmentalhealth** to access a wealth of online resources for this chapter – watch out for the margin icons throughout the chapter. If you are using the interactive ebook, simply click on the margin icon to go straight to the resource.

INTRODUCTION

The chapter introduces CBT by providing an overview of the history and development of CBT. The chapter will then take a skills and practice focus, the characteristics of CBT will be outlined, and then the structure and process of a CBT assessment, formulations and interventions will be presented.

Cognitive behavioural therapy (CBT) is an umbrella term that is used to describe a group of psychological therapies. Whilst there may be significant differences in the way the therapies are practised, they all focus on the interaction between an event, the thought processes (**cognitions**) a person has about the event and the subsequent behavioural and emotional consequences. The aim of CBT is to identify dysfunctional thoughts and behaviours that can maintain emotional problems by generating further distress, hindering the individual's ability to cope. The person is then assisted to try out strategies that may help them develop a more realistic appraisal of the situation, which, it is hoped, will facilitate **coping** and reduce distress. This may be via cognitive strategies, such as examining a person's thoughts from different perspectives, or it may be via behavioural strategies, such as behaviourally testing out a prediction to see if it is accurate.

THE ORIGINS AND DEVELOPMENT OF CBT

Modern CBT has its origins in behaviour therapy which is an approach to therapy based on the principles of learning theory, developed by scientists such as Ivan Pavlov (1849–1936) and Burrhus Skinner (1904–1990). Behaviourists argued that only directly observable phenomena could and should be studied scientifically. Prior to this, the dominant form of psychotherapy was psychoanalysis, an approach that originated from the work of Sigmund Freud (1856–1939). An essential component of psychoanalysis involves the exploration of the unconscious mind and behaviourists argued that processes that take place in a person's mind, which are not observable, are not amenable to scientific study. This led some researchers to question the validity of psychoanalysis (Eysenck, 1952). Conversely, Ivan Pavlov developed the theory of classical conditioning. Via a series of laboratory experiments, he demonstrated that animals can learn a new association with a stimulus, which can change their response to it. Pavlov observed that a dog would salivate (unconditioned response) when food was presented (unconditioned stimulus). He then rang a tuning fork just before the presentation of food and the dogs soon associated the ringing sound (conditioned stimulus) with the presentation of food, and salivated in response to the sound (conditioned response). The phenomena of classical conditioning demonstrated how a response can be generated by the association that is made with the stimulus, in this case a sound and food.

Operant conditioning

The second learning theory, known as operant conditioning, was developed by Thorndike (1911) and Skinner (1938). The principles of operant conditioning emerge from the observation that when an animal is rewarded with food after performing a behaviour, the frequency of the behaviour increases. Hence, the reward reinforces the behaviour. Two types of reinforcement were identified: first, positive reinforcement, which is the provision of a reward following a behaviour, serves to increase the frequency or strengthen the behaviour. An illustrative example of this would be a primary school teacher giving a pupil a sticker for concentrating well in class. The second type is negative reinforcement, which takes place when a behaviour increases or is strengthened as a result of taking away a feared stimulus. For example, when a person is worried about being anxious in a crowded supermarket (feared stimulus) they order their groceries to be delivered to their home. This removal of the potentially negative stimulus makes it more likely the person will continue to get their groceries delivered.

Behavioural therapies were successful, and proliferated, due to them following a line of scientific research that allowed them to demonstrate the effectiveness of the interventions. That said, a number of researchers and academics were unhappy as they believed that significant cognitive variables were being overlooked. For example, Meichenbaum (1975) argued that behaviour could change by altering the instructions that clients gave themselves, without the need for external reinforcement or conditioning.

Rational emotive therapy

In keeping with the premise that cognitions had a part to play in emotional disturbance, psychologist Albert Ellis developed rational emotive therapy (Ellis, 1962). He developed an ABC model of understanding emotional problems, whereby an activating event (A) was evaluated by belief (B), which then led to emotional and behavioural consequences (C). When his clients exhibited demanding beliefs, for instance 'I must never make mistakes', they were likely to experience unhealthy emotional and behavioural consequences such as **depression** and procrastination. Whereas the same activating event, if evaluated with a more flexible preference, for example 'I aim to get things right but mistakes can be part of the learning process', tended to result in healthy (but possibly still negative) emotions and adaptive behaviours.

Aaron T. Beck: cognitive therapy

Beck (1967) developed a cognitive model for understanding depression. He proposed that negative thinking in depression has its origins in early life experience that lead to the formation of, what he termed, core beliefs – for example, 'I am stupid' or 'other people are critical'. These core beliefs give rise to rules and assumptions that are developed by the person, and they may be adaptive or maladaptive. For example, 'If I work hard then I might succeed' may spur an individual to work hard when there is the risk of failure, whereas the assumption 'If I work hard then I will still fail' may increase the likelihood of avoiding the task or giving up.

These beliefs and assumptions are referred to as 'schemas'. Beck believed the content of an individual's schemas would provide clues as to the sort of events that could trigger depression. Consider the following illustrative example: a child who experienced rejection from a parent during childhood may believe themselves to be 'unlovable' and other people to be 'rejecting' (core beliefs). In an attempt to cope, they develop a rule such as 'If I keep someone happy then they might stay' and an assumption that 'If someone rejects me then it proves I'm unlovable'. These rules and assumptions would be likely to exert a strong influence on their behaviour towards others, and they are likely to acquiesce their own needs to keep people happy. When a critical life event occurs that matches their vulnerability, for example a relationship breakdown, they are likely to interpret this as proof they are unlovable. This could lead to depression and the production of negative automatic thoughts such as 'no one will love me'. This would then lead to further depressed **mood** and behaviours aimed at protecting them from rejection, such as avoiding social situations. Additionally, they may be hyper-vigilant for signs that they are likely to be rejected again, which may distort their perception, making it more likely they will interpret innocuous events as rejection. This model is illustrated in Figure 27.1.

In keeping with the scientific tradition of the behaviourists, cognitive therapy aimed to test the validity of both the cognitive model of emotional **disorders** and its effectiveness (Clark et al., 1999). Initially, the approach was developed for depression, but was extended as a means of understanding and working with a range of emotional disorders (Beck, 1967, 1976). In the years that followed, cognitive therapy integrated practices from behaviour therapy. This is illustrated by a treatment method for

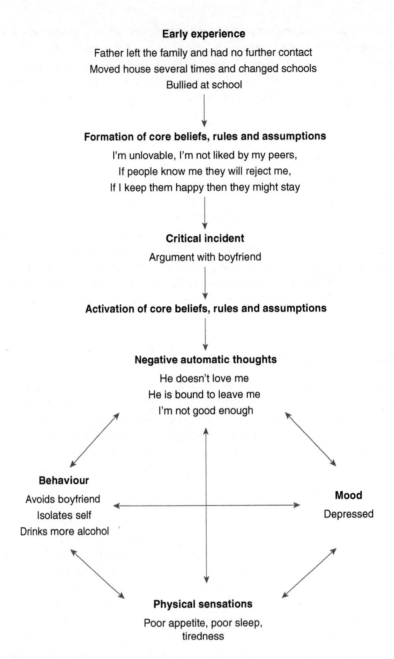

Early experience

Father left the family and had no further contact
Moved house several times and changed schools
Bullied at school

Formation of core beliefs, rules and assumptions

I'm unlovable, I'm not liked by my peers,
If people know me they will reject me,
If I keep them happy then they might stay

Critical incident

Argument with boyfriend

Activation of core beliefs, rules and assumptions

Negative automatic thoughts

He doesn't love me
He is bound to leave me
I'm not good enough

Behaviour

Avoids boyfriend
Isolates self
Drinks more alcohol

Mood

Depressed

Physical sensations

Poor appetite, poor sleep,
tiredness

Figure 27.1 Beck's model of depression

panic disorder developed by David Clark (1986). In this treatment, the catastrophic misinterpretation of the internal event that triggered the **panic attack** is identified, for instance an increased heart rate is interpreted catastrophically as 'I'm having a heart attack!' The likelihood of the heart attack explanation is considered alongside a more benign explanation, such as 'I'm anxious' or 'I'm hyperventilating'. Clark used behavioural exposure to the sensation (for example, jogging on the spot to temporarily raise the heart rate) to behaviourally test out whether the catastrophic or more benign explanation was the more accurate.

Since the 1980s, CBT models and treatment methods have been developed for a wide range of problems, including social anxiety (Clark & Wells, 1995), obsessive compulsive disorder (Salkovskis, 1985), generalised **anxiety** disorder (Wells, 1997; Borkovec & Newman, 1999), psychotic symptoms (Garety et al., 2001) and insomnia (Harvey, 2002). CBT is now one of the most widely researched and practised forms of psychotherapy.

PRINCIPLES OF CBT

Characteristics of CBT

As a psychotherapy, CBT has a number of key characteristics:

Problem oriented and goal focused: CBT aims to identify the problem (via assessment), make sense of the problem (via formulation) and identify an individual's goals and the strategies for overcoming or managing the problem and achieving goals.

Formulation driven: this is the use of a cognitive behavioural model to understand a problem. Formulations can be disorder specific, e.g. panic disorder (Clark, 1986). Some formulations are not disorder-specific, but help a person understand the maintenance of a problem, e.g. a five areas formulation (Figure 27.2). Longitudinal formulations incorporate historical events and their relationship with the current problem, e.g. Beck's formulation in Figure 27.1.

Active, directive and collaborative: good quality CBT involves **collaboration** and teamwork. The practitioner brings the knowledge of CBT, but the client knows most about themselves and which strategies they are most likely to use.

Scientific: CBT is underpinned by science, in that the approach is continually evaluated through empirical research. Also, CBT involves the scientific process of testing out thoughts via experimentation and the application of logic.

Time limited: CBT tends to be time limited, though the amount of time may vary considerably. As a general rule, recent problems of low severity take less time than chronic problems of high severity. Sessions may vary in length with some lasting 30 minutes and some lasting hours (e.g. exposure). But the therapy is not ongoing and open-ended.

Is CBT suitable for all people?

Safran and Segal (1990) developed an interview schedule to identify individuals who are most likely to benefit from CBT. Within the interview, there are a number of criteria that can be helpful to consider when assessing suitability for CBT:

- Can the person access their thoughts?
- Are they aware of different emotions and able to distinguish between them?
- Do they accept some personal responsibility for making changes?
- Do they accept the cognitive behavioural explanation of the problem?
- Are they able to stay focused in the session?
- Can they form a **therapeutic relationship** with the therapist?
- Are they able to form positive relationships with people in general?
- Are they optimistic about therapy?

Negative answers to the questions would indicate that CBT would take longer, or another approach would be more beneficial.

CASE STUDY 27.1

Panic scenario

Gina is 19 years old and over the last six months has experienced a number of panic attacks. She cannot attribute the attacks to anything and describes her home and work life as 'fine' prior to the onset of panic. The first episode happened six months ago, when she smoked cannabis at a party. This triggered racing heart, palpitations and dizziness. It felt like she was going to pass out. She experienced her second attack on a crowded bus on the way to work, with similar symptoms. Gina had a number of further episodes and frequently worries that she will experience another attack. She has been unable to work for the last few months, due to these concerns. As a result, she avoids public transport, crowds and places with no easy means of escape. When standing, she tries to keep her legs straight, avoids queuing and walks close to walls in case she needs to lean or sit down. She also tries to take deep breaths.

Depression scenario

Sam is 35 years old and is a first-year student at university, undertaking a degree in nursing. He is the youngest of three siblings, and whilst his older siblings did well at school, Sam struggled academically, achieving few qualifications. Sam went to work as a health care assistant. He was good at his job and was encouraged to apply for a nursing course. He attended college to gain the necessary qualifications to enable him to apply for nursing. It was at this point that Sam was assessed as having dyslexia. Over the next few years, Sam worked hard at college. He lacked confidence in his academic ability, but with support from his tutor he achieved the necessary grades and was accepted at a local university to study nursing. Sam enjoyed the practical side of the course but found the academic work difficult. His most recent essay did not pass and the experience was a significant blow to his confidence. Sam had really wanted to become a nurse but now believes he has been foolish, that he's stupid and should never have put himself in the position where he would expose his stupidity to others. He has been unable to face friends and family over the preceding weeks, has stopped going to his classes and has avoided looking at emails. As his mood has deteriorated, he has noticed he is drinking more alcohol, is not sleeping and is not taking care of himself well.

ASSESSMENT AND FORMULATION

The purpose of a CBT assessment is to gather enough information about the problem and what maintains it in order to develop a formulation that helps the person understand their problem. A clinician should start by asking a general open-ended question, for example 'Can you tell me about the problem(s) you have been having recently?' The clinician then moves the focus onto a specific example. This can be done by asking 'Can you tell me about a recent occasion where you felt depressed/anxious?' Padesky & Greenberger (1995) developed a simple five areas model for assessing and formulating problems which can be used in the assessment interview as a means of identifying the triggering situation and the associated moods, behaviours, negative automatic thoughts and physical symptoms. Figure 27.2 illustrates a five areas assessment and formulation for Sam.

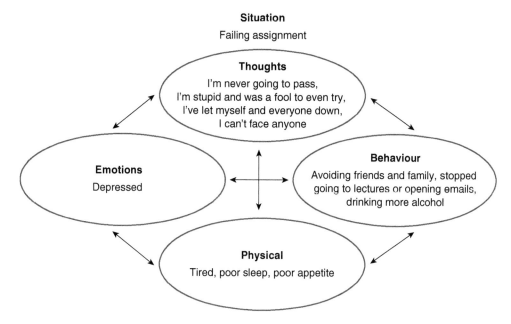

Figure 27.2 Sam's five areas formulation

In addition to the five areas, the assessment should also include questions to elicit the impact of the problem along with other elements that would be part of a standard mental health assessment (e.g. risk, medication, response to previous treatment). Once the assessment information has been gathered, the client's goals for therapy should be identified and these should be specific and measurable.

USE OF MEASUREMENT IN CBT

Measurement is an integral component, which begins in the assessment phase and is repeated throughout. There are a number of formal measures that can be used for assessment. They tend to be developed for particular problems and have good reliability and validity. Commonly used measures include the PHQ-9 (Kroenke et al., 2001), which measures the severity of depression symptoms, and the GAD-7 (Spitzer et al., 2006), which measures the severity of generalised anxiety disorder symptoms. Additionally, a number of informal measures are used in CBT, such as ratings of the intensity of a mood, recording the frequency of a thought or behaviour, or rating the conviction to a negative automatic thought.

I found it really interesting to look at how my PHQ 9 score changed over the course of therapy. It was helpful, because sometimes I'd think I'd not progressed very much and then I'd see that my scores were coming down and that helped spur me on. Of course there were times when my scores went up, and that helped me focus on using the techniques to help improve my mood or review the sort of pressures I was under and take action. In my final session it was great to see the graph showing how much I'd improved.

Maria, service user

THE THERAPEUTIC RELATIONSHIP

Bordin (1979) divided the therapeutic alliance into three components which were termed tasks, bonds and goals. Bordin believed that therapy would be successful if therapist and client had the same goal and agreed on the tasks that would be undertaken to achieve the goal. Moreover, a therapeutic bond could be best formed by demonstrating accurate empathy, genuineness and warmth. Bordin's model can be helpful to consider when the therapeutic alliance is not working well. Useful reflection questions include: Do we have the same goal? Do we agree on the tasks to reach the goal? Do we have a therapeutic relationship?

HOMEWORK

Beck (1976) argues that homework is an integral, not optional, part of CBT. There is some evidence to suggest that clients who undertake homework improve more than those who don't (Niemeyer & Feixas, 1990). Homework is an important part of helping someone become their own therapist, therefore careful consideration is given to the planning, implementation and evaluation of homework. All homework should have a clear rationale that links with the formulation. Clear instructions, in-session practice and a means of recording can all be helpful.

It is important to emphasise homework *completion* over homework *success*. On a final note, the name 'homework' can be off-putting to some, particularly if they have negative associations with school. So, homework can be re-named as, for example, 'between session practice'.

COGNITIVE INTERVENTIONS

Identifying cognitive distortions

Different cognitive distortions are associated with different disorders. For example, anxiety disorders are characterised by an overestimation of threat and an underestimation of the ability to cope; whereas depression is often characterised by negative thoughts about oneself, life conditions and pessimism about the future. Once a mood is activated, attention and memory can be drawn to experiences and events that are consistent with the mood. For example, if you are angry with a family member, you are more likely to remember their previous wrongdoings than occasions when they have been kind.

Helping people recognise whether they have distorted thinking is a technique used in the early phase of CBT. This is done by first providing information to the client on the sorts of cognitive distortions that exist, then reviewing the client's negative automatic thoughts to see if they fall within the categories.

Cognitive distortions include:

- all-or-nothing thinking – for example, seeing oneself as either a total success or a total failure
- overgeneralisation – for example, seeing a single negative event as a never-ending pattern of defeat
- mental filter – dwelling on the negative and ignoring the positives
- catastrophising (magnification) – blowing things out of proportion, for example an increased heart rate interpreted as a heart attack
- fortune telling – for example, predicting that things will go wrong
- personalisation – blaming yourself for something that was not your fault
- emotional reasoning – for example, you feel like a fool so therefore you must be one

- labelling – instead of saying you made a mistake, you call yourself a 'loser'
- mind reading – assuming you know what others are thinking.

Catching and modifying negative automatic thoughts

Negative automatic thought records

Negative automatic thoughts (NAT) are an appraisal of an event, they are negative and they pop into the mind automatically. For example, whilst revising for an upcoming examination a person may experience NATs such as 'I'm never going to pass'. Thought records can be used to modify NATs and develop realistic and helpful thoughts, which in turn reduce distress and promote coping behaviours. There are a number of steps in the process:

Step 1: Identify a situation that triggered the thought by answering the following questions: What was I doing? When did it happen? Where was I? Who was I with? These questions bring the memory into conscious awareness and allow easy access to the NAT.

Step 2: Identify the main emotion. At this point, it is important to note that emotions are described using one word, e.g. anxious, angry or depressed. If there a number of emotions, it can be helpful to use a different thought record for each, as it needs to be clear which emotion is associated with the NAT. Once the emotion is identified, rate the intensity of the emotion.

Step 3: Identify the NAT. Helpful questions include 'What went through you mind just before you started to feel...'; 'Did any memories or images come into your mind?' or, in the case of anxiety, 'What is the worst that could happen?' Once you have identified the NATs, identify the one that generates the most distress and circle it. This is called the *hot thought* and the remainder of the thought record will focus on this. Rating the current conviction to the thought provides a baseline to measure against once the exercise is complete.

Step 4: Look for evidence that supports the NAT. This provides insight into the sort of information the person is using to support their view.

Step 5: Look for evidence against the NAT. Questions that may be helpful include 'What would you say to a friend?', 'Would you still think this way if you weren't anxious?', 'Is there any evidence suggesting the thought isn't 100% true?', 'Is my negative automatic thought a biased thought?'

Step 6: Review the information collected at steps 4 and 5 and review the NAT. Does it need to change? If so, what would be a more accurate and helpful thought?

Step 7: Re-rate the intensity of the emotion.

Sam's thought record is provided in Table 27.1.

BEHAVIOURAL STRATEGIES

Behavioural activation is a strategy aimed at reducing negative reinforcement. For example, Sam is avoiding his family and friends because he thinks seeing them will be upsetting to him, and possibly them. So, when Sam receives a text inviting him to meet up with his fellow nursing students for an end-of-term drink, he worries that people will ask him about his work, or that he won't be able to put on a brave face. As a result, he declines the invitation and feels an immediate sense of relief that he

Table 27.1   Sam's thought record

Situation	Rate mood	NAT	Evidence for NAT	Evidence against NAT	New thought	Re-rate mood
Email telling me my essay didn't pass. I was on my own and it was two weeks ago	Depressed 80%	I'm never going to pass. I'm stupid. 90% rating of conviction	I didn't get many GCSEs at school. I find studying difficult	I did well when I went back to college. My tutor says they have confidence in me. Labelling myself as stupid is an opinion, not a fact	Getting something wrong doesn't mean I'm stupid, it can be part of the process of learning. 70% rating of conviction	Depressed 30% (but hopeful)

will be spared the upset. This is an example of negative reinforcement and it makes it more likely that Sam will respond the same way in the future. There are a number of different ways of undertaking behavioural activation, but the following is a straightforward series of steps that can be easy for clients to follow:

Step 1: Identify the current level of activity by asking the client to complete an activity diary, whereby they note the activity, when they did it and rate their mood at the time.

Step 2: Review the diary and look for associations between activity and mood, for example does mood improve when doing certain activities? Or being with certain people? When people are depressed, they often isolate themselves and withdraw from activities. This reduces the likelihood of a person experiencing positive reinforcement and results in the person feeling more depressed.

Step 3: Explain the role of reduced activity in the maintenance of depression and the rationale for a gradual increase in activity. It can be helpful to use the analogy of rehabilitation and **recovery** from physical injury.

Step 4: Identify activities that the person used to engage in, then rate each item in terms of its current difficulty. Turn this into three lists of activities: one easy, one medium and one difficult.

Step 5: Start including activity into the daily routine, beginning with the easiest, increasing the difficulty as the mood improves. Rate the impact on mood.

WHAT'S THE EVIDENCE? 27.1

Jacobson and colleagues (1996) compared three versions of CBT for depression. In the first version, the subjects received comprehensive CBT, including cognitive restructuring of negative automatic thoughts, dysfunctional assumptions and core beliefs, and behavioural activation. In the second version, the CBT focused on cognitive restructuring of negative automatic thoughts and behavioural activation. The third version just used behavioural activation. There was minimal difference in the level of improvement in all three conditions. This suggests that behavioural activation had the greatest influence on outcomes.

MAKING A DIFFERENCE 27.1

Nurses using behavioural activation

Ekers and colleagues (2011) completed a randomised controlled trial to examine the effectiveness of behavioural activation delivered by mental health nurses in the community who had no previous psychotherapy training. They were instructed on the practice of behavioural activation and received regular monthly clinical supervision. The results indicated that behavioural activation was a more effective treatment than the usual care.

GRADED EXPOSURE

Graded exposure is the therapeutic confrontation of a feared stimulus in order to learn that the stimulus is not dangerous which, in turn, reduces the anxiety. The approach is used for anxiety problems. The principle behind the approach is that when a person perceives a threat, the 'fight or flight' mechanism is activated. This results in a surge of adrenalin, the heart rate increases, blood flows to the muscles, breathing becomes more rapid and the urge to escape is overwhelming. Anxiety disorders occur when the threat is a 'false alarm' and there is an underestimation of the ability to cope. The instinct is to flee the situation. Once free, anxiety reduces rapidly and the opportunity to learn that the situation is not dangerous is missed. The practice of avoiding or escaping from **triggers** is an example of negative reinforcement and the next time a similar situation occurs, the person is likely to avoid or escape as a means of coping (see Figure 27.3). Graded exposure allows a person to become more familiar with and less anxious about the trigger. This process is called habituation and it provides the opportunity to realistically appraise the threat and develop a coping response.

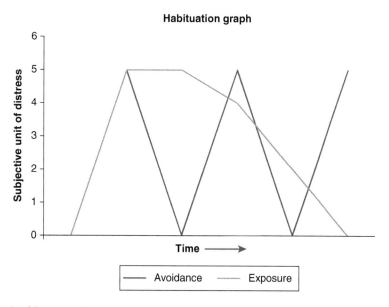

Figure 27.3 Avoidance and exposure

There are a number of steps to graded exposure: first, the fight, flight or freeze mechanism should be explained, alongside the role of escape and avoidance in maintaining the anxiety disorder. This provides the client with the reason for undertaking the exposure (Figure 27.3).

The second stage is to create a measure of anxiety that can be used to monitor changes in severity. This is referred to as the subjective unit of distress scale, or SUD. This can be represented as a number out of 10 on a scale where 0 is no anxiety and 10 is maximum anxiety. Alternatively, it could be represented visually, for example the point on a thermometer as in Figure 27.4 which shows an SUD for Gina who we met in Case Study 27.1.

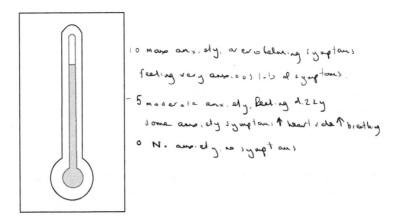

Figure 27.4 Gina's SUD thermometer

The next stage is to create a hierarchy of triggers, starting with the least anxiety-provoking and working up to the most anxiety-provoking.

There are four key principles to follow when setting up an exposure task:

1. The process should be **graded**, in that it should start with the easiest item on the hierarchy and work up to the most difficult; exposure should be challenging but not overwhelming.
2. The person will need to **experience anxiety** without avoiding or neutralising it with other safety behaviours. Otherwise, the anxiety will not reduce via habituation and the trigger will continue to produce distress.
3. The exposure should be **repeated** so that the task can be completed with relative ease.
4. The exposure task should be **prolonged** so that the individual stays with the anxiety long enough for the process of habituation to take place.

Table 27.2 Record of exposure

Situation/step on the hierarchy	SUD before	SUD during	SUD end	Comments (including skills used, difficulties experienced)
Catching the bus on my own, sitting near the front	7	6	1	I was nervous before I started, once the doors closed my anxiety went up and I felt dizzy, but this subsided. I told myself that I could do it and that my anxiety would go down and it started to reduce after about 5 minutes. It took about 15 minutes to feel OK.

Therapist-assisted exposure tends to be more successful than exposure that is undertaken for homework, as the therapist can provide encouragement and can model the best way to undertake the activity. Table 27.2 is an example of Gina's record of exposure.

BEHAVIOURAL EXPERIMENTS

The purpose of a behavioural experiment is to generate new information and insights via experimentation and observation. They can be used in a variety of ways and are most commonly used to test the validity of a formulation, to test out a NAT or to see whether an alternative thought is more accurate. For example, Sam could find out if other people view failing the same way as he does (see Table 27.3). Experiments are developed in collaboration with the client, and they follow on from discussions in the session. It can be important to document the experiment and the results, much as a scientist would plan, undertake and report on the findings of their experiments.

Behavioural experiments are powerful interventions that can help a person develop emotional insight. This is in contrast to cognitive restructuring where the insights tend to be intellectual. (For a full discussion on behavioural experiments, the theoretical basis and practical guidance, see Bennet-Levy et al., 2004.)

LATER STAGES OF CBT

One of the aims of CBT is that clients become their own therapist. By using a range of cognitive and behavioural strategies, the client becomes familiar with the types of interventions that provide most benefit. This is aided by the practice of keeping records in CBT, which serve as a review for what worked well and the progress towards therapeutic goals. As the client and therapist prepare for the

Table 27.3 Sam's behavioural experiment record

Date	Identify the thought/ assumption that is being tested and rate your conviction to it (0-100%)	Design the experiment. What will you do? Where will the experiment take place? What resources will you need?	What are the potential obstacles to this experiment? How can you overcome these?	What happened in the experiment and what did you learn? Has the conviction to the thought changed? 0-100%
12 Jan	'Failing can be an important part of learning how to do something new' 20%	My therapist will distribute a survey to 20 work colleagues asking: I. Have you ever failed at something you are now good at? II. Do you think failing in a task helped you learn how to do it correctly? We will review the results in the next session	Health professionals might say the 'helpful thing', rather than what they really think Survey people with different jobs	The responses varied but in general they all said it was normal to make mistakes and fail when learning something new. This has increased my confidence in the thought to 70%

end of therapy, it can be helpful to produce a relapse prevention plan, incorporating potential triggers, **early warning signs** of relapse and strategies for staying well. This is sometimes referred to as a *therapy blueprint*.

CHAPTER SUMMARY

This chapter has covered the following ideas:

- Cognitive behavioural therapy has its origins in both behavioural and cognitive psychology and maintains the same emphasis on the importance of evidence.
- CBT refers to a group of psychotherapies that focus on the link between thoughts, behaviours and emotions. They differ in emphasis but all tend to be problem focused and goal directed, use agenda setting and homework, and tend to be time limited.
- Effective CBT requires a good therapeutic relationship, a bespoke assessment and a formulation which is shared with the service user.
- There are a range of cognitive and behavioural strategies that can be used – the choice of intervention will be a result of the formulation, the evidence base and the preference of the service user.

BUILD YOUR BIBLIOGRAPHY

Books

- Loewenthal, D. & House, R. (eds) (2010) *Critically engaging CBT*. Maidenhead: Open University Press/McGraw-Hill. This book takes a critical review of CBT and encourages the reader to consider some of the debates around the practice of CBT.
- Westbrook, D., Kennerley, H. & Kirk (2011) *An introduction to cognitive behaviour therapy: Skills and applications*, 2nd edition. London. SAGE. This is a comprehensive introduction which covers the principles and practice of CBT. It is accessible to the novice practitioner and includes helpful demonstrations of CBT.

SAGE journal articles

FURTHER
READING:
JOURNAL
ARTICLES

Go to https://study.sagepub.com/essentialmentalhealth for further free online journal articles related to this chapter. If you are using the interactive ebook, simply click on the book icon in the margin to go straight to the resource.

- Bloch, S. (2004) A pioneer in psychotherapy research: Aaron Beck. *Australian and New Zealand Journal of Psychiatry*, 38(11–12), 855–867.
- Cohen, J. & Mannarino, A.P. (2008) Disseminating and implementing trauma-focused CBT in community settings. *Trauma, Violence, & Abuse*, 9(4), 214–226.
- Shawe-Taylor, M. & Rigby, J. (1999) Cognitive behaviour therapy: its evolution and basic principles. *The Journal of the Royal Society for the Promotion of Health*, 119(4), 244–246.

Weblinks

FURTHER
READING:
WEBLINKS

Go to https://study.sagepub.com/essentialmentalhealth for further weblinks related to this chapter. If you are using the interactive ebook, simply click on the book icon in the margin to go straight to the resource.

- British Association of Counselling and Psychotherapy introduction to CBT: www.babcp.com/Public/What-is-CBT.aspx
- Mind information about CBT: www.counsellingdirectory.org.uk/counsellor-articles/what-are-they-comparing-and-contrasting-the-three-main-counseling-approaches

ACE YOUR ASSESSMENT

Revise what you have learned by visiting https://study.sagepub.com/essentialmentalhealth. If you are using the interactive ebook, simply click on the tick icon to go straight to the resource.

- Test yourself with multiple-choice and short-answer questions and flashcards.

ONLINE QUIZZES & ACTIVITY ANSWERS

REFERENCES

Beck, A.T. (1967) *Depression: Clinical, experimental and theoretical aspects*. New York: Harper and Row.

Beck, A.T. (1976) *Cognitive therapy and the emotional disorders*. New York: International Universities Press.

Bennet-Levy, J., Butler, G., Fennell, M., et al. (2004) *Oxford guide to behavioural experiments in cognitive therapy*. Oxford: Oxford University Press.

Bordin, E. (1979) The generalizability of the psychoanalytic concept of the working alliance. *Psychotherapy*, 16, 252–260.

Borkovec, T.D. & Newman, M.G. (1999) Worry and generalised anxiety disorder. In P. Salkovskis (ed.) *Comprehensive clinical psychology* (vol. 6). Oxford: Elsevier. pp. 439–459.

Clark, D.A. (1986) A cognitive approach to panic. *Behaviour Research and Therapy*, 24, 461–70.

Clark, D.A. & Wells, A. (1995) A cognitive model of social phobia. In R.G. Heimberg, M.R. Leibowitz, D.A. Hope & F.R. Schneier (eds) *Social phobia: Diagnosis, assessment and treatment*. New York: Guilford Press.

Clark, D.A., Beck, A.T. & Alford, B. (1999) *Foundations of cognitive theory and therapy of depression*. New York: John Wiley.

Department of Health (1997) *The new NHS: Modern and dependable*. London: The Stationery Office.

Ekers, D., Richards, D., McMillan, J., et al. (2011) Behavioural activation delivered by the non-specialist: phase II randomised controlled trial. *British Journal of Psychiatry*, 198, 66–72.

Ellis, A. (1962) *Reason and emotion in psychotherapy*. New York: Lyle Stuart.

Eysenck, H.J. (1952) The effects of psychotherapy: an evaluation. *Journal of Consulting and Clinical Psychology*, 16, 319–24.

Garety, P., Kuipers, E.E., Fowler, D., et al. (2001) A cognitive model for the positive symptoms of psychosis. *Psychological Medicine*, 31, 189–195.

Harvey, A.G. (2002) A cognitive model of insomnia. *Behaviour Research and Therapy*, 40, 869–893.

Jacobson, N.S., Dobson, K.S., Trauax, P.A., et al. (1996) A component analysis of cognitive behavioural treatment for depression. *Journal of Consulting and Clinical Psychology*, 64(2), 295–304.

Kroenke, K., Spitzer, R. & Williams, J. (2001) The PHQ-9: validity of a brief depression severity measure. *Journal of General Internal Medicine*, 16, 606–613.

Meichenbaum, D.H. (1975) Self-instructional methods. In F.H. Kanfer & A.P. Goldstein (eds) *Helping people change: A textbook of methods*. New York: Pergamon. pp. 357–391.

Niemeyer, R.A. & Feixas, G. (1990) The role of homework and skill acquisition in the outcome of group cognitive therapy for depression. *Behavior Therapy*, 21, 281–292.

Padesky, C.A. & Greenberger, D. (1995) *Clinicians guide to mind over mood*. New York: Guilford Press.

Safran, J.D. & Segal, Z.M. (1990) *Interpersonal processes in cognitive therapy*. New York: Basic Books.

Salkovskis, P.M. (1985) Obsessive compulsive problems: a cognitive behavioural analysis. *Behaviour Research and Therapy*, 23, 257–283.

Skinner, B.F. (1938) *The behaviour of organisms: An experimental analysis*. New York: Appleton-Century.

Spitzer, R., Kroenke, K., Williams, J., et al. (2006) A brief measure for assessing generalised anxiety disorder: the GAD-7. *Archives of International Medicine, 166*, 1092–1097.

Thorndike, E.L. (1911) *Animal intelligence*. New York: Macmillan.

Wells, A. (1997) *Cognitive therapy for anxiety disorders: A practice manual and conceptual guide*. Chichester: Wiley.

PSYCHOSOCIAL INTERVENTIONS TO SUPPORT CARERS

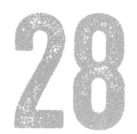

DOUG MACINNES, AMANDA FRANCIS AND ANNIE JEFFREY

THIS CHAPTER COVERS

- Defining a carer
- Mental health nursing and carers
- Concepts underpinning carer interventions
- Types of carer interventions
- New initiatives.

> "
>
> To care, and be cared for are both perspectives I have experienced, and the effect it can have on the balance and nature of any relationship. I was acutely ill for eight years and did not know myself and neither did my husband who kept insisting that he 'wanted his wife back', my youngest was eighteen months old, I feel I lost my four children's childhood and perhaps they felt the same. Photographs of them growing up are too painful to look at and I can't.
>
> When I was discharged, my then 19-year-old son had a psychotic breakdown and he became a dependent child, we camped in the living room evaporating his hallucinations and delusions, he having smashed up the house. I couldn't mend him; it was compounded by a sense of guilt that I had been so 'absorbed' in 'being mental' that it was my fault.
>
> I stopped being his mother and became his 'carer', anxiously scrutinising his every move, desperately afraid, and suffocating him. Desperate for him to recover, exhausted from reasoning with him. Realising why my husband had suffered carer breakdown. Sitting on the stairs at 2am as another room was broken, no one to help me, I called the police instead.
>
> Don't lose sight of love, because then it has to be found in anger and tears and hard words, as he delivered verbal slaps that stung. That now I could stop 'caring'. Three years on, he needed to breathe, so we both let go.
>
> **Amanda Francis, carer**
>
> "

Visit **https://study.sagepub.com/essentialmentalhealth** to access a wealth of online resources for this chapter - watch out for the margin icons throughout the chapter. If you are using the interactive ebook, simply click on the margin icon to go straight to the resource.

A survey conducted in 2011 indicated providing high quality information was the most important need identified by carers. Following this survey, a committed Carer Support Worker (CSW) was employed to work specifically with carers providing standardised information, specific advice and support to carers of service users.

I am the CSW and I can be contacted by telephone, by email, or meet in person at any of the Trust hospitals or the carer's own environment. It allows carers time to talk with someone about their own issues, concerns and frustrations. The CSW also acts as a liaison between carers, service users and health professionals, reducing the time taken for carers to get messages to people (key workers or their relative/friend) and receive messages in return.

I am bound by law and a professional code of conduct to a duty of confidentiality to service users and professionals working in mental health services, but by following correct policies and protocols this does not need to be a hindrance. It is often crucial to the ongoing wellbeing of both users and carers to share information.

The wellbeing of the carer can be vastly improved if encouraged to feel part of a team, receiving up-to-date information and invited to meetings where decisions are made about the future of their family member/friend. Without these measures in place, the carer may feel unable to continue giving the practical and emotional support that is so imperative to service users' mental wellbeing, recovery and rehabilitation.

Karen Tweedie, carer support worker

All happy families are alike; each unhappy family is unhappy in its own way. (Leo Tolstoy)

The above quotes give a lucid depiction of the experience of being a **carer** as well as the **value** of mental health nurses having an appreciation of the role that carers perform and the issues they face. This chapter focuses on the experiences of carers of people receiving mental health nursing care, the work undertaken to support and inform carers and the psychosocial approaches intended to support these carers.

DEFINING A CARER

The term carer is used in this chapter as it is the term used by most government agencies, third sector and charitable groups in the UK. There are some carers who dislike this term as it implies people have made a conscious decision to be a carer, and does not clearly differentiate between health professionals and family and friends providing an informal unpaid caring role. Some carers prefer the term caregiver. Many publications use the term family. Although family members are most likely to take on the caring support role, other people provide the main care and support in some cases. Most of the work (and research) examining the caring role has focused on the carers of older people, particularly those with **dementia**.

A more in-depth definition applied to carers of people using mental health services has been provided by Schene et al. (1990). One specific individual, the carer, assumes an unpaid and unanticipated responsibility for another, the client, who has health problems that are disabling and of a long-term nature, with no curative treatment available. Mental health problems mean the client is often unable to fulfil the normal reciprocal obligations that are considered part of normative adult relationships.

Carers in the UK

In the 2011 UK population census, over six and a half million people (approximately 10% of the population) identified themselves as being a carer. The charity Carers UK states that the majority of carers are female (58%) and that 60% of people will be carers at some point in their lives. At the time of writing (2016), carers providing unpaid care save the government an estimated £132 billion per year.

The impact of providing care has psychological, physical and social consequences for carers. Carers UK suggests that 48% give up work to provide care. Consequently, many carers struggle financially and there is a lack of contact outside of the caring relationship, with three-quarters of carers finding it hard to maintain relationships and social networks. Additionally, 80% of carers reported some form of mental distress because of their caring role – mainly **depression**. Almost a half of all carers reported that they did not think that wider society was aware of their role or cared about the difficulties they faced.

Carers of people with mental health problems

The Carers Trust reports that approximately 1.5 million people in the UK care for someone with a mental health problem. Most **service users** have ongoing contact with carers. Without carers, many people with a mental illness could not continue to live independently and the overall cost of community care would be much higher. In a scoping exercise, Lindon (2007) detailed the key issues faced by carers. These were:

- the unpredictability of caring for someone with a mental health problem
- the **stigma** of mental illness
- confidentiality and information-sharing conflicts with mental health professionals
- for some carers, the constant fear of a loved one's suicide
- the lack of specialised respite and/or 'sitting services'.

There is also significant evidence that those providing more hours of care were likely to have greater levels of mental distress (Smith et al., 2015).

CASE STUDY 28.1

The impact of living with a family member who has a diagnosis of severe and enduring mental illness

Mary is a 68-year-old woman whose 48-year-old son John was diagnosed as suffering from schizophrenia 28 years ago. During this time, John has been admitted to hospital eight times. On each occasion, he became distressed, did not sleep, eat or wash, and was convinced that people, including his mother, were trying to harm him.

Mary initially reduced her hours of employment working as a librarian at a local school but eventually took early retirement because she could no longer leave her son at home all day as she was concerned about leaving John alone in the house. Her salary loss meant the family finances significantly reduced. John would frequently leave electrical equipment or the gas cooker switched on.

(Continued)

In addition, he would often play music or pace around his room till the early hours, meaning that Mary would get very little sleep. Mary had gradually lost contact with her close circle of friends as she was embarrassed by John's behaviour and appearance, and rarely left the house for more than an hour because of her concerns about John. Mary and her husband often argue about the best way to cope with John's behaviour. They also worry about what will happen when they become too frail to care for John.

Questions

- What has been the impact of John's illness on Mary's life?
- What support could be offered to Mary and her husband by John's mental health nurse?

CASE STUDY 28.1 ANSWER

Historical influences on experiences of carers of people with mental health problems and perceptions by health professionals

Prior to the establishment of mental institutions, in the mid to late 1800s, the main caregiving role of a mentally ill person was undertaken by the family. However, with the development of large asylums, the service user became isolated from the family and the skills and experience of the family disappeared (Lefley, 1996). The separation of service users and families was later reinforced by psychodynamic theories and the **anti-psychiatry** movement which interpreted the patient–family relationship as destructive. These theories have not been supported by empirical evidence. However, they have influenced some health professionals in blaming carers for their role in the cause and development of mental health problems.

From the 1960s onwards, mental health policy has been geared towards caring for clients within community settings as opposed to in hospital and reuniting patients and their families. However, as Lefley (1996) points out, the problem with this approach is that carers had previously been excluded from involvement in their friends/relatives' care and were not prepared for this new role.

MENTAL HEALTH NURSING AND CARERS

Mental health nurses have a very important role to play in working with carers. Nurses often have most professional contact with carers of users receiving inpatient care or community care. Contact can take place informally such as carers visiting a ward, phoning up for advice, or meeting a carer when visiting the user in their home. More formal contact can be through situations such as care programme approach (CPA) meetings, **carer support** groups or family therapy sessions. This gives mental health nurses many opportunities to form positive collaborative relationships with carers.

A number of formal initiatives have guided the services provided to carers. The *National Carers Strategy* (DH, 2008) was published by the UK government and proposed that carers would be respected as expert care partners and have access to the services they need to support them in their caring role.

Carers in England and Wales have a legal entitlement to a carer's assessment. Eligibility for help is based on the risks of the impact of the caring role. Victor (2009) found some limited evidence of benefits in terms of emotional wellbeing, through carers being seen as giving themselves a chance to express their feelings and to be recognised and valued. Some carers were also able to access support services following the assessment.

The Triangle of Care approach was developed by carers and professionals to improve carer engagement in **acute** inpatient and home treatment services through an effective three-way partnership between service user, carer and clinicians, with all voices being heard. Six key standards were put forward:

- Carers are identified at first contact or as soon as possible thereafter.
- Staff are 'carer aware' and trained in carer engagement strategies.
- Policy and practice protocols regarding confidentiality and sharing information are in place.
- Defined posts responsible for carers are in place.
- A carer introduction to the service and staff is available, with a relevant range of information across the care pathway.
- A range of carer support services is available.

INFORMATION AND CONFIDENTIALITY

There is evidence that providing greater information improved carers' knowledge and use of services and was associated with greater satisfaction with services. MacInnes et al. (2013) found that carers rated access to quick and reliable information as the most important feature of a service. The National Institute for Health and Care Excellence (NICE) (2014) recommended that mental health professionals give family members and other carers written and verbal information about a diagnosis, about the role of different mental health teams and different services, about **recovery** and about how to get help in a crisis.

Victor (2009) suggests that a number of factors are important for carers when viewing information:

- the extent, layout and relevance of information
- staff manner
- whether staff follow up and resolve any queries
- ease of access to information
- whether the service is perceived as helpful.

It is well evidenced that the effective education of carers makes for a very positive impact on the wellbeing of both the service user and the carer themselves. However, this may mean that the carer is very aware of which intervention or service should be put in place for their loved one or family member, but that they do not have the power or position required to push this forward. This power instead lies with the practitioner responsible for the service user's care, who often has a high case load and may have had less time with the service user to come to the same conclusion as their carer. Carer input should, therefore, if the service user is agreeable, play a huge part in both decisions about treatment and the formation of care plans and as such a system should be put in place to enable the carer to contribute regularly, between appointments if required. It is of course important to ensure that the service user's wishes remain paramount and that they are never made to feel that their carer is part of a team separate to themself.

Heidi Turl, second-year mental health nursing student

CASE STUDY 28.2

The process of obtaining information and support from mental health services

Gayle is a single mother whose son Dwayne was admitted to a mental health inpatient unit for the first time following what Gayle was told was a psychotic episode. Before initially visiting Dwayne, Gayle was unsure about basic information, such as where she could park her car, the ward visiting times and whether she could bring in Dwayne's favourite food. When Gayle first visited the ward, she was unable to get any information about Dwayne's condition and progress as his key nurse was not on duty and no one else was sufficiently informed about Dwayne's care. However, the nurse in charge promised to inform the key nurse of Gayle's request for further information and also gave her a ward information leaflet giving practical details, phone numbers and website addresses. From these websites, she obtained some useful information about mental illness, medication and carer support. Over the next three weeks, Gayle was in regular contact with Dwayne's key worker and was able to address specific concerns, such as what may have caused his psychotic episode, the likelihood of her other two sons developing mental health problems, and her role at Dwayne's upcoming case conference.

Questions

- What do you think about Gayle's initial contact with the ward?
- Gayle asked questions about Dwayne's condition and progress. If you were Dwayne's key worker, how would you respond to Gayle?

CASE STUDY
28.2
ANSWER

CRITICAL THINKING STOP POINT 28.1

What is your understanding of the carer's role in helping people with mental health problems? What effect does caring have on their mental and physical wellbeing?

CONCEPTS UNDERPINNING CARER INTERVENTIONS

With an increasing number of service users living in the community, there has been a greater acknowledgement of the role that carers play in supporting service users and an awareness for health and social services to offer support to carers and to develop their skills and knowledge to support both themselves and their relative/friend. Smith et al. (2015) noted the importance of identifying the support needs of carers as soon as possible, to reduce the likelihood of poor mental and physical outcomes.

Expressed emotion, carer burden, carer attributions and caring are important concepts – they have been influential in the development of carer interventions focusing on the reduction of expressed emotion from high to low or the reduction in burden. They have also been used as outcomes to assess the efficacy of interventions.

Expressed emotion

Expressed emotion (EE) is a measure of the emotional temperature within the family. The level of EE has been mainly determined by undertaking a semi-structured interview, known as the Camberwell Family Interview, with carers and the service user. Initially, expressed emotion was rated on five dimensions: critical comments; hostility; emotional over-involvement; warmth; and positive remarks. The first three dimensions are considered the most important, and commonly the only three considered, with a family being rated as high EE if one of the three dimensions is above the predetermined threshold. High EE is predictive of user relapse and rehospitalisation. If none of the thresholds are achieved, then the family is rated as low EE.

However, there is concern that the description of high EE families has been perceived as a pejorative label, with families regarded by health professionals as responsible for the high EE within the household, and EE is inconsistent in different **cultures**. Many mental health services in the UK still prioritise high EE families for family interventions as, with limited resources, these families are viewed as being in greater need (Kuipers et al., 2010).

Carer burden

Carers encounter stressors that are either directly or indirectly related to the **illness**. These difficulties have traditionally been described as carer burden (Atkinson & Coia, 1995). Smith et al. (2015) report that high levels of stress for carers are associated with a reduction in the user's quality of life and an increase in the likelihood of exacerbating symptoms. However, there is no agreed standard instrument of carer burden, with different researchers often using different tools based on different underlying perceptions of the concept. Therefore, different studies may be assessing burden differently. Another limitation has been the lack of any positive caregiving experience, with Kuipers et al. (2010) recording that many carers report feelings of satisfaction and improved self-esteem.

Attributions

Carer attributions have also been used to support carers and assess intervention outcomes. If carers are critical, their attributions are more likely to lead to assertions that patients are substantially in control of, and therefore to blame for, negative events (Kuipers et al., 2010). This in turn relates to greater carer distress and negative evaluations of the caring role.

Coping

Lazarus (1993) describes different types of **coping** responses and proposes that appropriate coping depends on an accurate appraisal of situations, on one's resources and on how these are organised to respond to the situation. Therefore, using avoidant coping (i.e. wishing that the situation would go away or somehow be over with) may be useful for problems that resolve naturally, but not for those problems that are ongoing or worsening. Developing appropriate coping strategies is incorporated into many carer interventions.

There are associations between these different concepts, with carer burden strongly correlated with high EE, poor carer outcomes (increased stress, lower self-esteem) and less effective coping responses.

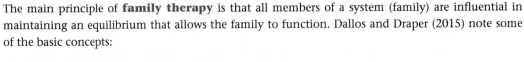

CRITICAL THINKING STOP POINT 28.2

Do you understand the main characteristics underpinning these concepts: expressed emotion, carer burden, attributions and coping?

TYPES OF CARER INTERVENTIONS

The most popular types of carer intervention have been categorised into three broad approaches: family therapy, **carer psychoeducation**, and carer support groups. These groups are categorised for ease of reference and clinicians often combine different approaches.

Family therapy

USEFUL FOR ASSIGNMENTS!

CASE STUDY:
RISK OF
DEVELOPING
MH PROBLEMS

The main principle of **family therapy** is that all members of a system (family) are influential in maintaining an equilibrium that allows the family to function. Dallos and Draper (2015) note some of the basic concepts:

- Families and other social groups should be considered as systems where the whole system is more than the sum of its individual parts.
- The operation of the family/carer system is governed by certain rules.
- Communication and feedback mechanisms are important to the functioning of the system.
- Events need to be understood as having a circular causality, where all members of the system play a part in changing how the whole system functions or resists change.

Family therapy sees the family group as the unit for study and treatment. Therapists see the problems of individuals in the context of the **environment**, especially the family. The therapy is concentrated on interpersonal processes, rather than on individual problems within the family.

Carer psychoeducation

In this approach, professionals provide information on issues surrounding the development and maintenance of mental health problems and current opinion on ways in which mental health problems could be alleviated or made worse. Sessions can be open or closed and are usually time limited. They can be focused on the carer of one service user or include multiple carers. The majority of interventions include both users and carers but carer-only groups are growing. Lucksted et al. (2013) state that carer psychoeducation:

- assumes that carers of individuals with mental illnesses need information, assistance and support
- combines informational, cognitive, behavioural, problem-solving, emotional, coping and consultation elements
- is created and led by mental health professionals
- includes content about illness, medication, and treatment management; services coordination; attention to all parties' expectations, emotional reactions and distress; assistance with improving family communication; structured problem-solving instruction, expanding social support networks and explicit crisis planning with professional involvement
- has content that is generally diagnosis-specific.

It is common for cognitive therapy approaches to be included to help carers develop coping responses.

Carer support groups

Support groups are normally professionally led with content based on research evidence (Duckworth & Halpern, 2014). They can be either time limited or ongoing, with carers coming to the sessions for the period they need. The groups are designed to help families get information about mental health, medication, self-care, mutual assurance, communication, problem solving and advocacy.

CASE STUDY 28.3

Involvement in a formal family intervention

Jasbir and his family were invited to attend a series of 6–8 family sessions arranged by the local mental health services to talk about his son Dev. This had been arranged through Dev's support team at the community mental health centre. The family went to the first session without any clear sense of what was expected of them. Once in the family session room, they met two people who introduced themselves as family therapists. Jasbir and his family did not understand the technical terms being used, but believed the therapists were there to support the family to help Dev, and were grateful for this help. During the first three sessions, Jasbir and the rest of his family became increasingly confused as to the purpose of the sessions. They were told where to sit and were usually asked to change seats once or twice a session. Individual members of the family were constantly asked to directly address Dev about their concerns, which some of the family (particularly Jasbir's daughter) found difficult. When other members of the family tried to support his daughter, the therapists would ask them to resist from interrupting the discussion. Outside of the session, the family met together and expressed concerns that they were being judged. Jasbir contacted the therapists' administrator to ask whether they could meet to discuss their concerns but were informed that the only discussions could be in the formal sessions. Jasbir and his family decided to terminate the sessions.

Questions

- What do you think made Jasbir and his family think they were being judged?
- What could the family therapy team do to make the experience more carer friendly?

CASE STUDY
28.3
ANSWER

WHAT'S THE EVIDENCE? 28.1

The effectiveness of carer interventions

Most carer interventions focus on service user outcomes, though there has been an increase in reports examining carer outcomes. This has included systematic reviews on: carers of users with psychosis, schizophrenia and bipolar disorder, where the user was not present at the intervention, brief family interventions for schizophrenia, bipolar disorder, family therapy for depression and psycho-education for siblings. Pharoah et al.'s (2010) systematic review examining the effectiveness of family interventions for people with schizophrenia found evidence that they decreased the frequency of relapse, reduced hospital admission and encouraged compliance with medication, though they didn't

(Continued)

reduce the length of service involvement. There is some limited evidence that the interventions improve levels of expressed emotion within the family. However, the main conclusions drawn from all of the above reviews was that there was only a limited number of relevant studies, generally of poor methodological quality, with different components of the intervention often not assessed separately, making it difficult to identify the effective part of any intervention programme. These systematic reviews of carer interventions indicate little or no benefit to the carers, though this is partly due to the lack of robust studies.

Victor (2009) reviewed a broader group of qualitative and quantitative studies examining carer support and psychoeducation groups for carers of people with a range of mental and physical health problems. The main findings were that carers gained additional knowledge about caring but there was little behavioural change in how they performed their role. Most carers also reported being satisfied with these groups and particularly targeted groups for carers from specific communities (i.e. people from a specific ethnic group or caring for someone with a particular health problem). The logistics of attending (frequency of meeting, topic coverage, location, time of meeting) as well as the characteristics of the other carers were also important in determining attendance.

Mental health nurses

A review of UK community mental health nurses indicated that they could effectively deliver a range of carer interventions to people diagnosed with **schizophrenia** (Curran & Brooker, 2007), while Macleod et al. (2011) reported that nurses providing community-based support reduced carer burden and increased coping skills. Victor (2009) reported that the most important skills required when working with carers were: good interpersonal skills, providing active assistance, being skilled and knowledgeable with regards to carer support, following up any agreed action, and maintaining contact.

The Thorn programme

The **Thorn programme** aimed to equip community psychiatric nurses to work effectively with people with severe mental health problems, and their carers. The programme utilised a stress vulnerability conceptualisation of **psychosis** and focused on case management, family intervention and the psychological management of psychotic symptoms. A national survey in 2007 found that there were over a thousand training places in England offering Thorn-style courses. Evaluations of the Thorn programme training were positive, though Couldwell and Stickley (2007) noted that community mental health nurses lacked the opportunities and support to implement the psychosocial skills acquired in training.

CRITICAL THINKING STOP POINT 28.3

What do you think are the strengths and weaknesses of different carer interventions? What role can mental health nurses play in delivering carer interventions?

MAKING A DIFFERENCE 28.1

We were completely unprepared for what to expect when our eldest son, Tom, came into contact with mental health services following a suicide attempt. We had tried numerous times to seek help which was not forthcoming, maybe partly due to several reasons, including our concerns not being listened to, patient confidentiality, our lack of knowledge concerning mental health services. When Tom became unwell, it felt as if the whole family was in crisis too. It would have been helpful to have included Tom's social network right from the very first meeting but this did not happen, and as with many families we felt we were battling against a coercive system which lacked any continuity of care – sent out of area due to lack of inpatient beds, passed from one service line to another, even within the crisis team no continuity, physical health and mental health dealt with separately. Despite NICE guidelines family therapy was not available. I found many mental health nurses very supportive, compassionate and helpful in trying to navigate the fragmented systems. Good communication skills were key.

I found it very useful to attend carers groups – an early intervention in psychosis group and a local Rethink carer group. Meeting with members of other families dealing with similar issues was very beneficial where we felt we could support one another. Being able to talk to others who were also feeling fear, guilt, shame and stigma helped us to deal with trying to care for our son, Tom.

Annie Jeffrey, carer

NEW APPROACHES

Peer-to-peer carer psychoeducation

Peer-to-peer psychoeducational interventions focus on carers providing the input to a standardised time-limited programme for other carers. Findings suggest that these groups help develop greater problem solving and better coping skills for carers (Lucksted et al., 2013, Duckworth & Halpern, 2014).

Open Dialogue

The **Open Dialogue** approach is an intervention where the majority of decision making is carried out in whole-system meetings involving the service user, carers and the extended social network, with as much as possible of the work undertaken in the user's home environment (Seikkula & Arnkil, 2014). All staff involved in the approach receive training in family, systems and related methodologies. There are few studies in this area so the current evidence on the impact for carers is limited.

Carer-focused workers

This role has focused on delivering basic information and support to carers with the facility to refer to specialist carer intervention services where necessary. A nurse-led, time-limited family service providing basic emotional support, advice and information was detailed by Radcliffe et al. (2012). There was positive feedback from the limited evidence available.

Carer breaks/respite care

There is very little evidence surrounding respite care, though Victor (2009) suggests that a break enables carers to stay in their caring role. A key factor as to whether carers will accept a break is their perception of the quality of the respite care on offer.

FACTORS TO CONSIDER FOR FUTURE CARER INTERVENTIONS

Carer empowerment

The Department of Health's (2008) stated aim is that carers are involved in all aspects of service design and delivery. However, Rowe's (2012) review of services shows poor engagement and communication by professionals, and carers struggling to cope. There is likely to be a future role for mental health nurses in supporting the development of carer empowerment.

Cultural competency

Cultural competency is now a core requirement for mental health professionals working with culturally diverse patient groups (Bhui et al., 2007). Victor (2009) noted that having carers from the same ethnic background together in support groups results in more positive outcomes. Mental health nurses will need to understand the belief systems and cultural sensitivities of specific groups of carers.

Demographic changes

Pickard (2015) notes that a key feature of population ageing in economically developed countries is the projected unprecedented rise in need for long-term care in the next two decades. There is considerable uncertainty over who will take on the existing role of older carers in the future. This may result in major changes in who becomes a carer and the caring role they are willing and able to perform.

New technologies

The NHS Confederation (2014) notes that there is a need for change in the way mental health services are designed and delivered regarding the use of technology. Reviews into carers of people with physical health problems report significant improvements in carers' outcomes. However, there has been limited work undertaken to examine how carers of people with mental health needs may benefit from this.

CRITICAL DEBATE 28.1

Carers would like relevant and immediate information and support. Case study 28.2 looked at some of the basic information requirements that carers have. However, as noted in the carer and practitioner voices at the start of the chapter, there are times when there are conflicts between what information the carer requires and what nurses are confident about sharing.

Lindon (2007) noted that information received by carers about their relative/friend's diagnosis, treatment and rehabilitation is where carers and professionals most often experience conflict. Individual interpretations and professional perceptions of patient confidentiality were consistently cited as a major barrier to ideal carer involvement in the care planning process, with dissatisfaction regarding requests for greater information making carers feel resentful and mistrustful of services (Cree et al., 2015).

For nurses, some of the difficulties about confidentiality and information sharing relate to ethical and legal obligations, with a breach of confidence potentially resulting in disciplinary or legal proceedings. Carers usually do not have a right to receive information from the clinical team (with the exception of where withholding information might put others at risk). This can only be done if the service user agrees to the information being shared. It should be noted that this duty of confidentiality also applies to information received from carers.

Cree et al. (2015) suggest that barriers are erected because of perceived rather than actual confidentiality issues, and these limit participation and dialogue between carers, users and professionals. Professionals are not always confident about where the limits of confidentiality lie, and further training about legal requirements may be beneficial. An alternative suggestion from Wynaden and Orb (2005) is for mental health services to introduce confidentiality procedures.

--- # CHAPTER SUMMARY ---

This chapter has covered the following ideas:

- Carers perform a major role in modern society. Approximately 10% of the UK population refer to themselves as carers with an estimated 1.5 million people caring for someone with a mental health problem. This caring role supports people with mental health problems to live in the community.
- Carers are likely to experience significant levels of distress and also have reduced social, employment, financial and leisure activities. Carers perceive that their role is not appreciated by society at large and can be dissatisfied by their contact with health professionals.
- There is some evidence that carer interventions increase carers' satisfaction with services and also their knowledge about mental health problems, potential ways of dealing with difficulties arising from their caring role, and of mental health services. However, there is a poor evidence base by which to evaluate the effectiveness of carer interventions. There is a need for more research on carer-focused interventions examining which interventions work for whom, where and when.
- Mental health nurses have a very important role to play in working with carers to assist in the care of service users and to alleviate the burdens and frustrations that carers have as part of their caring role. Mental health nurses are often the health professional that has most contact with carers. Carers are more satisfied and engaged with nurses (and services) with good interpersonal skills, who actively provide assistance and who are skilled and knowledgeable about carer support.
- Although the Department of Health has a stated aim that carers are involved in all aspects of the service design and delivery of mental health services, there is limited evidence that this occurs in practice.
- Mental health nurses have the opportunity to get involved in providing advice, support and training to carers either through involvement (as clinicians or researchers) in existing types of carer interventions or in areas where development in new types of carer intervention may occur. There is also a potential role for mental health nurses in the development of the carer voice.

BUILD YOUR BIBLIOGRAPHY

Books

- Lefley, H. & Wasow, M. (eds) (2013) *Helping families cope with mental illness.* Abingdon: Routledge.
- Lobban, F. & Barrowclough, C. (eds) (2009) *A casebook of family interventions for psychosis.* Chichester: John Wiley.
- Wilde, H. (2013) Working with families and carers. In I. Norman and I. Ryrie (eds) *The art and science of mental health nursing.* Buckingham: Open University Press. pp. 383-392.

SAGE journal articles

FURTHER
READING:
JOURNAL
ARTICLES

Go to https://study.sagepub.com/essentialmentalhealth for further free online journal articles related to this chapter. If you are using the interactive ebook, simply click on the book icon in the margin to go straight to the resource.

- Burns, T., Catty, J., Harvey, K., et al. & the ECHO Group (2013) Continuity of care for carers of people with severe mental illness: results of a longitudinal study. *International Journal of Social Psychiatry, 9*(7), 663-670.
- Crowe, A. & Lyness, K. (2014) Family functioning, coping, and distress in families with serious mental illness. *The Family Journal, 22*(2), 186-197.
- Polo-Lopez, R., Echeburia, E., Berry, K., et al. (2014) Piloting a cognitive-behavioral intervention for family members with individuals living with severe mental disorders. *Behavior Modification, 38*(5), 619-635.

Weblinks

FURTHER
READING:
WEBLINKS

Go to https://study.sagepub.com/essentialmentalhealth for further weblinks related to this chapter. If you are using the interactive ebook, simply click on the book icon in the margin to go straight to the resource.

- Carers Trust Professionals: https://professionals.carers.org - offers a wide range of resources and information for anyone who works with carers, including access to the Triangle of Care report
- Mind-psychosis information-contains reliable and up-to-date information about psychosis for family members and friends: www.mind.org.uk/information-support/types-of-mental-health-problems/psychosis/for-friends-and-family/#.WhsH6bp2vD4
- Rethink Mental Illness: www.rethink.org/home - links to the charity site which gives advice and information on mental health issues to services users, carers and professionals.

ACE YOUR ASSESSMENT

ONLINE
QUIZZES &
ACTIVITY
ANSWERS

Revise what you have learned by visiting https://study.sagepub.com/essentialmentalhealth. If you are using the interactive ebook, simply click on the tick icon to go straight to the resource.

- Test yourself with multiple-choice and short-answer questions and flashcards.

REFERENCES

Atkinson, J. & Coia, D. (1995) *Families coping with schizophrenia*. Chichester: John Wiley.

Bhui, K., Warfa, N., Edonya, P., et al. (2007) Cultural competence in mental health care: a review of model evaluations. *BMC Health Services Research*, 7, 15.

Couldwell, A. & Stickley, T. (2007) The Thorn Course: rhetoric and reality. *Journal of Psychiatric and Mental Health Nursing*, 14(7), 625–634.

Cree, L., Brooks, H., Berzins, K., et al. (2015) Carers' experiences of involvement in care planning: a qualitative exploration of the facilitators and barriers to engagement with mental health services. *BMC Psychiatry*, 15, 208.

Curran, J. & Brooker, C. (2007) Systematic review of interventions delivered by UK mental health nurses. *International Journal of Nursing Studies*, 44(3), 479–509.

Dallos, R. & Draper, R. (2015) *An introduction to family therapy: Systemic theory and practice*. Buckingham: Open University Press.

Department of Health (2008) *National carers strategy*. London: DH. Available at: www.gov.uk/government/publications/the-national-carers-strategy (accessed 19.11.17).

Duckworth, K. & Halpern, L. (2014) Peer support and peer-led family support for persons living with schizophrenia. *Current Opinion in Psychiatry*, 27(3), 216–221.

Kuipers, E., Onwumere, J. & Bebbington, P. (2010) Cognitive model of caregiving in psychosis. *British Journal of Psychiatry*, 196, 259–265.

Lazarus, R. (1993) Coping theory and research: past, present and future. *Psychosomatic Medicine*, 55, 234–257.

Lefley, H. (1996) *Family caregiving in mental illness*. Thousand Oaks, CA: Sage.

Lindon, D. (2007) *Carer support in forensic services: A scoping exercise*. London: Princess Royal Trust for Carers.

Lucksted, A., Medoff, D., Burland, J., et al. (2013) Sustained outcomes of a peer-taught family education program on mental illness. *Acta Psychiatrica Scandanavica*, 127(4), 279–286.

MacInnes, D., Beer, D., Reynolds, K., et al. (2013) The support needs of carers whose relative/friend is cared for by inpatient forensic mental health services. *Journal of Mental Health*, 22(6), 528–535.

Macleod, S., Elliott, L. & Brown, R. (2011) What support can community mental health nurses deliver to carers of people diagnosed with schizophrenia? Findings from a review of the literature. *International Journal of Nursing Studies*, 48, 100–120.

NHS Confederation (2014) *The future's digital: Mental health and technology*. London: NHS Confederation. Available at: www.nhsconfed.org/~/media/Confederation/Files/Publications/Documents/the-futures-digital.pdf (accessed 03.11.17).

National Institute of Health and Care Excellence (2014) Psychosis and schizophrenia in adults: Prevention and management. NICE guidelines (CG178). Available at: www.nice.org.uk/guidance/cg178 (accessed 03.11.17).

Pharoah, F., Mari, J., Rathbone, J., et al. (2010) Family intervention for schizophrenia. *Cochrane Database of Systematic Reviews*, 12, CD000088.

Pickard, L. (2015) A growing care gap? The supply of unpaid care for older people by their adult children in England to 2032. *Ageing and Society*, 35(1), 96–123.

Radcliffe, J., Adeshokan, E., Thompson, P., et al. (2012) Meeting the needs of families and carers on acute psychiatric wards: a nurse-led service. *Journal of Psychiatric and Mental Health Nursing*, 19(8), 751–757.

Rowe, J. (2012) Great expectations: a systematic review of the literature on the role of family carers in severe mental illness, and their relationship and engagement with professionals. *Journal of Psychiatric and Mental Health Nursing, 19*(1), 70–82.

Schene, A. (1990) Objective and subjective dimensions of family burden. *Social Psychiatry and Psychiatric Epidemiology, 25*, 289–297.

Seikkula, J. & Arnkil, T. (2014) *Open dialogues and anticipations: Respecting otherness in the present moment.* Tampere, FL: National Institute for Health and Welfare.

Smith, L., Onwumere, J., Craig, T., et al. (2015) Mental and physical illness in caregivers: results from an English national survey sample. *British Journal of Psychiatry, 205*(3), 197–203.

Victor, E. (2009) *A systematic review of interventions for carers in the UK: Outcomes and explanatory evidence.* London: Princess Royal Trust for Carers.

Wynaden, D. & Orb, A. (2005) Impact of patient confidentiality on carers of people who have a mental disorder. *International Journal of Mental Health Nursing, 14*, 166–171.

SELF-HELP AND PEER SUPPORT IN RECOVERY

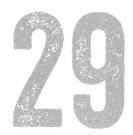

ALAN SIMPSON AND SUSAN HENRY

THIS CHAPTER COVERS

- Discussion of the context within which self-help and peer support take place
- Appreciation of the complexity of peer support roles
- Understanding of the need for organisational systems to support innovations
- Review of relevant research evidence
- The means by which peer support effects change and positive outcomes

---

In my experience as a service user, I have become accustomed to professionals trying to 'fix' and steer my recovery. This led to me feeling like I was broken with no hope or ability of living the life I wanted. However, in learning to accept myself with my condition and trying to hold myself accountable in a way that allows me to effectively live on my own terms, I have shaped my own recovery and now support others in doing so.

When I was introduced to the service users, having the words 'support worker' in my title, there was an expectation that I was there to 'do' things for them. But in peer support, the approach that we use in our role is 'being'. In being, I allow myself to be honest and acknowledge mental health issues without apologies. This allows service users to accept themselves based on their own personal narrative.

In group discussions, service users decide on the topics most relevant to them and we share our tools and stories of recovery. The sharing of our lived experience is then used by service users to self-advocate within ward rounds and care planning meetings. Working in this 'being' way enables the service user to redefine themselves beyond the limits of psychiatry, choosing how to manage their life as a whole individual rather than a service user alone.

This has had a positive effect on those who have engaged in peer support because we're peers: we get it!

Isha, peer support worker

INTRODUCTION

Self-help and **peer support** have played a part in the **recovery** of people with mental health problems and **addictions** for a very long time. This has often been provided informally and with little or no structured organisation. Individuals or groups of people with shared life experiences have found comfort, reassurance and confidence through sharing mutual experiences and providing support to one another in a variety of ways (Faulkner & Layzell, 2000). Mutual or peer support amongst users of mental health services also takes place informally within shared spaces such as inpatient wards or day centres and can include keeping each other safe (Quirk et al., 2004; Jones et al., 2010).

At times, the benefits of such informal support have led people to arrange more structured support or to organise local support groups or organisations, sometimes going on to link with others to create networks of shared knowledge and mutual empowerment. Self-help groups can be in the form of small independent user-led groups, self-help groups within larger organisations such as mental health charities Together, Mind and Rethink, or larger networks such as **Depression** Alliance, Bipolar UK and Hearing Voices Network. Similarly, there are long-standing groups and networks based on the 12 Steps programme, including Overeaters Anonymous, Alcoholics Anonymous and Narcotics Anonymous. Increasingly, self-help and peer support initiatives are being established for minority ethnic and marginalised groups (Faulkner & Kalathil, 2012), including people with mental health problems who are **lesbian**, gay, **bisexual** or **transgender**. With the growth of internet support and social media, people are increasingly turning to online groups that can provide flexibility and easy access alongside shared experiences, advice and support. The anonymity and intensity of online interactions can present its own challenges and often facilitation and moderation are useful (Faulkner, 2013).

HEARING VOICES NETWORK

The Hearing Voices Network offers information, support and understanding to people who hear voices and those who support them. Psychiatry traditionally refers to hearing voices as 'auditory hallucinations', but research shows that there are many explanations for hearing voices. Many people begin to hear voices as a result of extreme stress or trauma. The Network aims to:

- raise awareness of voice hearing, visions, tactile sensations and other sensory experiences
- give men, women and children who have these experiences an opportunity to talk freely about this together
- support anyone with these experiences seeking to understand, learn and grow from them in their own way.

The Network tries to achieve these aims by:

- promoting, developing and supporting self-help groups
- organising and delivering training sessions for health workers and the general public
- creating spaces to talk openly about experiences
- providing telephone information and regular newsletters. (Adapted from Hearing Voices Network: www.hearing-voices.org)

FIND OUT MORE

HEARING VOICES NETWORK

Mental health **service user/survivor** Alison Faulkner (2013) and colleagues acknowledge that the terms peer support, self-help and mutual support are often used interchangeably. Different groups place emphasis on different things, for example: learning and sharing strategies for dealing with particular symptoms or conditions, addressing social inclusion, taking part in campaigning or engaging in social activities. Seebohm et al. (2010) suggest that peer support and self-help groups are both characterised by mutual aid and reciprocity, but that different people or groups may prefer different terminology reflecting motivations or **culture**. Faulkner (2013) points out that the current political climate favours peer support, so groups may be pragmatically adopting this language to attract funding.

Self Help UK (see *Going further* at the end of the chapter) is an organisation that helps create, support and promote self-help groups. It suggests that people often find it useful to talk to others facing similar issues or experiences, whether that's dealing with a long-term medical condition, mental health problem or facing a life-changing experience like bereavement. Self-help groups are people who come together to offer and receive support.

People go to self-help support groups for many different reasons. Some simply want information and will then move on, while others may want to make sense of what is happening to them by sharing their experiences with those who have been through something similar.

Over the last decade, peer support has swiftly become established as a core component of modern mental health service provision in the UK and many other countries. Peer support includes support or services provided to people with mental health problems by other people who have experienced mental health problems themselves (Davidson et al., 2006). People with personal lived experience of mental distress, specific mental conditions and/or service use deliberately and constructively draw on these experiences to support and guide others in their recovery. Underpinning peer support is the concept of **co-production** and more equal relationships:

> Peer support is a system of giving and receiving help founded on key principles of respect, shared responsibility, and mutual agreement of what is helpful. Peer support is not based on psychiatric models and diagnostic criteria. It is about understanding another's situation empathically through the shared experience of emotional and psychological pain. (Mead, 2003: 1)

As outlined above, peer support has long been a component of support provided by many service-user-led organisations, charities and voluntary organisations working outside of statutory mental health services. Increasingly, however, many of these organisations are providing peer support as complementary services alongside or within governmental services. Faulkner (2013) identified a variety of initiatives in England across these various sectors, with peer workers providing social support, crisis support, advice and advocacy. And now peer workers are increasingly found in roles traditionally occupied by professional or support staff, such as case management, outreach work and providing support on discharge from hospital (Lawn et al., 2008; Pitt et al., 2013; Simpson et al., 2014).

Internationally, a wide range of peer support approaches have been enacted (Miyamoto & Sono, 2012; Myrick & del Vecchio, 2016). Peer support programmes and peer specialist roles have been developed and incorporated into state-run services in the USA (Sabin & Daniels, 2003; Clay et al., 2005; Bluebird, 2008; Kaufman et al., 2012), in Canada (Mental Health Commission of Canada, 2012), Australia (Centre of Excellence in Peer Support, 2011), New Zealand (MHC, 2012) and increasingly across Europe. The Scottish Recovery Network initiated some of the first peer support within UK mental health services (McLean et al., 2009). Training courses and certified programmes have been established alongside policies and procedures for the employment, support and payment of peer support workers (PSWs) in community and inpatient mental health services (Repper & Watson, 2012a; Gillard et al., 2013; Simpson et al., 2013).

In England, to some extent congruent with the ideological favouring of self-reliance, peer support is now included in government policy for mental health, such as *No Health Without Mental Health* (Department of Health, 2011), as one way in which people can be supported to manage their own mental health. The more critical Schizophrenia Commission (2012) also specifically recommended that all mental health providers explore opportunities to develop specific roles for peer workers. The promotion of peer support has been central to the work of the Implementing Recovery through Organisational Change (ImROC) programme, tasked with developing recovery-focused organisations (Shepherd et al., 2010; Repper et al., 2013). It is hard to credit that less than 30 years ago peer support was advocated almost solely on the radical wings of mental health service user movements (Chamberlin, 1978).

ROLE: WHAT DO THEY DO? PEER SUPPORT AND RECOVERY

The contribution of specific peer roles varies, depending on the requirements of employing organisations, the service users being offered the service and the settings in which peer support takes place (Gillard et al., 2014, 2015a). But the core **values** of acceptance, respect, empathy, support, companionship and hope typically underpin the sharing of experiences and ideas about how to cope with mental distress and promote recovery (Mead et al., 2001; also see Case studies 29.1 and 29.2).

Julie Repper and others at Nottingham have been at the forefront of developing and writing about peer support roles within mental health services in England (e.g. Repper & Watson, 2012a). Repper and Watson (2012b) studied the support provided by six peer support workers to 83 people over a six-month period, finding five broad types:

Emotional support involved finding out what a person was going through and sharing similar experiences, often using anecdotes, humour and sharing **coping mechanisms**. This appears to increase self-esteem and confidence for service users.

Practical support covers a wide range of interventions, including help in sorting out finances and welfare benefit entitlements; support accessing domestic violence or housing services; using public transport or encouraging and supporting engagement with education or training courses. Frequently, such support comes about through building relationships, enabling people to talk about their related fears and anxieties.

Social support involved encouraging service users to participate in or set up activities, such as sewing or horticulture classes, or discussing and sharing joint interests with peer workers such as music, poetry and art. Attending exhibitions or other events, or jointly attending women's groups or faith groups, or supporting contacts with family members were other activities that had a positive impact on developing social networks, motivation, confidence and self-esteem.

Support specific to care built on trusting relationships to help people access mental health services and better understand certain processes. Peer-to-peer discussions of medication and issues around care provision eased interactions with mental health staff during assessments, admissions and discharge. The peer support role, with increasing mutual understanding, also afforded exploration of early signs of relapse and how best to plan to mitigate or manage these.

Support specific to recovery was probably the most common type of support described by peer support workers, drawing on personal experiences to discuss and adapt methods of **coping** to guide service users through their own recovery. PSWs spent time working through recovery plans, explaining and reframing recovery language and ideas to better relate to individuals' personal experiences.

Similar interactions were reported in a study of peer support for people being discharged from hospital in east London (Simpson et al., 2014). Helpful support included face-to-face and telephone interactions and socialising (e.g. going for a coffee, to an exhibition or swimming); practical and emotional support that included reassurance and encouragement; mentoring, which included increasing life skills such as using a computer or emails, and building self-confidence; being a confidante through active listening; and sharing a mental bond or connection. Service users found peer workers to be respectful, encouraging and empathic and 'more like a friend' than a worker. They also valued their independence from the core clinical team (Simpson, 2013).

In a survey of peer support roles and activities in the USA, Salzer et al. (2010) found the most frequently reported role was sharing personal experiences and mutual aid. Peer workers also encouraged people to take more responsibility for their lives, focusing on health and wellness; addressing hopelessness; assisting in communications with service providers; providing education about **illness** management; and combating **stigma** in the community. Aside from peers providing emotional and practical support and aiding recovery, it has also been suggested that the very process of sharing experiences in common with others is empowering and has the potential to lead to a greater social and political awareness, and to campaigning and activism (Faulkner & Basset, 2010).

CASE STUDY 29.1

Working with transitions

Adele is based in the enhanced primary care team, working with service users who have been discharged from secondary mental health services and who are transitioning back to care under their GP. Adele provides 1-2-1 support meetings with service users in the community to discuss issues relating not only to their recovery but also to the feelings that come up when mental health support is being withdrawn. In these instances, Adele utilises her training and lived experience to provide reassurance, normalising anxious feelings that the transition evokes. She works with people to identify objectives related to all aspects of their life, including mental wellbeing.

Adele is also a service user who has recently been discharged from secondary care. Her meetings with service users provide opportunities for an exchange of ideas that assists both parties in their recovery journeys.

TRAINING AND ORGANISATIONAL SUPPORT FOR PEER SUPPORT ROLES

In Gillard et al.'s (2015a) comparative case studies of the implementation of peer support roles across a range of organisations and settings, a number of issues were identified as being universally important. These included a formal recruitment process and provision of training specifically designed for the peer worker role (Repper & Watson, 2012a; Simpson et al., 2013). These demonstrate that the role is a 'proper job' and allow opportunities to explore applicants' ability and willingness to draw on experiences or share recovery stories, whilst being sensitive to working with people who may not yet be able to talk about their experiences. Training is also an important element in the evolution of an occupational or work identity; a socialisation process whereby individuals identify with their 'professional' group, developing group norms and values (McNeil et al., 2013; Clarke et al., 2015).

Preparation of clinical teams and organisational support aligned with the expectations and values of PSWs is important. There can be a mismatch between peer workers working towards a recovery agenda and host organisations committed to more traditional medicalised psychiatry (McLean et al., 2009; Moran et al., 2013).

IMPORTANCE OF TRAINING

A core aspect of peer support is a robust training programme. All our Peer Support Workers (PSWs) must successfully complete training before they can formally provide peer support. Training provides PSWs with an opportunity to develop skills and learn, but it also allows facilitators to assess potential peer support workers.

Susan Henry, peer support coordinator

Many trainees are keen to 'give back' to mental health services and to support other service users so they do not have to experience difficulties previously faced by trainees. There is a real desire to make things right for users of mental health services. The training, however, encourages a more nuanced way of supporting peers. Instead of 'doing', the emphasis in the working relationship moves to simply 'being': completely opening oneself up to exploring and truly hearing the peers' personal narrative; the parts about mental health and treatment, and the parts about any other aspect of their life; the words that don't seem on the surface to be relevant and those so obviously imbued with intense meaning. This trust in exploring the narrative of other service users is with the explicit intention of supporting a process of recovery. With these complex skills tried and tested in a supportive training environment peer workers can begin to offer new approaches to support. With time, health care professionals can learn and begin to emulate the examples of relationship building demonstrated by those with a lived experience.

Susan Henry, peer support coordinator

CASE STUDY 29.2

Supporting staff

Shah is a PSW based in a specialist community mental health service, working with hard-to-reach service users who may also have additional complex needs, including a forensic history. He regularly attends ward rounds for the service users he is supporting. He works closely with the ward consultant and, using his lived experience, provides a service user perspective which encourages those involved in care review to take a holistic approach to the service users' mental wellbeing. Shah has direct experience of care on a PICU ward and under assertive outreach services. He uses this knowledge to offer insight into the complicated feelings that being sectioned might evoke, and how staff might best respond.

Shah's presence in ward rounds and his contributions to discussions have meant that service users' voices remain at the centre of discussions and that staff develop a deeper, more rounded understanding of mental health and treatment.

Gillard et al. (2015a) highlight some of the potential tensions around the introduction of peer support roles: professionalism and boundaries.

Being 'professional', as in working to a good standard, is valued but, for some, professionalism becomes associated with over-formalising the role or diluting some core qualities. For many, the peer role is about being different, about *not* being part of the establishment. Similarly, whilst the importance of peer workers maintaining certain boundaries is uncontroversial, there may be different understandings amongst teams about appropriate boundaries; regarding degrees of self-disclosure, for example. For some staff, retaining a certain distance is a key part of maintaining a 'professional' relationship. Such caution is often imbued in professional training and codes of practice, designed to protect both service users and staff (NMC, 2009; Griffith, 2013).

But peer workers are being asked to straddle tensions between drawing on lived experiences and mutuality and the expectation of a more formal professional–patient relationship. This is more akin to *friendship* – whilst not being friendship; as certain restrictions remain, such as not having sexual relationships with peers. In an interview study with recently employed PSWs, a complex situation was described where the peer workers were in 'a position of ambiguity and uncertainty' (Beech, 2011: 287), possessing a *liminal* identity (Turner, 1959, 1969), somewhere 'betwixt and between' the multiple roles performed in being service users, 'friends' and staff (Simpson et al., in press). Many of the rituals that usually lubricate journeys of occupational socialisation (Beech, 2011) may be more nuanced and complex for PSWs. Hence, attempts to 'professionalise' the role may be problematic, necessitating careful thought to ensure individuals' wellbeing and the future success of peer support initiatives. It is important that different beliefs and expectations of peer support roles are discussed within services where PSWs are becoming part of the team and that all staff are supported to constructively manage these tensions (Simpson et al., 2017). A trend towards formalisation and professionalisation of these roles raises concerns about the representativeness of those involved (Enany et al., 2013) or dilution of the original organic essence of community-based mutual support (Faulkner & Kalathil, 2012).

EVIDENCE FOR PEER SUPPORT

A number of positive outcomes of peer support in mental health services have been identified (Repper & Carter, 2011). Benefits for service users include: reduced hospital admissions; increased empowerment, social support and social functioning; empathy, acceptance and hope; and reduced stigma. Benefits for PSWs include: aiding continuing recovery; personal growth; development of skills and the therapeutic effect of helping others; and, for paid PSWs, the benefits of being employed (Faulkner & Bassett, 2010; Miyamoto & Sono, 2012; Walker & Bryant, 2013).

In a systematic review and meta-analysis of 18 randomised controlled trials of non-residential peer support interventions involving 5597 participants, Lloyd-Evans et al. (2014) drew cautious conclusions. The trial interventions were divided into mutual (reciprocal) peer support groups (n = 4), peer support services (n = 11) and peer-delivered mental health services (n = 3). There was substantial variation between trials in participants' characteristics and programme content, making comparisons difficult. Moreover, outcomes were often incompletely reported and there was little or no follow-up data, creating a high risk of bias. Conclusions stated that there was little evidence that peer support was associated with positive effects on hospitalisation, overall symptoms or satisfaction with services, but some evidence that peer support was associated with positive effects on measures of hope, recovery and empowerment at and beyond the end of the intervention. However, this was not consistent within or across different types of peer support.

Whilst accepting the paucity of well-designed studies and strong evidence for peer support, it is worth reflecting that the most positive outcomes identified in the above review concerned concepts that have been most clearly linked with peer support, such as hope, recovery and empowerment. Outcomes such as re-admission rates and reduction in symptoms are perhaps less directly influenced by mutual support and are more a target for and affected by a range of treatment and organisational factors, such as the availability of effective medications, psychological therapies and crisis support, or indeed impacted by prevailing socio-economic conditions.

In light of their findings, Lloyd-Evans et al. (2014) recommended that further peer support programmes should be implemented within the context of high-quality research projects in order to ensure that strong evidence is provided to support any claims for the effectiveness and further roll-out of peer support. This suggestion was echoed by the National Institute for Health and Care Excellence (NICE, 2014) in its treatment and management guidelines for adults with **psychosis** and **schizophrenia**.

A US systematic review assessed the level of evidence and effectiveness of peer support services delivered by people in recovery to those with serious mental illness or co-occurring mental and substance use **disorders** (Chinman et al., 2014). This review included a greater variety of studies than some earlier reviews (e.g. Pitt et al., 2013), which excluded quasi-experimental trials. It identified 20 studies, including 11 RCTs, across three service types: peers added to traditional services, peers in existing clinical roles and peers delivering structured education and self-management programmes such as Wellness Recovery Action Plans (WRAP) (Petros & Solomon, 2015). The quality of evidence for each type of peer service was deemed moderate, suggesting value in the consideration of effectiveness (Dougherty et al., 2014). Many studies had methodological weaknesses and outcome measures varied. Effectiveness varied by service type. A majority of studies in services where peers were added or where they delivered curricula showed improvement favouring peer support workers. Compared with professional staff, peer workers were better able to reduce inpatient use and improved a range of recovery outcomes. Just one study reported a negative impact. The effectiveness of peer workers in existing clinical roles like case management or assertive outreach was mixed. Chinman et al. (2014: 429) concluded that peer support services have demonstrated some 'notable outcomes' but future studies would need to be of better quality and focus.

The inclusion and exclusion criteria of different reviews determine the papers and results considered, and the quality of the included research should have a strong bearing on our consideration of the outcomes reported. In light of this, our best case scenario appears to be that there is moderate evidence for peer workers being added to existing services and teams to improve recovery-focused outcomes, and that peers delivering structured education and self-management programmes may be beneficial. However, as with many complex interventions, there remain major challenges in designing and delivering the highest quality research to provide rigorous evidence for peer support.

Claims have also been made for the cost savings of employing peer workers (Trachtenberg et al., 2013), albeit on the basis of very little data and even more limited methodology (Simpson et al., 2014). Whilst some studies suggest the potential for value for money of employing PSWs, this is not the same as showing statistical evidence of cost-effectiveness from a properly conducted cost-effectiveness analysis (Simpson et al., 2014).

MECHANISMS OF CHANGE IN PEER SUPPORT

The above review suggests that peer workers may well be having a positive impact on various outcomes for service users. Why might this be? With this in mind, Gillard et al. (2015b) drew on their study of peer support across a range of statutory and voluntary sector mental health services in England to model the change mechanisms underlying peer worker interventions.

Drawing on and analysing in-depth interviews with 71 peer workers, service users, staff and managers, the authors identified core processes within the peer worker role that were productive of change for service users supported by peer workers. The key processes were: (i) building trusting relationships based on shared lived experience; (ii) role modelling individual recovery and living well with mental health problems; and (iii) engaging service users with mental health services and the community:

(i) Building trusting relationships based on shared lived experience:

Peer workers build trusting relationships based on shared lived experience, first making a connection by talking about their lived experiences of mental health problems or of using services, enabling the peer worker and the service user to recognise a similar or shared experience. Next, the peer worker demonstrates an understanding of the service user's experiences based on their own lived experience, and in so doing validates the service user's experiences. Once the relationship is established, it seems important that peer workers allow people to initiate disclosure, rather than requiring it from them. Service users then often feel able to talk openly about their experiences and to listen to advice.

(ii) Role modelling individual recovery and living well with mental health problems:

Once a relationship is established, peer workers perform a role-modelling function, demonstrating their own recovery and ability to function well socially. This provides a sense of hope for the future – that peer workers have moved on from where service users currently see themselves. For some, the fact that the peer worker role is a job of work is important and being able to work in a caring role represents acknowledgement of the individual's usefulness and value. This acts as a powerful symbol of recovery. The role-modelling function also seems to challenge the internalised self-stigma often experienced by service users. It further supports increased self-care, resilience, empowerment and self-efficacy, enabling service users to take more control over their lives and to function better socially as a result.

(iii) Engaging service users with mental health services and the community:

Peer workers can act as a bridge between service users and other mental health professionals, extending trust across the clinical team and opening up discussions about difficult personal issues. Peer workers are also able to facilitate service users' engagement with the community, often by directly supporting people to attend activities outside of mental health services, breaking isolation and increasing the range and quality of social contacts people experience as a result.

These mechanisms are further explained by Gillard et al. (2015b) through the theoretical literature on role modelling and relationships in mental health services and explored in relation to some of the wider peer support literature. Social Comparison Theory (Festinger, 1955) describes the importance of comparing others with our own sense of self. By sharing lived experiences, peer workers first normalise those experiences for service users and then, where the peer worker is perceived as doing better by comparison, can promote feelings of hope and optimism for the future of the service user.

Bandura's (1977) Social Learning Theory suggests that significant others provide compelling role models of how to think, feel and act, determining motivation, behaviour and change. The individual pays attention to modelled behaviour that is relevant and has value, and is motivated to replicate this. Such processes, for example, may underpin the student nurse–mentor relationship. If an individual sees someone similar to them succeed, this can increase their own self-efficacy and self-esteem by empathic reinforcement (Bandura, 1997). So, by providing a socially and personally valued role, the peer worker shows a positive alternative to that of service user or patient.

Finally, many service users appear to have difficulties forming close relationships with family and friends and in establishing rapport with professional staff. This may often be underpinned by difficulties in early attachment and familial relationships. Gillard et al. (2015b) suggest that peer workers, through showing genuine understanding, validation and respect, might be able to form relational bonds with service users that underpin the therapeutic alliance (Bordin, 1979). This is important as therapeutic alliance has been shown to reinforce attachment to the mental health team (Catty et al., 2011) and predict engagement in treatment (McCabe & Priebe, 2004; Priebe & McCabe, 2006). If so, the added value that peer workers bring to enable such relationships may encourage engagement with wider mental health services and help explain some of the tentative positive outcomes reported above.

APPLICATION TO PRACTICE

Increasingly, mental health nurses and students will encounter, work alongside and liaise with peer workers in a range of settings. Peer support workers may be supporting and advocating for service users in various inpatient wards including forensic settings; supporting people in the transition between inpatient and community care, liaising with or being employed as part of home treatment, community or primary care mental health teams; or working to support people living at home, in supported accommodation or through a variety of mental health charities and voluntary sector or self-help organisations.

For some mental health staff, peer workers may be seen as threatening or slightly destabilising. On the one hand, they are most often working within a recovery model and extolling the value of lived experience of mental distress and service use to provide understanding, support and guidance and to promote recovery. This can be challenging to the more traditional professional–service user relationship where the expertise is seen to reside in the knowledge, training and wisdom of the health care professional and perhaps a more biomedical approach to care and treatment. Some staff may respond cautiously or even defensively to this new way of working. This may be particularly so in times of system reorganisation and financial pressures on services when jobs are being reduced or there is increased competition for limited resources. At such times, the introduction of peer workers may be seen as an economic threat to more expensive staff and, understandably, a professional protectionism may emerge (Simpson, 2013). At worst, indifference or even hostility may be shown to peer workers, which can damage relationships and create significant barriers to effective working (Bradstreet & Pratt, 2010).

However, most often mental health nurses and their colleagues embrace the involvement of peer workers and see the merits of including expertise through lived experience within or alongside the **multi-disciplinary team**, and quickly recognise the benefits this can bring to the engagement and recovery of service users. The evidence suggests that service users often like and value peer support workers and perceive greater empathy, understanding and respect from peer workers than they do from many professional staff. This can help create a more open and trusting relationship, which then empowers people to share their experiences and anxieties and to take more personal responsibility for recovery, building self-belief and self-efficacy, focusing on interests, strengths and recovery goals. By modelling recovery, peer workers imbue and raise hope.

So what should we do as mental health nurses and students? First, we should welcome and respect peer support workers and value what they can contribute in supporting service users in their recovery. We should aim to discover the peer support services that are available locally. We should point people towards such services and **advocate** for their greater involvement in service delivery, alongside the skills and expertise of mental health nurses and other professional staff who each bring their unique combination of personalities, knowledge, education, training and skills (Sainsbury Centre for Mental Health, 1997). Where required, we should encourage the development of local protocols and care pathways to improve access to and interactions between peer support and mainstream mental health services.

More than that, mental health nursing students can take the opportunity in their clinical placements to share information and ideas with peer support workers, aim to contact and visit local peer support services, seek out opportunities for role shadowing and participate in any joint training offered. There is much we can learn from peer support workers and there is much we can share and discuss to maximise the chances of effective recovery-focused working that enables people to achieve the hopes and goals they have for their futures.

CRITICAL DEBATE 29.1

Many people fear that becoming a peer support worker will be too stressful for people with personal experience of mental distress and service use and may lead to relapse. What factors should we consider to ensure the wellbeing of all staff, whether peer support workers, mental health nurses or others?

CHAPTER SUMMARY

This chapter has covered:

- The key concepts and overlaps between self-help and peer support
- Some of the self-help available for people with mental health problems
- Understanding the peer support role and what it offers
- A summary of the research evidence of the benefits of peer support
- An understanding of some of the limitations of the research evidence
- Possible psychological mechanisms underpinning peer support
- Some of the opportunities and challenges for mental health nurses and students in working in partnership with peer support workers.

BUILD YOUR BIBLIOGRAPHY

Books and reports

- Copeland, M.E. and Mead, S. (2004) *Wellness recovery action plan and peer support: Personal, group and program development.* Dummerston, VT: Peach Press. From the USA, but a very accessible book on some approaches to recovery-focused action plans and peer support.

- Faulkner, A. (2013) *Mental health peer support in England: Piecing together the jigsaw*. London: Mind. Available at: www.mind.org.uk/media/418953/Peer-Support-Report-Peerfest-2013.pdf. This report provides a very useful overview of self-help and peer support in England and is written in a very accessible style by a leading service user researcher.
- Watkins, P. (2007) *Recovery: A guide for mental health practitioners*. London: Churchill Livingstone. A smashing book written by an experienced mental health nurse explaining how to work with service users in a recovery-focused way.

SAGE journal articles

FURTHER
READING:
JOURNAL
ARTICLES

Go to https://study.sagepub.com/essentialmentalhealth for further free online journal articles related to this chapter. If you are using the interactive ebook, simply click on the book icon in the margin to go straight to the resource.

- Dark, F., Patton, M. & Newton, R. (2017) A substantial peer workforce in a psychiatric service will improve patient outcomes: the case for. *Australasian Psychiatry*, online.
- Deegan, P.E. (2005) The importance of personal medicine: a qualitative study of resilience in people with psychiatric disabilities. *Scandinavian Journal of Public Health*, 33(66 suppl.), 29–35.
- Scott, A. (2011) Authenticity work: mutuality and boundaries in peer support. *Society and Mental Health*, 1(3), 173–184.

Weblinks

FURTHER
READING:
WEBLINKS

Go to https://study.sagepub.com/essentialmentalhealth for further weblinks related to this chapter. If you are using the interactive ebook, simply click on the book icon in the margin to go straight to the resource.

- Rethink Mental Illness: Recovery: www.rethink.org/living-with-mental-illness/recovery – recovery means different things to different people. This site looks at what recovery can mean for some, the differences between types of mental health recovery, and some research and resources.
- Scottish Recovery Network: www.scottishrecovery.net/resource/welcome-to-our-new-website – a fantastic new website with lots of useful resources about recovery.
- Self Help UK: www.selfhelp.org.uk/home – Self Help UK is a unique organisation which helps create, support and promote self-help groups.

VEDEO
LINK 29

Video links

- Benefits of being in a self-help group: www.youtube.com/watch?v=LeO9t5SPNmA – people from independent self-help groups in Nottingham and Nottinghamshire talking about their experiences of being in a self-help group. People were asked for the reasons they attend a group and how it has helped change their lives. All the groups interviewed are supported by Self Help Nottingham.
- Peer2Peer: A route to recovery for people with mental illness through peer support training and employment (https://vimeo.com/151912074) is a short film that describes Peer2Peer, a European Union-funded partnership project to train people with lived experience of mental health problems to support others in their recovery.
- Shery Mead Intentional Peer Support: A personal retrospective at the Experts by Experience conference 2011: https://vimeo.com/36079409 – international author, trainer and peer support expert Shery Mead talks about her personal experiences.

ACE YOUR ASSESSMENT

Revise what you have learned by visiting https://study.sagepub.com/essentialmentalhealth. If you are using the interactive ebook, simply click on the tick icon to go straight to the resource.

ONLINE
QUIZZES &
ACTIVITY
ANSWERS

• Test yourself with multiple-choice and short-answer questions and flashcards.

REFERENCES

Bandura, A. (1977) *Social learning theory*. Englewood Cliffs, NJ: Prentice-Hall.

Bandura, A. (1997) *Self-efficacy: The exercise of control*. New York: Freeman.

Beech, N. (2011) Liminality and the practices of identity reconstruction. *Human Relations, 64,* 285–302.

Bluebird, G. (2008) *Paving new ground: Peers working in inpatient settings*. Alexandria, VA: National Technical Assistance Centre, National Association of State Mental Health Program Directors.

Bordin, E. (1979) The generalizability of the psychoanalytic concept of the working alliance. *Psychotherapy, 16,* 252–260.

Bradstreet, S. & Pratt, R. (2010) Developing peer support worker roles: reflecting on experiences in Scotland. *Mental Health and Social Inclusion, 14,* 36–41.

Catty, J., Cowan, N. & Poole, Z. (2011) Attachment to the clinical team and its association with therapeutic relationships, social networks, and clinical well-being. *Psychology and Psychotherapy, 85,* 17–35.

Centre of Excellence in Peer Support (2011) *The charter of peer support*. Hawthorn, VIC: Centre of Excellence in Peer Support.

Chamberlin, J. (1978) *On our own: Patient-controlled alternatives to the mental health system*. New York: Hawthorne Books.

Chinman, M., George, P., Dougherty, R.H., et al. (2014) Peer support services for individuals with serious mental illnesses: assessing the evidence. *Psychiatric Services, 65*(4): 429–441.

Clarke, C., Martin, M., de Visser, R., et al. (2015) Sustaining professional identity in practice following role-emerging placements: opportunities and challenges for occupational therapists. *British Journal of Occupational Therapy, 78,* 42–50.

Clay, S., Schell, B., Corrigan, P.W., et al. (2005) *On our own together: Peer programs for people with mental illness*. Nashville, TN: Vanderbilt University Press.

Davidson, L., Chinman, M., Sells, D., et al. (2006) Peer support among adults with serious mental illness. *Schizophrenia Bulletin, 32*(3), 443–450.

Department of Health (2011) *No health without mental health: A cross-government mental health outcomes strategy for people of all ages*. London: HMSO.

Department of Health (2012) *No health without mental health: Implementation framework*. London: HMSO.

Dougherty, R.H., Lyman, D.R., George, P., et al. (2014) Assessing the evidence base for behavioural health services: introduction to the series. *Psychiatric Services, 65,* 11–15.

Enany, N.E., Currie, G. & Lockett, A. (2013) A paradox in healthcare service development: professionalization of service users. *Social Science & Medicine, 80,* 24–30.

Faulkner, A. (2013) *Mental health peer support in England: Piecing together the jigsaw*. London: Mind. Available at: www.mind.org.uk/media/418953/Peer-Support-Report-Peerfest-2013.pdf (accessed 08.03.17).

Faulkner, A. & Basset, T. (2010) *A helping hand: Consultations with service users about peer support*. London: Together. Available at: www.together-uk.org/aboutus/peer-support (accessed 08.03.17).

Faulkner, A. & Kalathil, J. (2012) *The freedom to be, the chance to dream*. London: Together. Available at: www.together-uk.org/wp-content/uploads/2012/09/The-Freedom-to-be-The-Chance-to-dream-Full-Report1.pdf (accessed 08.03.17).

Faulkner, A. & Layzell, S. (2000) *Strategies for living: A report of user-led research into people's strategies for living with mental distress*. London: Mental Health Foundation.

Festinger, L. (1955) A theory of social comparison processes. *Human Relations, 7*, 117–142.

Gillard, S.G., Edwards, C., Gibson, S.L., et al. (2013) Introducing peer worker roles into UK mental health service teams: a qualitative analysis of the organisational benefits and challenges. *BMC Health Services Research, 13*(1), 188.

Gillard, S., Edwards, C., Gibson, S., et al. (2014) New ways of working in mental health services: a qualitative, comparative case study assessing and informing the emergence of new peer worker roles in mental health services in England. *Health Service Delivery Research*. 2 (19)

Gillard, S., Holley, J., Gibson, S.L., et al. (2015a) Introducing new peer worker roles into mental health services in England: comparative case study research across a range of organisational contexts. *Administration & Policy in Mental Health*, 42(6): 682–694.

Gillard, S.G., Gibson, S.L., Holley, J. et al. (2015b) Developing a change model for peer worker interventions in mental health services: a qualitative research study. *Epidemiology and Psychiatric Sciences, 24*(5), 435–445.

Griffith, R. (2013) Professional boundaries in the nurse–patient relationship. *British Journal of Nursing, 22*(18): 1087–1088.

Jones, J., Nolan, P., Bowers, L., et al. (2010) Psychiatric wards: places of safety? *Journal of Psychiatric and Mental Health Nursing, 17*(2), 124–130.

Kaufman, L., Brooks, W., Steinley-Bumgarner, M., et al. (2012) *Peer specialist training and certification programs: A national overview*. Austin, TX: University of Texas at Austin Centre for Social Work Research.

Lawn, S., Smith, A. & Hunter, K. (2008) Mental health peer support for hospital avoidance and early discharge: an Australian example of consumer driven and operated service. *Journal of Mental Health, 17*(5), 498–508.

Lloyd-Evans, B., Mayo-Wilson, E., Harrison, B., et al. (2014) A systematic review and meta-analysis of randomised controlled trials of peer support for people with severe mental illness. *BMC Psychiatry, 14*, 39.

McCabe, R. & Priebe, S. (2004) The therapeutic relationship in the treatment of severe mental illness: a review of methods and findings. *International Journal of Social Psychiatry, 50*, 115–128.

McLean, J., Biggs, H., Whitehead, I., et al. (2009) *Evaluation of the delivering for mental health peer support worker pilot scheme*. Edinburgh: Scottish Government Social Research.

McNeil, K.A, Mitchell, R.J. & Parker, V. (2013) Interprofessional practice and professional identity threat. *Health Sociology Review, 22*, 291–307.

Mead, S. (2003) *Defining peer support*. Available at: www.parecovery.org/documents/DefiningPeerSupport_Mead.pdf (acessed 08.03.17).

Mead, S., Hilton, D. & Curtis, L. (2001) Peer support: a theoretical perspective. *Psychiatric Rehabilitation Journal, 25*(2), 134–141.

Mental Health Commission (2012) *Blueprint II: Improving mental health and wellbeing for all New Zealanders – making change happen*. New Zealand: MHC.

Mental Health Commission of Canada (2012) *Changing directions, changing lives: The mental health strategy for Canada*. Calgary: Mental Health Commission of Canada.

Miyamoto, Y. & Sono, T. (2012) Lessons from peer support among individuals with mental health difficulties: a review of the literature. *Clinical Practice & Epidemiology in Mental Health, 8*, 22–29.

Moran, G.S., Russinova, Z., Gidugu, V., et al. (2013) Challenges experienced by paid peer providers in mental health recovery: a qualitative study. *Community Mental Health Journal, 49*, 281–291.

Myrick, K. & del Vecchio, P. (2016) Peer support services in the behavioural healthcare workforce: state of the field. *Psychiatric Rehabilitation Journal, 39*, 197–203.

National Institute for Health and Care Excellence (2014) *Psychosis and schizophrenia in adults: Prevention and management*. NICE Guideline (CG178). Available at: www.nice.org.uk/guidance/cg178 (accessed 08.03.17).

Nursing and Midwifery Council (2009) *Guidance on professional conduct: For nursing and midwifery students*. London: NMC.

Petros, R. & Solomon, P. (2015) Reviewing illness self-management programs: a selection guide for consumers, practitioners, and administrators. *Psychiatric Services, 66*, 1180–1193.

Pitt, V., Lowe, D., Hill, S., et al. (2013). Consumer-providers of care for adult clients of statutory mental health services. *Cochrane Database of Systematic Reviews, 3*, CD004807.

Priebe, S. & McCabe, R. (2006) The therapeutic relationship in psychiatric settings. *Acta Psychiatrica Scandinavica, 113*, 69–72.

Quirk, A., Lelliott, P. & Seale, C. (2004) Service users' strategies for managing risk in the volatile environment of an acute psychiatric ward. *Social Science and Medicine, 59*(12), 2573–2583.

Repper, J. & Carter, T. (2011) A review of the literature on peer support in mental health services. *Journal of Mental Health, 20*, 392–411.

Repper, J. & Watson, E. (2012a) A year of peer support in Nottingham: lessons learned. *The Journal of Mental Health Training, Education and Practice, 7*(2), 70–78.

Repper, J. & Watson, E. (2012b) A year of peer support in Nottingham: the peer support workers and their work with individuals. *The Journal of Mental Health Training, Education and Practice, 7*(2), 79–84.

Repper, J., Aldridge, B., Gilfoyle, S., et al. (2013) *Peer support workers: Theory and practice*. London: IMROC.

Sabin, J.E. & Daniels, N. (2003) Strengthening the consumer voice in managed care: VII. The Georgia peer specialist program. *Psychiatric Services, 54*(4), 497–498.

Sainsbury Centre for Mental Health (1997) *Pulling together: The future roles and training of mental health staff*. London: Sainsbury Centre for Mental Health.

Salzer, M.S., Schwenk, E. & Brusilovsiy, E. (2010) Certified peer specialist roles and activities: results from a national survey. *Psychiatric Services, 61*, 520–523.

Seebohm, P., Munn-Giddings, C. & Brewer, P. (2010) What's in a name? A discussion paper on the labels and location of self-organising community groups, with particular reference to mental health and black groups. *Mental Health and Social Inclusion, 14*(3), 23–29.

Shepherd, G., Boardman, J. & Burns, M. (2010) *Implementing recovery: A methodology for organisational change*. London: Sainsbury Centre for Mental Health.

Simpson, A. (2013) *The Eileen Skellern Lecture: Peers, professionals and politics – mental health nursing in an age of austerity*. London: City University, 12 June.

Simpson, A., Flood, C., Rowe, J., et al. (2014) Results of a pilot randomised controlled trial to measure the clinical and cost effectiveness of peer support in increasing hope and quality of life in mental health patients discharged from hospital in the UK. *BMC Psychiatry, 14*, 14–30.

Simpson, A., Oster, C. & Muir-Cochrane, E. (2017) Liminality in the occupational identity of mental health peer support workers: a qualitative study. *International Journal of Mental Health Nursing*, online. Available at: www.ncbi.nlm.nih.gov/pubmed/28548455 (accessed 12.08.17).

Simpson, A., Quigley, J., Henry, S.J., et al. (2013) Evaluating the selection, training, and support of peer support workers in the United Kingdom. *Journal of Psychosocial Nursing and Mental Health Services, 52*, 31–40.

The Schizophrenia Commission (2012) *The abandoned illness: A report by the Schizophrenia Commission.* London: Rethink Mental Illness.

Trachtenberg, M., Parsonage, M. & Shepherd, G. (2013) *Peer support in mental health care: Is it good value for money?* London: Centre for Mental Health and Mental Health Network/NHS Confederation.

Turner, V. (1959) *The ritual process: Structure and anti-structure.* Chicago: Aldine.

Turner, V. (1969) *From ritual to theatre: The human seriousness of play.* Chicago: Aldine.

Walker, G. & Bryant, W. (2013) Peer support in adult mental health services: a metasynthesis of qualitative findings. *Psychiatric Rehabilitation Journal, 36*, 28–34.

THERAPEUTIC COMMUNITIES, DEMOCRACY AND THE NEW RECOVERY MOVEMENT

30

JENELLE CLARKE, NICK MANNING, GARY WINSHIP AND SIMON CLARKE

THIS CHAPTER COVERS

- A definition of democratic approaches within mental health and an introduction to the core principles that underpin therapeutic communities (TCs)
- An exploration of some of the tensions and limitations of using TCs within a medical model
- An explanation of how a democratic approach works in practice within TCs
- An introduction to Enabling Environments (EE) and the New Recovery movement
- A critical reflection of how EEs and the New Recovery movement build on the TC approach.

> I would say that the therapeutic community approach is the most intensive treatment method we have at our disposal in the field of mental health today. Peplau talked about the 'other 23 hours' at Chestnut Lodge in the 1930s, in other words you can do intensive psychotherapy in an hour, but Peplau said what about if you do therapy across the whole day, at meal times, when we share tasks and so on? Since then a wide range of professionals have developed and adapted the TC model, sometimes with more elements of psychoanalysis, sometimes with more emphasis on ecology and social living, and other times with more emphasis on creative arts. But always the approach seeks to maximise client potential, with peer support and democratisation as key elements. I've trained in a number of modalities in the field, and I've worked across a range of different settings delivering ECT to CBT to DBT, but in the end I am convinced that the therapeutic community model is the greatest attainment in the history of psychiatry and mental health.
>
> **Gary Winship, mental health nurse and associate professor**

> It is like having a full-time job, it is. We have over 30 hours of therapy plus a week. Because quite often you have individual things like, for instance, today I've met with my key worker twice with an hour each so two hours I've had with her, aside from all the other stuff we do, and then meeting with yourself as well, so it's like a full-time job and it can be very draining at times. Especially when the community's going through difficult periods […] which has increased my sort of avoidant behaviours, but that's my stuff you know. Yeah, I think overall it's really beneficial, because it holds the mirror up to you, it has made me see the impact of my behaviour on other people and become horrified actually at what I've done to my family, to nurses looking out for me, to my partner, and that's obviously going to help me, prevent me from doing anything again. You know? I mean I'm sure it's not a 100% full-proof thing but it's definitely helping me to not do anything, act upon it, urges again, and I'm talking about them more. But you are on 24-hour call here so you can be woken up at any time of the night and I've been in meetings at 3 o'clock in the morning.
>
> **Alison, therapeutic community client**

INTRODUCTION

This chapter introduces democratic ways of working within mental health, specifically therapeutic communities (TCs), which are planned social **environments**, and the New **Recovery** movement, which includes participant involvement and social approaches to mental health. Claims that New Recovery represents a paradigm shift for mental health need to be tempered against the backdrop of TCs. The chapter begins by defining social approaches within mental health and introduces TCs, providing a brief history and current framework. You will learn how democracy works in practice within communities by exploring everyday life in TCs. By comparing the New Recovery movement with TCs, you will also be able to recognise the similarities of the approaches, including using wounded healers, flattened hierarchies, user involvement and cost-leaness. Other approaches to recovery are also considered here, including the traditions of **addiction** recovery approaches, Mutual Recovery, an arts-based approach to mental health, and Enabling Environments (EEs), an accredited award which recognises social principles that promote wellbeing. We propose a meta-recovery framework which organises and categorises the variety of recovery approaches. This meta-recovery model is presented as a guide for gauging which types of recovery approaches might be most suitable for which client population. By the end of the chapter, you will be able to reflect on the future of democratic approaches to mental health as we move forward.

DEMOCRACY IN MENTAL HEALTH CARE: INTRODUCING THERAPEUTIC COMMUNITIES

Democratic approaches to mental health care often recognise the importance of **service user** involvement within their therapy and therapy service. Current mental health policy in the UK particularly **values** service user empowerment and service user voice within mental health. This approach, such as that seen by the New Recovery movement, seeks to diminish the role of expert staff members, and proposes that education rather than therapy is central to the process of recovery. In order to achieve this learning, the responsibility for the administrative and therapy goals of a service are shared between service users and staff. Aspects of the service are also open to question, challenge and discussion by all members. It does not mean that staff members cease to have clinical responsibility for the wellbeing of service users, but that aims, definitions and notions of therapy are collaboratively and jointly agreed between staff and service users. New Recovery can be compared and contrasted with the progress of the therapeutic community movement which, over the last 60 years, has also been committed to changing the role of expert, user involvement and theoretical co-construction. But before comparing New Recovery and TCs, we will first introduce and explain the TC model of therapy.

Therapeutic communities (TCs) are planned social environments that see every social interaction in the life of the community as an opportunity for personal change. In keeping with a democratic approach, everyone in the community – both staff and service users – plays an active role in the therapeutic process. TCs recognise that social relationships can contribute to some forms of mental distress and, as such, they view networks as potentially helpful in restoring individual mental health (Boyling, 2011). Additionally, TCs seek to have an open, democratic environment whereby all aspects of community life are open to question by both staff and service users (Spandler, 2009). TCs mainly originated in hospital settings and have evolved into a variety of contexts: independent/voluntary communities, prisons, children's homes and day centres, addictions and learning disabilities. Communities focus on a range of issues, including **personality disorders**, eating disorders, alcoholism, gambling addiction, **psychosis**, drug addiction and a range of other personal and mental health related matters.

HISTORY OF THERAPEUTIC COMMUNITIES

Present-day adult mental health TCs can mainly be traced back to the period post-Second World War and two separate but related approaches. The first approach was that of Thomas Main, a psychiatrist at Northfield Military Hospital, who developed a social therapeutic model of treating traumatised soldiers returning from the war (Holmes, 2005). After concluding that one-to-one counselling interventions were ineffective, Main introduced the idea of using the whole hospital to therapeutically treat patients and, in doing so, found that hospital institutions could be therapeutic (Main, 1977). It was Main who coined the term 'therapeutic community' as an approach that defined a way of using all elements within the hospital community as potentially therapeutic. Institutions as therapeutic required giving clients a voice in their treatment, something that was unusual at the time, and supporting the staff to understand the suffering of service users, and equally, helping the service users understand the perspective of the staff. In other words, both groups had to work closely together to create a '**culture** of enquiry' to resolve daily interpersonal tensions within a community context (Main, 1977: 11). This was a significant shift that required staff to relinquish some power and adapt their role to respond directly to patient need. Importantly, it also deviated from the 'medical model' of mental health whereby the health professional knows best and the service user must comply with treatment (Main, 1980). By broadening the balance of power within the community, service users could openly question and challenge staff members. At the Cassel Hospital, this approach became known as psychosocial nursing (Barnes, 1968).

Taking a slightly different approach was Maxwell Jones, working at Mill Hill, then later the Belmont Hospital (renamed as the Henderson Hospital). Instead of the therapist at the centre of TCs, Jones emphasised social learning as a central feature (Jones, 1952). Jones (1968: 70) describes as 'social learning' that 'little understood process of change which may result from interpersonal interaction'. Thus, a tea and coffee break, lunchtime or smoking break are all considered potential therapeutic moments because of the social interactions that may occur within them. The two different approaches of Main and Jones prioritised a social, rather than a medical, model of mental distress. They did not ignore individual causes of distress, but they acknowledged that social environments and interpersonal relationships, such as traumatic events and abusive relationships, contribute to mental breakdown. This idea in many ways contradicted historic notions and practices of responding to mental distress. By using a social approach to treatment, both staff and patients work together to achieve personal change. Staff are expected to show their vulnerability and relinquish (some) professional power, whilst patients take an active role not only in their own therapy but also that of others.

CRITICAL THINKING STOP POINT 30.1

How do TCs differ from a medical model of mental health, and what can a social approach add to our understanding of mental distress and treatment?

CRITICAL
THINKING
STOP
POINT 30.1
ANSWER

VALUES OF THERAPEUTIC COMMUNITIES

Despite the diversity of TCs, they all share common values. Rapoport (1960) defined four common principles inherent in TCs based on his work at the Henderson Hospital (previously the Belmont Hospital): democratisation, permissiveness, communalism and reality confrontation. Like Main, Rapoport suggested that the community itself was the 'doctor', rather than an individual with specific psychiatric qualifications. The first principle, democratisation, suggests that both staff and clients should hold an equal share of power in regards to the TC's decision making. For staff, this requires that they relinquish some power so that service users can share in decisions around therapeutic and administrative processes. Permissiveness in a TC means tolerating behaviours and ways of interacting that may be considered 'distressing' or 'deviant' according to 'ordinary' standards (Rapoport, 1960: 58). Communalism identifies that the TC functions according to close interpersonal relationships whereby staff and clients mix freely together over meals, outings, meetings, etc. Lastly, reality confrontation means that clients are given continuous feedback as to how their behaviour impacts on others in order to challenge unhelpful self-beliefs and behaviours.

More recently, Haigh (2013) updated Rapoport's core principles to include five important 'experiences' to promote emotional health: attachment, containment, communication, inclusion and agency. Overlapping with Rapoport's original four principles, Haigh suggests that TCs promote a culture of belonging whereby troubling and distressing behaviours are contained. Communities should promote open communication between all members of the TC and everyone should feel equally included. The concept of agency extends Rapoport's democratisation to include negative forms of power and self-empowerment alongside shared decision making. Haigh's reconceptualisation of the principles of TCs not only updates them for modern practice, but, significantly, it also identifies belonging, inclusion and power (positive, negative and self-power) as key components to TCs alongside democracy, tolerance and open communication.

> I'd done CBT before, I didn't find that particularly helpful. But with as far as group therapy, no this was the first thing I'd done. I mean it's very beneficial though, it has been. It's very different because, I've like had one to one therapy and stuff like that but you're only getting feedback from one person and sometimes it can be a bit biased and stuff so here you're getting advice from people who have really been through stuff as well. So it's been yeah, I've learned a lot in the last year.
>
> **Ian, service user**

One of the key distinguishing values of TCs is that personal change is considered a social, rather than an individual, process. All community members, both staff and service users, together share the responsibility for the overall running of community life and for the community promoting an environment of therapeutic transformation. Such an approach means that therapy is continuously occurring within a TC. All aspects of life are open to question, interpretation, challenge and discussion as a community.

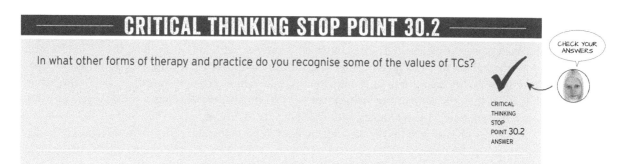

CRITICAL THINKING STOP POINT 30.2

In what other forms of therapy and practice do you recognise some of the values of TCs?

CHECK YOUR ANSWERS

CRITICAL THINKING STOP POINT 30.2 ANSWER

PERSONALITY DISORDERS AND THERAPEUTIC COMMUNITIES

CASE STUDY: JEAN

Whilst TCs are found in a variety of contexts, in adult mental health they have become particularly associated with treatment for those with a diagnosis of personality disorder. Personality disorder (PD) is characterised by a cluster of symptoms, including relational instability, risky behaviour including **self-harm** and suicide attempts, and emotional deregulation (Stalker et al., 2005). Perceptions regarding clinical treatment and effectiveness are mixed, and psychopharmacological treatments, in particular, show little evidence of treatment effectiveness (Gask et al., 2013). TCs have emerged as specialised treatment interventions for those with a diagnosis, in part because they acknowledge that social environmental factors, such as unhelpful life experiences, contribute to symptoms characteristic of PD (Johnson et al., 1999). With an emphasis on prosocial relation and group therapy as a staple of practice, TCs have been particularly effective in managing hostilities and providing a significant reduction in violence (Winship & Hardy, 2007).

Nonetheless, there are tensions with the treatment of PD within TCs. Whilst TCs have developed a more socially progressive approach to PD that views distress and symptoms as a logical response to experiences such as abuse and trauma, it does mean that TCs perpetuate the notion that PD is an **'illness'** that must be treated and contained by mental health professionals, reminiscent of the medical model of mental distress (Spandler, 2006). This is especially problematic as there are significant controversies surrounding the notion of PD as a diagnostic category (Pilgrim, 2001). Both theorists and service users have critiqued the notion and purpose of the diagnostic category of PD (Pilgrim, 2001; Kinderman et al., 2013). By accepting PD as an illness to be treated, it is much more difficult for TCs to critique notions of PD. Furthermore, in a social approach, TCs are also open to the critique that symptoms of PD are 'abnormal', and that TCs therefore regulate societal conceptions of normality (Spandler, 2006).

Whilst this chapter is not intending to challenge conceptions of PD, it must be acknowledged that TCs are not a 'gold' standard in confronting mental distress such as PD, despite their recognition that distress is rooted in earlier experiences. There are difficulties, tensions and contradictions within them that they have not adequately addressed as they juxtapose their social approach with a medical model.

Limitations and criticisms of the TC approach

In addition to some of the tensions involved in using a social approach within a medical model, TCs have faced several criticisms since the time of both Main and Jones. The **anti-psychiatry** movement of the 1960s and 1970s saw TCs adopt a permissive culture, such as in Kingsley Hall, led by R.D. Laing and Joseph Berke. However, during the 1980s and 1990s, the mainstream culture within mental health moved away from the permissiveness seen at communities such as Kingsley Hall and Paddington Day Centre. Prominent criticism of TCs emerged, including Ken Kesey's (1962) fictional account of life in a TC in *One Flew Over the Cuckoo's Nest*. His book was followed by Baron's (1987) study of Paddington Day Hospital, a London-based day community, which presents a particular narrative of how power is used within a TC. Baron argues that the TC's use of psychoanalysis imposed a negative self-view of clients that stifled any meaningful discussion and debate because service users' voices could be ignored in favour of staff psychoanalytic interpretations. Moreover, with no formal rules, the TC used a form of psychotherapy that was manipulative and ultimately destructive for the TC and its service users (Baron, 1987). Baron's account of Paddington was later reinterpreted by Spandler (2006), who argues that rather than the community being a bad TC, it highlights the tensions in using psychoanalysis, which uses interpretivist techniques, within democratic communities.

Rapoport's research and his four key principles of TCs also highlight that there are some contradictions between TC theory and TC practice (Whiteley, 2004). First, contradictions in the staff team as to what constitutes change could also create tension and confusion amongst the staff team and client group. Second, despite the declaration of equality, some clients could become overly dependent on staff members (Whiteley, 2004). Many of these tensions and difficulties continue to be a challenge for contemporary TCs. Additionally, like Paddington in Baron's account, there continues to be a gender imbalance, with a primarily dominant male TC lead with female nursing and support staff. This problem is also reflected in TC research, whereby white, male clinicians' voices, including those of Main, Jones, Rapoport, Whiteley, Kennard, Haigh and Hinshlewood, dominate the history and developments of TCs.

Nonetheless, TCs have evolved to reflect health policies and changes within mental health. For instance, present day TCs need to produce evidence-based research (Pearce et al., 2017) and compliance with audits and quality assurance standards (Kennard & Lees, 2012). In addition, since 2003, the Community of Communities (CofC), a project that is part of the quality assurance branch of the Royal College of Psychiatrists (2016a), has accredited communities as TCs. The accreditation process is rigorous, requiring careful justification as to how a particular community meets the TC criteria; communities must also apply for accreditation every three years. In between accreditation visits are annual peer reviews that are carried out by members of other accredited TCs.

CRITICAL THINKING STOP POINT 30.3

What are some of the tensions of using a social approach to mental health, when much of mental health is based within a medical model?

DEMOCRACY IN PRACTICE WITHIN TCS

Using a social approach to addressing mental health problems, such as personality disorder, is often challenging for both staff and service users as all aspects of everyday life are considered therapy. The question arises as to how life in a TC actually works in practice, particularly the role of client members in supporting one another. The excerpt below, from Clarke's (2015) ethnographic research with two TCs for individuals with a diagnosis of personality disorder, highlights how clients in a residential community supported each other during a mealtime:

Conversation around the table feels up beat. There is talk about Margaret's (Staff) dog, cooking, food, etc. Andrea eats very, very slowly whilst staring intently at all those around the table. She has a napkin in front of her with writing on it. I see that it says, 'I DO deserve to eat'. Staff later tell me that Tessa wrote it for her. This is because Andrea has voices telling her that the food is poison and that she doesn't deserve to eat. Yesterday Tessa had suggested cheerleading statements at dinner reminding her that she deserves to eat. Tessa said that eventually it will be helpful to put it in her own handwriting but for now, having a member of the community write it out may help [...] Andrea gets up to throw out her juice. She sits down and then asks Julie if she can have some of her fruit smoothie. Julie nods and brings the drink containers out of the fridge so Andrea can choose her flavour [...] At one point Anna moves down to sit near Andrea and speaks to hear in low, soft voices. I cannot hear what they were saying but Andrea manages to eat. (Residential TC, Winter 2013)

What is striking about this mealtime is the active role that service users play in helping one another through the meal. Service users do not wait for staff to step in with offers of support but, rather, are often the first ones to share their experiences, suggest solutions or offer encouragement to one another. By holding back and letting the service users respond first, staff are providing a safe space for service users to actively shoulder the responsibility of community life. However, this does not mean that staff members are silent, or do not offer any guidance or support to service users. For instance, during community meetings, which are often chaired by service users, staff members provide feedback, question service users and encourage them to discuss difficult and painful issues with the whole community.

This second short excerpt illustrates how tensions are discussed, though not always immediately resolved, during community meetings. All service users and often all available staff members attend community meetings in TCs, though this may vary from TC to TC. Service users chair meetings but everyone can provide feedback, raise questions, express concern and provide encouragement and support. In this community meeting, the discussion was around biscuits and whether over-eating and comfort eating should be monitored and challenged in the same way as under-eating:

Jessie explains she was very angry that the food shoppers bought biscuits. This turned into a big discussion about food with most people jumping in with opinions. Jessie is pushing for a ban on biscuits, whilst others of the group think it should be more measured, but also acknowledge that it's not fair to let others eat biscuits and challenge Jessie to eat. They acknowledge the inconsistency. But policing food doesn't seem to be what anyone really wants either. However, Jessie is feeling that she is being watched, told to eat, etc. No one pushes for a decision on a biscuit ban but rather staff members suggest that it continue to be discussed and explored in the coming days. (Day Community, Summer 2013)

Of note here is that service users can bring issues to the meeting and, in this case, suggest a new rule for the community. However, staff members resisted holding a vote or decision about a biscuit ban and instead suggested that the community as a whole continue to explore what food means to all members. Their approach also dovetailed with a life-skills session on food, cooking, shopping and portion sizes, whereby all aspects of service users' relationship to food, and food preparations, were discussed. Crucially, service users were not just learning about food, but also about negotiation, boundaries, consistency, and how to sit with and continue to openly discuss uncomfortable emotions, such as anger and frustration.

As staff and service users work together in the process of therapeutic change, it is important to acknowledge that this process is not linear and involves disruptions, successes and setbacks. Care then must be taken when interpreting an individual's change process in order not to dismiss setbacks as an indicator that change is not taking place. Change in TCs is closely linked with addressing troubling past and present events. Often, there is the recognition that these unhelpful past experiences continue to influence the present and manifest in difficulties with interpersonal relationships and managing social encounters. Within a community context, Castillo et al. (2013) identify that change occurs through certain stages. These stages are referred to as the 'hierarchy of progress' and include: feelings of safety and trust; care; belonging; knowledge of boundaries; containment and skills; hopes, dreams and goals; achievements and transitional recovery (Castillo et al., 2013: 268). Some of these stages have links with Haigh's (2013) five key principles of TCs that also refer to things such as containment, belonging and empowerment. For example, like Haigh, they identify that joining a community can be a daunting experience for a newcomer. Building a sense of safety and belonging are key to building a rapport that will enable honesty and social learning. However, Castillo et al.'s (2013) pyramid expands Haigh's principles through recognising that certain social processes, especially learning the boundaries, recognising achievements and having goals and dreams for life after the community, are important components during a process of change.

LEGACIES OF TCS: ENABLING ENVIRONMENTS AND THE NEW RECOVERY APPROACH

The history of progressive approaches in mental health care and the ethos of TCs do exist in other mental health environments. Recovery in the field of substance misuse dates back to the 1950s and has been the foundation of organisations such as Alcoholics Anonymous (AA) and Narcotics Anonymous (NA). There are a whole range of recovery programmes in the substance misuse and eating disorders field, such as concept houses in the UK, Twelve-Step or Minnesota Model rehabs, as well as a large network of correctional institutions in the USA closely allied to milieu therapy and TCs. The Safewards model, developed by Bowers (2014: 503), **advocates** that staff on **acute** units take an 'inquisitive' approach with patients, whereby they are attentive to patient distress, behaviours, needs and absences. Bowers' approach is reminiscent of Main's 'culture of enquiry' discussed above, which also requires staff to question and respond to patient need and conflict within the environment. Additionally, Star Wards (2006), developed by former service user Marion Janner, emphasises patient involvement in their treatment and in the running of the ward. Patient involvement at this level shares similar principles proposed by Jones (1952, 1968), particularly the principle of flattened hierarchy. The Star Wards model also advocates twice-daily community meetings and maximising the amount of quantity, and quality, of patient and staff interactions in order to foster healthy relationships. Though recognising the limitations of a TC approach on acute wards, Star Wards nonetheless calls for wards to run in a TC style (Star Wards, 2006). Social environments such as these advocate user involvement, group approaches and negotiation, as in TCs.

Closely associated with TCs is the Enabling Environments (EE) initiative. EEs have their roots within the TC movement, as members of the Royal College of Psychiatrists (RCP) recognised that some of the values and social perspectives of TCs exist within other contexts outside the framework of traditional TCs. Johnson and Haigh (2011) explain that the Community of Communities project, part of the RCP, set up a working group to explore how the core standards of TCs could be applied to other organisations. In order to be inclusive of how different settings may be applying TC-like principles, the working group specifically avoided the terms 'therapeutic' and 'community' in favour of 'Enabling Environments' (Johnson & Haigh, 2011). EEs then evolved into a three-year award accredited by the RCP.

Whereas TCs are held together by common psychosocial theories, EEs are joined by 'human values' that can be widely applied to a variety of contexts (Royal College of Psychiatrists, 2016b). These values include 10 core standards, shown in Table 30.1.

Table 30.1 Core standards of Enabling Environments

Belonging	The nature and quality of relationships are of primary importance
Boundaries	There are expectations of behaviour and process to maintain and review them
Communication	It is recognised that people communicate in different ways
Development	There are opportunities to be spontaneous and try new things
Involvement	Everyone shares responsibility for the environment
Safety	Support is available to everyone
Structure	Engagement and purposeful activily are actively encouraged
Empowerment	Power and authority are open to discussion
Leadership	Leadership takes responsibility for the environment being enabling
Openness	External relationships are sought and valued

Source: Royal College of Psychiatrists, 2016b

There are clear overlaps with the core values of TCs but, importantly, EEs are not mental health specific. As such, the application of EE values is much more broad than tends to exist within TCs. Johnson and Haigh (2011) state that EEs ambitiously aim to apply shared purposes that value a social and relational approach to interaction and work that would be shared across various settings, including areas of education, government, health, private business and the voluntary sector. To date, organisations accredited with the EE award include wards, day units, schools, supported accommodation, voluntary groups, faith communities and workplace settings (Royal College of Psychiatrists, 2016b). EEs also have links with Psychologically Informed Environments (PIEs), which is an initiative that applies a social approach to homelessness, and Psychologically Informed Planned Environments (PIPEs) that apply a psychosocial framework to high secure settings such as prisons.

Another new recent recovery method is the Mutual Recovery programme (Crawford et al., 2013), which has been funded to the tune of £1.5 million by the Arts & Humanities Research Council (AHRC). Mutual Recovery, while owing some of its impetus to the New Recovery movement, is distinguished by the fact that the process of recovery is arts-based rather than educative. The array of arts-based interventions for the Mutual Recovery programme includes music, clay making and creative writing, and the interventions are led by artists and practitioners but not therapists per se. In an off-shoot from the AHRC research, there are some other innovative workshop-based creative activities such as drumming, Capoeira (a Brazilian martial art), music and comedy workshops (Crawford et al., 2013).

We can also consider a more general model of psychosocial health recovery that covers an array of recovery-facing therapies, which are established traditions in psychiatric and mental health services – for example, social rehabilitation, occupational therapies and psychological interventions that are geared towards general principles of health recovery informed literature from the allied field of social psychiatry, and psychiatric rehabilitation (Winship, 2014). The TC approach to crisis intervention and recovery also offers a compatible frame for the emerging **Open Dialogue** (2016) model, which is currently breathing new life into psychosocial approaches to supporting people with mental health problems (Carter, 2015). The Open Dialogue approach, which is being mooted as a new avenue for mental health social work, seeks to support individuals in the context of their network of relationships.

Table 30.2 A meta-recovery framework

Traditional Recovery	Addictions Recovery
When: 1880s-present	**When:** 1930s-present
Brief: Based on models of rehabilitation for hospitalized patients (Benbow & Bowers, 1998). Social psychiatry (Jones, 1968), community psychiatry, group therapy, therapeutic communities (Dietrich, 1976; Hinshelwood & Manning, 1979), psychosocial interventions	**Brief:** Large international network of addictions recovery approaches, often using Therapeutic Community principles. Peer self-help group movement committed to recovery and sobriety. Later Narcotics Anonymous. Most addiction recovery programmes emphasize the importance of staged steps towards recovery, and the importance of peer relationships, prosocial encounters in therapy which addresses the antisocial compulsions of substance misuse. Many addiction recovery programmes employ people 'in recovery' as therapists, experts by experience.
Theoretical orientation: Clinical recovery: diminution of symptoms (Onken et al., 2007; Harvey & Bellack, 2009), industrial therapy units (Wells, 2006), biological model, often accompanied by pharmacological intervention, although some non-pharmaceutical approaches (e.g. Soteria, Arbours). A range of psychological therapies deployed.	**Theoretical orientation:** 12-Step, Milieu Therapy, Minnesota Model, Concept House approach, TCs, relapse prevention, replacement prescribing (route to detoxification), correctional institutions (US).
Client suitability: including involuntary and detained, patients suffering more acute or severe episodes requiring more intensive interventions, hospitalization, residential treatment or day hospitals, secure treatments, therapeutic prisons.	Clients: people suffering from drug and alcohol problems, also other compulsions such as eating disorders or gambling.
New Recovery	**Mutual Recovery**
When: 1990s-present	**When:** 2011-present
Brief: National Health Service, Psychiatry, Recovery Colleges, non-residential, private entrepreneurships (especially US).	**Brief:** Initially Arts & Humanities Research Council funded research (£ 1.5million to establish and trial research looking across a range of arts-based interventions) focusing on third sector, independent, non-residential services including arts centres, galleries, libraries.
Theoretical orientation: Education focused, anti-therapy, Recovery Colleges, consumer led, entrepreneurial, co-construction, with a focus on hope-inspiring relationships, both with peers and staff (Slade, 2009). Recovery features social inclusion, clients are 'valued as human beings' and where staff offer belief in the person's ability and potential. Changing practice including risk assessment and redefining user involvement (Boardman & Shepherd 2009). Socially focused-based approaches that included strategies for facilitating a befriending, health information, social skill and life skills and so forth, with a strong Rogerian underpinning (Repper & Perkins, 2003).	**Theoretical orientation:** Artists take the lead in programme design and delivery. Current programmes include; music, clay sculpting and creative writing, photography, drumming, Capoeira, digital storytelling, yoga, reading circles, performance arts workshops (e.g. comedy, poetry) (Crawford et al., 2013).
Client suitability: people who are able to voluntarily engage with recovery and educative approaches, clients with longer term conditions that require less intensive intervention.	Client suitability: people who are able to voluntarily engage with recovery and interested in arts-based approaches, clients with longer term conditions requiring less intensive intervention.

Source: Winship, 2016, reproduced under the terms of the Creative Commons Attribution License

Taken together, these domains of recovery can be represented as a quadrant (see Figure 30.2) which graphically offers a meta-recovery model or framework.

CRITICAL THINKING STOP POINT 30.4

How have therapeutic communities overlapped with other approaches within mental health, including addictions?

CRITICAL
THINKING
STOP
POINT 30.4
ANSWER

A CRITICAL REVIEW OF NEW RECOVERY: SIMILARITIES AND DIFFERENCES WITH TC PRACTICE

Like the TC movement, the recovery movement has its roots in the vision of a number of charismatic leaders. Perhaps one of the differences between the TC movement and the recovery movement is that the recovery movement has placed greater significance on leaders being people who have been in recovery. Indeed, being in recovery is not quite requisite to leadership in the New Recovery movement, but it plays a vital role. The recovery movement emerged in tandem with an era of mental health which saw a revitalised acknowledgement of the reality that many practitioners were indeed 'wounded healers'. Mike Shooter, who was president of the RCP (1998–2005), went public about his own depression that had taken him to the brink of suicide at one time (Crane, 2003). And Phil Burnard, one of the leading professors of mental health nursing in the UK, likewise went public about his **depression**. There might be some pause for reflection here because many therapeutic community practitioners have themselves been in therapy as part of their training, and, in most likelihood, therapy has been rather more of a necessity than a training requirement. It is certainly one of the strengths of the TC movement that it has been built on the principle of the co-construction of theories of mental illness and recovery, with an increasing role of clients involved in research and education. And, as we have seen, there has been a public acknowledgement of wounded healers, which has been an asset for the New Recovery movement.

And also like ... I think the whole point of it is, something for me is not being able to put myself in other people's shoes and being quite selfish [...] And I think it is just about, because I think you do connect more and you tend to like listen more and it's been harder for me to put myself in other people's positions as well. Especially like with the therapists, people just see them as like they have no kind of back-story, they're just therapists. And I see that with kind of people in here as well, so it's nice to get to know behind the scenes as it were. And getting to know what they're like now as well. Because some of them have overcome problems that I'm still going through, so getting to hear about that, even in social time ... Just generally like when we're cooking, how do I do this, how do I do this, and having someone go right, you've got to do this,

(Continued)

> tip this and pour this and it's like, ohhhh. And it's like training you up. And it's like passing the stick on as well. Because the person that taught me is now gone, but when the next person comes in, I can teach them how to do stuff, if they don't already know. It's kind of like teaching, it's continuously passing it down. So it's quite nice.
>
> **Alice, service user**

One of the features of the New Recovery approach is that is has been carved, to some extent, out of the more individualistic tendencies of social entrepreneurism. Pat Deegan's work in the USA is largely a private industry, and although more lately recovery is being moulded into the NHS, there can be no doubt that the recovery method seeks to diminish state intervention – that is to say, professional input is being replaced by a peer-facing workforce. The aim is explicitly to reduce costs, and it is therefore welcomed by those who have budgets to manage. New Recovery commentators tell us that they are setting out to challenge what they perceive to be the pessimism of other traditional approaches, that the focus is on resilience rather than vulnerability (Friedli, 2009) and that the inclination is therefore positively focused on the resources people have at their disposal, or an 'assets-based approach' (Burns, 2011). We might think of recovery, then, with its lean cost-effectiveness, as a paradigm fit for austerity. But, on the other hand, we might wonder whether this canny commodification of health and welfare, under the rubric of **social capital**, is an unnerving example of the unabashed march of capitalism into the territory of the public sphere. The New Recovery movement dismisses state health expertise and hammers a nail into the disappearing ideal that health professionals should be equally and freely available to help the many. We might say that the concept of recovery has been appropriated as a justification for evolving cheaper mental health services, with user-led and **carer**-focused models being unreasonably expected to fill the gaps where professional health intervention should otherwise be (Warner, 2004).

But the idea of cost-efficiency has always been at the heart of therapeutic communities, and in many ways TCs have led the way In privileging the role of the client, and therein diminishing the role of the professional. Maxwell Jones was criticised for hiring social therapists, but it was an ingredient of cost-efficiency. Arguably, there needs to be some closer scrutiny of the New Recovery approach as to its claims of cost-efficiency compared to other approaches, but also of its politics and **ethics**. New Recovery emerges from an entrepreneurial politics, which envisions a small-state approach, with its roots in US individualistic ideologies, with a number of charismatic champions who, by virtue of their claims to expertise by experience, carry forward the message. Additionally, the New Recovery movement has a different conception of self-help and self-organisation by replacing the role of professionals (Repper & Perkins, 2003). In contrast, whilst TCs collaboratively seek a flattened hierarchy, they can be seen to be rooted in a collective ideological approach (Winship, 2004). The recovery approach has been strong on the rhetoric of service user involvement, whereas TCs have developed the means to put principles into practice through the use of formal democratic structures and quality checks, including service audit and review (Winship, 2013).

One of the most significant differences between the New Recovery approach and TCs might be considered in terms of what we think of as 'soft' versus 'tough' recovery. Whereas New Recovery presupposes client cooperation, TCs seem more equipped to work with clients who are more reluctant to engage, such as service users with a diagnosis of personality disorder, who are often labelled 'difficult to treat'. TCs and New Recovery both value **peer support** in the therapeutic process, but it appears that TCs begin with the notion that social inclusion is not a given. Instead, TCs acknowledge that social isolation lies at the root of many mental health problems and there are any number of steps and approaches to help a client engage with peers. TCs are particularly able to support a client to work through resistance to social engagement and address conflict in a way that seems remote in the approach of New Recovery.

HOW DO TCS DIFFER FROM A MEDICAL MODEL OF MENTAL HEALTH AND WHAT CAN A SOCIAL APPROACH ADD TO OUR UNDERSTANDING OF MENTAL DISTRESS AND TREATMENT?

Moving forward: lessons from TCs

Family trees are essential to root one in the present, and set tenure for the future. Here, TCs have done rather well in mapping and archiving progress, and the Planned Environment and Therapy Trust (PETT) is a vital resource which manages the history of TCs, archiving documents and research. The TC movement has long since understood the precariousness of charismatic leaders, and has instead in recent years focused more squarely on proof of concept, but nonetheless the TC movement has a long and distinguished roll of honour – people past and present who created the identity of TCs. The New Recovery movement by contrast seems to be almost without family lineage. Appearing as an immaculate conception, without recourse to allied and influencing trajectories, it might well have inadvertently written itself into a vacuum. TCs have survived as a method through building alliances and sustaining an inclusive ambient network that can embrace a range of recovery approaches, including a method for communities operating a 'discovery-facing' approach in working with children and young people. New Recovery, and associated approaches, might do well to reflect on the way in which the TC movement has been a model of sustainability against the backdrop of phases and fashions in the field of mental health.

CRITICAL DEBATE 30.1

Whilst TCs have endured through decades of changes within mental health, there are far fewer of them in mental health services than in the 1960s and 1970s. Some have argued that TCs are too expensive and others have argued that TCs lack scientific evidence that demonstrates they are clinically 'effective' (Gask et al., 2013), making them difficult for commissioners to justify funding. Other approaches to addressing mental distress have become very popular within the health service, such as cognitive behavioural therapy and dialectical behaviour therapy, which are much more inexpensive than a TC-type approach. Nonetheless, Maughan et al. (2016) showed that TCs were able to generate savings in financial costs for clients, reducing clients' need for A&E attendance, crisis mental health appointments and secondary health care. These issues raise the question, do TCs, and democratic TC-type approaches, still have relevance within mental health care?

CRITICAL DEBATE 30.1 ANSWER

--- **CHAPTER SUMMARY** ---

This chapter has covered:

- What a democratic approach within mental health means
- What a TC is, its values and historical roots
- The limitations of the TC approach, particularly in relation to PD
- How TCs have influenced other democratic approaches, including the New Recovery movement
- The key similarities and differences between TCs and the New Recovery movement.

--- **BUILD YOUR BIBLIOGRAPHY** ---

Books

- Ballatt, J. & Campling, P. (2011) *Intelligent kindness: Reforming the culture of healthcare*. London: Royal College of Psychiatrists. Ballatt and Campling outline the importance of kindness and compassion which can work to foster positive therapeutic change and healthy working environments through a community and social approach.
- Lees, J., Manning, N., Menzies, D., et al. (2004) *A culture of enquiry: Research evidence and the therapeutic community*. Therapeutic Communities 6. London: Jessica Kingsley. This edited book brings together a wide range of perspectives on aspects of TC research to further develop the 'culture of enquiry' that is inherent in a TC framework.
- Spandler, H. (2006) *Asylum to action: Paddington Day Hospital, therapeutic communities and beyond*. London: Jessica Kingsley. Spandler explores some of the aspirations and conflicts of the early TC movement by using the case study of Paddington Day Hospital, and examines the current tensions in modern therapeutic community practices and mental health services in general.

SAGE journal articles

FURTHER
READING:
JOURNAL
ARTICLES

Go to https://study.sagepub.com/essentialmentalhealth for further free online journal articles related to this chapter. If you are using the interactive ebook, simply click on the book icon in the margin to go straight to the resource.

- Fussinger, C. (2011) 'Therapeutic community', psychiatry's reformers and antipsychiatrists: reconsidering changes in the field of psychiatry after World War II. *History of Psychiatry, 22*(2), 146–163. Fussinger outlines the achievements of reformist psychiatrists within therapeutic communities in the 1950s and how their ideas were used by anti-psychiatrists in the 1960s.
- Pearce, S. & Pickard, H. (2013) How therapeutic communities work: specific factors related to positive outcome. *International Journal of Social Psychiatry, 59*(7), 636–645. Pearce and Pickard provide a useful explanation of how TCs work and can foster positive therapeutic change.
- Stevens, A. (2012) 'I am the person now I was always meant to be': identity reconstruction and narrative reframing in therapeutic community prisons. *Criminology & Criminal Justice, 12*(5), 527–547. Stevens explores desistance and personal change within forensic therapeutic communities through an understanding of individuals changing their narratives.

Weblinks

Go to https://study.sagepub.com/essentialmentalhealth for further weblinks related to this chapter. If you are using the interactive ebook, simply click on the book icon in the margin to go straight to the resource.

FURTHER READING: WEBLINKS

- Centre for Social Futures (2016): www.institutemh.org.uk/x-about-us-x/our-centres/centre-for-social-futures – the Centre for Social Futures is based at the Institute of Mental Health (Nottingham) and is a collaboration of researchers, health professionals, service users and carers to promote a social approach to mental health recovery
- Community of Communities (Royal College of Psychiatrists) (2016): www.communityof communities.org.uk – the Community of Communities (CofC) is the accrediting and quality assurance organisation for therapeutic communities, and the website explains more about different types of TCs and EEs, and their core values and ethos
- Consortium for Therapeutic Communities (TCTC) (2016): www.therapeuticcommunities.org – the TCTC is a membership charity for TCs and the website contains useful links about TCs and research within communities.

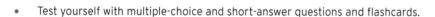

ACE YOUR ASSESSMENT

Revise what you have learned by visiting https://study.sagepub.com/essentialmentalhealth. If you are using the interactive ebook, simply click on the tick icon to go straight to the resource.

ONLINE QUIZZES & ACTIVITY ANSWERS

- Test yourself with multiple-choice and short-answer questions and flashcards.

REFERENCES

Barnes, E. (1968) *Psychosocial nursing: Studies from the Cassel Hospital*. London: Tavistock Publications.

Baron, C. (1987) *Asylum to anarchy*. London: Free Association Books.

Bowers, L. (2014) Safewards: a new model of conflict and containment on psychiatric wards. *Journal of Psychiatric and Mental Health Nursing, 21*(6), 499–508.

Boyling, E. (2011) Being able to learn: researching the history of a therapeutic community. *Social History of Medicine, 24*(1), 151–158.

Burns H. (2011) *Health in Scotland 2010: Assets for Health. Annual Report of the Chief Medical Officer 2010*. Edinburgh: The Scottish Government.

Carter, R. (2015) Open dialogue: a care model that could put mental health social work back on the map? *Community Care*. Available at: www.communitycare.co.uk/2015/02/12/open-dialogue-care-model-put-mental-health-social-work-back-map (accessed 26.09.16).

Castillo, H., Ramon, S. & Morant, N. (2013) A recovery journey for people with personality disorder. *International Journal of Social Psychiatry, 59*(3), 264–273.

Clarke, J.M. (2015) *Where the change is: everyday interaction rituals of therapeutic communities*. PhD thesis, University of Nottingham.

Crane, H. (2003) Depression. *BMJ, 326*, 1324–1325.

Crawford, P., Lewis, L., Brown, B., et al. (2013) Creative practice as mutual recovery in mental health. *Mental Health Review Journal, 18*(2), 44–64.

Friedli, L. (2009) *Mental health, resilience and inequalities*. Copenhagen: World Health Organization. Available at: www.euro.who.int/document/e92227.pdf (accessed 15.01.16).

Gask, L., Evans, M. & Kessler, D. (2013) Personality disorder. *British Medical Journal: Clinical Review, 347*, 28–34.

Haigh, R. (2013) The quintessence of a therapeutic environment. *The International Journal of Therapeutic Communities, 34*(1), 6–15.

Holmes, P.R. (2005) *Becoming more human: Exploring the interface of spirituality, discipleship and therapeutic faith community*. Milton Keynes: Paternoster Press.

Johnson, J.G., Cohen, P., Brown, J., et al. (1999) Childhood maltreatment increases risk for personality disorders during early adulthood. *Archives of General Psychiatry, 56*(7), 600–606.

Johnson, R. & Haigh, R. (2011) Social psychiatry and social policy for the 21st century: new concepts for new needs – the 'Enabling Environments' initiative. *Mental Health and Social Inclusion, 15*(1), 17–23.

Jones, M. (1952) *Social psychiatry*. London: Tavistock Publications.

Jones, M. (1968) *Beyond the therapeutic community: Social learning and social psychiatry*. New Haven, CT: Yale University Press.

Kennard, D. & Lees, J. (2012) A checklist of standards for democratic therapeutic communities. *The International Journal of Therapeutic Communities, 3*(2/3), 117–123.

Kesey, K. (1962) *One flew over the cuckoo's nest*. London: Penguin Books.

Kinderman, P., Read, J., Moncrieff, J., et al. (2013) Drop the language of disorder. *Evidence-Based Mental Health, 16*(1), 2–3. Available at: http://ebmh.bmj.com/content/16/1/2.short (accessed 02.08.16).

Main, T. (1977) The concept of the therapeutic community: variations and vicissitudes. *Group Analysis, 10*(2), S2–S16.

Main, T. (1980) Some basic concepts in therapeutic community work. In T. Main (ed.) *The therapeutic community*. London: Croom Helm.

Maughan, D., Lillywhite, R., Pearce, S., et al. (2016) Evaluating sustainability: a retrospective cohort analysis of the Oxfordshire therapeutic community. *BMC Psychiatry, 16*(285). Available at: https://bmcpsychiatry.biomedcentral.com/articles/10.1186/s12888-016-0994-3 (accessed 22.09.16).

Open Dialogue (2016) Home page. Available at: http://opendialogueapproach.co.uk (accessed 22.09.16).

Pearce, S., Scott, L., Attwood, G., et al. (2017) Democratic therapeutic community treatment for personality disorder: randomised controlled trial. *British Journal of Psychiatry, 210*(2), 149–156.

Pilgrim, D. (2001) Disordered personalities and disordered concepts. *Journal of Mental Health, 10*(3), 253–265.

Rapoport, R.N. (1960) *Community as doctor: New perspectives on a therapeutic community*. London: Tavistock Publications.

Repper, J. & Perkins, R. (2003) *Social inclusion and recovery*. London: Bailliere Tindall.

Royal College of Psychiatrists (RCP) (2016a) *Community of communities: A quality network of therapeutic communities*. Available at: www.rcpsych.ac.uk/quality/qualityandaccreditation/therapeuticcommunities/communityofcommunities1.aspx (accessed 02.03.16).

Royal College of Psychiatrists (2016b) *Enabling environments*. Available at: www.rcpsych.ac.uk/workinpsychiatry/qualityimprovement/ccqiprojects/enablingenvironments/introducingtheaward.aspx (accessed 02.03.16).

Spandler, H. (2006) *Asylum to action: Paddington Day Hospital, therapeutic communities and beyond*. London: Jessica Kingsley.

Spandler, H. (2009) Spaces of psychiatric contention: a case study of a therapeutic community. *Health & Place*, *15*(3), 672–678.

Stalker, K., Ferguson, I. & Barclay, A. (2005) 'It is a horrible term for someone': service user and provider perspectives on 'personality disorder'. *Disability & Society*, *20*(4), 359–373.

Star Wards (2006) *Practical ideas for improving the daily experiences and treatment outcomes of acute mental health inpatients*. London: Bright. Available at: www.horticulturaltherapy.info/documents/starwardsprogranandcsourbyquotepage28.pdf (accessed 02.02.16).

Warner, R. (2004) *Recovery from schizophrenia: Psychiatry and political economy*, 3rd edition. London: Routledge.

Whiteley, S. (2004) The evolution of the therapeutic community. *Psychiatric Quarterly*, *75*(3), 233–248.

Winship, G. (2004) Democracy in practice in 14 UK psychotherapeutic communities. *Therapeutic Communities*, *25*(4), 275–290.

Winship, G. (2013) Marcuse, Fromm and the Frankfurt School: reflecting on the history of ideas in therapeutic communities. *International Journal of Therapeutic Communities*, *34*(2/3), 60–70.

Winship, G. (2014) *A meta-recovery framework: positioning the 'New Recovery' movement and other recovery approaches*. Paper presented at the Royal College of Psychiatrist's Community of Communities Annual Forum, Brunei Gallery SOAS, London, May.

Winship, G. (2016) A meta-recovery framework: positioning the 'New Recovery' movement and other recovery approaches. *Journal of Psychiatric and Mental Health Nursing*, *23*, 66–73.

Winship, G. & Hardy, S. (2007) Perspectives on the prevalence and treatment of personality disorder. *Journal of Psychiatric & Mental Health Nursing*, *14*(2), 148–154.

PUBLIC MENTAL HEALTH: PREVENTION AND PROMOTION

31

RHIANNON CORCORAN AND ROSIE MANSFIELD

THIS CHAPTER COVERS

- The concepts and the importance of public mental health in terms of prevention of illness and promotion of wellness
- The distinction between the concepts of mental health and mental wellbeing
- An understanding that these constructs are important at both the individual and the community level
- The most established 'wider social determinants' of mental health and wellbeing – equity, social capital, poverty and urban living
- The promotion of wellbeing – the five ways to wellbeing and an awareness of the role that cooperation and prosociality play as fundamental determinants of public mental health and wellbeing
- The concept that mental health and wellbeing is related to the context in which we live
- The importance of place, space and community for mental health and wellbeing and the relationship of these issues to the 'urbanicity effect'.

"

Our places and spaces play a large part in our *'thrival'*; how we feel about ourselves, our world and our futures. These public places – buildings, streets, squares, parks, views, etc. – belong to us all, yet most public consultation for 'regeneration projects' only involves the public through questionnaires about pre-determined issues, or in formal public meetings where 'expert' panels lead managed discussions about pre-determined solutions. Some public engagement about our places does involve 'participatory exercises' but restrict people to choosing from 'palettes of materials or colours'. At best, it is information sharing, not a shared platform in the decision-making process.

A lack of trust lies at the heart of this. Design professionals and their clients believe they know best about how places should be developed, but often lack the real expertise needed to develop places for mental health and wellbeing. Their approach to community engagement is often one of *'managing expectations'*. Meanwhile, people typically feel that they are *'not listened to'*. If we are to progress towards making places that are better for us, those with the professional 'know-how' must increase their understanding of people's individual and community needs and respect their 'lived experience'.

(Continued)

"

“

'Living environment' practice begins by *designing with communities*. Knowledge of public mental health and wellbeing must replace untested theories of urban design. The place-making process should build the physical and social assets of places to provide learning opportunities, increase sense of belonging and ownership of place, and provide flexible spaces where people can come together in co-operation, action and celebration. If we can share and build our collective expertise of lived experience and professional know-how, we can produce self-generating future places for wellbeing.

Making Places that are Better for Us, Graham Marshall – Prosocial Place, landscape architect and urban designer

”

In this chapter, mental distress is framed as a public health issue. In particular, we consider the pathogenic impact of urban living and social inequalities. A notion of prosocial place is presented as an exemplar of efforts to prevent distress and promote individual and community wellbeing.

MENTAL HEALTH AND WELLBEING IS A PUBLIC HEALTH CONCERN

Mental wellbeing has many definitions, however a sense of agency, mastery and purpose in life has consistently been linked to life satisfaction and the promotion of good health. A mentally resilient individual tends to be someone who is connected and actively contributing to their community, who maintains positive, supportive relationships with others and who is likely to be 'feeling good and functioning well' (Aked et al., 2008). Individuals can more easily develop mental resilience when the communities and places that they live in are resilient too. We will be returning to the question of what we mean by a 'well' place later.

First of all, however, it is important to differentiate between mental wellbeing and mental **illness**. These two constructs are related but we should think of them as independent dimensions that feed into a holistic mental health state (Keyes, 2005). It is commonly assumed that mental health is merely the absence of mental illness. But, many individuals experience low mental wellbeing in the absence of a psychiatric diagnosis or 'psychiatric' symptoms. The state of low wellbeing is sometimes referred to as **'languishing'** (with high psychological wellbeing sometimes called 'flourishing'). Some practitioners believe that individuals with very low wellbeing have sub-threshold mental health difficulties. Equally important, low wellbeing should not necessarily be assumed of someone with a psychiatric diagnosis. There seems to be some overlap between **'recovery'**, however defined, and a state of relatively high psychological wellbeing. To illustrate the complex relationship between mental ill health and wellbeing, it has been found that there is a median prevalence rate of approximately 5% of the general population that experience psychotic symptoms, considerably more than the approximately 1% who receive any formal diagnosis (Van Os et al., 2009). Hearing voices, a traditionally accepted symptom of **psychosis**, is experienced by some people, both 'clinical' and 'non-clinical', as a supportive and positive experience that causes no distress, and is a source of wellbeing. In relation to recovery and wellbeing, a salutogenic as opposed to a pathogenic focus and a focus on capacity not incapacity are important. It is from this positively oriented standpoint that we can begin to clarify and address the social and environmental adversities that contribute to distress.

— WHAT'S THE EVIDENCE? 31.1 —

The capabilities approach was developed by economist and philosopher Amartya Sen in the 1980s. Sen (2005) understood poverty and disadvantage not simply as a lack of material possessions but also as a restriction of an individual's capability to flourish, or deprivation of opportunity. Sen is one of the most influential thinkers on equality and human rights, stressing the importance of understanding the causes and the consequences of them: 'Human ordeals thrive on ignorance. To understand a problem with clarity is already half way towards solving it' (Sen, 2008: iii).

Public health policy has increasingly focused on the promotion of personal wellbeing in recent years and, gradually, a more sophisticated understanding of the differences between **flourishing** and languishing, on the one hand, and mental health and ill health, on the other, is beginning to emerge. In terms of prevention and promotion, it is generally believed that by prioritising policies aimed at the prevention of mental health difficulties, by addressing the so-called *wider social determinants*, we can positively impact on the mental wellbeing of the whole population. Risk and protection factors are recognised from pre-natal to later life stages and from individual, family, community and population levels. Given that the determinants of mental ill health are complex and broad, stretching from individual characteristics to economic, societal and cultural factors, to achieve better population mental health and wellbeing, policies need to work across sectors, be far-sighted and be as universal as possible in their reach. Such policies need to address economic problems, 'toxic' physical **environments** and the promotion of **social capital** and reduction of social inequalities in an attempt to reduce the health and wellbeing inequalities gap.

MENTAL HEALTH AND WELLBEING: PARITY OF ESTEEM

Approximately 23% of the overall disease burden is accounted for by mental ill health. Despite this, there remains a disparity between mental and physical health care funding. The Department of Health's (2011) strategy paper, *No Health Without Mental Health* aims to address this inequity and, often through the valuable work of third-sector mental health organisations, this important issue is beginning to be looked at. The particular areas of focus of such third-sector organisations include:

- working towards fair funding mechanisms
- providing a good start in life
- improving physical health care for those with mental health difficulties
- raising awareness through funding campaigns like 'Time to Change'
- improving employment support for those with mental health difficulties
- improving access to services.

Some of these priorities coincide with the issues raised in mental health and wellbeing surveys in recent years across the country. However, the findings from surveys of public mental wellbeing demonstrate that the issues extend even further. They underline the important role of community and neighbourhood factors. For example, in the North West Mental Wellbeing Survey (Public Health England, 2013) factors that emerged as important in relation to low mental wellbeing were:

- living in a city
- feelings of isolation
- a sense of being unable to ask others for help in times of need
- an increased worry about money
- a decreased sense of belonging to a community
- reduced participation in organisations
- feeling unsafe outside the home.

Findings such as these strongly suggest that making a change 'at scale' to mental health and wellbeing needs direct action to address neighbourhood-level **inequality**, poverty, lack of social capital and the impoverished nature of some urban environments. The importance of improving the experience of living in cities is very clear when we are reminded that 82% of people in the UK live in cities (Public Health England, 2013). Inadequate social support and poorly managed fabric that characterise many of the UK's urban areas are known to be damaging for community living. Recent devolved nations' policy documents emphasise cross-sector working by stressing the importance of sensitive planning and promoting regeneration initiatives with a psychosocial focus that aim to improve community living experiences (Scottish Government, 2003; Welsh Government, 2015).

ADVERSITIES OF URBAN LIVING

The '**urban penalty effect**' refers to the robust set of epidemiological statistics that demonstrate poorer health in urban areas. This effect is thought to be a product of a high concentration of poor people in adverse physical and social environments (Freudenberg et al., 2005). Furthermore, urban sprawl, the fast, cheap development of peripheral areas of the city, has also been found to have negative impacts on health and the environment. In 1939 researchers in the USA first noted the link between urbanicity and specific psychiatric diagnoses with a per capita linear decrease in rates of **schizophrenia** and substance abuse from the densely populated, disorganised, inner-city regions of Chicago to the affluent, residential areas on the outskirts (Faris & Dunham, 1939). This pattern was later replicated in the UK, revealing higher rates of schizophrenia diagnoses in more central wards of Bristol, with segregation and social isolation thought to be important factors (Hare, 1956). Urban environments, defined in terms of their population size and density, have also been found to increase the risk of **depression** and **anxiety** (Peen et al., 2010). A recent meta-analysis found a 2.37 times greater risk of schizophrenia in urban environments compared to rural (Vassos et al., 2012). This phenomenon, where urban environments increase the risk of mental health difficulties, has been dubbed 'the **urbanicity effect**' (Giggs, 1986).

Some researchers have explained the urbanicity effect as a downward social drift of schizophrenia patients prior to the onset of psychosis (Murali & Oyebode, 2004). However, what is called a *dose-response relationship*, found between time spent in an urban area in childhood and the risk of developing schizophrenia, accounts for 15% of relevant cases (Pedersen & Mortensen, 2001). This alone suggests that social drift cannot be the only factor at work here. Interestingly, there are different findings for different diagnoses beyond schizophrenia and depression. For example, urbanicity findings in relation to bipolar **disorder** are far from clear, with some studies suggesting that the incidence and prevalence of bipolar disorder is not related to urban living (Sherazi et al., 2006).

CRITICAL DEBATE 31.1

While sociological, psychological and biomedical researchers draw similar conclusions about the effects of city living on mental health, the approaches contrast in terms of the risk factors identified at different life stages and across different levels, such as individual, family, community. For example, sociological explanations stress political, economic, social and environmental explanations and emphasise individual psychological processes and experiences rather less. Psychological research is predominantly cross-sectional and sometimes fails to prioritise sociological and political explanations. However, it does provide specific associations between place and psychological processes and experiences. Finally, the biomedical approach attempts to explain the risk of urban living at different life stages, for example pre-natal causes for adult mental health difficulties, but it tends to overlook socio-political determinants and life experiences. It is clear that each discipline, by itself, provides incomplete explanations of the urbanicity effect, and that a multi-disciplinary approach would provide a deeper understanding of this complex phenomenon.

Before reading on, try to come up with a list of as many risk factors as you can, that you think make cities potentially more distressing places to live than rural areas.

CRITICAL
DEBATE 31.1
ANSWER

Social and economic inequality is clearly linked to poor health outcomes (Wilkinson & Pickett, 2009). For a long time, scholars of urban design and geography have pointed to the benefits of well-planned city environments (Amin, 2006; Jacobs, 1961; Montgomery, 2013). From as early as the 1930s, sociologists were identifying the wider social determinants of mental health difficulties, stressing their prevalence in cities. This sociological research highlighted inequality and poor quality physical environments as risk factors. Sociologists viewed cities not just as a 'mosaic of social worlds' but as a 'landscape of uneven development with enormous discrepancies in the socio-economic and health conditions of its population' (Fitzpatrick & LaGory, 2003: 34). For these authors, cities were both places of chance and of risk, and they were seen to shape an individual's identity and experiences. Thus, it is now acknowledged that some of the 'urbanicity effect' resides in the perceived quality of the environment (Ellaway et al., 2009; Wang, 2004), such that those living in relatively poor quality or less well-resourced urban areas are exposed to an increased risk of depression, anxiety and paranoia (McKenzie et al., 2013). In the UK, 98% of the most deprived areas, with the highest indices of multiple deprivation, are found in cities and tend to be the areas where urban regeneration initiatives are focused (Department of Communities and Local Government, 2011). In support of this notion, physical characteristics, such as housing type and quality, impact on psychological wellbeing and influence perceived control, social support, risk of victimisation of crime and sense of belonging (Evans, 2003; Romans et al., 2011; Stafford et al., 2007).

CRITICAL THINKING STOP POINT 31.1

Opening your eyes to different places

Henry David Thoreau (American poet, journalist and philosopher, 1817–1862) asked:

'Could a greater miracle take place than for us to look through each other's eyes for an instant?'

CRITICAL
THINKING
STOP
POINT 31.1
ANSWER

THE SYMPTOMS OF MENTAL HEALTH EXIST IN CONTEXT

Some researchers and practitioners argue that discipline and diagnostic inconsistencies would disappear if symptoms of mental distress were understood in their real context and viewed as existing on dynamic continua. For example, paranoia and depression are closely related and are both objectively shown and subjectively experienced as part of a continuum with normal functioning (Freeman et al., 2005). Several related context-dependent, psychological processes are thought to underpin these continua. These include the anticipation and avoidance of social threat (Moutoussis et al., 2007). Depressed individuals, for example, have been shown to display biased implicit attention and attend longer to negative emotional stimuli in their environment (Auerbach et al., 2013). **Locus of control**, the extent to which individuals feel in control of their lives and outcomes (Rotter, 1966), appears to be another key process, where an external locus of control (i.e. control is experienced as coming from an external source) is associated with clinical and non-clinical depression, anxiety and paranoia, with more pronounced effects in more individualistic societies and ethnic minorities (Cheng et al., 2013). Consider the case of *Jane* below, who cites an incident in her childhood where she didn't have a say in what she did, reminding us that it isn't just health services that take control.

CASE STUDY 31.1

Jane's story: Having no say

What annoyed us was there was two good patches of land where the lads could have played a little game of football, (I'm saying the lads because we didn't play football), but all the time *NO BALL GAMES ALLOWED*, *NO BALL GAMES ALLOWED* and there was a top field ... *NO BALL GAMES ALLOWED.*

As kids we didn't have a say. Mum and dad were always arguing. Dad was a drinker but everybody loved Dad. But I didn't get the choice over who I could live with. Or I'd have well lived with my dad.

Yeah, mum and dad, they were always splitting up and we'd go to Grandma's and Grandma's was overcrowded and there wasn't enough room for us all, there wasn't enough space for us all to get a bath on a Sunday night for school.

SOCIAL ADVERSITY: RELATIVE POVERTY

Absolute poverty is an international standard that stays constant, changing only with the rate of inflation. It is usually expressed as an income measure that currently stands at around $1 a day. By contrast, **relative poverty** is multi-faceted, taking into account societal context and recognising the strong relationship between low income and social exclusion.

CRITICAL DEBATE 31.2

In 1979, Peter Townsend (1979: 45) defined poverty as follows:

Individuals, families and groups in the population can be said to be in poverty when they lack resources to obtain the type of diet, participate in the activities and have the living conditions

(Continued)

and amenities which are customary, or at least widely encouraged and approved, in the societies in which they belong.

What do you think is the relationship between mental ill health and poverty? Does poverty cause mental ill health? Does mental ill health cause poverty? Clearly, one can exist without the other – so what does it all mean?

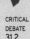

CRITICAL
DEBATE
31.2
ANSWER

Actually, relative poverty is predominantly calculated in terms of household income, which is adjusted by family size. The household income is compared to the median for that country, and households with incomes falling more than 60% below the median are judged to be in poverty. Critics of this calculation point out that a rise in unemployment will see a fall in median income within a country. As median income declines, so fewer household incomes fall below 60%. This gives the impression of reduced poverty that can only really result if the costs of essential goods and services fall.

IMPROVING MENTAL HEALTH AND WELLBEING AND CREATING RESILIENT URBAN COMMUNITIES: USING EVIDENCE ACROSS SECTORS

CASE STUDY:
JANE'S STORY

In recent years, people who work in different areas and researchers from different backgrounds have been getting together to try to gain a better understanding of the influence of the physical, social and economic characteristics of urban environments on the psychological processes that underpin wellbeing and mental health difficulties. For health and wellbeing professionals, *socially* sustainable environments are those that can promote mental health and wellbeing in their residents. The agreed understanding on sustainability among built environment professions is that we must reduce urban sprawl while trying to make dense living meet our needs. A balance must be struck between optimising social connections and facilitating the need to sometimes retreat into privacy.

The Community Wellbeing team of the What Works Centre for Wellbeing in the UK recently surveyed 315 professionals and practitioners working in the field of wellbeing. As part of this survey, respondents were asked to indicate what they believed was meant by the term community wellbeing: 62% of those who responded to this question believed that community wellbeing is about *strong networks of relationships and support between people in a community, both in close relationships and friendships, and between neighbours and acquaintances*; 35.1% believed that community wellbeing means *people feeling able to take action to improve things in, and influence decisions about, their community*; 30.4% considered that community wellbeing referred to *people's feelings of trust in, belonging to and safety in their community* (What Works Wellbeing, 2016).

GREEN SPACE AND WELLBEING

'**Green space**' is used to define a space situated within an urban area that is predominantly made up of grass, vegetation and trees, and is considered to have both aesthetic and recreational **value**.

With rapid urbanisation has come an increased concern about the loss of green spaces. With the UK moving closer towards the American model of a city, with a dense inner-city, greener suburb and an increase in the privatisation of public spaces, growing inequalities in terms of the quality and availability of urban green space are emerging. The idea that humans have an instinctual need to affiliate with nature is known as '**biophilia**', and evidence has even suggested that simply adding plants to a room can reduce stress and have psychological benefits (Bringslimark et al., 2009). However, some suggest the effects are mediated by the increased physical attractiveness of the room (Dijkstra et al., 2008). Increasing the amount of parks in cities has been linked to improved wellbeing and mental health outcomes (White et al., 2013) and green spaces have been found to buffer against stressful life events (Van den Berg et al., 2010). But growing evidence suggests that it is not the quantity but rather the quality, accessibility and perceived safety of green space that is important for physical and mental health (Lee & Maheswaran, 2011). This extends beyond the biophilia hypothesis, instead suggesting that the quality and management of green space is most important because it can change the use and perceptions of residents and visitors to the place, thus enabling social engagement.

It has also been found that white communities have 11 times more green space than ethnic minorities and this is undeniably accounted for by socio-economic and structural factors. One possible way forward that may address the inherent inequality issues in the use of quality green space is to reconsider how these spaces are managed. Increased scope for communities to utilise space in their neighbourhoods and to work alongside local authorities to improve the public realm and public spaces could improve residents' resilience, agency and mastery and their sense of belonging to and control over their neighbourhoods (Colding & Barthel, 2013).

CRITICAL THINKING STOP POINT 31.2

What do you think is meant by community wellbeing? Are there other important factors to consider when we think about what this means? How can the characteristics of spaces and buildings contribute to community wellbeing? What do you understand by the word community? Would a community that seems to be high in wellbeing be good for everyone?

In recent work, we have been considering what cross-sector working might look like. We have taken the evidence-based *Five Ways to Wellbeing* (Aked et al., 2008) as a starting point because we wanted to see if it was possible to use them to inform city place-making.

CRITICAL THINKING STOP POINT 31.3

Download the What Works Wellbeing (2016) paper at https://study.sagepub.com/essentialmental health to assist with the following task.

(Continued)

FIND OUT MORE

WEBLINK:
WHAT WORKS
WELLBEING

As a nurse, you will spend a lot of time talking to service users. But how much of this time is spent asking about their lives? Have you ever asked what has happened to them? What are their most important experiences? Where have they lived? What have they loved and hated? What are their thoughts about other people and society? Did they ever feel at home? Do they feel stigmatised? How many friends do they have? What kind of activities do they enjoy? What kind of schools/colleges did they go to? What was their favourite subject at school? Do they get on with their siblings? And so on.

These are all questions that relate to the 'wider determinants' of mental health and wellbeing. If you have these chats, see how the answers relate to the Five Ways to Wellbeing:

- Connect
- Give
- Take notice
- Keep learning
- Be active.

Also, think about what recommendations you might make to help the person make a change in their lives towards 'feeling good and functioning well'.

The Community Wellbeing team of the What Works Centre for Wellbeing asked UK professionals who work to promote wellbeing to give an example they knew of where high levels of community wellbeing existed. These are some examples of what they said (What Works Wellbeing, 2016):

A tower block in which the warden decided to help develop the previously unconnected residents into a community, including a conservatory, café, gardens, etc., based on the concept of the world's oldest residential towers in Yemen. The block went from having empty flats to a waiting list to move in.

A once run down, crime ridden area has been given a new sense of pride for the individuals to live in due to one street deciding to come together to do little things, i.e. plant flowers and shrubs and discourage their children throwing litter around, etc. It has made a huge difference over time and led to people appearing to smile more.

Spread & growth of 'Playing Out' activities. This is where streets are closed to traffic for short periods of time, but opened up to children and adults to play, talk, interact and socialise. This has the potential to increase exercise for children, reduce isolation and loneliness, allow neighbours to get to know one another, build trust, understanding, increase safety in that people look out for one another, and much more.

MENTAL HEALTH, ALTRUISM, AND COOPERATION: TOWARDS PROSOCIAL PLACES

The tendency to behave in an altruistic fashion shows large degrees of variability in our species, suggesting a role for environment. Indeed, evidence confirms that physical and social environments influence altruistic and cooperative tendencies, with the city appearing to be a context that makes these prosocial behaviours more difficult to establish and maintain. In more fine-grained analysis, it has been found that within a city, particular socio-economic factors further determine altruistic behaviour in cooperative exchanges, and that economic factors and the level of social capital in an area predict prosocial behaviours. Since it is both good for us to give and to receive acts of care from others, altruism is a trait that is fundamentally linked to the mental health and wellbeing of our species. Given its conditional relationship with the characteristics of place and community, it is easy to see how important it is for our future mental health and wellbeing to develop more prosocial cities designed to encourage an altruistic survival strategy (What Works Wellbeing, 2016).

CONCLUSION

This chapter has enabled us to consider the impact of our environment on our mental health and argues that the places and the circumstances in which people live their lives have a large impact on how they feel. City living can be detrimental to mental health and wellbeing and this is due to complex causes that include aspects of urban environments and structural economic issues. Prosocial places that are collaboratively designed with decent built environments and adequate green space, which foster egalitarian and positive social relationships, are better for people's wellbeing and health.

───── CHAPTER SUMMARY ─────

This chapter has covered the following ideas:

- Mental wellbeing and mental illness should be seen as related but independent constructs that contribute to a whole mental health state.
- Symptoms of mental distress should therefore be understood in their real context and viewed as existing on dynamic continua.
- Urban living is associated with an increased risk of mental distress known as the 'urbanicity effect'.
- Poverty, social deprivation and relative inequality in the UK are predictors of mental distress and low wellbeing, with the majority of the most deprived neighbourhoods existing in urban areas.
- Physical, social and economic characteristics of place act on psychological processes such as perceived threat and control, social support and trust, which are all known to underpin symptoms of depression, anxiety and paranoia.
- Evolutionary psychologists perceive these psychological processes, such as attention to threat and low trust, as adaptive responses to experiences and environments.
- The quality and management of green space predict the utilisation and social engagement benefits related to improved wellbeing. Increased scope for communities to utilise space in their neighbourhoods and to work alongside local authorities to improve the public realm and public spaces could improve residents' resilience, agency and mastery and their sense of belonging to and control over their neighbourhoods.

- Application of the evidence-based 'Five Ways to Wellbeing' to the planning and management of urban communities could be one way to decrease the adversities currently associated with city living, by increasing residents' sense of identity in, belonging to and control of the places they live.

BUILD YOUR BIBLIOGRAPHY

Books

- Baum, F. (2016) *The new public health*, 4th edition. Oxford: Oxford University Press. A comprehensive treatment of progressive models of public health, stressing globalisation and settings.
- Sennett, R. (2003) *Respect in an age of inequality*. New York: Norton. With reflections on urban life, Sennett explores how self-worth can be nurtured in spite of inequality; self-esteem needs to be balanced with concern for others; mutual regard and respect sustain bonds between people in the struggle against inequalities.
- Wilkinson, R.G. & Pickett, K. (2009) *The spirit level: Why more equal societies almost always do better*. London: Allen Lane. A classic text that demonstrates the detrimental effect of inequality on mental health and wellbeing, amongst other outcomes.

SAGE journal articles

FURTHER
READING:
JOURNAL
ARTICLES

Go to https://study.sagepub.com/essentialmentalhealth for further free online journal articles related to this chapter. If you are using the interactive ebook, simply click on the book icon in the margin to go straight to the resource.

- Amin, A. (2006) The good city. *Urban Studies*, *43*(5–6), 1009–1023.
- Burns, J.K., Tomita, A. & Kapadia, A.S. (2013) Income inequality and schizophrenia: increased schizophrenia incidence in countries with high levels of income inequality. *International Journal of Social Psychiatry*, *60*(2), 185–196.
- Ellaway, A., Macintyre, S. & Kearns, A. (2001) Perceptions of place and health in socially contrasting neighbourhoods. *Urban Studies*, *38*(12), 2299–2316.
- Luciano, M., De Rosa, C., Del Vecchio, V., et al. (2016) Perceived insecurity, mental health and urbanization: results from a multicentric study. *International Journal of Social Psychiatry*, *62*(3), 252–261.
- McKenzie, K. (2008) Urbanization, social capital and mental health. *Global Social Policy*, *8*(3), 359–377.

Weblinks

FURTHER
READING:
WEBLINKS

Go to https://study.sagepub.com/essentialmentalhealth for further weblinks related to this chapter. If you are using the interactive ebook, simply click on the book icon in the margin to go straight to the resource.

- Amartya Sen's Capability Approach – Internet Encyclopedia of Philosophy: www.iep.utm.edu/sen-cap
- The Centre for Urban Design and Mental Health: www.urbandesignmentalhealth.com
- Time to Change: www.time-to-change.org.uk

—————————— **ACE YOUR ASSESSMENT** ——————————

Revise what you have learned by visiting https://study.sagepub.com/essentialmentalhealth. If you are using the interactive ebook, simply click on the tick icon to go straight to the resource.

ONLINE
QUIZZES &
ACTIVITY
ANSWERS

- Test yourself with multiple-choice and short-answer questions and flashcards.

REFERENCES

Aked, J., Marks, N., Cordon, C., et al. (2008) *Five ways to wellbeing*. London: New Economics Foundation.

Amin, A. (2006) The good city. *Urban Studies, 43*(5–6), 1009–1023.

Auerbach, R.P., Webb, C.A., Gardiner, C.K., et al. (2013) Behavioural and neural mechanisms underlying cognitive vulnerability models of depression. *Journal of Psychotherapy Integration, 23*(3), 222.

Bringslimark, T., Hartig, T. & Patil, G.G. (2009) The psychological benefits of indoor plants: a critical review of the experimental literature. *Journal of Environmental Psychology, 29*(4), 422–433.

Cheng, C., Cheung, S.F., Chio, J.H.M., et al. (2013) Cultural meaning of perceived control: a meta-analysis of locus of control and psychological symptoms across 18 cultural regions. *Psychological Bulletin, 139*(1), 52.

Colding, J. & Barthel, S. (2013) The potential of 'Urban Green Commons' in the resilience building of cities. *Ecological Economics, 86*, 156–166.

Department of Communities and Local Government (2011) *Regeneration to enable growth: What government is doing to support community-led regeneration*. Available at: http://webarchive. nationalarchives.gov.uk/20120919132719/http:/www.communities.gov.uk/documents/ regeneration/pdf/1830137.pdf (accessed 13.08.17).

Department of Health (2011) *No health without mental health: Delivering better mental health outcomes for people of all ages*. London: DH.

Dijkstra, K., Pieterse, M.E. & Pruyn, A. (2008) Stress-reducing effects of indoor plants in the built healthcare environment: the mediating role of perceived attractiveness. *Preventive Medicine, 47*(3), 279–283.

Ellaway, A., Morris, G., Curtice, J., et al. (2009) Associations between health and different types of environmental incivility: a Scotland-wide study. *Public Health, 123*(11), 708–713.

Evans, G.W. (2003) The built environment and mental health. *Journal of Urban Health, 80*(4), 536–555.

Faris, R.E.L. & Dunham, H.W. (1939) *Mental disorders in urban areas: An ecological study of schizophrenia and other psychoses*. Chicago: University of Chicago Press.

Fitzpatrick, K.M. & LaGory, M. (2003) 'Placing' health in an urban sociology: cities as mosaics of risk and protection. *City & Community, 2*(1), 33–46.

Freeman, D., Garety, P.A., Bebbington, P.E., et al. (2005) Psychological investigation of the structure of paranoia in a non-clinical population. *The British Journal of Psychiatry, 186*(5), 427–435.

Freudenberg, N., Galea, S. & Vlahov, D. (2005) Beyond urban penalty and urban sprawl: back to living conditions as the focus of urban health. *Journal of Community Health, 30*(1), 1–11.

Giggs, J.A. (1986) Mental disorders and ecological structure in Nottingham. *Social Science & Medicine, 23*(10), 945–961.

Hare, E.H. (1956) Mental illness and social conditions in Bristol. *The British Journal of Psychiatry, 102*(427), 349–357.

Jacobs, J. (1961) *The death and life of great American cities.* New York: Vintage.

Keyes, C.L. (2005) Mental illness and/or mental health? Investigating axioms of the complete state model of health. *Journal of Consulting and Clinical Psychology, 73*(3), 539.

Lee, A.C.K. & Maheswaran, R. (2011) The health benefits of urban green spaces: a review of the evidence. *Journal of Public Health, 33*(2), 212–222.

McKenzie, K., Murray, A. & Booth, T. (2013) Do urban environments increase the risk of anxiety, depression and psychosis? An epidemiological study. *Journal of Affective Disorders, 150*(3), 1019–1024.

Montgomery, C. (2013) *Happy city: Transforming our lives through urban design.* London: Penguin.

Moutoussis, M., Williams, J., Dayan, P., et al. (2007) Persecutory delusions and the conditioned avoidance paradigm: towards an integration of the psychology and biology of paranoia. *Cognitive Neuropsychiatry, 12*(6), 495–510.

Murali, V. & Oyebode, F. (2004) Poverty, social inequality and mental health. *Advances in Psychiatric Treatment, 10*(3), 216–224.

Pedersen, C.B. & Mortensen, P.B. (2001) Evidence of a dose-response relationship between urbanicity during upbringing and schizophrenia risk. *Archives of General Psychiatry, 58*(11), 1039–1046.

Peen, J., Schoevers, R.A., Beekman, A.T., et al. (2010) The current status of urban-rural differences in psychiatric disorders. *Acta Psychiatrica Scandinavica, 121*(2), 84–93.

Public Health England (2013) *North West Mental Wellbeing Survey 2012/13.* With Centre for Public Health/Liverpool John Moores University. Available at: www.nwph.net/Publications/NW%20 MWB_PHE_Final_28.11.13.pdf (accessed 13.08.17).

Romans, S., Cohen, M. & Forte, T. (2011) Rates of depression and anxiety in urban and rural Canada. *Social Psychiatry and Psychiatric Epidemiology, 46*(7), 567–575.

Rotter, J.B. (1966) Generalized expectancies for internal versus external control of reinforcement. *Psychological Monographs: General and Applied, 80*(1), 1–28.

Scottish Government (2003) *The national programme for improving mental health and wellbeing: Action plan.* Available at: www.gov.scot/Publications/2003/09/18193/26508 (accessed 26.05.17).

Sen, A. (2005) Human rights and capabilities. *Journal of Human Development, 6*(2), 151–166.

Sen, A. (2008) Forward. In N. Akhavi (ed.) *AIDS sutra: Untold stories from India.* London: Vintage.

Sherazi, R., McKeon, P., McDonough, M., et al. (2006) What's new: the clinical epidemiology of bipolar disorder. *Harvard Review of Psychiatry, 14,* 274–284.

Stafford, M., Chandola, T. & Marmot, M. (2007) Association between fear of crime and mental health and physical functioning. *American Journal of Public Health, 97*(11), 2076–2081.

Townsend, P. (1979) *Poverty in the United Kingdom: A survey of household resources and standards of living.* London: Penguin Books.

Van den Berg, A.E., Maas, J., Verheij, R.A., et al. (2010) Green space as a buffer between stressful life events and health. *Social Science & Medicine, 70*(8), 1203–1210.

Van Os, J., Linscott, R.J., Myin-Germeys, I., et al. (2009) A systematic review and meta-analysis of the psychosis continuum: evidence for a psychosis proneness–persistence–impairment model of psychotic disorder. *Psychological Medicine, 39*(2), 179–195.

Vassos, E., Pedersen, C.B., Murray, R.M., et al. (2012) Meta-analysis of the association of urbanicity with schizophrenia. *Schizophrenia Bulletin, 38*(6), 1118–1123.

Wang, J. (2004) Rural–urban differences in the prevalence of major depression and associated impairment. *Social Psychiatry and Psychiatric Epidemiology, 39*(1), 19–25.

Welsh Government (2015) *Together for mental health: A mental health and wellbeing strategy for Wales*. Available at: http://gov.wales/topics/health/nhswales/mental-health-services/policy/strategy/?lang=en (accessed 26.05.17).

What Works Wellbeing (2016) *Voice of the user report: Communities evidence programme*. Available at: https://whatworkswellbeing.files.wordpress.com/2016/02/community-voice-of-the-user-report1.pdf (accessed 26/05/17).

White, M.P., Alcock, I., Wheeler, B.W., et al. (2013) Would you be happier living in a greener urban area? A fixed-effects analysis of panel data. *Psychological Science, 24*(6), 920–928.

Wilkinson, R.G. & Pickett, K. (2009) *The spirit level: Why more equal societies almost always do better*. London: Allen Lane.

PRIMARY MENTAL HEALTH CARE

32

NICK BOHANNON AND SUMAIYAA KHODA

THIS CHAPTER COVERS

- Definitions of primary mental health care (PMHC)
- The development of PMHC in the UK
- IAPT's contribution to PMHC
- The stepped care model
- Integration of physical and mental wellbeing in primary care settings.

> As a mental health nurse working in primary mental health care, there is an opportunity to work in a dynamic and integrative way with service users and service providers. In order to provide a holistic level of care, further training and knowledge on physical health illnesses will enhance treatment outcomes for service users. New developments such as the Improving Access to the Psychological Therapies programme has enabled patients to have access to evidence-based talking therapies, however this comes with its own challenges with high service demand and an increase in waiting lists for services. There is an opportunity to identify and trial innovative ways of practice such as group therapy with various services within primary care such as dentists and practice nurses.
>
> **Selina, mental health nurse**

> I was working in a job I had been in for 25 years when it all just seemed to come crashing down on top of me. I spent two months getting worse and worse on my own at home, and finally went to the doctor. He said I had depression and offered me medication but I didn't want that, so he sent me to see the mental health nurse at the surgery. I was OK going into the doctor's surgery because I had been going there for years. Talking helped, but what really made the difference was being helped to realise that I needed to make really small changes, and take baby steps every day and build them up. It worked, and while I was there I got to see my diabetic nurse too. I am glad to have got help at my doctors. It's just down the road and I probably wouldn't have gone anywhere else to be honest.
>
> **Gil, service user**

Visit **https://study.sagepub.com/essentialmentalhealth** to access a wealth of online resources for this chapter – watch out for the margin icons throughout the chapter. If you are using the interactive ebook, simply click on the margin icon to go straight to the resource.

INTRODUCTION

Primary care services provide the majority of care to people who have mental health problems and there is growing interest in service provision in this field. This chapter considers the policy drivers and clinical imperatives behind **primary mental health** care, the locations and organisation of services, the physical health needs of people with serious mental health problems and the opportunities that exist for making creative new links between services, communities and the people needing support for their mental wellbeing.

WHAT IS PRIMARY MENTAL HEALTH CARE?

Primary mental health care represents a diverse range of services with considerable regional variation. There is no standardised model of primary mental health care service, and this is reflected in the variety of approaches currently being taken. However, tucked away within the different approaches and complicated policy documents are two key strengths; first, agreement over what a good primary mental health care service should include seems to be emerging; and second, there is considerable opportunity for innovation in all sectors of primary mental health provision (see Figure 32.1). Community links, social prescribing, comprehensive **service user** involvement and a willingness amongst service providers to work jointly, are creating new and exciting opportunities. Also, services can be influenced by the needs of the population, for example social prescribing for areas in greater need of support due to poor housing or social deprivation.

The World Health Organization describes primary mental health services as providing first contact, accessible, continued, comprehensive and coordinated care (WHO, 2016). This definition is

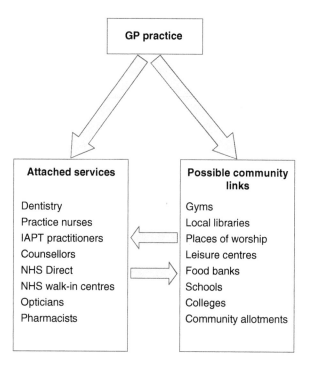

Figure 32.1 Typical primary health care team structure with example opportunities for community links in the UK

consistent with that offered by Bath and Wekerman (2015) who define primary health care as socially appropriate, universally acceptable, scientifically sound first-level care. They suggest that care should be delivered in a way that maximises community and individual self-reliance, and involves joint working with other sectors. In that way, services would be locally available, with easy access and easy self-referral processes, and would be integrated with other aspects of life that take place in the local community.

Of 2000 patients who attend a GP surgery:

352 will have a common mental health problem

8 will have psychosis

120 will have alcohol dependency

60 will suffer with drug dependency

352 will present with sub-threshold common mental health problems

120 people will present with sub-threshold psychosis

176 will have a diagnosis of personality disorder

125 will have a chronic long-term condition with comorbid mental illness

100 will have medically unexplained symptoms

That is approximately 1400 of 2000 people visiting their GP who may be negatively affected by their mental condition. (*Guidance for commissioners of primary mental health care services*)

Joint Commissioning Panel for Mental Health (JCPMH), 2013, Royal College of Psychiatrists

CRITICAL THINKING STOP POINT 32.1

How do you think the much reported 'one in four' description of the prevalence of mental illness in the population compares to the figures from the JCPMH?

THE DEVELOPMENT OF PRIMARY MENTAL HEALTH CARE IN THE UK

The National Health Service has underdone substantial changes in its structure and financing in the past 25 years. The introduction of the internal market required services that had previously been part of the wider NHS to become NHS trusts, and general practitioners to become fund holders who purchased services for patients from these NHS trusts. The *New NHS, Modern, Dependable* (DH, 1997) introduced primary care groups (PCGs) and those groups were able to apply to become primary care trusts (PCTs). Under the new system, the National Institute for Clinical Excellence (NICE) would identify national priorities and treatment protocols, and PCTs would encourage more accessible services through their purchasing power.

Concurrently, the move towards care in the community gained pace and, following concerns about public and patient safety, the care programme approach was developed to ensure smooth transition between services and improved coordination of care and support. Significantly for primary care, the National Service Framework for mental health (DH, 1999) emphasised the importance of a comprehensive and accessible primary care service for mental health care.

A further shift of considerable importance was seen with the document *No Health Without Mental Health* (DH, 2011a). The government now stressed the importance of local communities and the adoption of a life-span approach to service provision. It also clearly set out its intention for a more balanced system, with parity of esteem between mental and physical health services, in which mental and physical health outcomes were seen as equally important. The relationship between physical and mental health was now taken as a given.

No Health Without Mental Health sets out six key objectives:

- More people will have good mental health.
- More people with mental health problems will recover.
- More people with mental health problems will have good physical health.
- More people will have a positive experience of care and support.
- Fewer people will suffer avoidable harm.
- Fewer people will experience **stigma** and discrimination. (DH, 2011a)

No Health Without Mental Health offered a vision for improvement, suggesting that quality services depend on quality **commissioning**, and to that end guidance for commissioners of primary care services has been clarified and strengthened. The JCPMH asserts that mental health services should be managed as part of the primary care team working collaboratively with other services, and that those services should be mindful of the physical, psychological, social and spiritual components of mental health (JCPMH, 2013). The panel's guidance highlights the need for earlier detection of problems, better management of chronic **illness** and improved partnership working between the patient, extended team and local community support networks.

The current decade has seen increasing numbers of people seeking support for mental health problems and the numbers continue to rise (England, 2014). Currently, around 300 in every 1000 people will experience mental health problems every year, with 230 of those people visiting their GP. The number of working days lost to stress, **depression** and **anxiety** has increased by 24% since 2009 (Davies, 2014), with mental illness the largest single cause of disability, with it representing 28% of the national disease burden in the UK. It is also the leading cause of sickness absence, accounting for 70 million sick days in 2007 in the UK. Currently, services are stretched and access can be problematic; indeed, the Chief Medical Officer states in her annual report that there is a very significant overall treatment gap in mental health care in England, with about 75% of people with mental illness receiving no treatment at all. In addition to increasing demand, there is also a concurrent increase in the complexity of the care being delivered in the community. People are living longer and living with long-term or multiple conditions. A key response to this changing picture came with Improving Access to Psychological Therapies (IAPT).

WHAT'S THE EVIDENCE? 32.1

If the Chief Medical Officer is correct and up to 75% of people who have mental illness receive no treatment, why might that be? And how might that be improved?

THE CONTRIBUTION OF IMPROVING ACCESS TO PSYCHOLOGICAL THERAPIES (IAPT) IN PRIMARY CARE SERVICES

IAPT commenced in 2008 following the publication of *The Depression Report: A new deal for depression and anxiety disorders* (Layard et al., 2006). The report asserted that 40% of all disability was attributed to mental illness. The financial cost was estimated at £12 billion, while only 2% of NHS expenditure was invested in treatments for anxiety and depression. The Depression Report put forward a case for increasing resources for evidence-based interventions for anxiety and depression, and proposed investment in the development of teams of psychological therapists. The aim of the programme is consistent with the principles of primary care in that it emphasises early access into treatment. The treatment model was designed to offer patients access to a range of talking therapies for anxiety and depression in line with NICE guidelines. The publication of *No Health Without Mental Health* (DH, 2011a) and *Talking Therapies: A 4 Year Plan of Action* (DH, 2011b) drove IAPT services forward. By 31 March 2011, 142 of the 151 primary care trusts in England had a service from this programme in at least part of their area and just over 50% of the adult population had access to IAPT services (DH, 2012).

The most common forms of mental health condition treated in primary care are depression and anxiety, however, interestingly, only 24% of people in England with this diagnosis receive treatment for a common mental health problem (McManus et al., 2009). IAPT has been successful in offering evidence-based treatment to those who suffer with depression and anxiety, however the high demand for the service has led to increased waiting times in a significant number of areas (DH, 2012).

Practitioner roles in IAPT are in line with the stepped care model (see Figure 32.2). The staff generally consist of psychological wellbeing practitioners (PWPs) who work at step 2 and high-intensity therapists (HITs) who work at step 3. PWPs utilise facilitated self-help based on cognitive behavioural therapy (CBT) principles and carry large caseloads but offer brief, time-limited support (typically six sessions of about 30 minutes). HITs work at step 3 in the stepped care model and offer CBT for those with more chronic and severe problems. Length of treatment varies but is generally 12 sessions. Some services are expanding to offer a more diverse range of therapies, including interpersonal psychotherapy, couple's therapy for depression, and brief dynamic interpersonal psychotherapy. Around 30% of high-intensity therapists in the IAPT workforce are able to deliver these non-CBT therapies. In offering this range of therapies, IAPT services are ensuring that they are compliant with NICE guidelines (2004). IAPT workers have key performance indicators defined by NHS England, with the target currently set at 50% **recovery**. Prevalence and waiting times are also closely monitored. Recovery is determined using a minimum data set of standardised questionnaires including the Patient Health Questionnaire (PHQ-9) and Generalised Anxiety Disorder (GAD-7) (Spitzer et al, 2006)

CASE STUDY 32.1

Mike is a 60-year-old man who visits his GP and reports that he is struggling with poor sleep and has recently lost interest in the things he used to enjoy. Mike tells the GP that this started around two months ago and has been getting worse. He has never felt like this before and is unsure why he is feeling this way. The GP suggests that Mike may benefit from an appointment with the practice-based psychological wellbeing practitioner (PWP) and offers to do the referral. Mike agrees and attends the arranged assessment appointment. Mike reiterates what he said to his GP and also talks about feeling bad about himself. He explains that since retiring from work he has not felt himself. He has stopped seeing his friends as he does not feel he has anything to talk about with them. During the appointment, the PWP asks Mike to complete the PHQ-9 and GAD-7. He scores 15 on the PHQ-9 and 5 on the GAD-7, and she explains that his responses to the questionnaires indicate that he may be experiencing symptoms of depression. Mike is relieved to know there is a reason why he might be feeling this way. The PWP offers Mike some information on behavioural activation and goal setting and arranges a follow-up appointment for two weeks' time.

Questions

- Why might Mike be relieved to find out that he has depression?
- Usually, after an appointment with a PWP, the service user is given some homework to do. Here, Mike has some information to read. He will also be required to complete a thought diary. Some service users find that completing 'homework' is a struggle and are worried about getting it 'wrong'. How might we present such homework as possible and collaborative?
- Mike might have hoped that he would be prescribed an antidepressant. What is your opinion about medication? Is it better to try without?

In order for IAPT services to ensure access is improved and patients receive treatment in a timely manner, alternative methods of offering treatments are being considered. These methods include using online resources, telephone assessments and group sessions. An additional concern is that with the increased demand for IAPT services, there is less time for staff to focus on preventative and integrative approaches. The success of the service has also led to an increase in referrals of higher risk patients who traditionally may not have accessed services via primary care (DH, 2012). IAPT plays a role in a wider primary care mental health service, but cannot possibly cover all the aspects of mental health support needed within primary care.

CASE STUDY 32.2

Lyndsey is 18 years old and is studying art and fashion at university. Lyndsey has been falling behind with her work and has recently stopped attending lectures. Further to a meeting with her academic advisor, Lyndsey discloses that she is struggling to cope with the transition from home to university. Her academic advisor recommends she access her local university student support service. The mental health advisor at the university meets with Lyndsey who shares that she has not been eating meals regularly and has become increasingly obsessed with her weight. In order to cope, she has started to self-harm on her arms. The mental health advisor supports Lyndsey to self-refer to her local services and she is offered a telephone assessment within a week with a psychological wellbeing practitioner, who provides her with a menu of services from which she chooses to attend a group talk where she can learn more about all the treatment options. In the group talk, there are a number of services present who explain a number of treatment options available to Lyndsey. Lyndsey opts for the psychoeducation group which covers a number of topics such as stress and self-harm, which she relates to. She was also informed of other local services in her area, which included a list of activities available at her local leisure centre, and given a list of web-based applications she could use during her wait for the group, particularly in relation to eating difficulties and self-harm.

(Continued)

> ### Questions
>
> - Lyndsey has never self-harmed before. She is ashamed of her cuts, which are visible, and worried about going to the leisure centre because others might see them. What advice would you give her?
> - Identify the difference in the service user journey process for Lyndsey and Mike, who was discussed in Case study 32.1.
> - Can you see why it can be difficult to actually define primary mental health care?

STEPPED CARE

The recommended method of coordinating primary care services is a stepped care system (NICE, 2009). The stepped care model offers five levels of care, and clients move through treatments that are located on different steps until their needs are met. These interventions increase in intensity over progression through these steps and the system is designed to be self-correcting, in that the client's reaction to treatment is monitored and individuals are 'stepped up' to the next step if they do not respond to the treatment situated in their current step. For the stepped care model to work successfully, the transition of patients between the steps has to be smooth and timely. Patients can start treatment but clear referrals, back-referral and linkage systems should be implemented in consultation with health managers and health workers at all service levels (WHO & WONCA, 2008).

Patients who have physical health conditions are likely to present in various settings, such as a local pharmacy, practice nurse clinics, pre-natal assessments by health visitors, A & E liaison departments and dentistry services. These services form part of step 1 of the stepped care model.

Step 5: Inpatient care, crisis teams	Risk to life, severe self-neglect	Medication, combined treatments, ECT
Step 4: Mental health specialists including crisis teams	Treatment-resistant, recurrent, atypical and psychotic depression, and those at significant risk	Medication, complex psychological interventions, combined treatments
Step 3: Primary care team, primary care mental health worker	Moderate or severe depression	Medication, psychological interventions, social support
Step 2: Primary care team, primary care mental health worker	Mild depression	Watchful waiting, guided self-help, computerised CBT, exercise, brief psychological interventions
Step 1: GP, practice nurse	Recognition	Assessment

Figure 32.2 The stepped care model

Ami is a student nurse who is on placement at her local primary care service. She takes a call from Andy who is unsure which service he has been referred to following his course of cognitive behavioural therapy. Andy tells Ami that he suffers from debilitating symptoms of obsessive compulsive disorder (OCD) which he has had for 15 years and has tried various forms of medication and therapy over the years. There are occasions where it can take him up to 3 hours to leave the house, however he continues to function and works part time. He is currently eating very little due to fear of contamination. Andy regularly experiences thoughts that he cannot cope with feeling like this anymore. Ami agrees to make contact with services to identify which services are available for him. Ami makes contact with the therapist who Andy has just completed treatment with. She advises Ami that Andy has been 'stepped up' for further assessment and treatment as he has completed the maximum number of sessions as part of his treatment in step 3 services. Ami liaises with the local community mental health team who work within step 4 of the model. They confirm that Andy has been offered an assessment, however he doesn't meet the criteria for treatment within the service they offer. Andy has been discharged back to the care of his GP. They agree to explore alternative options for Andy and agree to give him a call.

Anonymous, mental health nurse

CRITICAL THINKING STOP POINT 32.2

Supporting a person who has greater need than step 3 services can meet, but doesn't meet the criteria for step 4, can be challenging for mental health nurses:

- What do you think is important about how you might manage this situation in practice?
- Which alternative services outside of the NHS may be helpful for Andy?

MENTAL AND PHYSICAL HEALTH

It is known that 69% of people experiencing depression in primary care initially present with physical symptoms (Simon et al., 1999), and 25% of people attending hospital emergency departments with **acute** chest pain actually have panic disorder (Huffman and Pollack , 2003). Research undertaken by the King's Fund on *Bringing Together Physical and Mental Health* (Naylor et al., 2016) identified high rates of mental health issues among those with long-term conditions (LTCs) such as cancer, diabetes or heart disease, and concluded that there is limited support available for the psychological aspects of physical health. Examples of this include during and after pregnancy, and poor management of 'medically unexplained symptoms' (MUS) such as persistent pain or tiredness. One factor for those who have poor physical and mental health can be lifestyle, some of which could be preventable with early recognition (Collins et al., 2013; Wand & Murray, 2008). In response to that situation, work streams have been planned and developed to support patients with long-term health conditions and medically unexplained symptoms as part of the IAPT programme.

The LTC/MUS work stream has now been added to the programme to extend the benefits of improved access to psychological therapies to people who have LTC and/or MUS. In February 2012, 15 services were selected as IAPT LTC/MUS pathfinder sites and they commenced work in April 2012. These sites are exploring and further developing the organisational, economic and quality arguments for increased integration of psychological support and physical health care. The results so far suggest that the majority of service users are satisfied and find materials helpful, however findings were limited due to the reduced completion of data set questionnaires and service user feedback. It is essential that data quality improves to make a stronger case for the IAPT LTC/MUS programme (De Lusignan et al., 2013).

Recent reports from the *Long-term Conditions Positive Practice Guide* (DH, 2008) confirm the importance of links to physical health services. An example of good practice is highlighted by Salford Pathfinder who have explored the needs of people with type 1 diabetes who are also experiencing depression and/or anxiety disorders by developing a suitable care pathway into the IAPT service. Staff who manage people with diabetes have been trained to screen for and identify common mental health problems, such as depression and anxiety, and to refer those patients to providers of psychological therapies.

CASE STUDY:
PTSD

Mental and physical health problems are frequently interwoven and current estimates suggest that approximately one quarter of people with physical illness develop mental health problems as a consequence of the stress of their physical condition (National Collaboration Centre for Mental Health, 2011). There is also an unacceptably large 'premature mortality gap' which sees people with mental illness dying up to 15–20 years earlier than those without, often from avoidable causes (Davies, 2014). The journey taken by a patient with a long-term condition is often one of loss, threat and uncertainty, which are established risk factors for anxiety and depression, which is itself associated with an increased risk of coronary heart disease (JCPMH, 2013). There are also social considerations to take into account. Practitioners in a primary care setting often have to be mindful of more than the presenting problem and its treatment. In essence, the solution has to fit the wider constraints of a person's life. Workers in primary mental health care are required to help with the presenting problem, while keeping the whole person in view and maintaining a broad sense of the person's life in a wide social context. Their family, friends, roles, and the contribution that they make to the lives of others are the cornerstones that keep the structure of the patient's life in place. Primary mental health care seeks to offer early detection and suitable assistance in a setting which minimises disruption to the overall balance of a person's life.

CASE STUDY 32.3

Rachel visited her GP for her annual medical review; her GP identified that her blood pressure and her Body Max Index (BMI) were over the recommended guidelines, suggesting she was overweight for her height. Her GP suggested she attend her local weight management programme. Rachel had tried to explain to her GP that the reason for her increase in weight was not her fault. Her GP dismissed this and suggested she attend the group. Rachel was reluctant to attend the programme, however agreed to go. The health trainer who had knowledge of the link between overeating and stress was able to identify that she had been overeating due to increased levels of stress, and provide her with appropriate information on a local programme, Stress control, which would enable her to learn coping strategies of how to manage stress and identify alternative coping strategies such as mindfulness and cognitive restructuring.

Some examples of how primary mental health care services have integrated with physical health care services are as follows:

- training in mental health and illness with chronic obstructive pulmonary disease nurses
- incorporating sessions on stress and mental health awareness on long-term conditions programmes
- co-delivering pain management sessions with services such as chronic pain and healthy lifestyle services
- volunteer health champions
- improving care pathways between physical and mental health services
- training for practice nurses and pharmacists in physical health services on early signs of poor mental health.

CRITICAL THINKING STOP POINT 32.3

- How else might services work collaboratively to provide integrated care for both physical and mental health?
- How confident do you feel working with clients with physical health needs?

CRITICAL DEBATE 32.1

- Think about the area that you live in. Where would you put mental health professionals so that they were truly accessible to the public? What times of day would you have them there? Which days would be best?
- Think about the people who live on your street. If they needed to get some support from a primary mental health service, what might make it difficult for them to do that? How could they be helped to get help?
- Think about what is good about 'community'. How could mental health care fit into that?

CONCLUSION

Primary mental health care provides the majority of mental health care to people living in the UK. Examples of high quality services do exist. In those services, the multiple ways to access the service are clear and straightforward, people are seen locally and quickly, at a time and place that suits them, and they receive expert intervention with appropriate follow-up. They are offered choices and provided with clear information to help them make decisions about their care. However, a high proportion of people who need a service like that do not get it. Many people with common mental health problems continue to suffer alone, or struggle on, thinking it is the only thing they can do.

Access to services remains a concern. Assessment and treatment are often only available during normal working hours, and there is more to do in order to reach people who are currently unsupported. Services could be offered in non-traditional community-based settings such as community centres, places of worship, colleges and social centres. Staff who work at those places could receive training to help with early identification and easy referral. It may be that short-term childcare assistance or **carer** respite would enable people to get to the help they need. Primary mental health care makes sense. It is close to the communities in which we live, linked in to wider social resources, and it reduces stigma and exclusion.

CHAPTER SUMMARY

Having read this chapter, you should now be able to:

- Define primary mental health care
- Give examples of the various settings in which it takes place
- Explain the contribution made to primary care services by IAPT
- Describe the stepped care model and a service user journey
- Provide examples of how physical and mental health services can work in a more integrative way.

BUILD YOUR BIBLIOGRAPHY

Books

- Collins, E., Drake, M. & Deacon, M. (eds) (2013) *The physical care of people with mental health problems: A guide for best practice.* London: SAGE. This accessible, practical text provides mental health practitioners with the core knowledge and skills they need to be able to care effectively for the physical health of those who have been diagnosed with mental illness.
- Gask, L., Lester, H., Kenderick, T., et al. (2009) *Primary care mental health.* London: Royal College of Psychiatrists. In this book, internationally respected authors provide a conceptual background and dispense practical advice for the clinician.
- Pryjmachuk, S. (2011) *Mental health nursing: An evidence based introduction.* London: SAGE. This is a practical, values- and evidence-based resource which focuses on all major mental health problems.

SAGE journal articles

FURTHER
READING:
JOURNAL
ARTICLES

Go to https://study.sagepub.com/essentialmentalhealth for further free online journal articles related to this chapter. If you are using the interactive ebook, simply click on the book icon in the margin to go straight to the resource.

- Borges, T., Miasso, A., Reisdofer, E., et al. (2016) Common mental disorders in primary health care units: associated factors and impact on quality of life. *Journal of the American Psychiatric Nurses Association, 22*(5), 378-386.
- Lamb, J., Bower, P., Rogers, A., et al. (2012) Access to mental health in primary care: a qualitative meta-synthesis of evidence from the experience of people from 'hard to reach' groups. *Health, 16,* 76-104.
- Wetherell, J., Kaplan, R., Kallenberg, G., et al. (2004) Mental health treatment preferences of older and younger primary care patients. *Int J Psychiatry Med, 34,* 219-233.

Weblinks

FURTHER
READING:
WEBLINKS

Go to https://study.sagepub.com/essentialmentalhealth for further weblinks related to this chapter. If you are using the interactive ebook, simply click on the book icon in the margin to go straight to the resource.

- IAPT: www.england.nhs.uk/mental-health/adults/iapt – supports the frontline NHS in implementing NICE guidelines for people suffering from depression and anxiety disorders. A gateway website to the NHS England programme
- The King's Fund: www.kingsfund.org.uk – an independent charity working to improve health and care in England. They help to shape policy and practice through research and analysis; develop individuals, teams and organisations; promote understanding of the health and social care system; and bring people together to learn, share knowledge and debate
- The Sainsbury Centre for Mental Health: www.centreformentalhealth.org.uk – works to improve the quality of life for people with mental health problems. It produces a number of publications, many of which are free to download.

GREAT FOR
REVISION

ACE YOUR ASSESSMENT

Revise what you have learned by visiting https://study.sagepub.com/essentialmentalhealth. If you are using the interactive ebook, simply click on the tick icon to go straight to the resource.

- Test yourself with multiple-choice and short-answer questions and flashcards.

ONLINE
QUIZZES &
ACTIVITY
ANSWERS

REFERENCES

Bath, J. & Wekerman, J. (2015) Impact of community participation in primary health care: what is the evidence? *Australian Journal of Primary Health, 21,* 2–8.

Collins, E., Drake, M. & Deacon, M. (eds) (2013) *The physical care of people with mental health problems: A guide for best practice.* London: Sage.

Davies, S.C. (2014) *Annual report of the chief medical officer 2013: Public mental health priorities – investing in the evidence.* London: Department of Health.

De Lusignan, S., Jones, S., McCrae, N., et al. (2013) *IAPT LTC/MUS pathfinder evaluation project interim report: The Improving Access to Psychological Therapies (IAPT) programme project report.* London: IAPT.

Department of Health (DH) (1997) *The new NHS, modern, dependable.* London: DH.

Department of Health (1999) *The national service framework.* London: DH.

Department of Health (2008) *Long-term conditions positive practice guide.* London: DH.

Department of Health (2011a) *No health without mental health: Delivering better mental health outcomes for people of all ages.* London: DH.

Department of Health (2011b) *Talking therapies: A four-year plan of action.* London: DH.

Department of Health (2012) *IAPT three-year report: The first million patients.* London: DH.

England, E. (2014) *The extraordinary potential of primary care to improve mental health.* Available at: www.rcgp.org.uk/clinical-and-research/clinical-resources/~/media/Files/CIRC/Mental%20

Health%20-%202014/RCGP-The-Extraordinary-Potential-of-Primary-Care-to-Improve-Mental-Health-June-2014.ashx (accessed 25.07.16).

Huffman, J.C. and Pollack, M.H. (2003) Predicting panic disorder among patients with chest pain: an analysis of the literature. *Psychosomatics*, 44(3), 222–236.

Joint Commissioning Panel for Mental Health (JCPMH) (2013) *Guidance for commissioners of primary mental health care services.* London: Royal College of Psychiatrists.

Layard, R., Clark, D., Bell, S., et al. (2006) *The depression report: A new deal for depression and anxiety disorders.* London: The Centre for Economic Performance's Mental Health Policy Group, LSE.

McHugh, P., Brennan, J., Galligan, N., McGonagle, C. & Byrne, M. (2013) Evaluation of a primary care adult mental health service: year 2. *Mental Health in Family Medicine*, 10, 53–59.

McManus, S., Meltzer, H., Brugha, T., et al. (2009) *Adult psychiatric morbidity in England 2007.* Leeds: NHS Information Centre for Health and Social Care.

National Collaboration Centre for Mental Health (2011) *Common mental health disorders: Identification and pathways to care.* London: Royal College of Psychiatrists.

National Institute for Health and Clinical Excellence (NICE) (2004) *Depression: Core interventions in the management of depression in primary and secondary care.* London: The Stationery Office.

National Institute for Health and Clinical Excellence (NICE) (2009) *Depression in adults: Recognition and management.* London: The Stationery Office.

Naylor, C., Das, P., Ross, S., et al. (2016) *Bringing together physical and mental health: A new frontier for integrated care.* London: King's Fund. Available at: www.kingsfund.org.uk/publications/physical-and-mental-health (accessed 09.08.17).

Simon, G.E., VonKorff, M., Piccinelli, M., et al. (1999) An international study in the relation between somatic symptoms and depression. *New England Journal of Medicine*, 341, 1329–1335.

Spitzer, R. L., Kroenke, K, Williams, J. B.W., et al. (2006). "A brief measure for assessing generalized anxiety disorder: The GAD-7". *Archives of Internal Medicine. 166* (10): 1092–7.

Wand, T. & Murray, L. (2008) Let's get physical. *International Journal of Mental Health Nursing, 17,* 363–369.

World Health Organization (WHO) (2016) *Main terminology.* Available at: www.euro.who.int/en/health-topics/Health-systems/primary-health-care/main-terminology (accessed 13.07.16).

World Health Organization and the World Organization of Family Doctors (WONCA) (2008) *Integrating mental health in primary care – a global perspective.* Geneva: WHO.

MEETING THE PHYSICAL HEALTH NEEDS OF MENTAL HEALTH SERVICE USERS

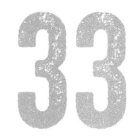

JACQUIE WHITE, SAMANTHA O'BRIEN, MEGAN BEADLE AND ANTHONY ACKROYD

THIS CHAPTER COVERS

- The higher than expected rates of physical health problems in users of mental health services, that lead to poor quality of life and a significantly shortened life span
- The complex interaction between biological, psychological, sociological and systems factors
- Physical health care as a core mental health nursing competence
- Barriers to assessment and intervention in primary and secondary care
- How mental health nurses can make a positive difference to the physical health of the service users they work with.

In my region the life expectancy of people with serious mental illness [SMI][1] is around 45 years of age. We took action to address this by providing annual health checks utilising the Health Improvement Profile [HIP] (Hardy et al., 2015). Our nurse led clinics provide lifestyle discussion and physical health checks, including full blood pathology, urinalysis, general observations and full body analysis. Our approach is engaging and motivational with the service being offered within primary care health centres (where our community mental health teams are based) or in the service user's [SU's] home to enable us to address social withdrawal and non-attendance.

(Continued)

Visit **https://study.sagepub.com/essentialmentalhealth** to access a wealth of online resources for this chapter – watch out for the margin icons throughout the chapter. If you are using the interactive ebook, simply click on the margin icon to go straight to the resource.

---

[1]SMI is usually defined as people with a diagnosis of schizophrenia, schizoaffective disorder, bipolar disorder or severe depression.

> We believe this intervention has to have real meaning so we work closely with primary care providers, commissioners and specialist services to provide relevant and timely interventions. The information from the HIP is shared with the GP, with a letter suggesting further investigations or referrals. We have negotiated fast-track access to dental services, smoking cessation and health trainers as well as using our own dietetic service.
>
> Since its conception our attendance rates have improved from the national average of 50% to 80%. We have detected common health issues such as glucose intolerance, renal issues, and hypertension to more sinister issues like cancers. Our findings show that 68% of our SUs have health issues that were not previously identified. This reinforces the real need and importance of the work we are doing.
>
> **Anthony Ackroyd, specialist clinical lead for a wellbeing health improvement service**

> I have had a diagnosis of serious mental illness for 21 years. The last 11 years though have been my biggest challenge, following being diagnosed with symphysis pubis dysfunction during my pregnancy. I had the front of my pelvis fused three years ago, however I still require crutches or a wheelchair. A major part of maintaining my mental health was visiting the gym, as this also helped manage the weight gain from psychiatric medication. However, all this has been taken away and instead I now have a life of constant chronic pain. This becomes worse during the colder months and can result in a deterioration in my mental health.
>
> Unfortunately, a small minority of staff have shown a poor understanding regarding how chronic pain impacts on my mental wellbeing and the challenges I face every day due to my physical disability, including poor sleep, social isolation, lack of independence and side-effects of strong pain medication. This makes an already difficult situation even worse.
>
> I fully support and value the ethos of service user recovery. However, at times I have been left with feelings of frustration when trying to explain the reason that I rest on my bed or sofa so much is due to chronic pain, which makes moving around agony, and that I need to pace myself. For this to be then interpreted as socially isolating myself demonstrates how much more work needs to be undertaken in order for staff across all areas to understand more how chronic pain or other long-term physical illnesses impact on individuals.
>
> **Sam, service user**

INTRODUCTION

It is a sad fact that many of the **service users** we work with experience physical health problems that significantly impact on their lives and their chances of a meaningful **recovery**. Most mental health nurses can recall service users who they have known and worked with who died in their 40s or 50s. Many of these service users did not die as a result of suicide, something we rightly work hard to regularly assess and intervene to prevent, but from preventable physical disease.

Large numbers of service users and their **carers** live with the consequences of long-term physical health problems and conditions that significantly impact on their ability to get on with and enjoy their lives. The way health services are set up and staff trained and expected to work within them creates many barriers to holistic (whole person) care. Individual service users may have to approach a number of different agencies to try to get their needs identified and met. They can experience **stigma** and discrimination from health professionals and services who fail to identify and respond appropriately to their physical health needs. This chapter outlines the importance of the integration of physical health care into the work of mental health nurses and services. It offers some potential solutions to the challenges faced by those who are striving to do this.

CHALLENGES

Users of mental health services have much higher than expected rates of physical health problems than people in the general population

The terms **comorbidity** and multimorbidity are used in the literature to describe people with coexisting diseases, **disorders**, conditions, **illnesses** or health problems. When only two of these are identified, the term 'dual diagnosis' is sometimes used, although this can be misleading because the person is likely to have a multitude of health problems and needs that require support, intervention and care.

It is estimated that 4.6 million people in England with a diagnosis of mental illness have a comorbid physical diagnosis (Naylor et al., 2012). The true figure is likely to be much higher because this data only represents people who have accessed health services and had their diagnosis identified and documented in their health record. It is also possible for mental and physical health problems to impact on people's lives without them meeting the criteria for formal diagnosis.

There is considerable overlap between mental and physical wellbeing, this overlap being relevant to the whole population and across the age spectrum. We know that people with long-term physical health conditions (e.g. diabetes, heart and respiratory disease) have higher than expected rates of psychological distress and mental illness. Rates of clinical **depression**, for example, are estimated to be 2 to 3 times higher than in the general population, with **anxiety** disorders at similar levels. Diabetes, heart and respiratory diseases are known risk factors for the development of cognitive impairment and **dementia**, with a greater risk when depression is also present. Not surprisingly, a recent systematic review highlighted very high rates of physical comorbidity in people with a diagnosis of dementia (Smith et al., 2014). The most commonly reported physical diagnoses were neurological disorders (96%), vascular disorders (91%), cardiac disorders (73%) and depression (59%). In SMI, a higher prevalence of physical comorbidity is seen in nearly every system organ class of the body, with the highest reported rates in cardiovascular and respiratory diseases (White, 2015).

The consequence of higher than expected physical health problems is poorer health-related quality of life and a significantly shortened life span

Health-related quality of life refers to the physical, psychological and social domains of health that can be considered to make up an individual's perception of their own health status (Testa & Simonson, 1996). Poorer physical and mental health-related quality of life as a consequence of comorbidity is associated with earlier than expected mortality (death).

Research has demonstrated a significantly reduced life expectancy for people with a range of mental illness diagnoses, representing one of the most significant public health challenges we face today. These types of studies use observational designs that follow up people over time to examine outcomes. One large cohort study in South London, which matched people admitted to mental health services with coroners' records, identified the shortest life expectancy in women with a diagnosis of schizoaffective disorder (17.5 years lost) and in men with a diagnosis of **schizophrenia** (14.6 years lost) (Chang et al., 2011). Suicide contributes to these statistics and (to a lesser degree) accidental death but both of these are more likely in the years immediately following diagnosis. When these causes of death are removed from the analysis, the importance of physical disease as a cause of early death is identified. The most significant one of these across all the studies undertaken so far is cardiovascular disease, causing 2.5–3 times more early deaths than for people in the general population.

Since the 1980s, life expectancy has been increasing in the general population but falling in the population of people with an SMI diagnosis. This 'mortality gap' appears to be linked to the transition from hospital to community care when large institutions closed in the late 1980s, and has been identified across the western world.[2] Public health campaigns that are continuing to make a significant impact on early mortality in the general population have not yet had the same impact on people with mental illness (e.g. smoking cessation campaigns).

The relationship between physical and mental health is complex and involves interaction between biological, psychological, sociological and systems factors

There are multiple risk factors that contribute to physical ill health and early mortality in people who access mental health services. These include those related to psychological and physical stress, symptoms, health behaviour, systems factors and the consequences of stigma and social exclusion. A simple sum of individual risk factors cannot determine the total risk faced by an individual as each risk interacts on a personal and system level to multiply the overall risk. All risks are potentially modifiable and present targets for intervention.

Physical and psychological stress is a state where homeostasis is threatened or there is a perception of threat. Stress is mediated through the hypothalamic–pituitary–adrenal axis and the sympathetic nervous system to impact on the body, brain and behaviour. A dysfunctional response to **acute** or chronic stress may lead to the development of inflammatory, metabolic and/or cardiovascular disorders (McEwen, 2006).

Hallucinations and **delusions** may theoretically increase the risk of physical ill health by making people avoid or take certain actions, by inferring protection or by distracting attention. Over-activity, hostility and impulsive behaviour may increase the risk of accident and injury, and all symptoms may result in a failure to attend to adequate self-care. Cognitive deficits and **negative symptoms** may reduce recognition or communication of physical symptoms or help-seeking behaviour. Depressed **mood** or **apathy** can impact on engagement, treatment or motivation to bring about behaviour change.

Sleep is a complex process that enables the brain to recover, reorganise and regenerate. Sleep of an adequate duration and quality is important for physical and mental health and improvements in sleep are early signs of recovery (Spiegelhalder et al., 2013). Insomnia is associated with fatigue, daytime sleepiness, poor concentration, irritability, memory loss, poor function, depression and a weakened immune system. Some psychiatric medications improve sleep duration and quality but can lead to

---

[2]In countries where people with mental illness are largely cared for in institutions, respiratory disease is the leading cause of death.

daytime sleepiness, and others (and many recreational drugs) impair sleep. Insomnia and oversleeping are associated with the development of diabetes and cardiovascular disease (Cappuccio et al., 2010).

Smoking behaviour is the largest modifiable risk factor for cardiovascular disease worldwide. The significant reduction in smoking seen in the general population in the developed world in recent years is not matched in SMI. Rates of around 50%, twice that of the general population, are reported (Vancampfort et al., 2013). This is despite good evidence that interventions, including nicotine replacement therapy (NRT), are just as effective in people with mental illness as for everyone else. A review of medication and information exchange at the preparation to stop stage is important because changes in smoking behaviour (even with NRT) and in the short term (e.g. during a hospital admission) can cause clinically significant medicine interactions (Medicines and Healthcare Products Regulation Agency & the Commission on Human Medicines, 2009).

Alcohol and substance use are common in mental health service users, and contribute to a worse prognosis and early mortality, including by suicide (Swofford et al., 2000). Choice of substance may be linked to availability, rather than preference. Cannabis is the most commonly used recreational drug after alcohol and, because it is commonly smoked with tobacco, the exact mechanism of effects on the cause, development of symptoms and progression/prognosis is difficult to determine. It certainly contributes to tobacco-related disease.

High doses of caffeine are readily available from the diet but also from popular 'high energy' drinks, often consumed with alcohol. Caffeine can enable a greater consumption of alcohol over longer periods of time by reducing the sedative effect. This can lead to a dangerous mix of risk-taking behaviour and disinhibition, because the person overestimates their ability to function. Excessive caffeine consumption is associated with insomnia and hostile/aggressive behaviour, particularly in acute mental health settings (Simmons, 1996). Restriction of caffeine may have unintended consequences as withdrawal can increase these behaviours.

Problems accessing, affording, cooking or understanding a healthy diet are all cited as barriers to eating healthily in surveys of the general population. Those people reporting existing health problems are more likely to report obesity and lower confidence in changing their current diet and exercise behaviour. Poor nutritional content, a lack of variety, overreliance on convenience foods and poor diet literacy have all been identified in people with schizophrenia (Hardy & Gray, 2012). Fluid intake can be impaired (or polydipsia may be present), leading to dehydration and/or electrolyte imbalance. There has been a recent focus on malnutrition in care **environments** associated with the elderly, but the quality of nutrition in residential environments for adults with SMI has received little attention.

The impact of prescribed medication is an important consideration. With respect to suicide, some **psychotropic medication** can be fatal in overdose (e.g. tricyclic antidepressants), while others substantially reduce suicide risk and rates (e.g. lithium). The risk of falls as a result of sedation side-effects are well documented in the elderly but can also contribute to accidents and injury in younger adults. The impact of antipsychotic medications on the risk of cardiovascular disease is highly controversial.

CRITICAL DEBATE 33.1

- Does antipsychotic medication damage physical health?

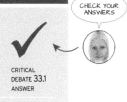

CHECK YOUR ANSWERS

CRITICAL DEBATE 33.1 ANSWER

The risk to individual service users extends beyond actions or omissions by individuals or specific professional groups to the system of care. There is a **culture** of risk assessment in mental health services in the UK that understandably focuses on the risk of suicide or potential harm due to violence or vulnerability to exploitation. A recent guide to risk assessment and management designed for mental health professionals did not include any assessment of previously unknown physical health risk (Hart, 2014).

Guidance highlights the importance of joint working with primary care to achieve optimal physical health care for mental health service users, known as collaborative or integrated care (National Collaborating Centre for Mental Health, 2014; National Institute for Health and Care Excellence, 2014). Cross-sectional surveys demonstrate that people with SMI attend primary care more frequently than the general population, have longer consultation times, and that these represent about two thirds of all their health contacts (Reilly et al., 2012).

A difference between the published prevalence (number of known cases in a population) and incidence (number of new cases) highlights considerable under-recognition, diagnosis and treatment of physical health problems in people with mental illness. For example, we know from large epidemiological studies that rates of heart disease in schizophrenia are 2.5–3 times higher than in the general population, but studies of primary care (GP) case registers of people with a schizophrenia diagnosis reveal rates nearer to 1.8 (Smith et al., 2013).

CASE STUDY:
PRIMARY
CARE

Stigma is a social construction that devalues or dehumanises people as a result of a distinguishing characteristic or label (Lauber, 2008). Mental health service users are amongst the most excluded groups in society. Stigma and social exclusion increase the likelihood of unemployment, poverty, social isolation and poor housing. These factors not only contribute to disease and mortality risk but interact with each other. For example, poverty may lead to inadequate nutrition and, along with poor transport links, reduce access to health care to treat the results. Even where there is contact with services and health professionals, being identified as 'mentally ill' may mean a failure to treat the whole person (Schulze, 2007). The term 'diagnostic overshadowing' has been used to describe a health interaction where the person assessing the person's needs responds only to what they would expect to be a symptom of their (recorded) primary diagnosis (Jones et al., 2008). For example, a person with dementia who is taken to see their GP by their husband due to an increase in **agitation** may be treated for the behavioural symptoms of dementia, rather than being referred for investigations to see if they are constipated and/or in pain. Self-stigma, where the person internalises common stereotypes about mental illness such as self-blame, may reduce help-seeking behaviour and/or the confidence to make positive changes to health behaviours (Watson et al., 2007).

Until 2014, GPs in England were paid to provide annual cardiovascular disease screening to people with SMI but this did not routinely take place and, where it did, was less frequent and less comprehensive than screening provided to people with other long-term conditions (Mitchell & Hardy, 2013). Low expectations of staff or 'therapeutic pessimism' may result in a culture of less engagement, investment of resources and intervention (Horsfall et al., 2010; Thornicroft et al., 2007). Once a physical comorbidity is diagnosed, people with mental illness receive fewer interventions and treatments than people with the same condition in the general population (Mitchell et al., 2009). Mental health service users may find it difficult to navigate the fragmentation of health services, i.e. the separation of psychiatric and medical services. Carers of people with SMI and the staff who work with them may themselves face negative attitudes that impact on collaborative care. Surveys of GPs and practice nurses report that many feel ill equipped to provide care for people with SMI (Lester et al., 2005). High caseloads, low contact time and problems with communication across service boundaries impair the ability of community mental health nurses to step in and perform this function (White, 2015). A radical change in service **commissioning** and design to deliver a real integration of services, at the point that an individual accesses them, has now been recommended (Naylor et al., 2016).

Physical health care as a core nursing competence

Mental health nurses are the largest group of health care professionals in contact with people with mental health problems. For mental health nurses, the challenge is to understand enough about the biological paradigm of health to assess and intervene positively to provide holistic care. There is a real opportunity to make a difference through existing contact and **therapeutic relationships** with service users. Mental health nurses can use their skills to listen to and assess service users, to support them to access and utilise services and interventions and to make changes to their health behaviours. Medicines management and physical health assessment and care are recognised as essential skills for all nurses (Nursing and Midwifery Council, 2010). Research indicates that where mental health nurses deliver this care, it is highly valued by service users and their carers:

In a political climate where many are crying out for parity of esteem, it seems ironic that within mental health services we don't seem to demonstrate the equality toward physical health that we would expect in return. Current pressures on services are clear, but in my experience basic physical health assessments are the first to be overlooked, making it difficult for student nurses to practise the skills they need and achieve competence and confidence.

Foundation anatomy and physiology modules begin by highlighting the influence of medications and lifestyle choices upon physical health, but without exposure to assessment and intervention in practice, a significant theory–practice gap remains. Students try to address this by utilising inpatient services to perform physical assessments to support learning during community placements but this is dependent on each student's motivation. More structured opportunities encompassing a training circuit are beneficial. A buddy system in the adult field could also help mental health nursing students to broaden their physical health knowledge (and adult students to broaden their mental health knowledge). Crossing traditional provider services boundaries would offer potential learning opportunities for both sets of students (and mentors). Regular simulated training exercises reminding students and mentors of the critical influence of physical–mental health could promote joint learning.

Megan, mental health nursing student

Current health policy focuses on assessment and intervention in both primary and secondary care

Current health policy in England focuses on assessment and intervention in primary or secondary care. However, confusion about who is responsible for physical care and problems communicating across services persist and present substantial barriers to effective care. The most significant impediments to improving the physical care and experience of service users and carers appear to be for those in the community, rather than inpatient mental health services. Many mental health services have implemented care pathways that include physical health assessment and intervention, driven by commissioning targets. Recent NICE guidance for **psychosis** states that annual health checks should take place in primary care, with access facilitated by the care coordinator or the responsibility transferred to primary care using the care programme approach (CPA) (National Collaborating Centre for Mental Health, 2014). This relies on the engagement of primary care clinicians with the CPA process, and service users being willing and able to access primary care. It also relies on GP services being able and willing to provide services for people with mental illness in the absence of financial incentives to do so.

Mental health nurses are keen to make a positive difference to the physical health of the service users they work with

Surveys indicate that mental health nurses (MHNs) regard physical health as an important part of their role, but deficits in clinical practice persist, hampered by a lack of knowledge, skills and resources and problems facilitating access to care across the primary–secondary care interface (Howard & Gamble, 2011; Nash, 2005, 2010; Robson & Haddad, 2012). This research largely represents MHNs working in inpatient settings, although the largest survey to date (n = 585) did not report any significant differences in the 30% of its sample who worked in community teams (Robson & Haddad, 2012).

WHAT'S THE EVIDENCE? 33.1

Screening or intervention?

At its core, the problem of comorbidity is one of a mismatch between a clinical reality in which medical conditions and mental health conditions are overlapping and interrelated, and a health care system in which the providers, clinics and treatments are separated. (Druss & Walker, 2011: 15)

Despite nearly a decade of practice guidance in the UK highlighting the need for physical health care in SMI, there is very little evidence that physical health screening or intervention is consistently taking place. A baseline audit of records on four randomly selected inpatient wards and one community mental health team in the largest UK mental health NHS trust identified 100% adult inpatients but only 22% community patients with a record of smoking status (Parker et al., 2012). Of the 62 inpatients who said they smoked, only 25% had a record of a conversation about risk and only one had been referred to smoking cessation services. For the five cardio-metabolic risk factors considered most important in SMI (body mass index, blood glucose, blood lipids, blood pressure and smoking status), the rate for a record of assessment of all five was a disappointing 33% (range 1%–77%) in the second National Audit of Schizophrenia (NAS) (Royal College of Psychiatrists, 2014).

There is evidence that interventions that are successful in the general population work just as well in people with mental illness (e.g. pharmacological treatments for smoking cessation). This is reflected in NICE guidance that recommends reference to the guidance for treatment of the specific comorbidity (e.g. type 2 diabetes). Despite numerous selective and systematic reviews of physical health interventions, authors have so far failed to find enough evidence to recommend specific interventions or health-screening methods. What is agreed is that future research should focus on collaborative and integrative ways of working to try to address the barriers to effective intervention. This is relevant to mental health nurses, many of whom undertake care coordination roles or (in inpatient settings) plan care that includes needs that have to be met by other service providers.

CRITICAL THINKING STOP POINT 33.1

In the absence of health-screening methods or interventions specifically recommended by authors of systematic reviews or NICE, what can mental health nurses safely use to guide their practice?

CRITICAL
THINKING
STOP
POINT 33.1
ANSWER

Even though evidence for a positive impact of physical health interventions specifically tailored to mental health service users is largely absent from the research literature, there is a growing body of good practice that can be shared and utilised. There is also a need for whole-system change, something mental health nurses can help to make a reality.

MAKING A DIFFERENCE 33.1

The vast majority of people with mental health problems access primary, not secondary, care services. Considering the increase in (physical and mental health) comorbidity in the population, everyone who comes into contact with a person seeking help or a service (wherever delivered) has an opportunity to act to improve the health outcomes of individuals, and, as a result, the wider population. This was promoted as an approach to improve public mental health and physical health in *Making Every Contact Count* (NHS Future Forum, 2012). In practice, it means that dentists should be able to engage someone in a health behaviour change conversation about smoking cessation, or a practice nurse seeing an elderly person to provide their influenza inoculation should be able to intervene just as appropriately if the person discloses low mood as they would if the person discloses shortness of breath, or a community mental health nurse visiting someone at home who has recently been discharged following a relapse of mania should have the skills to monitor blood pressure and take appropriate action if hypertension is identified. In secondary care, nurse-led clinics have the potential to engage mental health service users.

(Continued)

There are examples of mental health nurses adapting medication management clinics (previously used to administer long-acting antipsychotic injections and/or monitor clozapine) into 'wellbeing' clinics. Two examples are described in a publication about a nurse-led clinic in Scotland (Shuel et al., 2010) and at the beginning of this chapter. Commissioning is also making a difference in many areas where a national Commissioning for Quality and Innovation (CQUIN) target for 2015-16 specifically rewarded practice that assures regular health checks are delivered at identified intervals in the care pathway for SMI.

Core mental health nursing skills are of prime importance to both engage service users and actively listen to their needs, while maintaining an awareness of the likelihood of giving more attention to mental, rather than physical, health. Risk assessment should include family and personal history of metabolic and heart disease, the systematic assessment of current physical health parameters, health behaviours and the person's readiness to change. Education and supervision should be sought to develop and maintain skills in engaging service users and health behaviour change interventions (e.g. motivational interviewing). Maintaining skills in the competent assessment of vital signs and medicines management is important, and the use of an evidence-based systematic health assessment and improvement tool to support practice is recommended. Such tools act as an aide memoire as to which parameters to assess, how to interpret results and the recommended action when parameters are found to be out of normal range. As with many other areas of mental health nursing, establishing and building relationships with those who work in a range of other services and agencies will enable the service user to be assisted to access these, or the nurse to **advocate** their needs when they are unable to do so. Effective person-centred **care planning** can support this activity, as can lobbying for joined-up thinking through the commissioning process and the local development of services and integrated care pathways.

CHAPTER SUMMARY

This chapter has covered the following ideas:

- Physical and mental health are entwined but the design of health services has tended to separate the two, making it difficult for mental health service users to access truly holistic care.
- Physical comorbidity and early mortality in people who access mental health services is a significant public health challenge.
- Multiple risk factors contribute to physical ill health and early mortality.
- A simple sum of individual risk factors cannot determine the total risk faced by an individual as each risk interacts on a personal and system level to multiply the overall risk.
- All risks are potentially modifiable and present targets for mental health nursing intervention.
- Mental health nurses are uniquely placed to make a difference in this important area of practice by using core skills to listen to and engage service users, by challenging stigma and diagnostic overshadowing, conducting or improving access to health checks and supporting the implementation of interventions, particularly those associated with health behaviour change and medicines management.
- There are a range of tools and examples of good practice available to support this work that build on core mental health nursing skills, many of them designed and led by mental health nurses.

BUILD YOUR BIBLIOGRAPHY

Books

- Hardy, S., White, J. & Gray, R. (2015) *The health improvement profile: A manual to promote physical wellbeing in people with severe mental illness.* Keswick: M&K Publishing.
- Kurrle, S., Brodaty, H. & Hogarth, R. (2012) *Physical comorbidities of dementia.* Cambridge: Cambridge University Press.

SAGE journal articles

Go to https://study.sagepub.com/essentialmentalhealth for further free online journal articles related to this chapter. If you are using the interactive ebook, simply click on the book icon in the margin to go straight to the resource.

FURTHER READING: JOURNAL ARTICLES

- Deakin, B., Ferrier, N., Holt, R.I., et al. (2010) The physical health challenges in patients with severe mental illness: cardiovascular and metabolic risks. *Journal of Psychopharmacology, 24,* 1-8.
- Dursun, S., Dinan, T.G., Bushe, C., et al. (2005) Challenges in advancing mental and physical health of patients with serious mental illness. *Journal of Psychopharmacology, 19*(6 suppl.), 3-5.
- Young, S.L., Taylor, M. & Lawrie, S.M. (2015) 'First do no harm': a systematic review of the prevalence and management of antipsychotic adverse effects. *Journal of Psychopharmacology, 29,* 353-362.

Weblinks

Go to https://study.sagepub.com/essentialmentalhealth for further weblinks related to this chapter. If you are using the interactive ebook, simply click on the book icon in the margin to go straight to the resource.

FURTHER READING: WEBLINKS

- Physical health in SMI, a resource for primary care: http://physicalsmi.webeden.co.uk
- Rethink Physical Health Resources (includes the National CQUIN toolkit): www.rethink.org/phc
- Royal College of Psychiatrists physical health pages: www.rcpsych.ac.uk/mentalhealthinfo/improvingphysicalandmh.aspx

ACE YOUR ASSESSMENT

Revise what you have learned by visiting https://study.sagepub.com/essentialmentalhealth. If you are using the interactive ebook, simply click on the tick icon to go straight to the resource.

ONLINE QUIZZES & ACTIVITY ANSWERS

- Test yourself with multiple-choice and short-answer questions and flashcards.

REFERENCES

Baxter, A.J., Harris, M.G., Khatib, Y., et al. (2016) Reducing excess mortality due to chronic disease in people with severe mental illness: meta-review of health interventions. *The British Journal of Psychiatry, 208*(4), 322–329.

Cappuccio, F.P., D'elia, L., Strazzullo, P., et al. (2010) Quantity and quality of sleep and incidence of type 2 diabetes: a systematic review and meta-analysis. *Diabetes Care, 33*, 414–420.

Chang, C.-K., Hayes, R.D., Perera, G., et al. (2011) Life Expectancy at birth for people with serious mental illness and other major disorders from a secondary mental health care case register in London. *PLoS ONE, 6*, e19590.

Curtis, J., Watkins, A., Rosenbaum, S., et al. (2015) Evaluating an individualized lifestyle and life skills intervention to prevent antipsychotic-induced weight gain in first-episode psychosis. *Early Intervention in Psychiatry, 10*(3), 267–276.

De Hert, M., Detraux, J., Van Winkel, R., Yu, W. & Correll, C.U. (2012) Metabolic and cardiovascular adverse effects associated with antipsychotic drugs. *Nature Reviews Endocrinology, 8*, 114–26.

Druss, B.G. & Walker, E.R. (2011) Mental disorders and medical comorbidity. *Synthesis Project Research Synthesis Report, 21*, 1–26.

Gough, S.C.L. & O'Donovan, M.C. (2005) Clustering of metabolic comorbidity in schizophrenia: a genetic contribution? *Journal of Psychopharmacology, 19*, 47–55.

Hardy, S. & Gray, R. (2012) The secret food diary of a person diagnosed with schizophrenia. *Journal of Psychiatric Mental Health Nursing, 19*, 603–609.

Hardy, S., White, J. & Gray, R. (2015) *The health improvement profile: A manual to promote physical wellbeing in people with severe mental illness.* Keswick: M&K Publishing.

Hart, C. (2014) *A pocket guide to risk assessment and management in mental health.* Abingdon: Routledge.

Horsfall, J., Cleary, M. & Hunt, G.E. (2010) Stigma in mental health: clients and professionals. *Issues Mental Health Nursing, 31*, 450–455.

Howard, L. & Gamble, C. (2011) Supporting mental health nurses to address the physical health needs of people with serious mental illness in acute inpatient care settings. *Journal of Psychiatric and Mental Health Nursing, 18*, 105–112.

Jones, S., Howard, L. & Thornicroft, G. (2008) 'Diagnostic overshadowing': worse physical health care for people with mental illness. *Acta Psychiatrica Scandinavica, 118*, 169–171.

Lauber, C. (2008) Stigma and discrimination against people with mental illness: a critical appraisal. *Epidemiologia Psychiatria Sociale, 17*, 10–13.

Lester, H., Tritter, J.Q. & Sorohan, H. (2005) Patients' and health professionals' views on primary care for people with serious mental illness: focus group study. BMJ, *330*, 1122.

McEwen, B.S. (2006) Protective and damaging effects of stress mediators: central role of the brain. *Dialogues in Clinical Neuroscience, 8*, 367–381.

Medicines and Healthcare Products Regulation Agency & the Commission on Human Medicines (2009) Smoking and smoking cessation: clinically significant interactions with commonly used medicines. *Drug Safety Update, 3*, 9.

Mitchell, A.J. & Hardy, S.A. (2013) Screening for metabolic risk among patients with severe mental illness and diabetes: a national comparison. *Psychiatric Services, 64*, 1060–1063.

Mitchell, A.J., Malone, D. & Carney Doebbeling, C. (2009) Quality of medical care for people with and without comorbid mental illness and substance misuse: systematic review of comparative studies. *British Journal of Psychiatry, 194*, 491–499.

Nash, M. (2005) Physical care skills: a training needs analysis of inpatient and community mental health nurses. *Mental Health Practice*, *9*, 20–23.

Nash, M. (2010) Assessing nurses' propositional knowledge of physical health. *Mental Health Practice*, *14*, 20–23.

National Collaborating Centre for Mental Health (2014) *Psychosis and schizophrenia in adults: the NICE guideline on treatment and management.* Updated. Clinical Guideline No. 178. London: NICE.

National Institute of Health and Care Excellence (NICE) (2014) *Bipolar disorder assessment and management.* Clinical Guideline No. 185. London: NICE.

Naylor, C., Das, P., Ross, S., et al. (2016) *Bringing together physical and mental health: A new frontier for integrated care.* London: King's Fund. Available at: www.kingsfund.org.uk/publications/physical-and-mental-health (accessed 09.08.17).

Naylor, C., Parsonage, M., McDaid, D., et al. (2012) *Long-term conditions and mental health: The cost of co-morbidities.* London: King's Fund.

NHS Future Forum (2012) *The NHS's role in the public's health: A report from the NHS future forum.* London: NHS.

Nursing and Midwifery Council (NMC) (2010) *Essential skills clusters and guidance for their use* (guidance no. G7.15b). London: NMC.

Parker, C., McNeill, A. & Ratschen, E. (2012) Tailored tobacco dependence support for mental health patients: a model for inpatient and community services. *Addiction*, *107*, 18–25.

Reilly, S., Planner, C., Hann, M., et al. (2012) The role of primary care in service provision for people with severe mental illness in the United Kingdom. *PLoS One*, *7*, e36468.

Robson, D. & Haddad, M. (2012) Mental health nurses, attitudes towards the physical health care of people with severe and enduring mental illness: the development of a measurement tool. *International Journal of Nursing Studies*, *49*, 72–83.

Royal College of Psychiatrists (RCP) (2014) *Report of the Second Round of the National Audit of Schizophrenia (NAS) 2014.* London: Healthcare Quality Improvement Partnership.

Schulze, B. (2007) Stigma and mental health professionals: a review of the evidence on an intricate relationship. *International Review of Psychiatry*, *19*, 137–155.

Shuel, F., White, J., Jones, M., et al. (2010) Using the serious mental illness health improvement profile [HIP] to identify physical problems in a cohort of community patients: a pragmatic case series evaluation. *International Journal of Nursing Studies*, *47*, 136–145.

Simmons, D.H. (1996) Caffeine and its effect on persons with mental disorders. *Archives of Psychiatric Nursing*, *10*, 116–122.

Smith, D.J., Langan, J., Mclean, G., et al. (2013) Schizophrenia is associated with excess multiple physical-health comorbidities but low levels of recorded cardiovascular disease in primary care: cross-sectional study. *BMJ Open*, 3. e002808. doi:10.1136/bmjopen-2013-002808.

Smith, T., Maidment, I., Hebding, J., et al. (2014) Systematic review investigating the reporting of comorbidities and medication in randomized controlled trials of people with dementia. *Age and Ageing*, *43*, 868–872.

Spiegelhalder, K., Regen, W., Nanovska, S., et al. (2013) Comorbid sleep disorders in neuropsychiatric disorders across the life cycle. *Current Psychiatry Reports*, *15*, 364.

Swofford, C.D., Scheller-Gilkey, G., Miller, A.H., et al. (2000) Double jeopardy: schizophrenia and substance abuse. *American Journal of Drug & Alcohol Abuse*, *26*, 343.

Testa, M.A. & Simonson, D.C. (1996) Assesment of quality-of-life outcomes. *New England Journal of Medicine*, *334*, 835–840.

Thornicroft, G., Rose, D. & Kassam, A. (2007) Discrimination in health care against people with mental illness. *International Review of Psychiatry*, *19*, 113–22.

Tiihonen, J., Lonnqvist, J., Wahlbeck, K., et al. (2009) 11-year follow-up of mortality in patients with schizophrenia: a population-based cohort study (FIN11 study). *Lancet*, *374*, 620–627.

Vancampfort, D., Probst, M., Scheewe, T., et al. (2013) Relationships between physical fitness, physical activity, smoking and metabolic and mental health parameters in people with schizophrenia. *Psychiatry Research*, *207*, 25–32.

Watson, A.C., Corrigan, P., Larson, J.E., et al. (2007) Self-stigma in people with mental illness. *Schizophrenia Bulletin*, *33*, 1312–1318.

White, J. (2015) *Physical health checks in serious mental illness: A programme of research in secondary care.* Doctoral thesis, University of East Anglia.

PSYCHOPHARMACOLOGY FOR MENTAL HEALTH NURSES

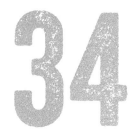

JENNIE DAY AND MICK McKEOWN

THIS CHAPTER COVERS

- The rationale for pharmacology knowledge for nurses
- An overview of one of the main groups of medications used in mental health – antipsychotics
- Indications, efficacy, adverse effects and clinical management of drugs used for the treatment of mental illness
- A review of the research evidence and clinical guidelines
- A consideration of medication from service users' perspectives and a practical framework to guide the effective use of medication to improve mental health outcomes
- A practical approach to management, assessing the benefits and adverse effects of medication from the perspective of the service user.

Like most decisions in life there were several reasons why I was so 'bad' at taking medication in the early years. Firstly, I scapegoated medication. Without the medication I would not be ill. I also really hated the tiredness. I had always taken physical and mental energy for granted so the sedative effects of antipsychotics made me feel very unlike myself indeed. My sense of self was knocked about enough by goblins without the collateral damage of medication side effects. When I was non-compliant I would have a period of renewed energy which I hugely enjoyed and felt far more in touch with myself – but at a cost, as I would rapidly construct an increasingly deranged world view built upon on all sorts of irrational links and significances. After a couple of days or so of mental flight and no sleep I would be exhausted and begin to shut down. At that point I would be so far from reality that restarting the medication was always a challenge, and it was something I couldn't do on my own. But those uncomfortable memories would fade and I would be tempted again and again by the remembrance of that first rush of life affirming energy – which I could access at will if I was prepared to skirt over the consequences.

Jane, service user

Visit **https://study.sagepub.com/essentialmentalhealth** to access a wealth of online resources for this chapter – watch out for the margin icons throughout the chapter. If you are using the interactive ebook, simply click on the margin icon to go straight to the resource.

'Doing the meds' can be one of the most stressful parts of the job. Most of the time it is uneventful; I situate myself in the treatment room and hand out the medications according to the prescription chart. However, it is such a dilemma when some of the service users tell me that they really don't want to take their meds and that they cannot tolerate the side effects of extreme tiredness and weight gain, for example. On other occasions I see people who have become reliant on various drugs such as tranquilisers and analgesia; I think that I could help them to get more comfortable, or help them gain a sense of calmness if I had the time. But the reality is that I am rushed off my feet and it is so much quicker to give them what they ask for. On the other hand, when I see the difference that medication can make to a person being tortured by their symptoms the tablets can seem to be miraculous. I cannot imagine how hard psychiatry must have been before the advent of contemporary psychotropic medication.

Laura Shorrock, ward manager

WHY DO NURSES NEED TO KNOW ABOUT PSYCHOPHARMACOLOGY?

Drug treatment of mental health conditions is commonplace but controversial. The medications used have many problems, including:

- lack of efficacy
- difficulty in effectively targeting treatments
- a plethora of adverse effects.

Most health professionals endorse the medical model of mental health and this can lead to an overestimation of the benefits and an underestimation of the adverse effects of medication. By developing a critical approach and by empathising with people who take medication, nurses will be more effective at empowering **service users** and bringing about the best outcomes for service users, even if this includes choosing not to take medication. By having a good critical understanding of the choices in medication available, nurses will be able to empower service users by listening to their views on medication, providing up-to-date information and enabling informed choices. This should include advocacy within clinical teams to prevent inappropriate choice and management of medication.

CHAPTER FOCUS

This chapter does not provide comprehensive information about medication and its management, partly for reasons of space and partly because information is constantly changing and it is practitioners' responsibility to keep up to date with that information. Most NHS hospital trusts have a medicines information pharmacist who is an invaluable source of independent evidence-based knowledge. Many trusts also produce their own prescribing guidelines and have a range of information leaflets for service users and families. This chapter will provide an overview of one of the main groups of medications used in mental health, **antipsychotics**, which illustrates some fairly general issues in medication management and its critique. This will cover the mechanism of action, efficacy, adverse effects and clinical management. As well as reviewing the research evidence and clinical guidelines, nurses are encouraged to consider medication from service users' perspectives, and a practical framework is offered to guide the effective use of medication to improve mental health outcomes. This includes assessing the benefits and adverse effects of medication from the point of view of the person taking it, to maximise wellbeing. The accompanying online resources at http://study.sagepub.com/essentialmentalhealth indicate relevant information sources and coverage of medications other than antipsychotics: antidepressants, **mood** stabilisers and anxiolytics/hypnotics.

The main focus is on the drug treatments, but it is equally important to consider the psychosocial and political context of the use of drugs in mental health. For example, the funding of mental health treatment and research has always been significantly lower than that for other conditions. Whilst mental health is estimated to account for 28% of the burden of disease in the UK, it accounts for only 13% of the NHS budget (BMA, 2017). In terms of funding, it yields a low proportion of money for charities and research compared to, for example, charities that raise funds for heart disease and cancer, and even animal charities. Although the **stigma** surrounding mental health has reduced, it is still present in society and this may influence people's choice of charitable donations. Whatever the cause, funding for research and health care for mental health has been disproportionately low for decades and the lack of choice of drugs that have good efficacy and low adverse effects may be a consequence of this disinvestment. We are still using drugs in mental health today that were developed in the 1950s, which would not happen in the treatment of physical conditions such as cancer or cardiovascular disease (Bentall, 2009).

In recent times, the prescribing of **psychotropic medication** has increased exponentially; in 1998 around 8 million antidepressants were prescribed and by 2015 this had increased to 61 million, nearly double the figure four years previously. This costs the NHS £285 million per year, which equates to £780,000 per day (Council for Evidence-based Psychiatry, 2015).

This massive increase in antidepressant prescribing coincides with burgeoning societal mental distress and a politics of austerity and cuts. The UK recession in 2008 led to increases in unemployment accompanied by substantial increases in suicide rates between 2008 and 2013 (Barr et al., 2015). The same period has seen about 10,000 additional suicides across Europe and North America (Reeves et al., 2014). Cuts to mental health services and welfare benefits are implicated in a proportion of these suicides. This context has contributed to the increased prescribing of psychotropics, which can be viewed as a panacea for social ills. It is also important to acknowledge that prescribing rates have clear social gradients, closely aligned with deprivation.

CRITICAL THINKING STOP POINT 34.1

Why do you think the prescribing of antidepressants has increased markedly since the turn of the century.

Why do you think the prescribing of antidepressants has increased so markedly in this period?

CRITICAL THINKING STOP POINT 34.1 ANSWER

(Continued)

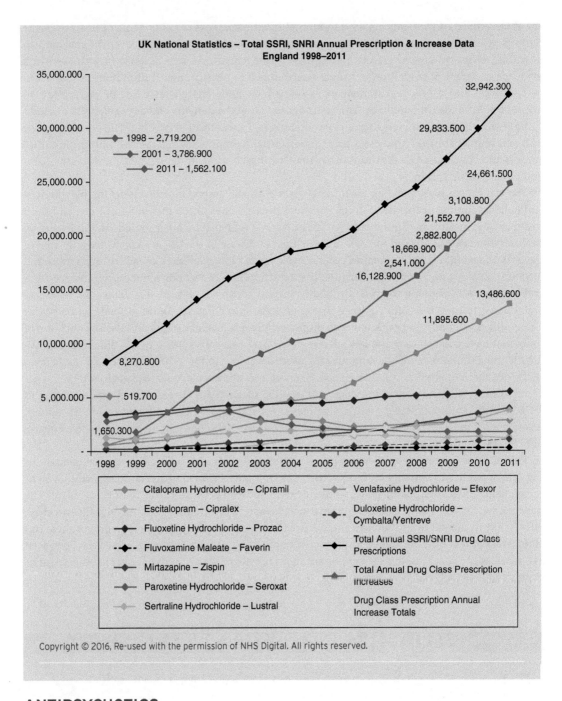

UK National Statistics – Total SSRI, SNRI Annual Prescription & Increase Data
England 1998–2011

- 1998 – 2,719.200
- 2001 – 3,786.900
- 2011 – 1,562.100

32,942.300
29,833.500
24,661.500
3,108.800
21,552.700
2,882.800
18,669.900
2,541.000
16,128.900
13,486.600
11,895.600
8,270.800
519.700
1,650.300

Legend:
- Citalopram Hydrochloride – Cipramil
- Escitalopram – Cipralex
- Fluoxetine Hydrochloride – Prozac
- Fluvoxamine Maleate – Faverin
- Mirtazapine – Zispin
- Paroxetine Hydrochloride – Seroxat
- Sertraline Hydrochloride – Lustral
- Venlafaxine Hydrochloride – Efexor
- Duloxetine Hydrochloride – Cymbalta/Yentreve
- Total Annual SSRI/SNRI Drug Class Prescriptions
- Total Annual Drug Class Prescription increases
- Drug Class Prescription Annual Increase Totals

ANTIPSYCHOTICS

Antipsychotics, formerly known as neuroleptics, and before that major tranquillisers, are prescribed for the treatment of **psychosis**. Antipsychotics are used widely in secondary and primary care, with 10.5 million antipsychotic items prescribed in general practice at a cost of £157.7 million in 2014 (Council for Evidence-based Psychiatry, 2015). It is important to be aware of how medications used in mental health were developed. For example, the first antipsychotic medication was chlorpromazine which was not initially developed for psychosis. In fact, it was an antihistamine drug in the early 1950s, used by the scientist Henri Laborit as a calming agent for surgical patients.

Laborit found the drug induced relaxation and indifference without sedation in surgical patients and suggested that it may be useful for psychiatry. At the time, the main treatments used in psychiatry were insulin shock treatment (giving people insulin until they went into a coma, causing permanent brain damage and death in some cases), water shock treatment, ECT and brain surgery, so it is perhaps surprising that Laborit initially found it hard to convince psychiatrists to try out chlorpromazine. Eventually, Jean Delay and Pierre Deniker carried out the first clinical trial on 38 patients in 1952. The drug was taken up in the USA after a visit from Deniker, and chlorpromazine is still in use today.

Following the discovery that antipsychotic drugs block dopamine receptors, this was developed as the main hypothesis for the mechanism of action. The theory is that an excess of dopamine in the brain leads to the development of psychotic symptoms such as **delusions** and **hallucinations**. This theory was based on the observation that clinical doses of antipsychotics correlated with potency to block D2 receptors in vivo, i.e. in test tubes (Seeman & Lee, 1975). Further to this, Creese et al. (1976) found a correlation between therapeutic potency and dopamine D2 blockade.

The dopamine theory was widely accepted for decades but, in fact, there was room for doubt. Dopamine blockade occurs within hours of taking an antipsychotic drug, but the drugs take weeks to work. Perhaps the biggest anomaly is that the binding of antipsychotics to dopamine receptors in brain-imaging studies does not correlate with therapeutic efficacy. So the receptors can be totally blocked but the person has no relief from symptoms. The biggest challenge to the theory was the insight that clozapine, a drug which has little effect on dopamine receptors, was shown to have improved effectiveness compared to other antipsychotics. This was the first time that an antipsychotic had been shown to possess superior efficacy to others, and instigated a flurry of psychopharmacological research into the receptors that clozapine did interact with, such as $5HT_2$ receptors.

Antipsychotics are not a homogenous group of drugs; there are quite big differences between them. There are two main sub-types of antipsychotics: the older drugs such as chlorpromazine that are known as typical or first-generation antipsychotics (FGAs) and the newer drugs such as aripiprazole that are known as the atypical or second-generation antipsychotics (SGAs). A list of the antipsychotic drugs available in the UK is presented in Table 34.1.

Table 34.1 Antipsychotic drugs available in the UK

Antipsychotics	
First generation	**Second generation**
Benperidol	Amisulpride
Chlorpromazine	Aripiprazole
Flupentixol	Clozapine
Fluphenazine	Lurasidone Hydrochloride
Haloperidol	Olanzapine
Levomepromazine	Paliperidone
Perphenazine	Quetiapine
Pericyazine	Risperidone
Pimozide	
Prochlorperazine	
Promazine	
Sulpiride	
Trifluoperazine	
Zuclopenthixol	

The main difference between the first- and second-generation antipsychotics is the side-effects profile, with the FGAs associated with a high burden of the movement-type side-effects know as extra-pyramidal side-effects, and the newer SGAs more likely to cause metabolic side-effects such as weight gain.

Antipsychotics are also available in the form of a depot injection (Table 34.2). There are two main types of depot injection: the older type where the drug is attached to a long chain and suspended in an oily solution and the newer type which has a more complicated mechanism and tends to be in an aqueous solution. In both cases, the solution is usually injected into the buttocks and the active drug is released slowly into the body over time, without the need to take oral medication. It is important to acknowledge the social and political context here.

Table 34.2 Antipsychotic medications available as depot injections

Depot antipsychotics	
First generation	**Second generation**
Flupentixol Decanoate	Aripiprazole
Fluphenazine Decanoate	Olanzapine Embonate
Haloperidol	Paliperidone
Zuclopenthixol Decanoate	Risperidone

CRITICAL THINKING STOP POINT 34.2

Why are depot injections available for antipsychotics but not for other groups of drugs such as anticonvulsants or antihypertensives?

CRITICAL THINKING STOP POINT 34.2 ANSWER

One of the biggest problems with antispychotics is that they have limited efficacy (Lieberman, 2007; Moncrieff, 2013; Samara et al., 2016). It is estimated that 20–30% of people experience no effects at all on their symptoms. Around a third of people will have a good response and symptoms will completely stop. It can usually take around six weeks to see an effect and may take several months for symptoms to stop. Another third of people will have a partial or ameliorative response, so, for example, they may feel less bothered about their symptoms, even though they occur as frequently. Some people say, for example, that their voices are quieter or that they previously heard three voices which have reduced to one, or that the voices have less distressing content. The problem is that it is not possible to predict who will respond. We also can't predict what type of symptoms respond to particular antipsychotics. In my experience, there is a strikingly positive view of the efficacy of antipsychotics amongst practitioners, yet research has shown that health professionals overestimate the benefits and underestimate the limitations of medication (Day et al., 1998; Finn et al., 1990; Hoffman & Del Mar, 2017).

CRITICAL THINKING STOP POINT 34.3

Prescribing antipsychotic medication is often a difficult balancing act between maximising efficacy and minimising adverse effects. If you were taking a medication, which box would you like to be in?

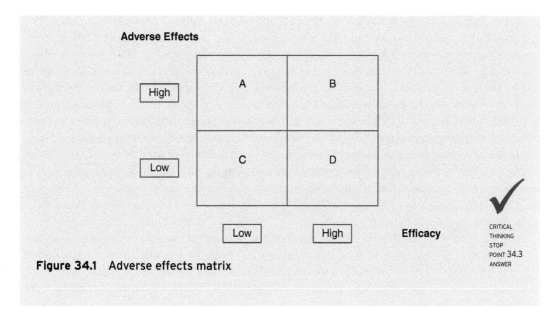

Figure 34.1 Adverse effects matrix

Conflict can arise between professionals and service users when there are different perspectives on the balance of positive and negative effects for individuals. Another problem is that, in practice, it can take a long time trying out different medications to achieve the best response and the lowest side-effects. This can leave service users dismayed by the whole process and a number of people have told me they felt like guinea pigs being tried out on different drugs. The only person who can really judge when the balance is right is the person taking the medication, and I have met some people who are prepared to tolerate the side-effects as the drug is the only one that has helped with symptoms, such as halting their voices. A crucial role for mental health practitioners is to not presume medication is working but to listen to service users and assess and record the efficacy of the medication and if necessary change it.

Research evidence from randomised controlled trials clearly shows that antipsychotics are associated with significantly lower relapse rates compared to placebo drugs in people with a diagnosis of **schizophrenia** who are discharged after an **acute** psychotic episode, as shown in Figure 34.2.

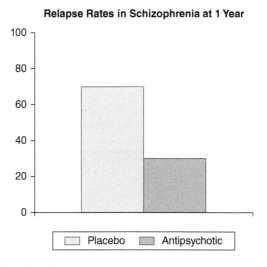

Figure 34.2 Relapse rates in schizophrenia

What is also clear, though, is that around 30% of people who take antipsychotics still have a relapse and that around 30% of people not taking medication do not relapse (e.g. Leucht et al., 2012); also, 20% of people who have a first episode of psychotic symptoms do not relapse again (Altamura et al., 2007). However, relapse whilst taking antipsychotics tends to be less severe and require lower doses of medication and fewer days in hospital (if required) to ameliorate, compared to relapse whilst not taking medication. In previous research, the response to antipsychotics has been found to be affected by: duration of untreated psychosis (Perkins et al., 2005), early response to treatment in the first two weeks (Samara et al., 2015), previous response (Kolakowska et al., 1985), presence of **negative symptoms** (Fenton & McGlassen, 1991), dosage and duration of treatment, not taking medication and comorbidities such as substance use (Carbon & Correll, 2014).

There are many problems with the evidence around antipsychotic response. First, many studies lump together symptoms under an umbrella diagnosis of schizophrenia. This doesn't tell us about the differential response of particular symptoms to medication, so, for example, we don't know what medication is most likely to be effective to, say, reduce paranoia. This is a major limitation and some research has indicated that there could be important differences. For example, one study found that delusions took longer to respond than hallucinations and response was related to the duration of untreated psychosis for delusions but not for hallucinations (Gunduz-Bruce et al., 2005).

Response has a narrow definition in many research studies; it is often focused on symptoms, for instance defined as a 20% reduction in validated measure (e.g. Positive and Negative Syndrome Scale (PANSS)). This isn't a large change and such measures neglect social functioning and quality of life, which most people would view as the most important aspect of response. It is vital to carry out assessments of subjective experience, symptoms, social functioning, quality of life and relapse before and after prescribing antipsychotics (or any mental health medication). This sounds basic but it is not routinely done in clinical practice. Ideally, the level of response should be recorded electronically in a way that could be easily accessed by service users and staff.

RESEARCH EVIDENCE

There are some landmark trials on antipsychotics that have an important bearing on clinical practice and guidelines, such as those produced by the National Institute for Health & Care Excellence (NICE). Large UK and US trials (respectively CUtLASS – Cost Utility of the Latest Antipsychotic drugs in Schizophrenias Study (Jones et al., 2006); and CATIE – the Clinical Antipsychotic Trial of Intervention Effectiveness) compared typical and atypical antipsychotics (Lieberman et al., 2005). The results questioned assertions that atypicals have a more favourable side-effect profile than typical antipsychotics and that they are less likely to cause or worsen negative symptoms. In fact, discontinuation rates and clinical response were no different between the groups, leading NICE to withdraw its recommendation to prescribe atypicals first line for psychosis. Time to discontinuation was longer for olanzapine compared to other antipsychotics, but this may be because a major side-effect of olanzapine is weight gain which takes longer to develop. The only antipsychotic that has improved efficacy compared to others is clozapine, but prescribing of this is limited to those with treatment-resistant schizophrenia due to the potentially fatal adverse reaction of agranulocytosis. Thus, the take-home message from this research evidence is that medication needs to be tailored to a person's individual needs.

ADVERSE EFFECTS

Antipsychotics interact with many different receptors in the body and their lack of specificity results in a high burden of side-effects for people who take them. Table 34.3 shows the main groups of side-effects associated with antipsychotics.

Table 34.3 Main groups of side-effects associated with antipsychotics

Extrapyamidal side-effects	Parkinsonian –	Rigidity Tremor Dyskinesias Expressionless face
	Acute dystonias	
	Akathisia	
	Tardive dyskinesia	
Anti-muscarinic side-effects	Dry mouth	
	Blurred vision	
	Constipation	
	Difficult micturition	
	Drowsiness	
Alpha-adrenergic	Postural hypotension – causing dizziness and fainting	
	Tachycardia, palpitations, ECG changes	
	Sexual dysfunction, especially reduced ejaculation	
	Sedation – less than histaminic effects	
Hormonal	Galactorrhoea	
	Gynaecomastia	
	Sexual dysfunction	
	Menstrual disturbances	
	Disturbance in body temperature regulation	
Cardiovascular	Orthostatic hypotension	
	Tachycardia	
	ECG changes – prolonged QT interval	
	Sudden death	
Allergic reactions	Urticaria	
	Exfoliative dermatitis	
	Contact sensitivity	
	Jaundice	
	Photosensitivity	
	Deposition of pigment	
Haematological	Agranulocytosis	
	Neutropenia	
	Haemolytic anaemia	

(Continued)

Metabolic	Hyperglycaemia
	Glucose intolerance/insulin resistance
	Diabetes
	Dislipidemia
	Weight gain
	Increased risk of cardiovascular disease
Miscellaneous	Peripheral oedema
	Insomnia
	Agitation
	Catatonia
	Neuroleptic malignant **syndrome**
Psychological	Neuroleptic induced deficit syndrome
	Dysphoria
	Depression

The extra-pyramidal effects result from a blockade of dopamine in the nigrostriatal pathway in the brain. The nigrostriatal pathway is a system of nerves that connects two parts of the brain: the substantia nigra and the striatum. This system is in balance due to the balance of two neurotransmitters – dopamine and acetylcholine – and is responsible for motor functions, i.e. movement of the body. When antipsychotics block dopamine in this pathway, this produces extra-pyramidal side-effects which are physical, as listed in Table 34.3, including Parkinson's-type symptoms and abnormal involuntary movements such as pill rolling tremor and twitching of the legs. The tragedy of these side-effects is that they **affect** people's appearance and the physical effects can be mistaken for symptoms of mental health conditions and can be stigmatising.

As a group of drugs, antipsychotics have a wide range of side-effects and some of these have adverse effects on health and can, in rare cases, be fatal. In addition, many of these side-effects can have a significant impact on a person's quality of life. For example, sexual dysfunction can have a negative impact on wellbeing and relationships and service users and health professionals may find it difficult to discuss the issue. Dry mouth can mean that someone feels the need to drink; this can be a problem if the drink contains a high amount of caffeine, which can increase stimulation and **anxiety** and disturb sleep, or sugar, causing weight gain and dental decay. There are practical solutions for many of these adverse effects, such as using a dry mouth spray or reducing the dose or changing the drug. The most important thing a health professional can do is *listen* to people when talking about side-effects and, more importantly, *take action to reduce side-effects*. There is a tendency for professionals to downplay side-effects and to not know what to do about them, but there are many simple practical interventions that can result in a much improved quality of life, so it is imperative to be proactive. This includes a systematic approach to and regular monitoring of side-effects using a validated assessment tool, for example the Glasgow Antipsychotic Side-effects Scale (GASS; Waddell & Taylor, 2008) or the Liverpool University Neuroleptic Side Effect **Rating Scale** (LUNSERS; Day et al., 1995).

When antipsychotics are stopped, particularly if this is done too quickly, they have distinct withdrawal effects, which can include nausea, vomiting, diarrhoea, restlessness, anxiety, mood disturbances, dizziness, insomnia, fatigue, malaise, myalgia, diaphoresis, rhinitis, paresthesia, GI distress, headaches, nightmares and movement **disorders**. It is thought that some of these effects occur due to the change in the blockade of receptors on discontinuation of the drugs. For example, there is a distinct effect of cholinergic rebound which causes many of these symptoms when muscarinic (acetylcholine) receptors are no longer blocked on discontinuation. There is very little research on this and few guidelines on how exactly antipsychotics should be withdrawn, apart from saying that it should be done 'gradually and slowly' and they should not be stopped abruptly. The most conservative method is advisable, with a recommendation to reduce the dose by a small percentage (e.g. 10–20%) every few months, carefully monitoring for withdrawal effects and prodromal symptoms.

CRITICISMS OF PSYCHOPHARMACOLOGY

The history of the development of psychopharmacological treatments coincided with the beginnings of the retraction of the asylum system, hence it has typically been claimed that medications such as antipsychotics were responsible for emptying the asylums (see Gelder et al., 2006). The true story, however, is much more complicated (Scull, 1977) and the use, and alleged over-use, of such prescriptions has been vociferously contested by critical practitioners and survivors (Breggin, 1991; Weitz, 2011). The journalist, Robert Whitaker (2010a, 2010b; Whitaker & Cosgrove, 2015), for example, has forensically analysed the evidence base and argues that the science actually makes a case for considering antipsychotic medication to be the cause of chronic serious mental health conditions. Similarly, the evidence for the efficacy of antidepressants is fairly equivocal, with some claims that there is no effect at all, or that psychological therapies are of equivalent **value** or superior (Gartlehner et al., 2016; Huhn et al., 2014; Moncrieff, 2015; Spijker et al., 2013). Regardless of whether individuals experience improved mental health as a consequence of psychiatric drugs, there is plentiful evidence of harmful physical health effects implicated in increased morbidity and mortality amongst mental health service users (Mitchell & Malone, 2006; Robson & Gray, 2007), so much so that radical critics consider these treatments to be iatrogenic (Breggin, 1991; Burstow, 2015). The evidence for the efficacy of minimal medication treatments such as Soteria (Calton et al., 2008; Mosher, 1999) or **Open Dialogue** (Anderson, 2002) further adds to the critique of the value of psychopharmacology. Whitaker has been so possessed by the startling evidence stacking up against psychiatric medication that he started the *Mad in America* Foundation to campaign on this territory (www.madinamerica.com).

CASE STUDY: COMMUNITY PSYCHIATRIC NURSE

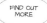

FIND OUT MORE

MAD IN AMERICA

A prominent critic of psychopharmacology from a clinical perspective is Joanna Moncrieff (2013, 2015). She argues persuasively that the distinction between treatment effects and side-effects is a false one, and that drugs should be considered simply on the basis of their psychoactive effects rather than any alleged targeting of a known disease process: the so-called drug-centred model of action (Moncrieff & Cohen, 2009; Moncrieff et al., 2013). This standpoint is interesting, as it allows for an appreciation of the actual idiosyncratic effect of drugs; the same drug can have different effects for different people, and the relationship of effect to dose can also vary between people. Hence, we can begin to distinguish between people for whom particular drugs work and those for whom no drugs are of benefit, and be more honest with people about *how* we think the drugs work. For example, the main effect of antipsychotics is sedation, and this may be helpful for some people without getting into labyrinthine, and perhaps misguided, explanations about dopamine response. Critics have argued that the dopamine theory of antipsychotic drug action has been the most continually revised in the history of hypotheses (Bentall, 2009; Bentall et al., 1988), and the growing evidence for the role of trauma in the causation of psychosis also accounts for dopamine disturbances (Read et al., 2014).

Moncrieff (2006) and others (Cohen et al., 2008; Healy, 2004; Rose & Abi-Rached, 2013) have also been vociferously critical of the incestuous connections between large pharmacological companies and the politics of **neo-liberalism** and social control: the problematics of so-called Big Pharma. This critique also includes disquiet over inadequacies in the science of pharmacological research. A failure to publish negative findings is criticised, thus skewing an appreciation of medication towards more positive results, and blatantly fraudulent research can also be a problem (Davies, 2013; Goldacre, 2012).

MEDICATION-FREE SERVICES AND COMING OFF MEDICATION

> My journey with medication began at the age of 14 when I was admitted to an adult psychiatric ward and over the years I have been prescribed old and new antipsychotics, with periods of high doses. Over the years I have had an uneasy relationship with medication. At times I have felt I need it, or at least some of it, but some of it I really don't like. I have had periods when I have been compelled to take medication and others when the care team have supported me to reduce or cease certain prescriptions. Recently, I decided to stop taking medication all together and although most people would advise doing this with appropriate support and supervision, I just stopped one day. I would say it was akin to withdrawing from illegal drugs and went on for weeks but I persevered. I believe it's a person's choice to take or not take medication, and if it works for you that's fine. But for me it made sense to try and come off. I now have no medication and have discovered that natural sleep instead of chemical sleep is a truly restful experience. I have more energy, am fitter, and have lost most of the excess weight I put on. I am now 43 and feel that the medication I was on only served to keep me dumbed down and manageable. I am also helping to teach nurses and clinical psychologists about medication and side effects.
>
> **Fiona Edgar, service user**

In Norway, service users have had a right to *medikamentfritt behandlingstilbud*, that is, medication-free treatment, since an order issued in 2015 by the Ministry of Health. This resulted from campaigning by a number of service user groups highlighting the controversies over the evidence base for psychiatric drugs, and particular objections to forced treatment by antipsychotics. In Tromsö in the Arctic Circle, there is a whole ward now devoted to treatment without drugs or helping people come off psychiatric medication safely (Hakansson, 2017). In other regions of the country, the services have been less responsive to the edict and only reserve a few beds for this approach, typically focusing on withdrawing antidepressants rather than antipsychotics. Critics have remarked that the relatively tawdry compliance by services has been a result of a backlash orchestrated by the psychiatric establishment. This has necessitated ongoing campaigning and public debates regarding the evidence for and against medication, and contributors have notably included Jaakko Seikkula, the founder of Open Dialogue (Whitaker, 2017).

The **survivor** movement has demanded for a long time that people should have the right to refuse psychiatric medication and receive support to come off long-term prescriptions (Lehmann, 2004). A number of critical practitioners and researchers have also made a case for providing services to assist people to safely stop taking psychiatric medication (see Read, 2009). Across the world, there are a number of alternative services and resources that exist to help in this regard, and some of these are user-controlled (e.g. Simpson, 2016). The Icarus Project, for example, has published a harm-reduction guide to coming off psychiatric drugs (Hall, 2012). Its notion of harm reduction takes into account an ethos of self-determination and striking a balance between risks and benefits, without being assertively pro or anti medication. In the UK, the Sunrise Project operates a non-judgemental, peer-to-peer co-counselling model that engages with people's experiences and feelings, in the belief that these are numbed by psychiatric drugs, which is ultimately not helpful (Simpson, 2016).

CONCLUSION

This chapter has provided a critical review of the use of mental health medication with a focus on antipsychotics and, to an extent, evaluated the psychosocial aspects of prescribing medication in mental health. If medication is used, it should be used with a critical approach and, most importantly, with the subjective experience and wellbeing of the service user as the goal for treatment outcomes. This can only be achieved by listening to service users and acting to maximise the benefits and minimise the adverse effects of medication. It is important to acknowledge that medication can be ineffective or only partially effective and has serious and sometimes life-threatening side-effects. It is crucial to minimise and hopefully avoid side-effects that have a detrimental effect on quality of life, relationships and the ability to work. Reflecting on Fiona's experience of medication, how much was she listened to and what would you have done to improve her experience? Should she have been prescribed medication at all?

CHAPTER SUMMARY

This chapter has covered:

- A critique of one major form of medication treatment: antipsychotics
- Key aspects of research evidence regarding efficacy
- The role of the mental health nurse in relation to medication, including the importance of assessment of subjective responses and attitudes towards treatment
- Information about drug withdrawal and possibilities of promoting this as an option for individuals not helped by medication, or expressing this choice.

BUILD YOUR BIBLIOGRAPHY

SAGE journal articles

Go to https://study.sagepub.com/essentialmentalhealth for further free online journal articles related to this chapter. If you are using the interactive ebook, simply click on the book icon in the margin to go straight to the resource.

FURTHER READING: JOURNAL ARTICLES

- Allison, L. & Moncrieff, J. (2014) 'Rapid tranquillisation': an historical perspective on its emergence in the context of the development of antipsychotic medications. *History of Psychiatry*, 25(1), 57-69.
- Moncrieff, J. (1999) An investigation into the precedents of modern drug treatment in psychiatry. *History of Psychiatry*, 10(40), 475-490.
- Taylor, M., Cavanagh, J., Hodgson, R., et al. (2012) Examining the effectiveness of antipsychotic medication in first-episode psychosis. *Journal of Psychopharmacology*, 26(5 suppl.), 27-32.

Weblinks

Go to https://study.sagepub.com/essentialmentalhealth for further weblinks related to this chapter. If you are using the interactive ebook, simply click on the book icon in the margin to go straight to the resource.

FURTHER READING: WEBLINKS

- Icarus Project: http://theicarusproject.net/
- Moncrieff, J. & Cohen, D. (2009) How do psychiatric drugs work? *British Medical Journal*, 338: www.mentalhealth.freeuk.com/howwork.pdf
- Peer statement on medication optimization and alternatives: http://bit.ly/h1T3Fk

- Take These Broken Wings: Recovery from Schizophrenia without Medication – film: www.iraresoul.com/dvd1.html
- Robert Whitaker's blog pages, Mad in America: www.madinamerica.com/author/rwhitaker
- Psychotropic Drugs Directory http://psychotropicdrugdirectory.com
- Maudsley Prescribing Guidelines: http://maudsley-prescribing-guidelines.co.uk
- BNF: www.bnf.org
- Electronic Medicines Compendium: www.medicines.org.uk/emc

———— ACE YOUR ASSESSMENT ————

ONLINE
QUIZZES &
ACTIVITY
ANSWERS

Revise what you have learned by visiting https://study.sagepub.com/essentialmentalhealth. If you are using the interactive ebook, simply click on the tick icon to go straight to the resource.

- Test yourself with multiple-choice and short-answer questions and flashcards.

REFERENCES

Altamura, A.C., Bobo, W.V. & Meltzer, H.Y. (2007) Factors affecting outcome in schizophrenia and their relevance for psychopharmacological treatment. *Int Clin Psychopharmacol, 22*, 249–267.

Anderson, H. (2002) In the space between people: Seikkula's open dialogue approach. *Journal of Marital and Family Therapy, 28*, 279–281.

Barr, B., Kinderman, P. and Whitehead, M. (2015) Trends in mental health inequalities in England during a period of recession, austerity and welfare reform 2004 to 2013. *Social Science & Medicine, 147*, 324–331.

Bentall, R.P. (2009) *Doctoring the mind: Is our current treatment of mental illness really any good?* London: Allen Lane.

Bentall, R.P., Jackson, H.F. & Pilgrim, D. (1988) Abandoning the concept of 'schizophrenia': some implications of validity arguments for psychological research into psychotic phenomena. *British Journal of Clinical Psychology, 27*(4), 303–324.

Breggin, P. (1991) *Toxic psychiatry: A psychiatrist speaks out.* New York: St Martin's Press.

British Medical Association (BMA) (2017) www.bma.org.uk/news/2017/february/mental-health-budgets-cut (accessed 16.09.17)

Burstow, B. (2015) *Psychiatry and the business of madness: An ethical and epistemological accounting.* New York: Palgrave Macmillan.

Calton, T., Ferriter, M., Huband, N., et al. (2008) A systematic review of the Soteria paradigm for the treatment of people diagnosed with schizophrenia. *Schizophrenia Bulletin, 34*(1), 181–192.

Carbon, M. & Correll, C.U. (2014) Clinical predictors of therapeutic response to antipsychotics in schizophrenia. *Dialogues Clin Neurosci, 16*, 505–524.

Cohen, C.I., Timimi, S. & Thompson, K.S. (2008) A new psychiatry? In C.I. Cohen & S. Timimi (eds) *Liberatory psychiatry: Philosophy, politics and mental health.* Cambridge: Cambridge University Press.

Council for Evidence-based Psychiatry (2015) *Latest prescription data shows consumption of psychiatric drugs continues to soar.* Available at: http://cepuk.org/2015/04/10/latest-prescription-data-shows-consumption-psychiatric-drugs-continues-soar (accessed 26.05.17).

Creese, I., Burt, D.R. & Snyder, S.H. (1976) Dopamine receptor binding predicts clinical and pharmacological potencies of antischizophrenic drugs. *Science, 192*, 481–483.

Davies, J. (2013) *Cracked: Why psychiatry is doing more harm than good*. London: Icon Books.

Day, J.C., Kinderman, P. & Bentall, R. (1998) A comparison of patients' and prescribers' beliefs about neuroleptic side-effects: prevalence, distress and causation. *Acta Psychiatrica Scandinavica, 97*(1), 93–97.

Day, J.C., Wood, G., Dewey, M., et al. (1995) A self-rating scale for measuring neuroleptic side-effects: validation in a group of schizophrenic patients. *Br J Psychiatry, 166*, 650–653.

Fenton, W.S. & McGlassen, T.H. (1991) Natural history of schizophrenia subtypes II: positive and negative symptoms and long-term course. *Arch Gen Psychiatry, 48*, 978–986.

Finn, S.E., Bailey, J.M., Schultz, R.T., et al. (1990) Subjective utility ratings of neuroleptics in treating schizophrenia. *Psychological Medicine, 20*(4), 843–848.

Gartlehner, G., Gaynes, B.N., Amick, H.R., et al. (2016) Comparative benefits and harms of antidepressant, psychological, complementary, and exercise treatments for major depression: an evidence report for a clinical practice guideline from the American College of Physicians. *Annals of Internal Medicine, 164*(5), 331–341.

Gelder, M., Harrison, P. & Cowen, P. (2006) *Shorter Oxford textbook of psychiatry*. Oxford: Oxford University Press.

Goldacre, B. (2012) *Bad pharma: How drug companies mislead doctors and harm the public*. London: Fourth Estate.

Gunduz-Bruce, H., McMeniman. M., Robinson, D.G., et al. (2005) Duration of untreated psychosis and time to treatment response for delusions and hallucinations. *American Journal of Psychiatry, 162*, 1966–1969.

Hakansson, C. (2017) Visiting the medication free psychiatric ward in Tromsö. Blog. Available at: http://extendedroom.org/en/visiting-the-medication-free-psychiatric-ward-in-tromso (accessed 03.05.17).

Hall, W. (2012) *Icarus Project & Freedom Centre*. Available at: http://theicarusproject.net/resources/publications/harm-reduction-guide-to-coming-off-psychiatric-drugs-and-withdrawal (accessed 03.05.17).

Healy, D. (2004) *Let them eat prozac: The unhealthy relationship between the pharmaceutical industry and depression*. New York: New York University Press.

Hoffman, T.C. & Del Mar, C.D. (2017) Clinicians' expectations of the benefits and harms of treatments, screening, and tests: a systematic review. *JAMA Intern Med, 177*, 407–419.

Huhn, M., Tardy, M., Spineli, L.M., et al. (2014) Efficacy of pharmacotherapy and psychotherapy for adult psychiatric disorders: a systematic overview of meta-analyses. *JAMA Psychiatry, 71*(6), 706–715.

Jones, P.B., Barnes, T.R., Davies, L., Dunn, G., Lloyd, H., Hayhurst, K.P., et al. (2006) Randomized controlled trial of effect on quality of life of second- vs first-generation antipsychotic drugs in schizophrenia: cost utility of the latest antipsychotic drugs in schizophrenia study (CUtLASS 1). *Arch Gen Psychiatry, 63*, 1079–1087.

Kolakowska, T., Williams, A.O., Ardern, M., et al. (1985). Schizophrenia with good and poor outcome. I. Early clinical features, response to neuroleptics and signs of organic dysfunction. *British Journal of Psychiatry*, 146, 229–239.

Lehmann, P. (ed.) (2004) *Coming off psychiatric drugs: Successful withdrawal from neuroleptics, antidepressants, lithium, carbamazepine and tranquilizers*. Berlin: Peter Lehmann Publishing.

Leucht, S., Tardy, M., Komossa, K., et al. (2012) Antipsychotic drugs versus placebo for relapse prevention in schizophrenia: a systematic review and meta-analysis. *Lancet, 379*, 2063–2071.

Lieberman, J.A. (2007) Effectiveness of antipsychotic drugs in patients with chronic schizophrenia: efficacy, safety and cost outcomes of CATIE and other trials. *The Journal of Clinical Psychiatry, 68*(2), e04.

Lieberman, J.A., Stroup, S., McEvoy, J.P., et al., for the Clinical Antipsychotic Trials of Intervention Effectiveness (CATIE) Investigators (2005) Effectiveness of antipsychotic drugs in patients with chronic schizophrenia. *N Engl J Med, 353*, 1209–1223.

Mitchell, A.J. & Malone, D. (2006) Physical health and schizophrenia. *Current Opinion in Psychiatry*, *19*(4), 432–437.

Moncrieff, J. (2006) Psychiatric drug promotion and the politics of neoliberalism. *The British Journal of Psychiatry*, *188*(4), 301–302.

Moncrieff, J. (2013) *The bitterest pills: The troubling story of antipsychotic drugs*. New York: Springer.

Moncrieff, J. (2015) Antidepressants: misnamed and misrepresented. *World Psychiatry*, *14*(3), 302–303.

Moncrieff, J. & Cohen, D. (2009) How do psychiatric drugs work? *British Medical Journal*, *338*, 1535–1537.

Moncrieff, J., Cohen, D. & Porter, S. (2013) The psychoactive effects of psychiatric medication: the elephant in the room. *Journal of Psychoactive Drugs*, *45*(5), 409–415.

Mosher, L.R. (1999) Soteria and other alternatives to acute psychiatric hospitalization: a personal and professional review. *The Journal of Nervous and Mental Disease*, *187*(3), 142–149.

Perkins, D.O., Gu, H., Boteva, K., et al. (2005) Relationship between duration of untreated psychosis and outcome in first-episode schizophrenia: a critical review and meta-analysis. *American Journal of Psychiatry*, *162*, 1785–1804.

Read, J. (2009) *Psychiatric drugs: Key issues and service user perspectives*. Basingstoke: Palgrave Macmillan.

Read, J., Fosse, R., Moskowitz, A., et al. (2014) The traumagenic neurodevelopmental model of psychosis revisited. *Neuropsychiatry*, *4*(1), 65–79.

Reeves, A., McKee, M., Gunnell, D., et al. (2014) Economic shocks, resilience, and male suicides in the Great Recession: cross-national analysis of 20 EU countries. *The European Journal of Public Health*, 25(3):404-409.

Robson, D. & Gray, R. (2007) Serious mental illness and physical health problems: a discussion paper. *International Journal of Nursing Studies*, *44*(3), 457–466.

Rose, N.S. & Abi-Rached, J.M. (2013) *Neuro: The new brain sciences and the management of the mind*. Princeton, NJ: Princeton University Press.

Samara, M.T., Dold, M., Gianatsi, M., et al. (2016) Efficacy, acceptability, and tolerability of antipsychotics in treatment-resistant schizophrenia: a network meta-analysis. *JAMA Psychiatry*, *73*(3), 199–210.

Samara, M.T., Leucht, C., Leeflang, M.M., et al. (2015) Early improvement as a predictor of later response to antipsychotics in schizophrenia: a diagnostic test review. *American Journal of Psychiatry*, *172*, 617–629.

Scull, A.D. (1977) *Decarceration: Community treatment and the deviant – a radical view*. Englewood Cliffs, NJ: Prentice-Hall.

Seeman, P. & Lee, T. (1975) Antipsychotic drugs: direct correlation between clinical potency and presynaptic action on dopamine neurons. *Science*, *188*, 1217–1219.

Simpson, T. (2016) The sunrise project: helping adults recover from psychiatric drugs. In J. Russo & A. Sweeney (eds) *Searching for a rose garden: Challenging psychiatry, fostering Mad Studies*. Waystone Leys: PCCS Books. pp. 152–159.

Spijker, J., van Straten, A., Bockting, C.L., et al. (2013) Psychotherapy, antidepressants, and their combination for chronic major depressive disorder: a systematic review. *The Canadian Journal of Psychiatry*, *58*(7), 386–392.

Waddell, L. & Taylor, M. (2008) A new self-rating scale for detecting atypical or second-generation antipsychotic side effects. *Journal of Psychopharmacology*, *22*, 238–243.

Weitz, D. (2011) Struggling against psychiatry's violation of human rights. *Asylum: the Magazine for Democratic Psychiatry*, *18*(4), 14–18.

Whitaker, R. (2010a) *Anatomy of an epidemic: Magic bullets, psychiatric drugs and the astonishing rise of mental illness in America*. New York: Broadway Paperbacks.

Whitaker, R. (2010b) *Mad in America: Bad science, bad medicine, and the enduring mistreatment of the mentally ill*, 2nd edition. Cambridge, MA: Basic Books.

Whitaker, R. (2017) *The door to a revolution in psychiatry cracks open*. A MIA report: Norway's health ministry orders medication-free treatment. Mad in America blog, 25 March. Available at: www.madinamerica.com/2017/03/the-door-to-a-revolution-in-psychiatry-cracks-open (accessed 03.05.17).

Whitaker, R. & Cosgrove, L. (2015) *Psychiatry under the influence: Institutional corruption, social injury, and prescriptions for reform*. New York: Springer.

NON-MEDICAL ALTERNATIVES FOR CRISIS CARE

35

HELEN SPANDLER AND MICK McKEOWN

THIS CHAPTER COVERS

- Non-medical alternatives to crisis admissions
- The impact of hospital admissions for service users
- The case for service user controlled alternatives
- A therapeutic community inspired model and its potential benefits
- The role of the mental health nurse in providing information about the alternatives to crisis admission for service users and their families.

" For me a crisis would often end up with a hospital admission, and more medication! This was awful for my family and friends and added to our trauma, but there didn't seem to be an alternative. It was a terrible time for us. Eventually I was referred to a therapeutic community, where being helped through a crisis was totally different.

The main thing was that people were able to sit with you while you experienced really destructive thoughts and feelings – they sat with the risk. The therapists didn't panic, they wanted to know what it was about. In the community, there is no 'them and us' and the members become therapists to each other, no one person held the power of knowledge, it was something shared and thought about together. So, when you were in crisis people understood what was and wasn't helpful because they had their own experience to draw on.

There is something very healing about what we called 'the knowing nod', to not be on your own with what was in your head, or feel judged or dismissed as 'attention seeking'. There was opportunity to learn from everyone's crisis, as well as how to be responsible for yourself and other members; to trust and be trusted. Once you start connecting with people you don't want to betray their trust or trigger them, you learn to be trusted and you value that.

A mental health worker asked me recently if people ended up self-harming more. It wasn't like that, if you came in after self-harming, or were planning to do something risky you'd be challenged and often you just didn't want to let others down, so you struggled to find other ways of dealing with it, with the support of the community. It "

Visit **https://study.sagepub.com/essentialmentalhealth** to access a wealth of online resources for this chapter – watch out for the margin icons throughout the chapter. If you are using the interactive ebook, simply click on the margin icon to go straight to the resource.

wasn't all cosy chats and tea – it could be hard to receive a blunt challenge, but somehow it was contained no matter how heated it might get and there was always tomorrow to work it out a bit more. Gradually you come to understand where your crisis fits in the context of your history and the context of your life now. All the time the therapists were there to help and guide us, nudging us toward finding the meaning behind our feelings or behaviour.

I haven't had a crisis that is not containable since. It was a transformative experience for me and my family. I think you internalise all those conversations and confrontations and find a different perspective, and new ways to manage your own legacy of early trauma. The safety and rhythm of space and time living alongside each other allows for something new to be created within you that can last – if you want it to. For me, it was the collaborative nature of the community – the combined expertise of the professionals and those with lived experience that made this possible.

Jane Wackett, service user

When I qualified as a registered mental health nurse in 2011, austerity was already biting, resulting in this Swiss cheese of a mental health service that we see today. Incidents of mental health problems are increasing whilst the safety net shrinks. Neoliberalism seems to be heaping responsibility on those who experience mental health difficulties, ironically coinciding with high profile debates around stigma and inequality. I've observed with growing disillusionment how seemingly well intentioned government rhetoric remains just that.

Since qualifying as a nurse, I've always had a degree of internal dissonance about nursing practice, particularly concerning the medical model and coercive care. Despite growing dissatisfaction with psychiatric approaches there is, I feel, a lack of critical perspective. I've watched with interest innovations such as Finland's Open Dialogue and more recently, Norway's drug free treatment wards. My faith in psychiatric medicine is almost non-existent, reflected beautifully in Robert Whitaker's book, *Anatomy of an Epidemic*. As the revolving door continues to spin, I believe the dominance of the medical model needs to be challenged in a meaningful way.

In recent talks I have been having with some like-minded and equally exhausted and frustrated colleagues, we have discovered joint aspirations to create our 'dream service'. It's almost comical, patient choice of treatment has been a high priority, yet where is this choice? We believe the time is ripe for a fully coproduced service which comprises a therapeutic facility and space, integrating service users with the local community. This would offer the opportunity of small business start-ups which would hopefully grow organically from some of the treatment options, including an open dialogue service, an outreach service for supporting people in the community, alongside promoting mutual support in educational settings and workplaces. More complementary approaches may include: nutrition, yoga and meditation, aromatherapy massage, singing and music, art, horticulture and the like. The facility would be collectively cared for and decorated using people's own art, for instance. A relaxing café and lounge would serve all from the community with workshops and employment opportunities for the

(Continued)

> service users, and a crisis space provided. Meanwhile, targeted educational and self-help groups would offer a more traditional approach alongside talking therapies. A commitment to democratic service design would extend to democratic service delivery and ongoing research and the continuing advancement in our understanding of, and ability to provide, acceptable and meaningful care and support.
>
> **John Marsden, mental health nurse**

INTRODUCTION

Whatever we think about the language of 'mental illness' or **'disorder'**, mental distress and fragmentation is a very real problem for many people. It requires collectively organised and compassionate responses. Arguably, this response ought to consist of a plural range of options and alternatives, not just biomedical psychiatry. Much has been written about how some 'developing' countries have better mental health **recovery** rates than many 'developed' countries (like the UK and the USA). For example, World Health Organization studies report greater recovery rates from **schizophrenia** in parts of the developing world (Hopper et al., 2004). Some attribute this discrepancy to differential diagnostic practices and definitions of recovery. Others argue that developing countries rely less on western medicine and medications which may actually induce chronicity (Whitaker, 2010), and recovery rates in the West may even be decreasing, despite the introduction of new **antipsychotics** (Warner, 2004). Arguably, the improved recovery rates in parts of the global south may result from a greater *plurality* of support and treatments, including those rooted in a person's own frameworks and belief systems (Halliburton, 2004). For example, in South India some people are able to access western medicine, but also more traditional healing systems such as Ayurvedic and other holistic-based treatments. In other words, whilst by no means an ideal system, services may not be dominated by one overarching ideology of treatment such as biomedical psychiatry.

The critique of narrow, biomedical psychiatry has persuasively been made elsewhere, including within the pages of this book, so we will not revisit these here. Suffice to say that whilst statutory mental health services are not uniform and include a range of diverse practices and interventions, they tend to be dominated by a bio-psychiatric model which uses high levels of **compulsion, coercion, restrictive practices** and an overreliance on medication as standard. Despite widespread policy rhetoric in favour of holistic approaches and biopsychosocial service provisions, the diversity of care and treatment is limited (Read, 2005).

For example, the majority of people in the UK who experience a severe mental health crisis (such as serious **self-harm**, a suicide attempt or a psychotic breakdown) are likely to be hospitalised and/ or medicated, sometimes against their will. Unfortunately, whilst some people do report some benefit, psychiatric units are usually the worst places for people in serious crisis – they tend to be risk averse, medicalised, controlling and have few therapeutic opportunities on offer. Despite pockets of good practice, if anything, this situation has deteriorated over recent years, due to pressure on services, staff and clients. In turn, this has meant that the use of coercive powers to detain and treat is actually on the rise.

A significant number of people who experience **psychosis** do not benefit from medication (a category known as 'persistent neuroleptic non-responders'); some may benefit as much, if not more, from minimal medication alternatives, and others may recover anyway with adequate social support (Warner, 2004). Yet, despite studies suggesting that medication is not always essential for good outcomes in the treatment of people exhibiting first-episode psychosis or 'schizophrenia-like' illness, drug-free strategies are rarely, if ever, considered by modern psychiatric services (Calton & Spandler, 2009; Spandler & Calton, 2009). This has provoked many practitioners, family members and **service users** to call for alternatives. It is fair to say that ever since its inception, the user/**survivor** movement has consistently argued for alternatives for people in crisis.

Historically, alternatives have emerged from time to time and, despite many positive outcomes, they have proved hard to sustain over time. Of course, what is regarded as the 'medical model' is a relatively recent development, and a range of alternative forms of support and care have existed prior to, and during, the dominance of the bio-psychiatric model. Hence, there are numerous examples of alternative approaches to care and support, too many to describe here, so we will restrict ourselves to presenting a selection, mostly in the UK. A fantastic guide to international alternatives can be found in the edited collection *Alternatives beyond Psychiatry* (Stasny & Lehmann, 2017), which explores the diverse ways that people have developed to support themselves and each other, without recourse to diagnosis, psychiatrisation and overreliance on medication.

Although the examples we give are diverse, they share certain characteristics that distinguish them from much of mainstream practice, typically involving:

- a commitment to *be with* and *work alongside* people who are distressed or disturbed, rather than manage or control their 'symptoms'
- an attempt to make sense of seemingly unintelligible speech or irrational thinking and behaviour, rather than seeing them merely as symptoms of an underlying disease or **illness**
- working within the person's own preferred framework of understanding (this might be cultural, psychosocial, political and/or spiritual), rather than imposing on them particular 'expert' medically informed explanations
- an emphasis on dialogue rather than didactic communication
- attention to the therapeutic potential of different types of place and space, beyond hospital
- an appreciation of the underpinning psychosocial causes of distress, especially trauma, abuse and oppression
- **values** such as pro-sociality, sense of community, cooperation, compassion, comradeship, mutuality and reciprocal living, honesty, humility, transparency, equality, respect and self-awareness.

This list is by no means exhaustive and there will always be a debate about what constitutes 'alternatives'. Some alternatives might exist, or be taken up, within mainstream services and some so-called alternatives may mimic more conventional approaches in practice. They are not a panacea. Trying to understand and support someone going through a serious mental health crisis is never easy. In addition, many individual mental health practitioners develop good relationship-based support in very traditional psychiatric contexts and damaging work can be carried out in projects badged as alternatives. Any alternative is problematic if it becomes ideologically driven and seeks to impose alternative understandings on people, however well-meaning. Of course, some people may prefer more medical understandings and frameworks and this should be respected. Therefore, the distinction between 'mainstream' and 'alternative' may not be easy to sustain in practice. Nevertheless, there are some appealing and promising examples of organised alternatives that mental health nurses should be aware of.

Alternatives are necessary for three main reasons. First, they potentially address many service users' dissatisfaction with an overreliance on hospitalisation, medication and the iatrogenic harm these interventions may cause. Second, the emphasis on developing meaning and understanding makes these initiatives more likely to have a long-lasting impact and effect, as they may involve more radical personal learning and change (rather than the 'revolving door' **syndrome** we frequently see in mental health services). Third, increasing the range and diversity of different approaches will benefit more people, providing greater choice and autonomous control.

Unfortunately, these examples are quite rare and certainly not widely available. They could certainly be replicated, and developed according to context, to enable alternatives to be more widely accessible. At the very least, they might help the minority who are able to access them, and may help to influence mainstream practices. More than this, for a truly plural set of alternatives to flourish, current levels of alternative provision need to be substantially expanded and appropriately resourced.

SURVIVOR-CONTROLLED CRISIS HOUSES

From the early days of the service user movement, users and survivors have tried to organise their own alternatives to the mental health system. Judi Chamberlin's *On Our Own: Patient-Controlled Alternatives to the Mental Health System* (Chamberlin, 1978), initially published in the USA, has been very influential in inspiring alternatives. In the 1970s and early 1980s, the London Mental Patients Union ran a housing project in Hackney and Wanstead, which included 'crash pad' emergency accommodation where people going through a crisis could stay and be supported by other residents (http://studymore.org.uk/mpu.htm). There have been numerous similar initiatives since then. Unfortunately, they have been hard to sustain, partly because they have usually been entirely self-funded or rely solely on unpaid volunteers. Survivor-controlled alternatives can take a range of forms (Stasny & Lehmann, 2017).

One of the most successful projects is the Leeds survivor-led crisis service which has provided an alternative to hospital admission and statutory provision for people in **acute** mental health crisis since the late 1990s. Although not residential, it provides a variety of support and sanctuary in the evenings, at night-time and weekends in a home-like **environment**. It provides support to a range of clients and has gained a considerable reputation for supporting people who self-harm (Noad & Butlin, 2013; Venner, 2009).

The recently published *Searching for a Rose Garden* (Russo & Sweeney, 2016) presents a number of survivor-controlled practice alternatives that range across forms of **peer support**, including support for women with alcohol problems, trauma-informed care, support for coming off psychiatric drugs, advocacy for supported decision making and culturally sensitive support. Whilst the authors recognise that there are few actual examples of user-led crisis services – the 'rose garden' remains elusive – they make the important point that users and survivors should be supported to find their own alternatives, on their own terms, which work for them.

One of the editors, Jasna Russo (2016: 60), argues that it is 'still a revolutionary act when we stop being "cases to be managed" and "problems to be solved", and take the lead in defining support and generating knowledge about madness'.

THERAPEUTIC COMMUNITIES

Therapeutic communities (TCs) have a reputable and long history as alternatives. Most notably, the Quaker-inspired York Retreat was seen as a more humane alternative to the asylum system during the 19th century. Indeed, for a time TCs were seen as an accepted part of the range of psychiatric practice, if not necessarily universally available. The original TCs were residential units grounded in a psychosocial group-based intervention, where the process of personal growth and recovery is brought about by the relationships and interactions between staff and service users, notably through the facilitation of peer support. In effect, the community itself is seen as the main therapeutic ingredient and there is typically at least one daily meeting of all members of the community to discuss the day-to-day functioning and relationships within the community. TCs have had particular success with people who tend to express their distress behaviourally, through their relationships with others – for example, people struggling with **addictions** and people diagnosed with '**personality** disorders'. However, the ethos of therapeutic communities can be utilised across a variety of settings and client groups.

Therapeutic communities provide the physical and relational space to model more equitable democratic communication which can aid understanding and recovery. The popularity of TCs within mainstream services has waned in recent decades, but certain key figures have worked hard to ensure that their democratising features are not lost altogether (Haigh & Pearce, 2017). For example, the 'enabling environments' programme aims to ensure that various places, such as inpatient wards, aspire to organisational approaches that exhibit important characteristics of TCs, even if they fall short of being a fully-fledged therapeutic community (Johnson & Haigh, 2011). The core standards of enabling environments refer to the collective of staff and service users as 'participants' or 'members', and include:

- an emphasis on the nature and quality of relationships between participants, and all participants being equally valued
- all behaviour, even disruptive behaviour, being viewed as meaningful
- all participants sharing responsibility for the environment
- efforts made to recognise and even out power imbalances; importantly, power and authority have to be accountable and open to discussion
- purposeful activity and engagement being encouraged, especially planned and spontaneous creativity
- clear and transparent decision making
- formal and informal rules and expectations being made clear, unless there is good reason for ambiguity. (Johnson & Haigh, 2011)

A promising extension of therapeutic communities and enabling environment practices is seen in some 'greencare' initiatives. These include nature and the natural world as an integral part of therapeutic programmes (Haigh & Lees, 2017): for example, therapeutic horticulture, animal-assisted interventions, care farming and wilderness camping. Attempts are being made to develop a TC-inspired whole social system approach in the town of Slough, incorporating multiple levels of support with ecological and sustainability initiatives (Haigh, 2012).

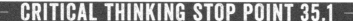

CRITICAL THINKING STOP POINT 35.1

CHECK YOUR
ANSWERS

Reflect on the mental health services you have experience of. To what extent do they possess the features of an enabling environment?

CRITICAL
THINKING
STOP
POINT 35.1
ANSWER

SOTERIA

In the 1960s and 1970s, notable **anti-psychiatry** practitioners such as Laing (Kingsley Hall, Philadelphia Houses, London) and Cooper (Villa 21, Shenley Hospital, Hertfordshire) attempted to organise residential alternatives to mainstream psychiatry based on therapeutic community principles for people diagnosed with schizophrenia. A common point of departure was the assumption that experiences usually viewed as symptoms could be better understood as a meaningful dimension of people's lives rather than reduced to an illness. Thus, the emphasis was on providing high levels of relational support, with staff prepared to be alongside individuals who were going through so-called psychotic experiences, with minimal interference and a relative disinclination to treat with medication. Despite being seen as 'failures' by mainstream psychiatry, and the fact that they were often affected by the sometimes wayward ideas and practices of particular charismatic individuals, they had some success and have been developed in a variety of ways since.

For example, the Soteria model was developed by Loren Mosher (1996, 1999) in the USA after he was inspired by visiting Kingsley Hall. Soteria shares a foundation in the TC movement with some similarities in its identifying 'critical elements', which involve: an emphasis on therapeutic milieu, an affinity for lay person staffing, the preservation of personal power, social networks, communal responsibilities and a commitment to minimal use of antipsychotic medication. It is not ideologically driven or anti-medication – sometimes medication is used in the short term, especially minor tranquillisers to aid sleep, but long-term use of antipsychotics is avoided wherever possible. Staff are supported to 'be with' and 'do with' the service users, using a particular 'phenomenological' approach to relating, that aims to understand individuals' experiences of psychosis by looking for meaning in that which might at first seem bizarre or unintelligible.

The Soteria model has been researched using methods acceptable to the mainstream scientific community, including controlled trials, and these have been systematically reviewed (Calton et al., 2008). The results show that Soteria has been at least as successful in terms of outcomes as standard approaches. Indeed, the 'minimal medication/maximum support' approach offered by the Soteria paradigm may be more responsive to patients' own priorities. Thus, it has proved very popular amongst many service users and practitioners internationally.

Whilst the UK doesn't have any Soteria Houses yet, the Soteria Network in the UK has campaigned for Soteria-informed approaches which draw on a wide range of creative and innovative practices, and has developed ideas about practices like 'mindful companionship', informed by radical ideas of mindfulness, to intensively support people experiencing extreme states of mind in various ways. The Soteria Network is attempting to establish Soteria Crisis Houses in Bradford and Brighton.

CRITICAL THINKING STOP POINT 35.2

What do you think the challenges are for mental health staff working in places like Soteria Houses which use minimal or no medication?

CRITICAL
THINKING
STOP
POINT 35.2
ANSWER

MAYTREE SANCTUARY

The Maytree Suicide Respite Centre is a London-based, short-term residential space for people who are experiencing suicidal thoughts and behaviour. It provides brief respite, usually a five-day stay, away from a person's usual environment, to get support from a team experienced in supporting people through suicidal crisis without judgement and with compassion and warmth. It is the only place of its kind in the UK and fills a gap in services between the medical support of the NHS and the helplines and drop-in centres of the voluntary sector.

It has been positively evaluated in a follow-up study of people who stayed in the sanctuary (Briggs et al., 2007). Despite small numbers participating, the evaluators noted that the findings were striking. For these guests, their stay not only helped reduce levels of suicidal feeling, intent and threat but also represented a significant moment of transformational change in their lives. In other words, it acted as a turning point for them, promoting understanding and learning. This finding relates to the idea that suicidal thoughts and feelings may be seen as a crisis of the self, full of opportunity, despite its risks (Webb, 2010). In *Thinking about Suicide*, David Webb, a suicide survivor, argues that suicidal thoughts and feelings may be a genuine and authentic human experience that should be honoured and respected as real, legitimate and important. He maintains that the healing of any crisis of the self begins with telling our stories, so we need to create safe story-telling spaces to talk about suicidal feelings (Webb, 2010). Organisations like the Maytree provide just these kinds of healing and learning opportunities.

SLI EILE FARM

The Sli Eile Farm was set up in Ireland by the parent of a service user dissatisfied with the support offered in mainstream services, especially locked wards and high levels of medication. The farm provides a place for supported living where people experiencing mental distress can feel safe, accepted, and find the support to recover and live more independently. There is only room for a small number of residents but there are plans to expand and create a fully working therapeutic farm. At present, residents are involved in a cooperative approach to participation in the everyday work tasks required to support living on the farm: cooking, cleaning and shopping, extending to working in a small bakery that sells bread to local businesses. The initiative is connected to Critical Voices Network, Ireland (CVNI) which itself supports critically minded service users, **carers**, practitioners and academics who want to see an alternative, non-biomedical mental health system, and runs annual conferences to this end in Cork, at which residents at Sli Eile are regular participants (Sapouna & Gijbels, 2016).

OPEN DIALOGUE

Emerging from a service-wide reorganisation in Western Lapland, Finland, the **Open Dialogue** approach represents a pragmatic transformation of publically provided care away from inadequacies in the reigning bio-psychiatric approach. In its early years, it transformed the dominant approach to supporting people who experience psychosis in the region. As such, it represented a large natural experiment, able to compare the outcomes achieved with what had gone before and mainstream approaches elsewhere, with remarkable results. Latterly, Open Dialogue has been combined with peer support approaches (Peer Support Open Dialogue) and subject to robust study; versions of the approach are currently being evaluated by trial-designed studies in the UK (Razzaque & Stockmann, 2016) and New York (Pope et al., 2016).

Characteristics of Open Dialogue include a labour-intensive commitment to support and an equivalent commitment to: honest communication with service users and their families or social networks who meet together, tolerance of uncertainty, and minimal paperwork and documentation. The mental health crisis is seen as not just located in the person allegedly 'mentally ill' but in the 'whole system' of which the person is a part. This isn't about blame, but about developing better communication amongst members of the person's social network; about underlying difficulties and how to better deal with crises when they arise. Though the practice of Open Dialogue preceded research and theory development, the underpinning theory stresses critical sociological ideas concerning democracy, and dialogic communication, drawing on the work of Mikael Bakhtin (Seikkula & Arnkil, 2014).

Whilst there is much excitement about this approach in the UK, and a number of mental health trusts are piloting the approach, there are some concerns. For example, there is the worry that service users might be coerced into conversations with family members who may have contributed to their difficulties in the first place (abuse, neglect and domestic violence often being precursors to mental health crisis, especially for women). Including a person's social network seems sensible, given that difficulties are usually relational and contextual, not just individual. However, this underscores the need for people to choose and self-define their own networks and level of involvement themselves, a task never easy when in crisis. Others have raised concerns that these approaches will be co-opted, professionalised and watered down by being adopted in mainstream services. Nevertheless, we are encouraged by these developments and think they are worth further investment and investigation.

SPIRITUAL COMMUNITIES

Some collectives provide crisis support within their own spiritual frameworks which might make sense to some people. Sometimes these are fused with therapeutic community ideals. For example, Lothlorien is a small, modern residential therapeutic community situated in a quiet rural setting in south-west Scotland. It has been running successfully since 1989. Though not a religious community, Lothlorien mixes the usual commitment to egalitarian, democratic empowerment with Buddhist values of compassion and tolerance. In addition, the Spiritual Crisis Network provides support to those who may wish to see their crisis as a 'spiritual emergency' replete with opportunities for spiritual growth and understanding, rather than an illness (see Clarke, 2010).

It is worth noting that whilst the anti-psychiatry therapeutic communities were heavily criticised, many of their components have continued or resurfaced in different ways over the years. For example, R.D. Laing's use of yoga and meditation was sneered at by many, but these more holistic or spiritual ideas continue to inform alternatives and, to some extent, have been taken up in mainstream practice (with the rise of pursuits like mindfulness). In addition, one of the pioneers of Peer Support Open Dialogue has developed more spiritually informed approaches to mental health care (Razzaque, 2014).

THE ROLE OF MENTAL HEALTH NURSES

CASE STUDY:
NON-MEDICAL
ALTERNATIVES

There are many lessons to draw from these initiatives. For example, it is worth noting the numerous common factors in these approaches, which feature again and again and re-emerge in different ways – such as community, mutuality and democracy.

However, the main issue we focus on here is the role of mental health nurses in developing and supporting alternatives. The possibilities for transformed services implicit in the various alternatives suggest that large numbers of appropriately skilled staff working intensively would be required for wholesale adoption. Mental health nurses, given their numbers within the total workforce, their close working proximity to service users, and their expressed affinity for relationship-based support, are perhaps well placed to support alternative forms of care. On occasion, nursing staff have even developed their own alternative models of care (e.g. Barker, 2001).

Because of prevailing power structures, most nurses work in services and systems that are not of their design in the first place, nor do they expect to have much say in how they may be redesigned for the future. Because of this, nursing exists in a state of disempowerment which, albeit not the same as service user disempowerment, is still disabling and alienating. This is especially the case for nurses trying to reconcile progressive personal values with the conflictual and coercive reality of day-to-day practice. As such, the idea of alternative forms of care should be appealing to the nursing workforce as well as to service users and survivors.

That said, nursing is also complicit in most of the highlighted failings in services and has largely accommodated itself to a subordinate role under psychiatry. Indeed, radical service users and survivors are often explicitly committed to a complete break with the mainstream, including nurses, preferring to articulate and organise alternatives without interference from the established order, or at the very least in selective **collaboration** with trusted allies (Russo & Sweeney, 2016).

Indeed, many of these alternative initiatives favour lay staff over professionals, and this may well be an impediment to nurses assuming much of a role. It is entirely appropriate that many alternative services or sources of support would be user-led and cautious about employing staff with previous professional identities and psychiatric training. However, as Jane's narrative at the beginning of this chapter illustrates, training, awareness and experience – as well as good supervision – are also desirable in being able to offer appropriate specialist support and preventing burnout and compassion fatigue. In addition, there is nothing to stop mental health nurses, many of whom may well have experienced mental health crises themselves, taking the initiative in developing alternatives alongside service users. Another reason why mental health nurses might support moves for alternative services is the political framing of their work and client group. Within a neo-liberal policy backdrop, nurses have to work in increasingly cash-starved services, perhaps most acutely felt in inner-city inpatient care, with excessive staff turnover and sickness, overuse of agency staff, high bed occupancy, few opportunities for relational care and overemphasis on physical security (McKeown et al., 2013).

All of this is compounded by a parallel turn in society – the exaggeration of risk aversion in social and public policy arenas, and most obviously in mental health services (Slemon et al., 2017). This combination of factors results in ever increasing numbers of people subject to compulsion, and justifies policies replete with problems for progressively minded practitioners and service users alike. Within this political climate, creative alternatives are perpetually marginalised precisely because they are alternatives to dominant orthodoxy, and are thus seldom taken up wholesale by public services. Nevertheless, if nursing as an occupational group can become more constructively politically engaged, then a common cause for pursuing alternative forms of care could be the basis for alliances with critical service user and survivor activists. If a key question is how to organise services so that progressive values can manifest, then at least one set of solutions lies in supporting alternatives to current orthodoxies.

CRITICAL THINKING STOP POINT 35.3

Specifically, nursing staff can take a number of steps to support alternatives:

- Find out about available alternatives in your local area and nationally (some are able to support people outside their area).
- Make sure service users and their families and friends are aware of them.
- Consider referring or supporting self-referrals.
- Work alongside service users to help prepare for any future crises to enable them to better use alternatives in the future (e.g. utilise various advance planning tools, advance directives, crisis cards).
- Support and regularly communicate with your local user group and local advocacy services, including **Independent Mental Health Advocates** (IMHAs).
- Make alliances with services users and survivors and take joint action to support their cause (e.g. in defending valued services or campaigning for crisis alternatives).

Take a moment to reflect on these points. Make a list of the challenges and opportunities for working in this way within mainstream services. Do you think there is anything else mental health nurses can do to support the choice of alternatives?

CRITICAL THINKING STOP POINT 35.3 ANSWER

We have made the case elsewhere that alliances between workers and service users are required to help transform mental health services and construct alternatives (e.g. McKeown et al., 2013). However, an important question remains over whether all parties agree that this is a worthwhile goal and, if so, what form 'alternatives' should take. More radical service users and survivors may not care to work with psychiatric nursing staff because of a lack of trust, born out of a history of harm experienced at the hands of services. Staff who are invested in current services may also be reluctant to join an alliance calling for radical change. We have argued that a necessary first step for forming constructive alliances is to establish genuine dialogue *outside* current services (Spandler & McKeown, 2017). Here, staff and ex-service users or psychiatric survivors could get together to hear each other's perspective – of either trying to give or receive crisis support – without interruption or judgement. Both parties would be freed from the need to 'do' anything or 'treat' anyone, and able to think imaginatively and critically about the ways services are usually delivered. This may help to heal prior hurt experienced by service users or staff in the system, develop trust and greater understanding of service failings. More than this, in the process of dialogue, we could learn from past mistakes and consider new and creative ways of supporting people through crisis.

CONCLUSION

Various alternatives to mainstream mental health services exist. These have been developed over the years by service users, carers and progressive practitioners. The extent to which such alternatives are available is limited and part of their appeal is that they represent something different from services that appear to rely too heavily on **medical treatments**. The task of ensuring more widespread availability, or transforming psychiatry so that the alternative approaches become much more part of the mainstream, is likely to be difficult. To some extent, this requires new forms of politics and a rapprochement between mental health care workers and critical survivors and service users.

CHAPTER SUMMARY

This chapter has covered:

- Discussion of a range of alternatives to crisis admissions
- Consideration of hospital admission as a risk-averse model that may not be in the best interests of the service user
- Therapeutic community approaches to care and treatment and how core principles can transfer to other settings
- The role of the mental health nurse in providing information about the alternatives to crisis admission for service users and their families.

BUILD YOUR BIBLIOGRAPHY

Books

- Foot, J. (2015) *The man who closed the asylums: Franco Basaglia and the revolution in mental health care.* New York: Verso Books. An excellent biography of Basaglia, the psychiatrist who fought to transform the Italian mental health system.

- Mosher, L.R., Hendrix, V. & Fort, D.C. (2004) *Soteria: Through madness to deliverance.* Bloomington, IN: Xlibris. An engaging introduction to the Soteria approach.
- Russo, J. & Sweeney, A. (2016) (eds) *Searching for a rose garden: Challenging psychiatry, fostering Mad Studies.* Wyastone Leys: PCCS Books. A marvellous statement of the importance for service users and survivors of being in control of their own knowledge production and alternative services.

SAGE journal articles

Go to https://study.sagepub.com/essentialmentalhealth for further free online journal articles related to this chapter. If you are using the interactive ebook, simply click on the book icon in the margin to go straight to the resource.

FURTHER READING: JOURNAL ARTICLES

- McGeachan, C. (2014) 'The world is full of big bad wolves': investigating the experimental therapeutic spaces of R.D. Laing and Aaron Esterson. *History of Psychiatry, 25*(3), 283-298.
- Mosher, L.R., Vallone, R. & Menn, A. (1995) The treatment of acute psychosis without neuroleptics: six-week psychopathology outcome data from the Soteria project. *International Journal of Social Psychiatry, 41*(3), 157-173.
- Soyez, V. & Broekaert, E. (2005) Therapeutic communities, family therapy, and humanistic psychology: history and current examples. *Journal of Humanistic Psychology, 45*(3), 302-332.

Weblinks

Go to https://study.sagepub.com/essentialmentalhealth for further weblinks related to this chapter. If you are using the interactive ebook, simply click on the book icon in the margin to go straight to the resource.

FURTHER READING: WEBLINKS

- Asylum Magazine online: www.asylumonline.net – Asylum: the magazine for democratic psychiatry is a brilliant source of radical mental health ideas written in a down-to-earth style, with great art, cartoons, poetry and much more
- Critical Voices Network, Ireland: www.cvni.ie
- Maytree House: www.maytree.org.uk – is described above and is a registered charity supporting people in suicidal crisis in a non-medical setting
- Soteria Network: www.soterianetwork.org.uk

ACE YOUR ASSESSMENT

Revise what you have learned by visiting https://study.sagepub.com/essentialmentalhealth. If you are using the interactive ebook, simply click on the tick icon to go straight to the resource.

ONLINE QUIZZES & ACTIVITY ANSWERS

- Test yourself with multiple-choice and short-answer questions and flashcards.

REFERENCES

Barker, P. (2001) The Tidal Model: developing an empowering, person-centred approach to recovery within psychiatric and mental health nursing. *Journal of Psychiatric and Mental Health Nursing, 8*(3), 233–240.

Briggs, S., Webb, J., Buhagiar, J., et al. (2007) Maytree: a respite centre for the suicidal – an evaluation. *Crisis: The Journal of Crisis Intervention and Suicide Prevention, 28*(3), 140–147.

Calton, T. & Spandler, H. (2009) Minimal-medication approaches to treating schizophrenia.*Advances in Psychiatric Treatment*, *15*(3), 209–217.

Calton, T., Ferriter, M., Huband, N. & Spandler, H. (2008) A systematic review of the Soteria paradigm for the treatment of people diagnosed with schizophrenia. *Schizophrenia Bulletin*, *34*(1), 181–192.

Chamberlin, J. (1978) *On our own: Patient-controlled alternatives to the mental health system*. New York: McGraw-Hill.

Clarke, I. (ed.) (2010) *Psychosis and spirituality*, 2nd edition. Oxford: Wiley.

Haigh, R. (2012) The philosophy of greencare: why it matters for our mental health. *Mental Health and Social Inclusion*, *16*(3), 127–134.

Haigh, R. & Lees, J. (2017) Democratic therapeutic communities in the 21st Century. *Asylum: the magazine for democratic psychiatry*, *24*(3), 10–11.

Haigh, R. & Pearce, S. (2017) *The theory and practice of democratic therapeutic community treatment*. London: Jessica Kingsley.

Halliburton, M. (2004) Finding a fit: psychiatric pluralism in South India and its implications for WHO studies of mental disorder. *Transcultural Psychiatry*, *41*(1), 80–98.

Hopper, K., Harrison, G., Aleksander, J., et al. (2004) *Recovery from schizophrenia: An international perspective*. Madison, CO: International Universities Press.

Johnson, R. & Haigh, R. (2011) Social psychiatry and social policy for the 21st century: new concepts for new needs – the 'Enabling Environments' initiative. *Mental Health and Social Inclusion*, *15*(1), 17–23.

McKeown, M., Jones, F. & Spandler, H. (2013) Challenging austerity policies: democratic alliances between survivor groups and trade unions. *Mental Health Nursing*, *33*(6), 26–29.

Mosher, L.R. (1996) Soteria: a therapeutic community for psychotic persons. *The Psychotherapy Patient*, *9*(3–4), 43–58.

Mosher, L.R. (1999) Soteria and other alternatives to acute psychiatric hospitalization: a personal and professional review. *The Journal of Nervous and Mental Disease*, *187*(3), 142–149.

Noad, M. & Butlin, H. (2013) Embracing the self, holding the hurt: self-harm in a survivor led service. In C. Baker, C. Shaw & F. Filey (eds) *Our encounters with self-harm*. Monnmouth: PCCS Books

Pope, L.G., Cubellis, L. & Hopper, K. (2016) Signing on for dirty work: taking stock of a public psychiatry project from the inside. *Transcultural Psychiatry*, *53*(4), 506–526.

Razzaque, R. (2014) *Breaking down is waking up*. London: Watkins Publishing.

Razzaque, R. & Stockmann, T. (2016) An introduction to peer-supported open dialogue in mental healthcare. *BJPsych Advances*, *22*(5), 348–356.

Read, J. (2005) The bio-bio-bio model of madness. *The Psychologist*, *18*(10), 596–597.

Russo, J. (2016) Towards our own framework: or reclaiming madness, part two. In J. Russo & A. Sweeney (eds) *Searching for a rose garden: Challenging psychiatry, fostering Mad Studies*. Waystone Leys: PCCS Books. pp. 59–68.

Russo, J. & Sweeney, A. (eds) (2016) *Searching for a rose garden: Challenging psychiatry, fostering Mad Studies*. Wyastone Leys: PCCS Books.

Sapouna, L. & Gijbels, H. (2016) Social movements in mental health: the case of the Critical Voices Network Ireland. *Critical and Radical Social Work*, *4*(3), 397–402.

Seikkula, J. & Arnkil, T. (2014) *Open dialogues and anticipations: Respecting otherness in the present moment*. Tampere, FL: National Institute for Health and Welfare.

Slemon, A., Jenkins, E. & Bungay, V. (2017) Safety in psychiatric inpatient care: the impact of risk management culture on mental health nursing practice. *Nursing Inquiry*, *24*(4), e12199.

Spandler, H. & Calton, T. (2009) Psychosis and human rights: conflicts in mental health policy and practice. *Social Policy & Society, 8*(2), 245–256.

Spandler, H. & McKeown, M. (2017) Exploring the case for truth and reconciliation in mental health services. *Mental Health Review Journal, 22*(2), 83–94.

Stasny, P. & Lehmann, P. (2017) *Alternatives beyond psychiatry.* Berlin: Peter Lehmann Publishing.

Venner, F. (2009) Leeds survivor led crisis service: survivor-led philosophy in action. *A Life in the Day, 13*(2), 28–31.

Warner, R. (2004) *Recovery from schizophrenia: Psychiatry and political economy,* 3rd edition. London: Routledge.

Webb, D. (2010) *Thinking about suicide: Contemplating and comprehending the urge to die.* Ross-on-Wye: PCCS Books.

Whitaker, R. (2010) *Anatomy of an epidemic: Magic bullets, psychiatric drugs, and the astonishing rise of mental illness in America.* New York: Crown.

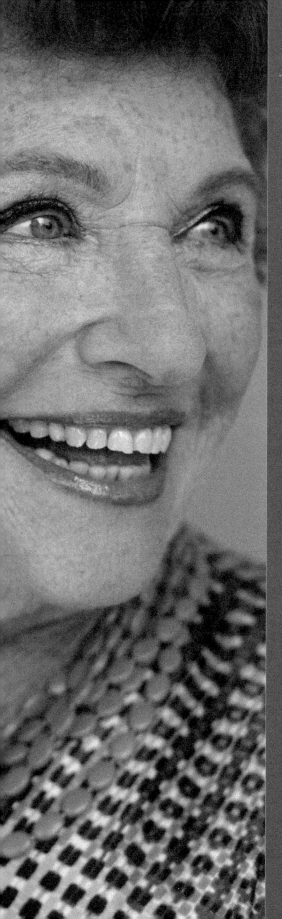

PART D TAILORING CARE TO PEOPLE WITH SPECIFIC NEEDS

DEMENTIA: ASSESSMENT AND CARE APPROACHES

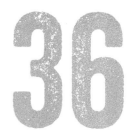

DAVID PULSFORD

--- **THIS CHAPTER COVERS** ---

- What dementia is
- Philosophies of care for people with dementia and their families and the qualities needed of carers
- Diagnosis and support in the early stage of dementia – the role of memory assessment services
- Community mental health nursing for people with dementia and their family carers
- Residential care for people with dementia.

> The provision of supportive therapeutic interventions and development of relationships is key to the work of nurses in helping families cope with the many changes and difficulties that dementia as a long-term condition may bring. Nurses often support people with complex and multiple needs. This support is wide ranging and can include assisting with difficulties with adjusting to diagnosis; significant changes in the mental and physical health of the person with dementia; family carer stress anxiety and depression; managing risk and supporting transitions in care.
>
> **Rachel Thompson, Admiral Nurse**

> As carers we needed an experienced member of staff who cared about Dad's welfare and who could empathise with the family's ongoing trauma and distress, who behaved in a professional and sensitive manner and led by example being a good role model for the rest of the staff. An individual who instilled confidence, someone we could trust to answer our questions honestly or could find out the answers for us if they didn't know. Although dying from dementia can be a long drawn out process, for our family it was no less traumatic than had Dad died suddenly, the distress just lasted longer and took its toll on us all.
>
> **Sally Frey, family carer**

Visit **https://study.sagepub.com/essentialmentalhealth** to access a wealth of online resources for this chapter – watch out for the margin icons throughout the chapter. If you are using the interactive ebook, simply click on the margin icon to go straight to the resource.

INTRODUCTION

There are growing numbers of people living with **dementia**. Despite this, dementia does not always seem to receive the attention and resources of other health issues. Care of people with dementia is often not the first choice of career for student mental health nurses. However, people with dementia and their families benefit greatly from skilled and empathic mental health nursing care and they can be highly rewarding to work with. In this chapter, we will consider dementia as a medical condition, review care philosophies for people with dementia and their families, and outline best practice in mental health nursing care in a range of care settings.

WHAT IS DEMENTIA?

Dementia is a condition that results from disease of the brain. In medical terms, it is a *syndrome*, that is, a collection of clinical features that can result from a number of different disease processes. There are over 100 types of dementia, most extremely rare. A significant feature of most types of dementia is that they are progressive (the person will deteriorate over time) and they are terminal conditions – the person will die of dementia, if they do not die of another **illness** before they reach the advanced stage of dementia.

The overall clinical features that a person with dementia may experience are:

- memory problems: often (but not always) the first sign of dementia is that the person becomes more forgetful, or finds it harder to learn new things
- cognitive difficulties: many cognitive (intelligence-based) abilities will decline; these include information processing, attention, *executive function* (the ability to sequence information or carry out complex tasks) and decision making
- language difficulties: in the early stages, the person may understand language but may find it hard to express themselves verbally; in the later stages, the person may lose the ability to understand language
- changes in manner or behaviour: the combined effects of the memory, cognitive and language difficulties may lead to changes in the way the person expresses feelings and interacts with the world, or with others. Sometimes other people will find the person's manner or behaviour difficult; for example, a previously equable person may become more anxious or restless and even aggressive in some situations. Some people may want to do things that will put them at risk of harm, while others may become more placid than usual and may appear to be apathetic or unmotivated
- difficulties with carrying out the activities of daily living: as cognitive difficulties increase, the person will need increasing assistance with nutrition and hydration, dressing and keeping clean; in the later stages, the person may have difficulties with toileting and may become incontinent
- psychiatric symptoms: many people with dementia experience periods of **depression** and some may have other psychiatric symptoms, such as **hallucinations** or delusional ideas
- physical decline: as stated above, dementia is a terminal condition and in the advanced stage the person may decline physically, to the point where they may need total nursing care.

This is a broad list of clinical features, but people with dementia will present in very different ways, due to several factors. The type of dementia they have will be one factor; some types of dementia have different features to others, particularly in the early stages. How far the condition has progressed is also an issue. Clinicians recognise three very broad stages of dementia – early, moderate and advanced. The clinical features of dementia tend to become more pronounced as the person moves through these stages. Another factor is the person's life history; often, the best way to understand and interact with a person with dementia is through knowing about their life before they contracted the condition, as their manner and behaviour often reflect aspects of their past lives. Finally and most importantly, the quality of care that the person receives will have a big influence. As the condition progresses, people with dementia become more and more reliant on others and will be particularly affected by how others regard them and interact with them.

DEMOGRAPHICS OF DEMENTIA

There are around 850,000 people living with dementia in the UK at the present time. If no medical preventative or cure is found, this figure is likely to increase to over 2 million by 2050. Dementia is predominantly a condition of older people and its prevalence increases exponentially with age: roughly 1% of people aged 65 will have dementia, rising to 6% of those aged 75 and 20% of 85-year-olds. At the same time, around 42,000 people have *young-onset dementia*, where the condition manifests itself before the age of 60.

Women are slightly more likely than men to have dementia. The majority of people with dementia are in the early stage of the condition (55.4%), with 32.1% in the moderate stage and 12.5% in the advanced stage (reflecting the fact that many people with dementia will die of other age-related conditions before they reach the advanced stage). Around 25,000 people with dementia are from black, Asian and minority ethnic groups and their numbers are predicted to increase at a greater rate. Also rising are the numbers of people with learning difficulties and dementia.

Finally, the majority of people with dementia (around 67%) live in 'the community', in most cases supported by a family member or other informal **carer**. Around 240,000 people with dementia live in care homes.

The source for these figures is *Dementia UK: Update* (Alzheimer's Society, 2014).

MEDICAL ASPECTS OF DEMENTIA

As previously stated, dementia results from brain disease. The most common *late-onset dementias* (conditions that manifest after the age of 60) are:

- Alzheimer's disease: a neuro-degenerative condition that leads to atrophy of the cerebral cortex and progressive difficulties in cognitive functioning
- vascular dementia: a group of conditions primarily caused by disease of the blood vessels that supply the brain, leading to the person experiencing a series of *transient ischaemic attacks* (mini-strokes) that progressively damage brain tissue
- dementia with lewy bodies: another degenerative condition linked to Parkinson's disease.

Rarer, but more common than previously thought, are the *young-onset dementias*, that manifest before the age of 60. Alzheimer's disease is still the most common young-onset dementia and other significant conditions include:

- fronto-temporal dementia: a degenerative condition that initially **affects** the frontal and temporal lobes of the cortex, leading to changes in manner and behaviour and executive function difficulties
- Huntington's disease: a genetically influenced condition in which cognitive difficulties are accompanied by movement difficulties caused by damage to motor-nerve pathways
- alcohol-related dementia: long-term alcohol abuse may directly lead to dementia, or may cause *Korsakoff's syndrome*, which is triggered by vitamin B deficiency.

In addition, other neurological conditions can lead to dementia, including Parkinson's disease, multiple sclerosis and muscular dystrophy, among many much rarer diseases.

TREATMENTS FOR DEMENTIA

There are currently no **medical treatments** that will prevent or reverse any type of dementia. Three drugs are available (donepezil, rivastigmine, galantamine) that may slow the progression of some types of dementia, such as Alzheimer's disease, for a few months, if given in the early or moderate stages. A further drug, memantine, may influence the manner and behaviour of some people with more advanced dementia. Clearly, none of these drugs are 'magic bullets' and it is likely that dementia will be with us for many years to come.

PREVENTION OF DEMENTIA THROUGH LIFESTYLE FACTORS

The good news is that there is growing evidence that the risk of contracting the most common types of dementia (Alzheimer's disease and vascular dementia) may be reduced through lifestyle factors. Two broad areas have been researched. First, ongoing 'intellectual' and social activity may be protective. Those who keep their minds active may be at reduced risk, or may delay the onset of dementia. Any kind of 'intellectual' activity will do, such as reading, doing puzzles, learning new things, playing musical instruments, and so on. The slogan 'use it or lose it' is sometimes used to highlight the need to keep the brain active. Social stimulation may also be protective and there is growing evidence that those who experience depression may have an increased risk of dementia.

Second, reducing vascular risk factors may help. It is becoming clear that both Alzheimer's disease and vascular dementia are cardiovascular conditions and those who have conditions such as hypertension, high cholesterol, type 2 diabetes and a history of heart disease and stroke are at increased risk of dementia. This has led to the slogan, 'what is good for the heart is good for the brain'. Lifestyle factors such as maintaining a normal body weight, not smoking, drinking in moderation, eating a 'Mediterranean' diet and (in particular) maintaining physical activity and exercise may all reduce the risk of dementia as well as other cardiovascular conditions.

For more information about medical aspects of dementia, see the many clear, peer-reviewed and regularly updated factsheets on the Alzheimer's Society website (www.alzheimers.org.uk).

USEFUL FOR ASSIGNMENTS!

CASE STUDY: SUPPORT & THERAPEUTIC CARE

PHILOSOPHIES OF CARE FOR PEOPLE WITH DEMENTIA

In the past, dementia was regarded simply as a progressive and untreatable condition and people with dementia were thought of in a negative way. A popular textbook for mental health nurses in the 1970s baldly stated, 'the outlook [in dementia] is hopeless' (Minski, 1972). The lot of many people with dementia was to be admitted to 'psychogeriatric' wards in large psychiatric hospitals where care regimes were described as 'minimal warehousing' (Robb, 1984). This medicalised, nihilistic view of dementia has come to be known as the *standard paradigm*.

Attitudes began to change during the 1990s, through the influence of theorists such as Tom Kitwood, who set out a comprehensive *person-centred* philosophy of dementia, to contrast with the standard paradigm (Kitwood, 1997). He noted (as we have above) that how a person with dementia presents is not simply a function of neurological impairment but is also influenced by psychosocial factors, including the person's life history, their physical and mental health and the quality of care that the person receives. For Kitwood, the aim of dementia care should be to assist the person with dementia to maintain *personhood*, wellbeing and a good quality of life. To this end, carers should recognise that the person's behaviour is meaningful and that behaviour that carers find difficult is an expression of 'poorly communicated need' (Stokes, 2000).

Table 36.1 contrasts the basic principles of Kitwood's person-centred philosophy with the standard paradigm. For a brief, clear and critical account of Kitwood's ideas, see Adams (1996).

Table 36.1 The standard paradigm and Kitwood's person-centred philosophy contrasted

	Standard paradigm	Person-Centred paradigm
People with dementia are:	Ex-people, as a result of the deficits caused by neurological damage	People like ourselves, with a capacity for feelings and for experiencing well- and ill-being
Dementia is:	The consequence of central nervous system disease, which progressively destroys the individual's personality and identity	A form of disability, which will affect the person in a unique way, due to the interaction of: life history; the disease process and the quality of care the person receives
Interactions between carers and people with dementia are:	I-It (I am a person, you have lost your personhood)	I-Thou (I will go the extra mile to help you maintain your personhood)
The goals of nursing care are:	To provide a safe environment; to give physical care in a competent way	To maintain and enhance personhood, and a sense of wellbeing. Safety and good physical care are of no value to the individual if personhood is lost
Behaviours that others find difficult are:	Random expressions of neurological damage. Carers should use tranquillising drugs and physical restraints to eliminate such behaviours	Primarily attempts at communication related to need. Carers should try to understand the message and find some way of meeting the underlying need

A (rather unfair) criticism of Kitwood is that he has underplayed the role of the family and other informal carers in assisting the person with dementia to maintain personhood and quality of life. This has led to the philosophy of *relationship-centred care* (Nolan et al., 2004), set out diagrammatically in Figure 36.1. This philosophy encourages professionals to assess the dynamic relationship between the person with dementia and their family members. It also regards family members as equal partners in the care process, with their own care needs and much to offer to professionals in terms of

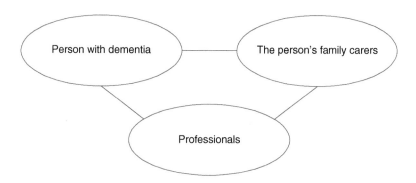

Figure 36.1 Relationship-centred care

Source: Nolan et al., 2004

their knowledge of the person and (often) their willingness to continue to assist with caregiving, even when the person has entered residential care.

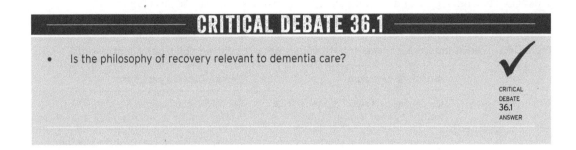

CRITICAL
DEBATE
36.1
ANSWER

ACHIEVING PERSON-CENTRED AND RELATIONSHIP-CENTRED CARE - QUALITIES NEEDED BY CARERS OF PEOPLE WITH DEMENTIA

Brooker (2004) conceptualises person-centred and relationship-centred care in the form of a formula, under the acronym VIPS:

- V: *Valuing* people with dementia and those who care for them
- I: Treating people as *individuals*
- P: Looking at the world from the *perspective* of the person with dementia
- S: A positive *social* **environment** in which the person living with dementia can experience relative wellbeing.

In order to achieve these conditions, carers (professionals and family members) need particular personal qualities (Pulsford et al., 2016), as set out in Figure 36.2.

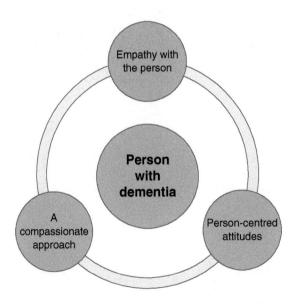

Figure 36.2 Qualities needed by a carer (professional or family) of a person with dementia

Empathy with the person

As Brooker (2004) points out, it is necessary for carers to see the world from the perspective of the person with dementia, as their perspective may be very different from that of the carer. As well as having different feelings and values, the person is viewing the world through the filter of their cognitive difficulties. These are likely to lead the person to have an increasingly restricted and simplified perspective as the condition progresses. Carers must try to see the world through the person's eyes and interpret the person's manner and behaviour in terms of their meaning for the person, using:

> *person-centred attitudes*: carers must embrace the philosophies of person-centred and relationship-centred care and must *want* to put these principles into practice

> *a compassionate approach*: this quality combines the carer's personal manner with their skills at delivering individualised care. The carer's manner should be reassuring, open and reaching out to the person. As set out in the case studies included in this chapter, creativity is often needed to find appropriate care solutions to individual needs.

MENTAL HEALTH NURSES AND PEOPLE WITH DEMENTIA

Mental health nurses may work with people with dementia and their families in a range of settings, including memory assessment services, community mental health teams, hospital-based assessment units and care homes. Their role embraces specialised assessment, care interventions for the person and their carers, advice giving to families and other professionals, and care management, including leadership and supervision of junior staff who deliver day-to-day care. We will consider the main care settings in which mental health nurses work, and highlight best practice in nursing care for people with dementia and their families.

DIAGNOSIS AND SUPPORT IN THE EARLY STAGE OF DEMENTIA: THE ROLE OF MEMORY ASSESSMENT SERVICES

As student nurses, you will be used to taking unseen examinations. You will recall the **anxiety** that exams generate – will my memory and intelligence be equal to the task? Imagine, however, that you had to take an examination, the result of which would determine whether or not you had a degenerative and terminal neurological disease. That, in effect, is what people being assessed for possible dementia have to undergo. Those carrying out cognitive assessments (and this is often a role for mental health nurses) should be aware of this and ensure that they use sensitivity and empathy when interacting with the person and their family members.

DIAGNOSIS OF DEMENTIA

Many people with dementia never have a formal assessment of their condition, but there are many advantages of a proper assessment and diagnosis (Department of Health, 2009). Diagnosis gives the person and their family an understanding of what is happening and allows them to try to come to terms with the condition and make plans for the future, including possibly making an ***advance directive***, setting out the person's care wishes for when they lack the capacity to make decisions. Diagnosis gives access to treatment and care services, and early support for families may enhance their ability to care for the person at home, reducing the need for residential care.

NICE guidelines on dementia (National Institute for Clinical Excellence, 2006) state that diagnosis should only be made following history taking, cognitive and mental state examination, physical examination and a review of medication to identify any drugs that may impair cognitive functioning. A number of cognitive and mental state **assessment tools** are available, administered by a professional and involving a range of memory and cognitive tasks for the person to fulfil.

MEMORY ASSESSMENT SERVICES

Universal provision of memory assessment services (as they tend to be called – sometimes abbreviated to MAS) is a feature of the *Prime Minister's Challenge on Dementia 2020* (Department of Health, 2015). The recommended functions of a MAS should include making the diagnosis well, breaking the diagnosis well to the person with dementia and their family and providing directly **appropriate treatment**, information, care and support after diagnosis.

Memory assessment services have developed in individual ways in different parts of the country and models of good practice have been published (Banerjee et al., 2007; Hean et al., 2011). Mental health nurses are often integral to the **multi-disciplinary team** that makes up a MAS. They need an understanding of the tools that are integral to assessment and high quality interpersonal skills to conduct the assessment in a skilled fashion. Nurses should have the ability to offer information and support following diagnosis, to both people with dementia and their families, in individual and group settings. There is evidence, however, that in some places the MAS has become little more than a 'diagnosis factory' and a setting for the short-term prescription of anti-dementia drugs, with the role of the nurse reduced to little more than administering cognitive assessments (Abley et al., 2013). People with early dementia and their carers (particularly those not suitable for anti-dementia medication) may be left more or less unsupported, with instructions to return to their GP if a crisis occurs (Samsi et al., 2014).

CASE STUDY 36.1

Assessing and diagnosing dementia

Martin is 74 and Joan is 72. They have been together for five years, both having previously been divorced. Both are retired and between them have several children and grandchildren. For the past couple of years, Martin has found it increasingly difficult to remember things. They put it down to 'getting on a bit' and laugh about it, but recently Martin's memory problems have got worse and he has on occasion done risky things, such as forgetting to shut the front door when going out and getting lost on familiar car journeys. He has also been forgetting the names of his children and grandchildren. Joan has become increasingly worried and, with some difficulty, persuaded Martin to talk to his GP, who carried out a brief assessment and referred Martin to a memory assessment service.

On the day of the appointment, Joan was full of anxiety. Martin put on an unconcerned air, but Joan could tell that he was worried too. The cognitive testing was carried out by a mental health nurse, who had a calm, friendly and reassuring manner, offered Martin encouragement and tried to put him at ease. Martin's medical history was taken by a doctor and he had a physical examination.

At a later appointment, the doctor and nurse broke the news to Martin and Joan that Martin was in the early stage of Alzheimer's disease. Although Joan had feared that this was the case, the news was still a shock to her and she found it hard not to cry. Martin understood what the doctor said and asked some questions about the condition but did not appear to react very strongly. Martin was prescribed aricept.

After the meeting with the doctor, the nurse spent time with Martin and Joan, answering Joan's questions and giving her some leaflets with more information. They were put in contact with a dementia care advisor, who would be their first point of contact for advice and further referrals, and they were given details of a local dementia café, which they could both attend for social support and further advice. Martin was invited to attend a cognitive stimulation group (Spector, 2003). The couple were also encouraged to talk with each other about the future, while Martin retained awareness of his condition, and to consider taking steps to make an advance directive and for Joan to acquire lasting power of attorney for Martin's affairs.

Question

- What factors might influence Martin and Joan's reaction to Martin's diagnosis?

CASE
STUDY 36.1
ANSWER

COMMUNITY MENTAL HEALTH NURSING FOR PEOPLE WITH DEMENTIA AND THEIR FAMILY CARERS

Two-thirds of people with dementia live in 'the community', either alone or with family members or in a *supported living* setting. Family members are in most cases called upon to act as informal carers, becoming the first line of support and care for the person. The philosophy of relationship-centred care implies that professionals should work with family carers as much as with the person with dementia (we will use the term 'family carers' for anyone who takes on a caring or supportive role, recognising that sometimes a person's carer may not be a family member). For those living in the community, this approach can make the difference between the person remaining at home and entering residential care.

People with dementia and their family carers have many needs that professionals such as community mental health nurses (CMHNs) can assist with. In the early stage of dementia, the person may retain considerable awareness of their condition and their growing difficulties (Clare et al., 2011). They may benefit from counselling approaches to help come to terms with their condition and techniques to help them retain their cognitive abilities and compensate for their difficulties. As the condition progresses, they may need assistance to remain active and to meet their social and daily living needs. Family carers may benefit from education regarding the nature of dementia and specific training in caring principles and techniques. It should not be assumed that a family member knows instinctively how to care for their relative. They may be assisted by written resources, such as the many helpful factsheets produced by the Alzheimer's Society or one of the growing number of books written for carers (e.g. Pulsford & Thompson, 2012). Carers may find it especially hard to cope with the person's manner and behaviour, particularly if the person behaves in ways that put themselves at risk, or if the person is sometimes hostile or apathetic (Donaldson, 1997). Family carers may also need emotional support and signposting to other services, such as **peer support** groups or services to assist with practical or financial issues.

CMHNs may take on the role of key worker or care manager for a person with dementia and their family carers. Some may take on the specialised role of an *Admiral Nurse*. Admiral Nurses are specialist dementia nurses who give practical and emotional support to family carers, as well as the person with dementia. They are able to take on complex cases. Rather like Macmillan Nurses, they are supported by a charity, *Dementia UK* (www.dementiauk.org/what-we-do/admiral-nurses). A number of research-based accounts and evaluations of the work of CMHNs and Admiral Nurses have been published, to identify best practice and also areas where CMHNs could make a more positive contribution, if they possessed the more specialised skills of Admiral Nurses (Keady et al., 2004, 2007; Moniz-Cook et al., 2008; Quinn et al., 2012).

CASE STUDY 36.2

A community mental health nurse assists a person with dementia and his family carer

Robert Hall is 65 and was diagnosed with Alzheimer's disease two years ago. He is cared for by his wife, Susan. Robert was a high-ranking civil servant who had to take early retirement when his condition became apparent. He is now in the moderate stage of the condition. Robert has been referred to a day centre run by Age UK, so that he has the opportunity to socialise and keep occupied while Susan has a break from caring. He is collected from home by a volunteer driver.

Robert insists on taking his briefcase with him, believing that he is being driven (as he used to be) to an important meeting. Susan gets upset at this, saying to Robert, 'You don't need that now - you're not going to work any more, don't you remember?' This leads Robert to become upset in turn and to refuse to get into the car. Sometimes, he will shout at Susan and even lash out at her.

Susan expressed her frustration about the briefcase to Janice, the community mental health nurse who was Robert's care coordinator. Janice gently and respectfully encouraged Susan to see the situation from Robert's perspective. His dementia had progressed to the point where he sometimes muddled memories of the past with the present. His belief that he was going to work was an expression of his need for self-esteem and to feel that he had a purpose. Surely it was better for Robert to take his briefcase to the day centre (which he enjoyed attending) than to argue about it. At the same time, Janice empathised with Susan's feelings and the sense of loss that the briefcase represented - that her husband was not the person he used to be. Janice used counselling skills to help Susan talk about her feelings and to carry on the difficult process of coming to terms with Robert's condition.

Question

- What ethical issues may arise from this scenario?

✓

CASE STUDY
36.2
ANSWER

Another important area in which CMHNs are making an increasing contribution is as part of *liaison services*, which have been established to provide specialised advice and support to professionals working with people with dementia in general hospitals (Sheehan et al., 2013) or in care homes (Hughes et al., 2013).

While CMHNs may make a considerable contribution, resource constraints and the sheer numbers of people with dementia living in the community mean that people with dementia and their families may need to access more informal sources of support. Charities such as the Alzheimer's Society or Age UK offer a range of supportive services, including support groups, dementia care advisors, dementia cafés and day care and respite services. Former prime minister David Cameron's Challenge on Dementia also aimed to promote more community-based support as an example of the 'Big Society', with initiatives such as *Dementia Friends* and *Dementia-friendly Communities* (Department of Health, 2015).

MAKING A DIFFERENCE 36.1

The dementia-friendly communities initiative

Many people with dementia (and their family carers) experience *social exclusion* - the feeling that they are not part of their local community and are constrained from meeting their needs to socialise and make a contribution to society. As a response to this, the Alzheimer's Society is promoting the concept of *Dementia-friendly Communities* (Alzheimer's Society, 2013). This initiative aims to encourage local authorities, businesses and local community groups to become more enabling towards people with dementia. An analogy can be made with the way that people with physical disabilities are today much more accepted and accommodated by society and enabled to live fulfilling and independent lives. Dementia-friendly communities are those in which people with dementia would have the same level of acceptance and support.

Becoming dementia-friendly involves raising awareness of the condition and the needs of people with dementia and their families. Organisations are encouraged to give their staff training in recognising and understanding dementia and how to interact with a person with dementia. Acceptance is also needed to reduce the stigma that people with dementia may experience. Mental health nurses may play a role in promoting dementia-friendly communities through education and facilitating community involvement, and also through leading by example in promoting positive attitudes towards people with dementia:

> Sometimes in the evening my Mum and Dad would wander to the local pub and they'd have a drink and people would make a fuss of my Mum and that was good for Dad, it got him out of the house and my mum would respond - even when she didn't have any conversation she would smile at people. For him it was trying to keep a bit of normality in the changing situation.
>
> Sheila, daughter of a person living with dementia

RESIDENTIAL CARE FOR PEOPLE WITH DEMENTIA

The majority of people with advanced dementia end their days in a care home. At present, over 240,000 people with dementia live in care homes and two-thirds of care home residents have dementia (Alzheimer's Society, 2014). In the UK, care homes are classified as either residential homes or nursing homes. As the name implies, nursing homes must have registered nurses among their staff. Virtually all continuing care beds for people with dementia are today in care homes, mainly run by independent sector companies, with a smaller number run by local authorities and third-sector providers. Continuing care is classed as 'social care', meaning that state funding is means tested and limited and residents and their families may have to pay significant amounts towards the fees.

Key activities of registered nurses working in care homes include assessing residents' mental and physical health needs and planning and implementing appropriate interventions, liaising with families and informal carers and other services, ensuring that legal requirements under the Mental Health and Mental Capacity Acts are fulfilled, and providing leadership and supervision to the care assistants who provide the bulk of direct care. **Care planning** may involve finding creative responses to residents' manner and behaviour when these are perceived by others to be difficult, based on the assumption that such behaviour reflects 'poorly communicated need' (Stokes, 2000).

CASE STUDY 36.3

Marjorie Richards has moderate dementia and has recently come to live in a care home. She has quite profound cognitive difficulties and limited language abilities. She retains some self-care abilities and attempts each morning to get herself dressed, but frequently gets muddled, picking inappropriate clothes and putting them on in the wrong order. She will then throw her clothes on the floor. If care staff try to correct her errors, she will resist and sometimes lash out at them.

Marjorie's family told care staff that she has always been very proud of her appearance and took a great deal of trouble to ensure that she was dressed immaculately. The care staff sensed that Marjorie's behaviour resulted from her feelings of frustration at her lack of understanding of her situation and an inability to meet her needs for independence in self-care and for looking her best. They consequently adopted a daily approach of offering Marjorie a choice of two dresses to wear each morning, by showing her both dresses together and using simple, clear language to ask her to choose one. They assisted her by handing her items of clothing in the correct order for getting dressed properly, while offering calm and simple verbal prompts. Marjorie was able to dress herself successfully using this approach and appeared more contented as a result.

Question

- How could the care home staff justify the extra time it took to implement this care plan with Marjorie?

CASE STUDY
36.3
ANSWER

A few years ago, the Alzheimer's Society published a major report into care homes for people with dementia (Alzheimer's Society, 2007). The report concluded that, 'The excellent care provided by some homes makes a huge difference to their residents' quality of life. Carers hugely **value** the efforts of staff who provide this level of care'. However, the report also stated that, 'Many homes are still not providing the level of person centred care people with dementia deserve'. Key problems identified included the provision of activities and occupation, treating residents with dementia with dignity and respect, and the relationship between care home staff and relatives/friends, implying also a lack of relationship-centred care. The quality of care in care homes is strongly linked to the leadership of the registered manager or nurse-in-charge (Bowman, 2009). The need for nurses working in and managing care homes to possess person-centred and relationship-centred values and caring qualities is clear.

WHAT'S THE EVIDENCE? 36.1

The use of antipsychotics as a response to behaviour that others find difficult

A report by the All-Party Parliamentary Group on Dementia (APPG, 2008) highlighted what it regarded as the excessive use of antipsychotic medication as a response to behaviour that care home staff found difficult. What is the evidence for and against the use of antipsychotics and what are the alternatives?

Corbett et al. (2014) have succinctly discussed the issues. They conclude that the evidence that antipsychotics are effective in modifying the behaviour of people with dementia is limited, with only a modest clinical benefit for risperidone in reducing **aggression**. At the same time, the negative side-effects of antipsychotics, including increased rates of cognitive decline and cardio-vascular events, are well documented. Corbett et al. (2014) point out that there are no drug-based alternatives to antipsychotics and doctors may find themselves under pressure to prescribe them, from family members or care home staff. They report that prescriptions of antipsychotics have reduced since the APPG report, but believe that there is still considerable 'off licence' prescribing.

There is, Corbett et al. (2014) assert, evidence that other approaches can reduce levels of behaviour that others find difficult. Getting to know the person well and trying to interpret the person's behaviour in terms of its meaning for them is important. Sometimes, agitated or aggressive behaviour results from unidentified pain, and analgesics can help (Corbett et al., 2012). A range of psycho-social interventions have been researched and found to be helpful, including simply spending quite brief periods of time with the person in activities that the person enjoys (Testad et al., 2014). NICE guidelines (National Institute for Clinical Excellence, 2006) state that antipsychotics should only be used as a last resort and mental health nurses should familiarise themselves with evidence-based alternatives to drug treatments.

Here, one student nurse gives her advice to other students on caring for a person with dementia:

Sit down with them, smile, introduce yourself. Don't worry if the conversation doesn't come easily or you don't feel like you're achieving anything – you are achieving a connection with that person, which is more important than anything else right now.

Go to where the person is. Don't expect them to chase after your point or read your mind. Be polite. Respect them. Be aware of when you feel they may not have understood – they may be too embarrassed to ask you to explain or repeat yourself. If they want to tell you something, listen actively. If they want to ask questions, answer them. If they want to play a game, sing, hold your hand, walk, laugh or cry – let them. Share the experience with them. Bring all your humanness and enjoy their company as a fellow person.

If they spill something, don't tut – help them. If they become incontinent, don't look disgusted – help them. If they cry and scream and walk about all day looking for the cat that died years ago, be gentle and look for what they need from you.

When you don't know what to do, or what to give them, give them your compassion. Sit down with them, smile and tell them you're here to help them.

Jonathan Crane, mental health nursing student

CONCLUSION

People with dementia are among the most vulnerable members of society. At the same time, working as a mental health nurse with people with dementia and their families can be highly rewarding, as the contributions of nurses in a range of care settings can make a big difference. Dementia care is subject to many resource constraints as governments try to keep costs down, as the numbers of people with dementia rise, and, to some extent, shift the cost burden from the state to families. The need for skilled and empathic mental health nurses to specialise in dementia care has never been greater.

CHAPTER SUMMARY

This chapter has covered:

- The syndrome of dementia and conditions that lead to dementia
- Philosophies of care for people with dementia and their families
- The role of the mental health nurse in the assessment and diagnosis of dementia
- The role of the mental health nurse in supporting people with dementia and their families in community settings
- The role of the mental health nurse in supporting people with dementia and their families in residential care settings.

BUILD YOUR BIBLIOGRAPHY

Books

- Brooker, D. & Lillyman, S. (2013) *Dementia care* (Nursing and Health Survival Guides). Abingdon: Routledge. Ideal for quick reference, this pocket-sized guide puts all the crucial information on caring for patients with dementia at your fingertips.
- Downs, M. & Bowers, B. (eds) (2014) *Excellence in dementia care: Research into practice*, 2nd edition. Maidenhead: Open University Press. An up-to-date evidence-based textbook with an international perspective.
- Kitwood, T. (1997) *Dementia reconsidered: The person comes first*. Maidenhead: Open University Press. An overview of Kitwood's thinking about dementia care, published shortly before his death.

SAGE journal articles

FURTHER
READING:
JOURNAL
ARTICLES

Go to https://study.sagepub.com/essentialmentalhealth for further free online journal articles related to this chapter. If you are using the interactive ebook, simply click on the book icon in the margin to go straight to the resource.

- Manthorpe, J., Samsi, K. & Rapaport, J. (2014) Dementia nurses' experience of the Mental Capacity Act 2005: a follow-up study. *Dementia*, 13(1), 131–143. A qualitative study of CMHNs who specialise in dementia care to explore their understanding of the Mental Capacity Act and how it influences their clinical decision making.
- Oppikofer, S. & Geschwinder, H. (2014) Nursing interventions in cases of agitation and dementia. *Dementia*, 13(3), 306–317. A research study that examined the effectiveness of simple interventions carried out by nurses to reduce agitation in people with dementia in care homes.
- Quinn, C., Clare, L., McGuinness, T., et al. (2012) Negotiating the balance: the triadic relationship between spousal caregivers, people with dementia and Admiral Nurses. *Dementia*, 12(5), 588–605. An in-depth analysis of how individual Admiral Nurses worked with people with dementia and their family carers.

Weblinks

Go to https://study.sagepub.com/essentialmentalhealth for further weblinks related to this chapter. If you are using the interactive ebook, simply click on the book icon in the margin to go straight to the resource.

- Dementia UK: www.dementiauk.org – a charity that supports Admiral Nurses
- Royal College of Nursing dementia project: www.rcn.org.uk/workingwithus/corporate-relations/dementia-partnership-project – contains a range of information about ongoing work at the RCN on dementia care with supporting information plus lots of other useful resources.

FURTHER
READING:
WEBLINKS

ACE YOUR ASSESSMENT

Revise what you have learned by visiting https://study.sagepub.com/essentialmentalhealth. If you are using the interactive ebook, simply click on the tick icon to go straight to the resource.

- Test yourself with multiple-choice and short-answer questions and flashcards.

ONLINE
QUIZZES &
ACTIVITY
ANSWERS

REFERENCES

Abley, C., Manthorpe, J., Bond, J., et al. (2013) Patients' and carers' views on communication and information provision when undergoing assessments in memory services. *Journal of Health Services Research and Policy, 18*(3), 167–173.

Adams, T. (1996) Kitwood's approach to dementia and dementia care: a critical but appreciative review. *Journal of Advanced Nursing, 23*, 948–953.

Adams, T. (2010) The applicability of a recovery approach to nursing people with dementia. *International Journal of Nursing Studies, 47*, 626–634.

All-Party Parliamentary Group (APPG) on Dementia (2008) *Always a last resort: Inquiry into the prescription of antipsychotic drugs to people with dementia living in care homes.* London: TSO.

Alzheimer's Society (2007) *Home from home: A report highlighting opportunities for improving standards of dementia care in care homes.* London: Alzheimer's Society.

Alzheimer's Society (2013) *Building dementia-friendly communities: A priority for everyone.* London: Alzheimer's Society.

Alzheimer's Society (2014) *Dementia UK: Update.* London: Alzheimer's Society.

Banerjee, S., Willis, R., Matthews, D., et al. (2007) Improving the quality of care for mild to moderate dementia: an evaluation of the Croydon Memory Service model. *International Journal of Geriatric Psychiatry, 22*(8), 782–788.

Bowman, C. (2009) Nursing homes: quality reflects leadership. *British Medical Journal, 339*, 550.

Brooker, D. (2004) What is person-centred care in dementia? *Reviews in Clinical Gerontology, 13*, 215–222.

Clare, L., Markova, I., Roth, I., et al. (2011) Awareness in Alzheimer's disease and associated dementias: theoretical framework and clinical implications. *Aging and Mental Health, 15*(8), 936–944.

Corbett, A., Burns, A. & Ballard, C. (2014) Don't use antipsychotics routinely to treat agitation and aggression in people with dementia. *BMJ, 349*, g6420.

Corbett, A., Husebo, B., Malcangio, M., et al. (2012) Assessment and treatment of pain in people with dementia. *National Review of Neurology, 12*(8), 264–274.

Department of Health (2009) *Living well with dementia: A national dementia strategy.* London: DH.

Department of Health (2015) *Prime minister's challenge on dementia 2020.* London: DH.

Donaldson, C. (1997) The impact of the symptoms of dementia on caregivers. *British Journal of Psychiatry, 170*, 62–68.

Gavan, J. (2011) Exploring the usefulness of a recovery-based approach to dementia care nursing. *Contemporary Nurse, 39*(2), 140–146.

Hean, S., Nojeed, N. & Warr, J. (2011) Developing an integrated memory assessment and support service for people with dementia. *Journal of Psychiatric and Mental Health Nursing, 18*, 81–88.

Hughes, J., Hedley, K., Harris, D., et al. (2004) The practice and philosophy of palliative care in dementia. *Nursing & Residential Care, 6*(1), 27–30.

Hughes, S., O'Hara, P. & Higgins, R. (2013) Promoting positive practice in mental health liaison. *Journal of Dementia Care, 21*(5), 26–28.

Keady, J., Ashcroft-Simpson, S., Halligan, K., et al. (2007) Admiral nursing and the family care of a parent with dementia: using autobiographical narrative as grounding for negotiated clinical practice and decision-making. *Scandanavian Journal of Caring Science, 21*, 345–353.

Keady, J., Woods, B., Hahn, S., et al. (2004) Community mental health nursing and early intervention in dementia: developing practice through a single case history. *International Journal of Older People's Nursing, 13*(6b), 57–67.

Kitwood, T. (1997) *Dementia reconsidered: The person comes first*. Maidenhead: Open University Press.

Minski, L. (1972) *A practical handbook of psychiatry for students and nurses*. London: Heinemann.

Moniz-Cook, E., Elston, C., Gardiner, E., et al. (2008) Can training community mental health nurses to support family carers reduce behavioural problems in dementia? An exploratory pragmatic randomised controlled trial. *International Journal of Geriatric Psychiatry, 23*, 185–191.

National Institute for Health and Care Excellence (NICE) (2006) *Dementia: Supporting people with dementia and their carers in health and social care*. NICE guideline no. CG42. London: NICE.

Nolan, M., Davies, S., Brown, J., et al. (2004) Beyond person-centred care: a new vision for gerontological nursing. *Journal of Clinical Nursing, 13*(3a), 45–53.

Pulsford, D. & Thompson, R. (2012) *Dementia: Support for families and friends*. London: Jessica Kingsley.

Pulsford, D., Duxbury, J. & Carter, B. (2016) Personal qualities necessary to care for people with dementia. *Nursing Standard, 30*(37), 38–44.

Quinn, C., Clare, L., McGuinness, T., et al. (2012) Negotiating the balance: the triadic relationship between spousal caregivers, people with dementia and Admiral Nurses. *Dementia, 12*(5), 588–605.

Robb S. (1984) Behaviour in the environment of the elderly. In A. Yurick, B. Spier, S. Robb & N. Ebert (eds), *The Aged Person and the Nursing Process*. Norwalk: Appleton-Century-Crofts.

Samsi, K., Abley, C., Campbell, C., et al. (2014) Negotiating a labyrinth: experiences of assessment and diagnostic journey in cognitive impairment and dementia. *International Journal of Geriatric Psychiatry, 29*, 58–67.

Sheehan, B., Lall, R., Gage, H., et al. (2013) A 12-month follow-up study of people with dementia referred to general hospital liaison psychiatry services. *Age and Ageing, 42*(6), 786–790.

Spector, A., Thorgrimsen, L. Woods, B.O., et al. (2003) Efficacy of an evidence-based cognitive stimulation therapy programme for people with dementia: randomised controlled trial. *British Journal of Psychiatry, 183*, 248–254.

Stokes, G. (2000) *Challenging behaviour in dementia: A person-centred approach*. London: Speechmark.

Testad, I., Corbett, A., Aarsland, D., et al. (2014) The value of personalised psychosocial interventions to address behavioural and psychological symptoms in people with dementia living in care home settings: a systematic review. *International Psychogeriatrics, 26*, 1083–1098.

CHILD AND ADOLESCENT MENTAL HEALTH CARE

37

MADDIE BURTON, LAURA BAKER AND KAREN M. WRIGHT

THIS CHAPTER COVERS

- Child and adolescent mental health services (CAMHS)
- Typical child and adolescent mental health problems and disorders
- Typical interventions
- Connecting attachment theory, risk and resilience theories with mental health
- The transition to adult mental health services.

> " As a CAMHS nurse practitioner and previously a family nurse within Family Nurse Partnership the importance of thinking and working systemically cannot be underestimated. The child or young person must be thought of in relation to their family and the systems (school and other services) that they interact with. This way of working supports the family to enable change and underpins all approaches/interventions within Child and Adolescent Mental Health Services.
>
> **Denisse Levermore, CAMHS nurse** "

> " In my time coming in and out of both CAMHS and other healthcare services I have had different experiences. The better staff treat me with respect and do not judge or patronise me. They are understanding and empathic about my reasons for self-harming and treat me with kindness. At other times, I have had almost the opposite and staff have made me feel even worse that I already did to start with. This makes me want to avoid services if I can help it. I don't want to be treated as a 'problem' or a 'condition' – I just want to be treated as a person.
>
> **Abbie, patient** "

Visit **https://study.sagepub.com/essentialmentalhealth** to access a wealth of online resources for this chapter – watch out for the margin icons throughout the chapter. If you are using the interactive ebook, simply click on the margin icon to go straight to the resource.

INTRODUCTION

Contemporary times and policies have an unarguably detrimental effect on wellbeing so it would be unsurprising if this did not extend to children. This chapter presents a person-centred ethos towards supporting children experiencing mental distress and intervening *carefully* with them and their families. Policies and practitioners navigate a tricky balance between meeting needs and taking care not to over-extend the reach of psychiatry into people's lives. The chapter focuses on meeting needs. Critical commentators from within services caution us to also be aware that the socio-economic factors that undermine mental health are also entwined with the creeping medicalisation of distress, and we need to be vigilant not to overdo diagnosis and pharmacological responses to childhood distress (see Timimi, 2010).

CHILD AND ADOLESCENT MENTAL HEALTH SERVICES (CAMHS)

The *No Health without Mental Health* strategy (Department of Health, 2011b) cited that over half of lifetime mental health problems begin to emerge by age 14, and three-quarters by the mid-20s. Multi-disciplinary teams, focusing on these needs of young people, include psychologists, psychotherapists, social workers, play therapists, doctors, paediatricians and psychiatrists as well as nurses, make up CAMHS. Additionally, school nurses support children and young people with emotional and psychological difficulties (Bohenkamp et al., 2015; NHS Benchmarking Network, 2013), despite their lack of mental health training. This has been recognised by the Royal College of Nursing as an important issue and the College has asked for countrywide standardised mental health training (Brown, 2015).

Much of the policy, strategy and practice guidance referred to in this chapter is specific to England. Although the challenges are common across the UK, Wales, Northern Ireland and Scotland have devolved powers and they subsequently developed their mental health policy and practice with some distinct variations. For example, the Welsh Government has made it a requirement of local authorities to provide access to school-based counselling services for children and young people aged between 11 and 18 and for pupils in Year 6 of primary school. This followed a number of suicides of younger people in Bridgend, South Wales in 2007–2008 and was already a recommendation made by the Children's Commissioner for Wales in her earlier Clywch Inquiry Report (Welsh Government, 2011). The Children's Commissioner for England has recently made similar recommendations for England based, in part, on the responses and evaluation of provision in Wales (Ward, 2016). Young Minds has a useful overview of CAMHS policy and services in the UK (Young Minds, 2016a).

CAMHS was commissioned and established following the *Together we Stand* health advisory service report (Department of Health, 1995). CAMHS also encompasses care for children and young people with neurodevelopmental presentations such as attention deficit hyperactivity **disorder** (ADHD) and autistic spectrum conditions/disorders (ASC/D), many of whom will also experience comorbidities such as **anxiety** or **depression**. The CAMHS model is known as the Tiered model:

Tier 1: includes professionals working at the primary level of care, so, for example, the universal settings of health, education, social care and the criminal justice system.

Tier 2: includes professionals working in services related to those in Tier 1. These would include child psychologists, community mental health nurses and paediatricians.

Tier 3: includes more specialised services and professionals – for example, child and adolescent psychiatrists, psychologists, psychotherapists, family, speech and language, art, music and drama therapists and nurses.

Tier *3 and a half*: these tend to be home treatment/hospital at home teams for more severe presentations such as deliberate **self-harm** or eating disorders. [For a time, Laura (co-author and **service user**) was looked after by this sort of service, as you will hear about, where nurses visit daily.]

Tier 4: includes specialised inpatient units and outpatient teams including all of the above Tier 3 professionals cited.

The complexity of the Tiers model is criticised in the *Future in Mind* paper (Department of Health, 2015) and is, in part, being addressed through the Children and Young People Improving Access to Psychological Therapies (CYP IAPT) project which commenced in 2012. CYP IAPT is based on and followed the earlier IAPT for adults and older age model, but with a different agenda. CYP IAPT works with existing CAMHS to:

- improve access to CAMHS, and the partnership with children, young people, families, professionals and agencies
- build capability to deliver positive and measurable outcomes for children, young people and families
- increase the choice of evidence-based treatments available.

It is a rolling model with service transformation at the heart, with the voices of children and young people being instrumental in this process. There is an also an emphasis on improving the skills of professionals in the Tier 1 or universal settings workforce, to improve the mental health and wellbeing of children and young people. Key concerns are enhancement of the **therapeutic relationship** with children and families and a focus on collaborative practice. Already 'self-referral' – the ability of a parent or child to refer themselves into CAMHS without needing a professional referral to access the service – has started (CYP IAPT, 2012). This major service transformation is set to continue in line with *Future in Mind* (DH, 2015) and *The Five Year Forward View for Mental Health* (NHS England, 2016). However, it is not without problems, including a target of 60% coverage by 2015 in England, so transformation is patchy and, in a time of budget restraints and cuts to services, is being challenged. It is worth remembering that CAMHS has an allocation of only 6% of the total mental health budget (House of Commons Health Committee, 2014, points 80 and 86).

CRITICAL THINKING STOP POINT 37.1

- CAMHS are divided into Tiers 1-4. Who benefits from this most? Services? Young people and their families?
- There is now a focus to improve the skills of workers in universal settings (Tier 1), in terms of early recognition, help and support. What skills should be prioritised, in your opinion?

CHILD AND ADOLESCENT MENTAL HEALTH

Prevalence

The National Service Framework for Children, Young People and Maternity Services (2004) identified that 10% of 5–15-year-olds had a diagnosable mental health disorder. That is equivalent to three children in every classroom in every school in Britain. A further 15% have less severe problems and remain at an increased risk of future mental health problems (Department for Education, 2015: 34). *Future in Mind* (DH, 2015) acknowledged that one in 10 children needs support for mental health problems. These figures are based on the B-CAMHS survey last commissioned and published over 12 years ago, in 2004. There has been no full-scale study since then. This has been criticised as now being long overdue by the Royal College of Paediatrics and Child Health (2014).

ORIGINS, FORMULATION AND INTERPRETATIONS

As mentioned, over half of lifetime mental health problems (excluding **dementia**) begin to emerge by age 14, and three-quarters by the mid-20s. Up to 80% of adults with depression and anxiety disorders first experience them before the age of 18 (DH, 2011a, 2015). Many mental health problems have origins in childhood (Dogra et al., 2009). An accepted view is that mental health and ill health arise from a context of variables including biological factors such as genetics and brain development, which will include early childhood experiences, psychological variables that include **coping mechanisms** and how these then interact in relation to either adverse or positive environmental circumstances or experiences. It is important to consider and be mindful of the different view between traditional adult mental health and children's mental health in that most presenting mental health conditions are medicalised in adult services. But in CAMHS, in addition, they are about an interpretation of behaviours considered to be beyond accepted normal behaviour. So these are always thought of from a psychological perspective. It therefore makes sense to consider a biomedical and psychosocial approach in both understanding mental health and the treatment of mental health problems over the life span.

Children and young people can experience the same mental health problems as adults. The difference, which is important to understand, is the requirement to think about these presentations within the context of the developmental phase.

PROBLEMS AND CONDITIONS

The most common mental health problems for children and young people are conduct disorders, ADHD, anxiety, depression and autistic spectrum conditions (Murphy & Fonagy, 2012). Other significant mental health disorders include: eating disorders, such as **anorexia nervosa**, attachment disorder, post-traumatic stress disorder, self-harm, suicidal behaviours, **mood** changes, behaviour changes, relationship and attachment difficulties, substance misuse, changed eating patterns, isolation and social withdrawal and somatic disorders. Somatising features (physical symptoms with psychological origins) include, for example, headaches, enuresis and encopresis (faecal soiling), tummy aches and sleep disturbances, often present in in younger children.

SEE ALSO
CHAPTER 38

Anorexia nervosa, self-harm and suicidal behaviour in children and young people are also common presentations to CAMHS and some of the most concerning. Many young people will experience more than one of these, as comorbidities are commonplace (see also Chapter 38).

Depression

CASE STUDY:
'LISA'
REFERRED TO
CAMHS

Depression is now recognised as a major public health problem in the UK and worldwide. It accounts for 15% of all disability in high-income countries. In England, one in six adults and one in 20 children and young people at any one time are affected by depression and related conditions, such as anxiety. According to the International **Classification** of Diseases (ICD 10) (WHO, 2010) and the Diagnostic Statistical Manual (DSM-5) (APA, 2013), depression is characterised by an episodic disorder of varying degrees of severity characterised by depressed mood and loss of enjoyment, persisting for several weeks. There must also be a presence of other symptoms, including: depressive thinking, pessimism about the future, suicidal ideas and biological symptoms such as early waking, weight loss and reduced appetite (Harrington, 2003; NICE, 2013).

The criteria is similar for children and adults but with important differences (Keenan & Evans, 2009). With children and young people, developmental perspectives and context are highly relevant, as already discussed. For example, eating and sleeping disturbances often present as potential symptoms, but these would be common in childhood anyway. Tearfulness and crying have a very different meaning and incidence in childhood compared with adulthood. It is not uncommon to feel depressed at times. It is also important to 'normalise' sadness as a passing human condition. If sadness becomes persistent over time, this would be different and a cause for concern (Burton et al., 2014).

Anxiety

Anxiety, it must be remembered, is normal. Anxiety becomes pathological when the fear is out of proportion to the context of the life situation, and in childhood when it is out of keeping with the expected behaviour for the developmental stage of the child (Lask, 2003). It is also one of the most common mental health problems, with an estimate that 300,000 young people in Britain have an anxiety disorder (Royal College of Psychiatrists, 2014). For example, separation anxiety would be considered normal for infants (leaving a primary **carer**) but less so for a teenager. In a relatively short time span, in comparison to the full length of human life, children move from a state of limited emotional understanding to becoming complex individuals. The number and complexity of emotional experiences, together with the modulation of human expression, increase with age. It is therefore not surprising that some children and young people are easily overwhelmed and experience emotional disorders, which, if they persist, are debilitating and require intervention.

There are many variations of anxiety and children can experience anxiety in some of the following ways: worries, **phobias**, separation anxiety, panic disorder, post-traumatic stress disorder and obsessive compulsive disorder. Thinking about the above variations in how anxiety is expressed, it is useful to consider a developmental perspective, as there are different fears for different years. In infancy, if secure attachment is accomplished, fear of separation from the caregiver diminishes. Separation anxiety usually begins in the pre-school years any time after the attachment period but typically in late childhood/early adolescence. Performance anxiety can emerge in late childhood and social anxiety in adolescence. During adolescence, autonomy and independence are major developmental challenges, endeavouring to balance a compliance with rules with expressing independent autonomy. It is normal to experience conflict to some level, but the challenge posed by emerging autonomy can trigger or exacerbate interpersonal problems that require negotiation with the accompanying anxiety (Royal College of Psychiatrists, 2014; Young Minds, 2016b).

TYPICAL INTERVENTIONS

Child and adolescent mental health sits within a medical and psychological diagnostic model. Children and young people, as already identified, tend to receive a diagnosis if an assessment reveals this to be appropriate. This will be a primarily medical interpretation but the approach both to interpretation and treatment is one which considers all factors, including psychological and sociological. Proposed interventions need to be both biopsychosocial and person centred. The humanistic, person-centred approach developed by Carl Rogers (1957), and further developed by Prever (2010), details working with children and young people. It is very important to remain 'child focused' and to be in a position that maintains and supports the child or young person from an appropriately developmental position.

Age-appropriate approaches require the avoidance of 'adult' terminology, including the replacement of terms such as 'client' or 'service user' with 'child and young person'. In CAMHS, as discussed previously, a person-centred approach considers the child and young person in relation to their context of family. Whilst the family can be seen as part of the problem, it is important to avoid a blaming stance and to also see the family as a resource for change.

Interventions and therapeutic approaches in Tiers 2–4 usually include: play therapy, art therapy, parent–infant psychotherapy, under-5s work, **cognitive behaviour therapy**, individual work, family work, parenting work and **family therapy**. There will often be a combination model of a psychological and pharmacological intervention and approaches. Laura's interventions, as part of her treatment, also included her family, as above, and are discussed next.

Integrating psychological care in Tier 1 universal settings such as Children's Centres offers timely and supportive community-based interventions which can work as a preventative and protective strategy. School-based counselling is an available and accessible form of psychological therapy for young people in the UK, with approximately 70,000–90,000 young people accessing services per year (British Association for Counselling and Psychotherapy, 2013). *Future in Mind* (DH, 2015) suggests a whole-child and family approach, with a move away from thinking purely clinically about child mental health and an emphasis on prevention, early intervention and **recovery**. Other whole-school approaches include 'circle time' for younger children. In addition, nurture groups, peer mentoring and buddy systems offer important opportunities to build on children and young people's resilience factors, and therefore mitigate risk factors.

Counselling and psychotherapy for children and young people are very different from the traditional adult approaches and need to be developmentally appropriate, individualised, flexible and creative. The young person's context or system also requires attention as they are interrelated, and one cannot function in isolation of the other. Children and young people are usually one part of a wider family and are often relatively powerless to change their situation unless their family is supportive of the changes. Typically, a young person may be receiving age-appropriate support individually but ideally and, if possible, this would also be alongside parent and family work (Burton et al., 2014).

CRITICAL THINKING STOP POINT 37.2

- Finding the appropriate model of treatment from a 'tool kit' of resources and interventions is paramount, and not the other way round of fitting the person to a model.
- Approaches have person-centred care at the heart which also considers the young person and family context with varied treatment approaches.
- Supportive interventions in universal settings (Tier 1) can act as a protective factor and improve resilience to mental ill health.

ATTACHMENT THEORY, RISK AND RESILIENCE THEORIES AND LINKS TO MENTAL HEALTH

Attachment theory

You are introduced to attachment theory within the context of this chapter as attachment is crucial to understanding relationships that begin before birth and extend throughout the life span. Emotional and mental health problems and disorders originate within a context of relationships and inherited characteristics, together with the role that risk and resilience factors articulate with these. Those who have experienced significant maltreatment exhibit clinical symptoms of post-traumatic stress disorder (PTSD) (National Scientific Council on the Developing Child, 2004: 3). Early environmental experiences are critical to the maturation of the brain. Nature's potential can only be realised if it is facilitated by nurture (Schore, 2005: 205).

All of us are born into a context of relationships and what is going on within that context at the time, and babies' brains develop with another important person in their life. Becoming a *person* involves a large investment by others early in life and an emerging sense of self as reflected back to us through the eyes and minds of others. As Music (2011: 7, 24) described:

> a person's sense of self arises from being in the minds of others, without which it simply does not develop ... and that one's sense of self is socially and co-constructed ... human life develops from the delicate interplay of nature and nurture, the meeting of a bundle of inherited potentials and the cultural, social and personal influences of the adults in an infant's life.

Donald Winnicott focused on emotional life and the meaning and formative effects of early relationships, stressing the primary significance of the nature and quality of the relationship between the self and another. Winnicott (1956) termed the phrase 'good enough mothering', meaning if parenting is just that, an optimal developmental outcome could be realised. Winnicott still has resonance and meaning today.

Attachment is a biologically driven behaviour as important as food and nutrition and essential for survival. John Bowlby's post-Second World War studies of 'maternal deprivation' led to his attachment theory, which concluded that children use adults as a safe haven and secure base from which the world can be explored (Bowlby, 2008/1988). *Attachment quality* is an important aspect of development and is a predictor of all lifetime relationships. Emotional care is equal to physical care (Goldberg et al., 2000). An infant's principal caregiver will become the attachment figure. The attachment system becomes activated when under distress or threat which in turn initiates attachment behaviours. The attachment figures' response to the infant is crucial and thus how the infant is helped or not helped to feel safe. If attachment behaviours, such as crying, do not achieve a response, the attachment system remains activated as a survival mechanism and so there is less time for other developmental opportunities such as play and social interaction. So, for children exposed to ongoing neglect, abuse and rejection, there is less time for play and developing relationships. If the parent's caregiving system can be activated by the child, then the child's attachment system can be de-activated. The long-term effects of neglect, abandonment and prolonged separation should not be underestimated (Howe, 2011).

WHAT'S THE EVIDENCE? 37.1

Working with and supporting children, young people and their families in varied ways have at their heart the humanistic 'person-centred' approach. Have a look at the following articles which demonstrate some of the therapeutic approaches and ways of working in CAMHS:

Jack, A., Lanskey, C. & Harvey, J. (2015)
Roberts-Collins, C. (2016)
Southwell, J. (2016)

WHAT'S THE
EVIDENCE? 37.1
ARTICLES

(Continued)

How do you feel these varied approaches maintain at their heart 'person-centred' work with children and young people?

The role of 'risk and resilience'

The nature and process of risk and resilience are an important consideration. The risk and resilience model in terms of the likelihood of developing a mental health problem was explained by Pearce (1993) in *Together we Stand* (DH, 1995: 23). The three areas of risk he identified were:

(i) environmental/contextual
(ii) the family
(iii) the young person/child themselves.

Examples of risk include negative experiences in the **environment** such as poverty, disaster, violence or being a refugee or asylum seeker. Precipitating factors in the family include early attachment difficulties, domestic abuse, parental conflict and parental mental **illness**. When working with adults in mental health services, be mindful of what needs their children may have. This may include collaborative working with CAMHS. For the young person, areas of risk include neurodevelopmental difficulties and conditions, physical illness and genetic influences. The flip side is the consideration of resilience factors which mitigate risk. Having and acquiring resilience can shield against stress and adverse life events. Relevant factors include: secure attachments, self-esteem, familial compassion and warmth and family stability, having a skill or a talent. Despite major adversity and overwhelming odds, many young people cope well. The key is *resilience* which acts as a protective factor. Rutter (1985, 2006) described this as a dynamic evolving process. Positive experiences that improve resilience can mitigate or offset genetic factors and poor early experiences. Many young people can survive adverse childhoods through personal strength which can be further strengthened through experiencing difficulties (Joslyn, 2016). Studies have led theorists to suggest that each child inherits characteristics which make them both vulnerable (risk factors) and resilient (protective factors).

TRANSITION FROM CAMHS TO ADULT SERVICES

CASE STUDY 37.1

The transition from CAMHS to adult mental health services can feel like a metaphorical void that you fall into. I went from seeing a consultant once a week and a community psychiatric nurse (CPN) every day when I was 17 to being offered an appointment with a consultant once every three months after my 18th birthday. This undoubtedly led to a regression in my stage of recovery. There was no handover to adult services and no information given to myself or my family about the new service, so we were effectively 'starting from scratch', though in a service with an entirely different model of working which had no continuity from my previous years of treatment. Poor communication between services and different styles of service impede the ability to provide cohesive services. It seems to be a postcode lottery in the way transition is managed and at what age it takes place. The transition period can lead to gaps in care with young people being placed on waiting lists or failing to meet the severity thresholds for adult services. These problems with transition can often lead to young people completely falling off the radar of services.

Laura's experience demonstrates the difference in service provision between CAMHS and adult mental health services (AMHS). In addition, there are variables that impact the transition from CAMHS to AMHS, including the postcode lottery and particular conditions. For example, the Early Intervention in **Psychosis** Service has a typical age range of 14–35 and therefore provides a relatively smooth transition. Conversely, with young people who have an autistic spectrum condition (ASC), one service stops at 18 and another starts at 18 with no overlap to manage the transition process. Problems encountered for a young person moving to an entirely different model of care at an **acute** and critical time are clearly illustrated (RCN, 2013). There are parallels with the social care sector where, upon reaching 18, young people in care move out of the care system. In both cases, these are highly vulnerable individuals who need a safety net and model of joined-up working to protect them. Using the age of 18 as a cut-off point for receiving appropriate support is a fairly clumsy system. Ideally, cases should be decided on an individual basis, with consideration given to what is the best service for that individual at that point in time.

The importance of being able to access flexible, needs-based care, having a designated lead professional to ensure a smooth transition between services, and advance planning for transition was highlighted in the National CAMHS Review (DH, 2008). NHS Choices (2016) has useful guidance for CAMHS provision and age limits. Some services, but again this is patchy, are moving to an upper age limit of 25. Forward Thinking Birmingham (2016) is an example of such a service change.

REFLECTION POINT 37.1

- How does Laura's case demonstrate the biomedical and psychosocial approach in both the interpretation of her symptoms and treatment interventions during her care in CAMHS?
- How did Laura's treatment and approach in understanding her condition differ between CAMHS and AMHS? Transition from CAMHS to AMHS is a critical point. Do you have any ideas about how this process could be improved?

CRITICAL DEBATE 37.1

Now that you have read the chapter, consider the following points:

Children and young people who have a parent with mental illness are at a much higher risk of developing a mental health problem themselves. Children and young people often become 'invisible' in families where adults are receiving attention from other professionals. As a mental health nurse, most of you will be working with and supporting adults:

WHAT'S THE EVIDENCE?
37.1 ARTICLES

(Continued)

- How will you ensure the children and young people associated with these adults remain visible?
- What steps will you take to make sure this happens?
- Why is this important?

What other agencies could you be working collaboratively with as best practice to meet this need?

CHAPTER SUMMARY

This chapter has covered:

- The significance of childhood experiences leading to greater understanding of the people you are working with and helping
- Consideration of children and young people as the other vulnerable family members if you are working with the adults in a family
- Working in CAMHS from a biomedical and psychosocial perspective with children, young people and families being a 'window of opportunity' for getting appropriate diagnosis and treatment, so that conditions can be treated and resolved without persisting into adulthood where often successful treatment and recovery become prolonged; it also demonstrates a holistic model for all mental health practice across the life span.

BUILD YOUR BIBLIOGRAPHY

Books

- Burton, M., Pavord, E.& Williams, B. (2014) *An introduction to child and adolescent mental health*. London: SAGE.
- Campbell, S., Morley, D. & Catchpole, R. (2016) *Critical issues in child and adolescent mental health*. London: Palgrave.
- Claveirole, A. & Gaughan, M. (eds) (2011) *Understanding children and young people's mental health*. Chichester: Wiley-Blackwell.
- Dogra, N. & Leighton, S. (eds) (2009) *Nursing in child and adolescent mental health*. Maidenhead: Open University Press.

SAGE journal articles

FURTHER READING: JOURNAL ARTICLES

Go to https://study.sagepub.com/essentialmentalhealth for further free online journal articles related to this chapter. If you are using the interactive ebook, simply click on the book icon in the margin to go straight to the resource.

- Gale, F. & Vostanis, P. (2003) The primary mental health worker within child and adolescent mental health services. *Clinical Child Psychology and Psychiatry*, 8(2), 227-240.
- Ronzoni, P. & Dogra, N. (2012) Children, adolescents and their carers' expectations of child and adolescent mental health services (CAMHS). *International Journal of Social Psychiatry*, 58(3), 328-336.
- Timimi, S. (2010) The McDonaldization of childhood: children's mental health in neo-liberal market cultures. *Transcultural Psychiatry*, 47(5), 686-706.

Weblinks

Go to https://study.sagepub.com/essentialmentalhealth for further weblinks related to this chapter. If you are using the interactive ebook, simply click on the book icon in the margin to go straight to the resource.

FURTHER
READING:
WEBLINKS

- Association for Child & Adolescent Mental Health: www.acamh.org.uk – a multi-disciplinary membership association and valuable resource for those engaged in child and adolescent mental health and its associated specialities
- Mental Health Foundation's Fundamental Facts about Mental Health (2015) www.mentalhealth.org.uk/sites/default/files/fundamental-facts-15.pdf – has interesting statistics for the whole of the UK
- MindEd: www.minded.org.uk – a free educational resource on children and young people's mental health for all adults
- Young Minds: www.youngminds.org.uk – the voice for young people's mental health and well-being.

GREAT FOR
REVISION

——— ACE YOUR ASSESSMENT ———

Revise what you have learned by visiting https://study.sagepub.com/essentialmentalhealth. If you are using the interactive ebook, simply click on the tick icon to go straight to the resource.

ONLINE
QUIZZES &
ACTIVITY
ANSWERS

- Test yourself with multiple-choice and short-answer questions and flashcards.

REFERENCES

American Psychiatric Association (APA) (2013) *Diagnostic statistical manual* 5th *edition* (DSM-5). Available at: http://psychiatry.org/psychiatrists/practice/dsm (accessed August 2015).

Bohenkamp, J.H., Stephan, S.H. & Bobo, N. (2015) Supporting student mental health: the role of the school nurse in co-ordinated school mental health care. *Psychology in the Schools*, *52*(7), 714–727. Available at: http://onlinelibrary.wiley.com/doi/10.1002/pits.21851/pdf (accessed 08.16).

Bowlby, J. (2008/1988) *A secure base*. London: Routledge.

British Association for Counselling and Psychotherapy (BACP) (2013) *School-based counselling: what it is and why we need it*. Available at: www.bacp.co.uk/admin/structure/files/pdf/11791_sbc_may2013.pdf (accessed 08.15).

Brown, J. (2015) School nurses need better mental health training. *Children and Young People Now*. Available at: www.cypnow.co.uk/cyp/news/1153192/school-nurses-%E2%80%98need-better-mental-health-training%E2%80%99 (accessed 11.16).

Burton, M., Pavord, E. & Williams, B. (2014) *An introduction to child and adolescent mental health*. London: Sage.

Children and Young People's (CYP) Improving Access to Psychological Therapies (IAPT) (2012) Newsletter, December. Available at: www.iapt.nhs.uk/silo/files/cyp-iapt-newsletter-3-december-2012.pdf (accessed 08.15).

Department for Education (2015) *Mental health and behaviour in schools*. Available at: www.gov.uk/government/uploads/system/uploads/attachment_data/file/416786/Mental_Health_and_Behaviour_-_Information_and_Tools_for_Schools_240515.pdf (accessed 08.15).

Department of Health (1995) *Together we stand: Commissioning, role and management of CAMHS*. Health advisory service report. London: HMSO.

Department of Health (2008) *Children and young people in mind: the final report of the national CAMHS review*. Available at: http://webarchive.nationalarchives.gov.uk/20081230004520/publications.dcsf.gov.uk/eorderingdownload/camhs-review.pdf (accessed 08.15).

Department of Health (2011a) *Talking therapies: a four-year plan of action*. A supporting document to 'No health without mental health': a cross-government mental health outcomes strategy for people of all ages. Available at: www.gov.uk/government/uploads/system/uploads/attachment_data/file/213765/dh_123985.pdf (accessed 08.16).

Department of Health (2011b) *No health without mental health: A cross-government mental health outcomes strategy for people of all ages*. Available at: www.dh.gov.uk/en/Publicationsandstatistics/Publications/PublicationsPolicyAndGuidance/DH_123766 (accessed 08.15).

Department of Health (2015) *Future in mind: Promoting, protecting and improving our children and young people's mental health and wellbeing*. Available at: www.gov.uk/government/uploads/system/uploads/attachment_data/file/414024/Childrens_Mental_Health.pdf (accessed 08.15).

Dogra, N., Parkin, A., Gale, F., et al. (2009) *A multidisciplinary handbook of child and adolescent mental health for front-line professionals*, 2nd edition. London: Jessica Kingsley.

Forward Thinking Birmingham (2016) *What is Forward Thinking Birmingham?* Available at: https://forwardthinkingbirmingham.org.uk/Teens (accessed 11.16).

Goldberg, S., Muir, R. & Kerr, J. (2000) *Attachment theory: Social, developmental, and clinical perspectives*. London: Routledge.

Harrington, R. (2003) Depression and suicidal behaviour. In *Child psychology and psychiatry: An introduction*. Oxford: The Medicine Publishing Co.

House of Commons Health Committee (2014) *Children's and adolescents' mental health and CAMHS: Third report of session 2014–15*. Available at: www.publications.parliament.uk/pa/cm201415/cmselect/cmhealth/342/342.pdf (accessed 11.16).

Howe, D. (2011) *Attachment across the lifecourse: A brief introduction*. Basingstoke: Palgrave Macmillan.

Jack, A., Lanskey, C. & Harvey, J. (2015) Young offenders' and their families' experiences of mental health interventions. Journal of Children's Services, 10(4), 353–364.

Joslyn, E. (2016) *Resilience in childhood: Perspectives, promise and practice*. London: Palgrave Macmillan.

Keenan, T. & Evans, S. (2009) *An introduction to child development*. London: Sage.

Lask, B. (2003) *Practical child psychiatry: The clinician's guide*. London: BMJ Publishing Group.

Murphy, M. & Fonagy, P. (2012) Mental health problems in children and young people. Ch. 10 in *Annual report of the chief medical officer 2012: Our children deserve better – prevention pays*. Available at: www.gov.uk/government/uploads/system/uploads/attachment_data/file/252660/33571_2901304_CMO_Chapter_10.pdf (accessed 11.16).

Music, G. (2011) *Nurturing nature's attachment and children's sociocultural and brain development*. Hove: Psychology Press.

National Institute for Health and Care Excellence (2013) *Depression in children and young people*. Quality standard QS48. Available at: www.nice.org.uk/guidance/qs48 (accessed 11.16).

National Scientific Council on the Developing Child (2004) *Children's emotional development is built into the architecture of their brains*. Working Paper No. 2, Center on the Developing Child, Harvard University, USA. Available at: www.developingchild.net (accessed 08.15).

National Service Framework for Children, Young People and Maternity Services (2004) *The mental health and psychological wellbeing of children and young people*. Standard 9. Available at: www.gov.uk/government/uploads/system/uploads/attachment_data/file/199959/National_Service_Framework_for_Children_Young_People_and_Maternity_Services_-_The_Mental_Health__and_Psychological_Well-being_of_Children_and_Young_People.pdf (accessed 08.15).

NHS Benchmarking Network (2013) *CAMHS benchmarking report*. Available at: www.rcpsych.ac.uk/pdf/CAMHS%20Report%20Dec%202013%20v1(1).pdf (accessed 11.16).

NHS Choices (2016) *Child and adolescent mental health services* (CAMHS). Available at: www.nhs.uk/NHSEngland/AboutNHSservices/mental-health-services-explained/Pages/about-childrens-mental-health-services.aspx (accessed 11.16).

NHS England (2016) *Health and high quality care for all, now and for future generations: Children and young people*. Available at: www.england.nhs.uk/mentalhealth/cyp (accessed 10.16).

Prever, M. (2010) *Counselling and Supporting Children and Young People: A Person-centred Approach*. London: Sage.

Roberts-Collins, C. (2016) A case study of an adolescent with health anxiety and OCD, treated using CBT: single-case experimental design. Journal of Child and Adolescent Psychiatric Nursing, 29(2), 95–104.

Rogers, C. (1957) The necessary and sufficient conditions for therapeutic change. *Journal of Consulting Psychology, 21*, 95–103.

Royal College of Nursing (RCN) (2013) *Lost in transition: Moving young people between child and adult health services*. Available at: https://www2.rcn.org.uk/__data/assets/pdf_file/0010/157879/003227_WEB.pdf (accessed 11.16).

Royal College of Paediatrics and Child Health (2014) *Making the UK's child health outcomes comparable to the best in the world: A vision for 2015*. Available at: www.rcpch.ac.uk/system/files/protected/news/RCPCH%20Child%20Health%20Manifesto%20WEB.pdf (accessed 11.16).

Royal College of Psychiatrists (2014) *Worries and anxieties: Helping children to cope – information for parents, carers and anyone who works with young people*. Mental health and growing up factsheet. Available at: www.rcpsych.ac.uk/healthadvice/parentsandyouthinfo/parentscarers/worriesandanxieties.aspx (accessed 11.16).

Rutter, M. (1985) Resilience in the face of adversity: protective factors and resistance to psychiatric disorders. *British Journal of Psychiatry, 147*, 589–611.

Rutter, M. (2006) Implications of resilience concepts for scientific understanding. *Annals of the New York Academy of Science, 1094*, 1–12.

Schore, A. (2005) Back to basics: attachment, affect regulation and the developing right brain – linking development neuroscience to pediatrics. *Pediatrics in Review, 26*(6), 204–217.

Southwell, J. (2016) Using 'expressive therapies' to treat developmental trauma and attachment problems in preschool-aged children. Children Australia, 41(2), 114–125.

Timimi, S. (2010) The McDonaldization of childhood: children's mental health in neo-liberal market cultures. *Transcultural Psychiatry, 47*(5), 686–706.

Ward, H. (2016) *Put counsellors in all schools, says children's commissioner*. TES. Available at: www.tes.com/news/school-news/breaking-news/put-counsellors-all-schools-says-childrens-commissioner (accessed 08.16).

Welsh Government (2011) *Evaluation of the Welsh school-based counselling strategy: Final report*. Available at: www.ncl.ac.uk/cflat/news/documents/wagesfinalreport.pdf (accessed 08.16).

Winnicott, D.W. (1956) Primary maternal preoccupation. In *Through paediatrics to psychoanalysis*. London: Hogarth Press and The Institute of Psychoanalysis. pp. 300–305.

World Health Organization (2010) *International classification of diseases* (ICD-10). Geneva: WHO. Available at: www.who.int/classifications/icd/en (accessed 08.15).

Young Minds (2016a) *CAMHS policy in the UK*. Available at: www.youngminds.org.uk/training_services/policy/camhs_in_the_uk (accessed 11.16).

Young Minds (2016b) *About anxiety*. Available at: www.youngminds.org.uk/for_parents/worried_about_your_child/anxiety/dealing_anxiety (accessed 11.16).

CARE OF PEOPLE WITH EATING DISORDERS

KAREN M. WRIGHT, MADDIE BURTON AND LAURA BAKER

THIS CHAPTER COVERS

- Eating disorders: what they are and who suffers
- What we can learn from the experience of service users and practitioners
- Caring for people with eating disorders in CAMHS and adult services and the transition between the two
- Understanding the Maudsley Method to help young people and their families
- The challenges for nurses
- The *reluctant service user*
- What helps and what hinders.

> **"** When you do see somebody recovering, it is so immensely rewarding, because you know that it's such a mammoth task and this work is so emotionally draining. It feels like you can't do anything right sometimes, so, if I could give one piece of advice to nurses new to this work, I would say 'persevere'. It's those glimmers of hope that keep me going. If I gave up every time they gave up, we wouldn't get anywhere! But sometimes it's hard to convince them that we are not fighting *them*, we are fighting *their illness*, that's the hardest part.
>
> **Lorna, SEDU ward manager** **"**

> **"** Young people with eating disorders I have worked with over the past 20 years have often said to me: 'you don't understand what this feels like'. Now that I have a fair bit of knowledge and experience in the field I can confidently tell them, 'you're absolutely right'.
>
> Although eating disorders are typically complex, often dangerous and at times very misunderstood, I can safely say that I do not grow tired of meeting teenagers and families affected by this type of illness and I do my best to listen and help.
>
> I hold in mind that an eating disorder can be overcome, recovery is possible and treatment and facilities are improving all the time.
>
> **Dan, ward manager, CAMHS Tier 4 Eating Disorders Unit** **"**

Visit **https://study.sagepub.com/essentialmentalhealth** to access a wealth of online resources for this chapter – watch out for the margin icons throughout the chapter. If you are using the interactive ebook, simply click on the margin icon to go straight to the resource.

> I was diagnosed with anorexia nervosa at age 12. My problems began around the time of transition to secondary school, a significant life event. I also experienced parental illness, a family history of anorexia and I also had selective mutism and a neurodevelopmental condition, which was undiagnosed at the time and so was untreated. I started to drastically reduce my dietary intake and my Body Mass Index (BMI) dropped to a dangerously low level. My mother took me to the GP and I was immediately admitted straight into Tier 4 specialist inpatient services, as my condition was life threatening. I spent 6 months in Tier 4 receiving different interventions including physical stabilisation and re-feeding. Psychological interventions included group therapy, holistic therapy and psychotherapy. I was discharged to Tier 3 community CAMHS and received weekly cognitive behavioural therapy and family work, however after nine months my condition had deteriorated significantly and again needed inpatient services. There were no beds available immediately and by the time one became available I was in multi organ failure. I then spent almost three years in hospital and underwent many interventions including art therapy, CBT, family therapy and speech and language therapy. It was during this stay that I was diagnosed with autism. I was discharged to a Tier 3.5 service where I received hospital at home care up until my 18th birthday when services came to an end and I was transitioned to adult services.

Laura Baker, service user

This chapter is shaped by the experiences of four people: Laura (a **service user** in **recovery** and co-author), Rachelle (who was a service user in a specialist eating **disorder** unit [SEDU] at the time of writing), Lorna (an adult SEDU ward manager) and Dan (a CAMHS Tier 4 Eating Disorders Unit manager). We attempt to combine experience with theory and practice to provide you with an insight into how to care authentically and in an evidence-based way. We focus on care across the life span, so look at both young people and adults.

EATING DISORDERS

Eating disorders are thought to **affect** over 725,000 people in the UK. **Anorexia nervosa**, which the chapter mainly focuses on, has the highest mortality rate of any psychiatric condition (BEAT, 2015; Treasure & Alexander, 2013). The teenage years are the most common age of onset (BEAT, 2015), with seven girls in every thousand affected by an eating disorder (RCP, 2013). Figures for bulimia are 1% although bulimia is rare under 12 with an average onset of 15–18 years compared to 15 years for anorexia. With approximately 0.3%–0.5% of the population up to 18 developing anorexia nervosa, it is nevertheless a relatively rare condition. Gender ratio is female–male 4:1 for under 12 years and 9:1 for the age range 13–18 years (Cullen, 2011: 153).

The most recent statistics demonstrate that 20% of anorexia nervosa sufferers die prematurely, 46% fully recover, 33% improve and 20% remain chronically ill. Similar research into bulimia suggests that 45% make a full recovery, 27% improve considerably and 23% suffer chronically (BEAT, 2015).

Anorexia comprises a complex set of experiences that are best made sense of from a multi-factorial perspective that does not favour any single causative mechanism. It is generally considered that eating disorders, as with other psychological disorders and mental **illnesses**, arise from a combination of biological/medical, psychological and social or environmental factors, as discussed above. It is the articulation and interrelation of these overlapping theories, together with various risk and resilience factors, as a combination, which lead to an understanding and interpretation of the causes of eating disorders; it is not about a single application of a model (Burton, 2014).

CRITICAL THINKING STOP POINT 38.1

Laura had an undiagnosed neurodevelopmental condition which existed prior to developing anorexia. Consider this in relation to risk/resilience and also the impact this may have on presentation and treatment.

Individuals suffering with eating disorders are not exempt from other mental health problems and it is common to observe co-occurrence with **depression**, **personality** disorder, obsessive compulsive behaviours and suicidality (Strober, 2010). Furthermore, physical problems such as osteoporosis, cardiovascular and gastrointestinal abnormalities are also common, particularly in adults who have struggled with anorexia from adolescence to adulthood (Fairburn & Harrison, 2003).

Laura's experience bears this out:

I have suffered a great deal of physical complications from anorexia since my illness began as a child, including gastroparesis, irregular menstruation, cardiovascular problems and multi-organ failure as well as anxiety and depression in fluctuating degrees of severity. This highlights the complexity of eating disorders and the many comorbid conditions and complications that can occur alongside and/or as a result of a severe eating disorder.

It takes a skilled workforce to address the multifaceted nature of these service users' needs, develop empathic approaches and establish positive **therapeutic relationships** (Strober, 2010). The gravity of concern about the vulnerability and fragile nature of those with eating disorders is largely underpinned by an **acute** awareness of the many physical complications involved and the elevated morbidity that exists, particularly with anorexia nervosa (Arcelus et al., 2011).

CRITICAL THINKING STOP POINT 38.2

Given the complexity of the needs of the person with anorexia (physical and psychological), does basic mental health nurse education really prepare a nurse to work in SEDUs/Tier 4 CAMH EDUs? Think about the needs of the nurse working in this service and what skills they need. List them. Are these covered in your curriculum? If not, how can you learn the required skills? What/who can inform you?

REFLECTION POINT 38.1

It is common practice nowadays in CAMHS eating disorder inpatient settings to have a mixed staff team of mental health nurses and children's nurses. This helps address the multi-faceted problems of the service user group and enables a richer skill and knowledge mix in the multi-disciplinary team, so that it is best equipped to meet the needs of this population.

Who suffers?

Anorexia has always been considered a predominantly female disorder, borne out by the statistics, nevertheless boys and young men do develop anorexia which practitioners also need to be mindful of. Recent research suggests a strong genetic link and predisposition and demonstrates that anorexia nervosa is not a lifestyle choice but rather an inherent gene which is most probably present and becomes vulnerable when exposed to other factors (Lask et al., 2012). Other factors would include psychological attributes with perfectionism implicated as both a risk and a maintaining factor (Fairburn & Harrison, 2003; Wade & Tiggeman, 2013). Typically, young people with anorexia often have 'perfectionist' traits and can be academically high achievers, but they often have low self-esteem and find it difficult to express or externalise negative emotions (Dhakras, 2005). Anorexia nervosa is not a disease of the middle classes, as is sometimes thought, and crosses all cultural and social backgrounds. There is increasing global recognition of the condition, especially in countries experiencing economic change alongside the changing roles of women in these countries (Cullen, 2011). It is interesting to note that in areas of the world where food is in short supply, eating disorders are virtually unknown (Lawrence, 2008).

CASE STUDY:
ANOREXIA

Heenan (2005b), writing from a feminist perspective, discusses the role of European consumer **culture** in the promotion of insecurities in women, their diet and their **body image**. She argues that the woman with an eating disorder has a perceived need to transform herself, and this is accompanied by the much needed sense of control, enabling her to translate her insecurities into bodily concerns. The inference is therefore that eating disorders are socially produced – a way in which women express themselves in our western society – and hence a product of social and societal interactions (Heenan, 2005a). Media and societal attitudes towards thinness are often cited as 'reasons' but they are not reasons in isolation; rather, they can act as contributing factors or **triggers**. Other predisposing factors centre on the negotiation of transitional points, for example the negotiation of adolescence in combination with an adverse life event such as bereavement, parental divorce or sexual abuse, together with a psychological vulnerability (Burton, 2014).

EATING DISORDER SERVICES

Clinicians struggle to find specialist care for adults, children and young people due to the poor availability and accessibility of specialist services, a situation which is referred to as the 'postcode lottery of UK eating disorder services' (Escobar-Koch et al., 2010: 558; Marsh & Campbell, 2016). Clinicians then struggle, again, to gain funding, as some of the UK specialist provision is in the private sector. Those services that do exist tend to use low body weight as a criterion for admission and general practitioners (GPs) act as the 'gatekeepers' to specialised treatment in the UK.

WHAT'S THE EVIDENCE? 38.1

Early treatment is particularly important for those with or at risk of severe emaciation and such patients should be prioritised for treatment. (NICE, 2017: 1.2.2)

The NICE guidance (2017) states that we should admit a person to hospital for medical stabilisation when they have severe electrolyte imbalance, severe malnutrition, severe dehydration or signs of incipient organ failure, to provide a structured, symptom-focused treatment regimen

(Continued)

with the expectation of weight gain, careful monitoring of the service user's physical status and psychological treatments that focus on eating behaviour and attitudes to weight and shape (NICE, 2017).

The NICE guidelines (2017) also state that 'children and young people with an eating disorder may also present with faltering growth (for example, a low weight or height for their age) or delayed puberty [1.2.7]' and 'Do not use single measures such as BMI or duration of illness to determine whether to offer treatment for an eating disorder [1.2.8]'.

This recent publication now supports the decision of GPs, described in Green et al.'s study (2008) that showed that the weight of the service user at GP consultations did not make a significant difference to their decision to refer to specialist services. The report goes on to recommend that BMI barriers should be removed from all services and be replaced with a comprehensive physical and mental health assessment (BEAT, 2016). Weight is a symptom of the mental illness, anorexia nervosa, so it is impossible to assess the severity of the mental health and distress based purely on physical markers. Care has to be individualised as there are so many unique variables. For example, in Laura's case there is a big difference between her presenting with a low BMI following on from 17 years of **acute** and chronic phases, meaning she has multiple associated physical problems, and a newly presenting case. Despite these problems, there are some who recover without any care and treatment, seemingly spontaneously; they do not enter the health care system but can be considered to be clinically recovered (Vandereycken & Devidt, 2011).

Day services are limited, so when service users are admitted to a specialist ED unit, they tend to be those diagnosed with 'anorexia nervosa', as they are clinically underweight and initial concerns focus on weight restoration. Diagnostic and assessment criteria differ for adults and children with eating disorders as they are at different developmental stages. Inpatient specialist eating disorder services provide 24-hour, around-the-clock care for severely malnourished service users. Hence, re-feeding and the establishment of a healthy weight is usually the primary goal. National guidelines have been provided for both children and adults, called MARSIPAN[1] and junior MARSIPAN (Royal College of Psychiatrists, 2014). Treatment is also offered for other medical problems and management of behaviours which may compromise treatment, such as food avoidance and concealment, exercising, falsifying weight and excessive water drinking (RCP, 2014). Additionally, for children, the provision of family interventions and the involvement of other family members in treatment are encouraged (NICE, 2017).

'THE RELUCTANT SERVICE USER'

The NICE guidance highlights the problem that 'service users with anorexia nervosa are notoriously reluctant to have treatment' (NICE, 2017: 58), making these service users some of the most challenging and resistant to treatment because they are not ready for active change (Treasure, 2004). Kaplan and Garfinkel (1999: 665) also use the word 'reluctant' to refer to both service users and clinicians: service users can seem unwilling to give up the disorder and clinicians may struggle to find sufficient motivation to treat them, and staff burnout is high. The word 'reluctant' is used frequently when referring to a service user's decline of engagement in services, as well as in Nordbø et al.'s use of the phrase 'reluctance to recover', referring to the enduring nature of the condition and the service user's wish to retain their anorexia (Nordbø et al., 2012).

---

[1]MARSIPAN stands for the Management of Really Sick Patients with Anorexia Nervosa.

Laura explains that, for her, it is the eating disorder that is 'reluctant', rather than the person:

Being in the grip of an eating disorder is like a paradox; on one hand you are desperate for help to be free of the illness and on the other hand accepting treatment is the scariest thing as it forces you to confront everything you fear the most. It's important to remember that as much as the eating disorder resists treatment, the person suffering from the illness is often desperate for help.

Service users believe they are coerced, persuaded or threatened by family, friends and health workers, which may cause an antagonistic relationship to develop with those who try to help them (Goldner, 1989). MacSween (1996) argues that service users suffering from AN believe that thinness will provide a solution to their unhappiness (MacSween, 1996: 38). Serpell et al. (1999) assert that anorexia nervosa is highly valued by the sufferer and so acceptance of treatment threatens ownership of their anorexia. Paulson-Karlsson et al. (2006) discuss the issue of treatment resistance, in relation to adolescents with anorexia, due to the service user's reluctance to admit the seriousness of their condition. Any attempts to feed and to promote weight gain are in direct conflict with these views and people with anorexia will go to extreme lengths to prevent their attempts to lose weight being thwarted (Cassell & Gleaves, 2006). Treatment resistance in anorexia nervosa is complex and influenced by personality traits, behavioural and neurobiological factors and the severity of the psychopathology of the eating disorder (Halmi, 2013).

Like Laura, many eating disorder sufferers have a long history of admissions, some of them for prolonged periods of time, and many involuntary (RCP, 2013), as people with anorexia will regularly refuse treatment, if they can. Institutionalisation is clearly a risk in such situations, especially where there is limited change in their condition, and hence inpatient care could actually be harmful (NICE, 2017). Once admitted, a named nurse or key worker will be assigned to them who they are unlikely to know, have no choice about and they may 'resent the imposition' (Hewitt et al., 2009: 68). At this stage, clear objectives need to be set for the admission and reviewed at least monthly.

Attempts to treat very low BMI[2] clients who are steadily losing weight and becoming increasingly physically vulnerable often result in the use of legal powers, thus imposing treatment on people who deny that they are unwell and so decline voluntary treatment. Although the Mental Health Act 1983/2007 in England and Wales allows for compulsory treatment of service users with eating disorders, Kim et al. (2008: 88) discuss 'empowerment' as an important factor in the therapeutic alliance, adding: 'the patient develops confidence and becomes a partner in the decision-making process'.

Yet, the reality is often that the treatment plan requires the anorexic service user to surrender their goal to eat less and strive for thinness, in favour of compliance; thus, if not formally 'detained', they are still, effectively, 'involuntary'. Whilst sufficient weight gain remains the primary goal of eating disorder services, the service users do not want to eat; they do not want to put on weight; they do not consider themselves to be ill and they may appear deceptively well, for example they are often extremely energetic right up to a physical collapse (Cassell & Gleaves, 2006; RCP, 2014). Hence, persuading people to accept and engage in care is a challenge and many sufferers 'drop out' of care.

'DROP-OUT' FROM SERVICES, CARE AND TREATMENT

'Drop-out' rates from eating disorder services are high and service users report low satisfaction with treatments that are often lengthy, expensive and of limited efficacy (Ryan et al., 2006). Studies relating to treatment drop-out tend to focus on aspects such as weight at admission, diagnosis, characteristics

---

[2] a BMI of less than 15.

of the service user, family **environment**, treatments offered and co-occurring conditions, rather than the context of care (Campbell, 2009; Mahon, 2000; Wallier et al., 2009). But, as Wallier and colleagues report, 'Future research should consider whether the therapeutic alliance of the patient and her family to clinicians predicts dropout, as we believe that a good therapeutic alliance will also relate to treatment completion' (Wallier et al., 2009: 646).

Seidinger et al. (2011) cite the service user's difficulty in intrapersonal relationships and the therapeutic alliance as significant issues affecting drop-out rates. These insights further reinforce the rationale for research into how relationships are played out within these services. We can speculate that high levels of **ambivalence** about treatment will influence a decision to opt out of treatment, but there is very little high quality evidence about why (DeJong et al., 2012; Mahon, 2000; Zeeck & Hartmann, 2005). Drop-out from a treatment programme is often associated with lack of engagement or motivation to engage with treatment. Service users who reluctantly engage with treatment that is in conflict with their own view of their health and wellbeing may take an early option to leave that treatment. However, this ultimately results in halted recovery and a poor prognosis, as service users who leave treatment early ('drop out'[3]) are unlikely to recover independently (DeJong et al., 2012).

The high drop-out rate is somewhat predictable when we acknowledge the lack of agreement between the nurse and the service user around the task and goals of the therapy (Fairburn & Harrison, 2003; Pereira et al., 2006). If we consider this from Szasz's (2007) perspective, that we all have a right to bodily and mental self-ownership, then conflict can be seen as inevitable as the individual relinquishes their personal beliefs and choices in favour of **adherence** to the treatment goals. Goldner suggests that service users are coerced, persuaded or threatened by family, friends and nurses, and consequently an antagonistic relationship develops due to the service user's intense fear of gaining weight (Goldner, 1989). Service users may have a strong need to be self-determining, a distrust of nurses and a reluctance to give up control, but are ultimately compliant rather than concordant.[4] Their beliefs about themselves remain unchanged but are often dismissed as delusional, irrational and as such lacking in insight. As soon as the service user is discharged, Goldner says that the service user will revert to the behaviours that originally brought about their weight loss and admission, thus becoming known as a 'revolving door' service user as re-admission occurs (Langdon et al., 2001). Ironically, slow progression may also be attributed to the nurses' reluctance to upset the service user by challenging their perspective (Goldner, 1989).

THE MAUDSLEY METHOD

The Maudsley Method (Treasure et al., 2007) is a specific model developed and practised at the Maudsley Hospital in London and at specialist centres throughout the world. The Maudsley Method is not family therapy as such but is a *family-based treatment*, hence it is largely focused on children and young people with eating disorders. It integrates principles and skills from many of the major schools of **family therapy** and is suitable for adolescents where there is less than three years' duration of anorexia nervosa (Maudsley Parents, 2013). This approach, adopted by Treasure (2013), is

---

[3]Although the term 'drop-out' is frequently used, some authors such as Sly (2009) and Vandereycken and Devidt (2010) view it as pejorative and call for new, less pejorative terms for those who do not complete treatment.

[4]Compliance is defined as: 'The extent to which the service user's behaviour matches the prescriber's recommendations.' However, the use of this term is declining as it implies lack of service user involvement. 'Concordance' is predominantly used to describe the situation where the worker and the service user agree therapeutic decisions that incorporate their respective views.

underpinned by a motivational style that is designed to encourage and stimulate service users to maintain their attendance and engagement with services and so thus reduce 'drop-out' (Prochaska et al., 1992). It is frequently used within Tier 3 and 4 CAMHS in conjunction with re-feeding programmes both in Tier 3 and 4 services. NICE guidelines state that families be provided with education and information on the nature and risks of the eating disorder and how it is likely to affect them, as well as the treatments available and their likely benefits and limitations. It is also suggested that eating disorder-focused family therapy should be offered (NICE, 2017). This would include both treatment approaches and family therapies.

The approach is separated into three phases:

Phase 1: Re-feeding the service user

The family is tasked with helping the child to gain weight and restore healthy eating practices. Modelling empathy and understanding, the therapist encourages the parents to take control of their child's food intake through empathic but firm instruction. Family meals are taken at the clinic and the therapist observes the family's typical interaction patterns around eating. Parents take charge of the mealtime and siblings are encouraged to align themselves more with their sister, showing their understanding of how hard it is for her. This is an important part of the work, using Minuchin's structural ideas to help the family to form appropriate parental and sibling subsystems. This phase can last up to 12 or more weeks as the family adjust to their roles and ensure that the child is regaining weight and developing healthier eating patterns. The therapist takes note of family interactions that are unhelpful. Parent and sibling subsystems are reinforced and attention is paid to any attempts to criticise the child or to any strong emotion expressed about the child's eating. When parents criticise or get emotional with their child, it is reframed or *externalised* as the anorexia taking control. They are reminded that the anorexia is the one to blame, not the child nor the parents. The Maudsley Method thus presents 'externalising' as a really important feature of managing and treating young people with anorexia nervosa to prevent the blaming of the service user and/or their family. Often **carers** cannot understand, and ask 'why can't you just eat?' It must be remembered that food refusal is a symptom of the disease process and one the service user will have an ongoing struggle with, such is its power.

Phase 2: Negotiating for a new relationship

Once the service user has regained weight and accepts her parents' demands that she eat, the therapist encourages the parents to start to give back some of the control over eating to their daughter. The therapist still supports the parents in their attempts to feed their daughter but they are encouraged to feel more confident about their ability to deal with difficult situations that might arise. The therapist facilitates negotiations between parents and daughter so that she can start to take more responsibility for her mealtime behaviour. If there are any significant problems, Phase 1 is revisited. Family concerns and issues that have had to take a back seat are now discussed with the therapist and healthy family functioning is emphasised.

Phase 3: Adolescent issues and termination

This phase is commenced once the adolescent reaches 90–100% of ideal weight and has appropriate control over food intake. The focus is taken off the re-feeding process and the adolescent's identity and individuality are explored in detail for the first time. Throughout Phases 1 and 2, the therapist has helped the family to restructure more appropriate boundaries so that their child can now continue to develop individuality in an appropriate way. Her healthy development had previously been impeded by the control exerted by the anorexia. A wide variety of adolescent issues are explored and worked through with the family, including separation, peer relationships and sexuality. The parents are also encouraged to give up attitudes and skills that were appropriate at earlier stages in their child's life and to spend more time together as a couple. If particular problems arise, the parents are advised to seek couple therapy in order to deal with their own issues. It is not always the case that a strong parenting team leads to a happier marriage (Maudsley Parents, 2013; Rhodes, 2003).

The Maudsley Method is particularly suited to working with children and adolescents due to the pivotal role of the family. It is less well accepted in adult services. In adult services, 'externalising' is often seen as unhelpful; it can create tension between health care staff as the eating disorder 'takes the blame' when hostility and abuse are targeted at staff members, which makes them feel vulnerable when caring for this group of clients. The construction of the anorexic voice/identity has some utility as it provides an entity on which to attribute the anorexic behaviours and the angst, but this mechanism has been blamed for subsequent fractures in the relationship. Workers are unsure about whom they are relating to, and the 'bad' behaviours, such as emotional and expletive communication around mealtimes or weigh times, are attributed to the anorexic identity and therefore not owned by the 'real' person. Nurses with insight understand that the battle is with the disorder not them, hence resilience and a constant reminder of their duty of care are prerequisites for this work (Wright & Shroeder, 2016).

For adults, it is suggested that couple-based interventions might be preferable to family therapy and also that cognitive behavioural therapy (CBT) be offered to the individual (Gilbert, 2014). The success of therapy rests on the services user's continued active engagement with treatment. Vandereycken and Devidt (2010) purport that if we *listen* to our service users more, it might not prevent drop-out from treatment, but it may prevent people from prematurely stopping therapy. Below, Rachelle talks about the way nurses behave that makes her feel at home and welcome. Different settings influence the ways in which people communicate and behave, dependent on social factors and how these occur within the built environment, due to considerations such as available space and privacy (Bandura[5], 1977; DeVito, 1991).

WHAT HELPS AND WHAT HINDERS? LED BY RACHELLE'S STORY

Rachelle was an in-service user in an adult Specialist Eating Disorder Unit (SEDU). At the time of writing, she kindly offered an insight into her experience, knowing that she might be able to enable learner nurses to better understand her and her experience:

> I was around 16, in my last year in school. I didn't like my body, but I thought that was normal for a teenager. It wasn't an obsession. I just decided to lose weight. But it spiralled, the thoughts became intrusive, they wouldn't go away and eventually took control. When I wasn't controlling my eating, I coped in other ways, like self-harming and over-dosing. I didn't like myself. It's all a blur now. I've wasted my teenage years. Before I came into hospital was the worst time in my life. My mum thought that I was going to die. I was scared. I didn't want to die, but I felt that my body was giving up on me. I couldn't walk up the stairs. My skin hurt. I couldn't lie down without being in pain.

---

[5]Bandura's social learning theory, more recently known as 'social cognitive theory', can be described as 'the impact of observing other people's behaviour on one's own behaviour' (Odgen, 2003: 29) and is rooted in child development theory. Bandura claimed that people learn by observing others and adopt patterns of behaviour that are fitting within their group, particularly in institutional settings, such as a hospital or an education establishment.

I asked Rachelle: 'If you could go back and advise the 16-year-old you, what would you say?' This was her response:

> Please open up and tell someone ... don't keep doing it; I always think that if I'd told someone when I was 16, I wouldn't be here [in hospital] right now.

We learn so much from understanding what service users feel and experience. Rachelle felt able to offer some suggestions:

> Karen: What are the important things that the nurses do?
>
> Rachelle: It helps a lot when they are positive. It's easy to be negative here. When the nurses are happy and jokey it's good. It's good when they ask us how we feel, they let me get it out. They always know what to say. They are really caring. They give me a hug, make me feel welcome, they make it feel like 'home'.
>
> Karen: What is the most important thing?
>
> Rachelle: With this illness it's easy for people to say the wrong thing and we are so sensitive. So please don't make comments about how we look, or about our food.
>
> Karen: What would you ask nurses NOT to do?
>
> Rachelle: Don't be distant. Don't behave like it's just a job. Don't be unapproachable.

There is an acceptance that the workers want different things to the service users, so there is an expectation of conflict – conflict that, in some ways, can be resolved by being helped to battle not with the person, but with the *illness*. Here, Rachelle and Laura have generously shared their experience in order to find a position of mutual acceptance and understanding.

CHAPTER SUMMARY

This chapter has covered:

- What we mean by 'eating disorders' and the seriousness of these conditions; this chapter has focused primarily on anorexia nervosa due to the complexity and life-threatening nature of this eating disorder and the impact on the sufferers and their families
- What we can learn from Laura and Rachelle, their experiences of anorexia and also of their transition from CAMHS to adult mental health services; nurse managers from both adult and child and adolescent health services have also shared their perspectives on working in this specialist field
- The Maudsley Method and its utility, particularly in CAMHS
- The challenges for nurses working in this field
- How to empower and engage the reluctant service user.

This is a complex and vast field, so we would strongly advise you to look further and utilise the resources that you are signposted to below.

———— BUILD YOUR BIBLIOGRAPHY ————

Books

- Fathallah, J. (2006) *Monkey taming*. London: Definitions. This book is one of the few biographical accounts that strikes the right balance for the student nurse who is trying to gain insight into the experience of anorexia, from onset to recovery.
- Grilo, C. & Mitchell, J.E. (2010) *The treatment of eating disorders: A clinical handbook*. New York: Guilford Press. A sound textbook that covers all the basics and so much more.
- Knightsmith, P. (2015) *Self-harm and eating disorders in schools: A guide to whole-school strategies and practical support*. London: Jessica Kingsley. Although this text is aimed at staff in educational settings, it is a really useful guide. If you are working with children and young people with eating disorders, you will most likely be working collaboratively with staff in their school settings.
- Williams, G. (2002) *Internal landscapes and foreign bodies: Eating disorders and other pathologies*. London: Karnac. This text offers a fascinating psychoanalytic view of eating disorders and thus provides a wider breadth of understanding of the origins, maintenance and resistance of eating disorders.

SAGE journal articles

FURTHER
READING:
JOURNAL
ARTICLES

Go to https://study.sagepub.com/essentialmentalhealth for further free online journal articles related to this chapter. If you are using the interactive ebook, simply click on the book icon in the margin to go straight to the resource.

- Hatmaker, G. (2005) Boys with eating disorders. *Journal of School Nursing*, 21(6), 329.
- Lyckhage, E.D., Gardvik, A., Karlsson, H., et al. (2015) Young women with anorexia nervosa: writing oneself back into life. *SAGE Open*, March, 1–8.
- Withrow, R.L. & Shoffner, M.F. (2006) Applying the theory of work adjustment to clients with symptoms of anorexia nervosa. *Journal of Career Development*, 32(4), 366–377.

Weblinks

FURTHER
READING:
WEBLINKS

Go to https://study.sagepub.com/essentialmentalhealth for further weblinks related to this chapter. If you are using the interactive ebook, simply click on the book icon in the margin to go straight to the resource.

- BEAT: www.b-eat.co.uk/support-services
- Royal College of Psychiatrists (RCP) website has a range of materials pivotal to the care of the person with an eating disorder, including the 'MARSIPAN' guidelines: www.rcpsych.ac.uk/useful resources/publications/collegereports/cr/cr189.aspx
- SEED: www.seedeatingdisorders.org.uk

———— ACE YOUR ASSESSMENT ————

ONLINE
QUIZZES &
ACTIVITY
ANSWERS

Revise what you have learned by visiting https://study.sagepub.com/essentialmentalhealth. If you are using the interactive ebook, simply click on the tick icon to go straight to the resource.

- Test yourself with multiple-choice and short-answer questions and flashcards.

REFERENCES

Arcelus, J., Mitchell, A.J., Wales, J., et al. (2011) Mortality rates in patients with anorexia nervosa and other eating disorders: a meta-analysis of 36 studies. *Archives of General Psychiatry*, *68*(7), 724–731.

Bandura, A. (1977) *Social learning theory*. Englewood Cliffs, NJ: Prentice-Hall.

BEAT (2015) *Eating disorder statistics*. Available at: www.b-eat.co.uk/about-beat/media-centre/information-and-statistics-about-eating-disorders (accessed 02.17).

BEAT (2016) *Eating disorder sufferers turned away for specialist treatment*. Available at: www.b-eat.co.uk/about-beat/media-centre/press-releases/5354-eating-disorder-sufferers-turned-away-for-specialist-treatment (accessed 02.17).

Burton, M. (2014) Understanding eating disorders in young people. *Practice Nurse*, *25*(12), 606–610.

Campbell, M. (2009) Drop-out from treatment for the eating disorders: a problem for clinicians and researchers. *European Eating Disorders Review*, *17*, 239–242.

Cassell, D. & Gleaves, D.H. (2006) *The encyclopaedia of obesity and eating disorders*. New York: Infobase Publishing.

Cullen, G. (2011) Eating disorders. In A. Claveirole & M. Gaughan (eds) *Understanding Children & Young People's Mental Health*. Chichester: Wiley-Blackwell. pp. 149–164.

DeJong, H., Broadbent, H. & Schmidt, U. (2012) A systematic review of dropout from treatment in outpatients with anorexia nervosa. *International Journal of Eating Disorders*, *45*, 635–647.

DeVito, J.A. (1991) *Human Communication*. New York: Harper Collins.

Dhakras, S. (2005) Anorexia nervosa. In M. Cooper, C. Hooper & M. Thompson (eds) *Child and Adolescent Mental Health Theory and Practice*. London: Hodder-Arnold. pp. 156–163.

Escobar-Koch, T., Banker, J.D., Crow, S., et al. (2010). Service users' views of eating disorder services: an international comparison. *International Journal of Eating Disorders*, *43*(6),549–559.

Fairburn, C.G. & Harrison, P.J. (2003) Eating disorders. *The Lancet*, *361*(9355), 407–416.

Gilbert, G. (2014) The origins and nature of compassion focused. *The British Journal of Psychology*, *53*(1), 6–41.

Goldner, E. (1989) Treatment refusal in anorexia nervosa. *International Journal of Eating Disorders*, *8*(3), 297–306.

Green, H. , Johnson, O., Cabrini, S., et al. (2008) General practitioner attitudes towards referral of eating-disordered patients: a vignette study based on the theory of planned behaviour. *Mental Health in Family Medicine*, *5*(4), 213–218.

Halmi, K.A. (2013) Perplexities of treatment resistance in eating disorders. *BMC Psychiatry*, *13*: 292.

Heenan C. (2005a) A Feminist psychotherapeutic approach to working with women who eat impulsively. *Counselling and Psychotherapy Research*, *5*(3), 238–245.

Heenan, M.C. (2005b) 'Looking in the Fridge for Feelings': The Gendered Psychodynamics of Consumer Culture. In J. Davidson, L. Bondi & M. Smith (eds) *Emotional Geographies*. Burlington, VT and Aldershot: Ashgate.

Hewitt, J., Coffey, M. & Rooney, G. (2009) Forming, sustaining and ending therapeutic interactions. In P. Callaghan, J. Playle & L. Cooper (eds) *Mental health nursing skills*. Oxford: Oxford University Press. pp. 63–73.

Kaplan, A.S. & Garfinkel, P.E. (1999) Difficulties in treating patients with eating disorders: a review of patients and clinical variables. *Canadian Journal of Psychiatry*, *44*, 665–670.

Kim, S.C., Kim, S. & Boren, D. (2008) The quality of therapeutic alliance between patient and provide predicts general satisfaction. *Military Medicine*, *173*(1), 85–90.

Langdon, P., Yagüez, L., Brown, J., et al. (2001) Who walks through the 'revolving-door' of a British psychiatric hospital? *Journal of Mental Health*, *10*(5), 525–533.

Lask, B., Frampton, I. & Nunn, K. (2012) Anorexia nervosa: a noradrenergic dysregulation hypothesis. *Medical Hypotheses*, 78(5), 580–584.

Lawrence, M. (2008) *The anorexic mind*. London: Karnac.

MacSween, M. (1996) *Anorexic bodies: A feminist and sociological perspective on anorexia nervosa*. London: Routledge.

Mahon, J. (2000) Dropping out from psychological treatments for eating disorders: what are the issues? *European Eating Disorders Review*, 8, 198–216.

Marsh, S. & Campbell, D. (2016) *Clean eating trend can be dangerous for young people, experts warn. The Guardian*. Available at: www.theguardian.com/society/2016/oct/01/clean-eating-trend-dangerous-young-people-food-obsession-mental-health-experts (Accessed 16.09.2017).

Maudsley Parents (2013) *Family-based treatment of anorexia nervosa: The Maudsley approach*. Available at: www.maudsleyparents.org/whatismaudsley.html (accessed 03.17).

National Institute for Health and Care Excellence (NICE) (2017) *Eating disorders: Recognition and treatment* NICE Guideline (NG69). London: NICE. Available at: www.nice.org.uk/guidance/ng69 (accessed 27 May 2016).

Nordbø, R.H.S., Espeset, E.M.S., Gulliksen, K.S., et al. (2012) Reluctance to recover in anorexia nervosa. *European Eating Disorders Review*, 20, 60–67.

Ogden, J. (2003) *The Psychology of Eating: From Healthy to Unhealthy Behaviour*. Blackwell, Oxford.

Paulson-Karlsson, G., Nevonen, L. & Engstrom, I. (2006) Anorexia nervosa: treatment satisfaction. *Journal of Family Therapy*, 28, 293–306.

Pereira, T., Lock, J. & Oggins, J. (2006) Role of therapeutic alliance in family therapy for adolescent anorexia nervosa. *International Journal of Eating Disorders*, 39, 677–684.

Prochaska, J.O., DiClemente, C.C. & Norcross, J.C. (1992) In search of how people change. *American Psychologist*, 47, 1102–1114.

Rhodes, P. (2003) The Maudsley Model of family therapy for children and adolescents with anorexia nervosa: theory, clinical practice, and empirical support. *Australian and New Zealand Journal of Family Therapy*, 24(4), 191–198.

Royal College of Psychiatrists (RCP) (2013) *Anorexia and bulimia*. Available at: www.rcpsych.ac.uk/expertadvice/problems/eatingdisorders/anorexiaandbulimia.aspx (accessed 15.08.17).

Royal College of Psychiatrists (RCP) (2014) *MARSIPAN: Management of really sick patients with anorexia nervosa*. College Report CR189. Available at: www.rcpsych.ac.uk/usefulresources/publications/collegereports/cr/cr189.aspx (accessed 15.08.17).

Ryan, V., Malson, H., Clarke, S., et al. (2006) Discursive constructions of 'eating disorders nursing': an analysis of nurses' accounts of nursing eating disorder patients. *European Eating Disorders Review*, 14, 125–135.

Seidinger, F.M., Garcia, C., Böttcher-Luiz, F., et al. (2011) Dropout in the treatment for anorexia nervosa and bulimia: a systematic review from the international databases. *European Psychiatry*, 26, 738.

Serpell, L., Treasure, J., Teasdale, J., et al. (1999) Anorexia nervosa: friend or foe? A qualitative analysis of the themes expressed in letters written by anorexia nervosa patients. *International Journal of Eating Disorders*, 25, 77.

Sly, R. (2009) What's in a name? Classifying 'the dropout' from treatment for anorexia nervosa. *European Eating Disorders Review*, 17, 405–407.

Strober, M. (2010) The chronically ill patient with anorexia. In C.M. Grilo & J.E. Mitchel (eds) *The treatment of eating disorders*. New York: The Guilford Press.

Szasz, T. (2007) *Coercion as cure*. Piscataway, NJ: Transaction Publishers.

Treasure, J. (2004) Eating disorders. *Medicine, 32*(8), 63–66.

Treasure, J., Smith, G. and Crane, A. (2007) *Skills-based Learning for Caring for a Loved One with an Eating Disorder*. London: Routledge.

Treasure, J. & Alexander, J. (2013) *Anorexia nervosa: A recovery guide for sufferers, families and friends*. London: Routledge.

Vandereycken, W. and Devidt, K. (2010) Dropping out from a specialized inpatient treatment for eating disorders: the perception of patients and staff. *Eating Disorders 18*(2):140–147.

Wade, T.D. & Tiggeman, M. (2013) The role of perfectionism in body dissatisfaction. *Journal of Eating Disorders 1, 2*. Available at: https://jeatdisord.biomedcentral.com/articles/10.1186/2050-2974-1-2 (accessed November 2016).

Wallier, J., Vibert, S., Berthoz, S., et al. (2009) Dropout from inpatient treatment for anorexia nervosa: critical review of the literature. *International Journal of Eating Disorders, 42*, 636–647.

Wright, K.M. & Shroeder, D. (2016) Turning the tables: the vulnerability of nurses treating anorexia nervosa patients. *Cambridge Quarterly, 25*(2), 219–227.

Zeeck, A. & Hartmann, A. (2005) Relating therapeutic process to outcome: are there predictors for the short-term course in anorexic patients? *European Eating Disorders Review, 13*(4), 245–254.

CARE OF INDIVIDUALS WHO SELF-HARM OR EXPERIENCE SUICIDAL FEELINGS

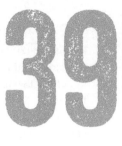

39

KAREN JAMES AND ISAAC SAMUELS

THIS CHAPTER COVERS

- The meaning of self-harm
- Developing a practice of ongoing reflection
- A narrative approach to working alongside people who have challenges around self-harm
- The relationship between self-harm, suicidal feelings and suicide
- Talking about suicidal feelings.

> At first I think I really didn't understand why people wanted to self-harm to actually do things to make themselves suffer. I found it scary. But I've nursed lots of different people with lots and lots of different reasons and histories and dynamics and backgrounds. So you come to really know the people individually. You spend a lot of time learning about their lives and what's troubled them, and what's brought them to the situation they're in.
>
> **Helen, mental health nurse**

> As somebody that has had challenges and support needs around my self-harming behaviour, I feel it is vital that people are not only supported to manage this taboo area of mental health, but additionally are supported to make sense of their self-harm and how they plan to manage this ongoing challenge. Just because I don't self-harm everyday doesn't mean that I don't have challenges around the feelings that I now recognise as part of my self-harming cycle. People who self-harm are seen very differently from those in recovery from addiction; there is an assumption that you either self-harm or you don't, but for me, it is a constant battle and is never far away from the reality of my day. What has made a difference is when people have seen it as a daily challenge, and have supported me in a way that has been less stigmatising and more accepting of my needs.
>
> **Catherine, service user**

INTRODUCTION

In this chapter, we present a person-centred, **narrative approach** to supporting people who self-harm, drawing on current research evidence in this area, alongside the lived experiences of people who have self-harmed and the practitioners who have supported them. We'd like to acknowledge Sharon Wolf and David W. Gorski who have shared their personal narratives in this chapter.

THE MEANING OF SELF-HARM

Self-harm is a very complex behaviour that can hold a number of different meanings for one person, which can change during different times in their life. UK clinical guidance defines self-harm as any 'act of intentional self-poisoning or self injury, irrespective of the extent of suicidal intent' (National Institute for Health and Clinical Excellence, 2011: 4). However, there is no commonly accepted definition of 'self-harm' and these behaviours will be understood in different ways by different people. Take Jay, for example: Jay is on an **acute** ward and is cutting her legs. She calls this a 'self-management strategy', whilst her care-coordinator calls it 'self-harm'. People are likely to hold different perspectives of self-harm based on their individual and cultural beliefs, education, professional identity and life experience: Jay's care-coordinator understands that her self-harm is a **coping** strategy, but her partner views it as an 'attention-seeking behaviour'. Her brother is fully aware that her self-harming has nothing to do with suicide, whilst her mum believes it is an attempt to take her own life. As a nurse, it is important to be mindful of these complexities in terms of how self-harm is understood (and the wider social context of the person you are supporting), as this can present additional challenges to someone who will be managing their self-harm within the context of their relationships. A central part of your role is to support individuals to identify and share their *own* experiences of self-harm and the meaning behind their behaviour. One way you can do this is by using a personal narrative approach, which we explain in more detail below.

Current research suggests that the most common method of self-harm used within our communities is cutting, although people also often self-harm by self-poisoning, hitting themselves or banging their head (Moran et al., 2012). Other methods reported in research include strangulation, burning and the insertion of foreign objects into the body (for example, putting a paperclip under the skin). Women, young people and people who have experienced trauma during childhood, such as neglect, emotional, physical or sexual abuse, are more at risk of self-harm. Jay would describe self-harm as a behaviour, not a mental health challenge, but from a clinical perspective around 90% of people who self-harm meet the criteria for a psychiatric diagnosis (Haw et al., 2001). Research has found that this is most often **depression** and **anxiety** (Klonsky et al., 2003). Self-harm is one of the criteria for diagnosis of borderline personality **disorder** (sometimes referred to as emotionally unstable **personality** disorder), however most people who self-harm will not meet the criteria for this diagnosis (Haw et al., 2001). Other challenges that someone who self-harms might experience include alcohol and substance misuse and suicidal ideation.

People will have very individual experiences of their relationship with self-harm and, as a nurse, it is essential that you understand their personal narrative. For example, Jay self-harms because it helps her to manage feelings of frustration, anger and inner tension. Research suggests that the most common reason for self-harm is to manage emotional distress, and laboratory studies have found that physical pain can help to reduce negative emotions (Haines et al., 1995; Niedtfeld et al., 2010). For around half of people who cut themselves, seeing blood is also important (Glenn & Klonsky, 2010). Blood can symbolise the release of unwanted feelings from the body, or can help to relieve periods of **depersonalisation**, where people enter a dream-like state and feel disconnected from their physical selves:

'when I'm having a flashback I cut myself and seeing the blood helps me to feel in control again.'

In these cases, seeing blood can help people become fully conscious again. Another common meaning of self-harm is 'self-punishment':

'I feel bad and not worthy of love and care, so when people show me they care I burn myself to punish myself for being bad.'

Research has found that between 10% and 83% of people say they self-harm for this reason (Briere & Gil, 1998; Herpertz, 1995). This can be a response to extreme feelings of low self-worth, or a re-enactment of past abuse. For **survivors** of abuse, self-harm can be a way of coping with feelings of being 'bad' or contaminated inside, by allowing people to remove this part of themselves. Self-harm can also be used as a way of communicating with others, or to change their behaviour:

'When I poison myself and I become ill this shows people around me that I am suffering'; '

The scars from my self-harming are a signal to people that I am vulnerable and they should tread lightly around me.'

For example, in a survey of young people who self-harmed, 67% said they did so to have an impact on others (Scoliers et al., 2009). For some people, self-harm can be a way of communicating their distress when they feel unable to express this pain in words, or believe that they will not be heard.

APPROACHES TO WORKING IN PARTNERSHIP WITH PEOPLE WHO SELF-HARM

Developing a practice of ongoing reflection

Reflective practice is a way of studying your own experiences to improve the way in which you work. An important part of the process of supporting people who self-harm involves identifying the beliefs and **values** that you hold, or the policies or practices within the **environment** where you are working, which may be in conflict with the needs of the person you are supporting. A process of active reflection can help to ensure that these factors do not influence your practice in an unhelpful way. This process takes time, and so it is important that you allow time for reflection during your day. Some approaches which aid reflective practice include using a reflective journal or speaking with your peers about your experiences, for example in reflective staff groups or during supervision.

Reflecting on what you bring to the therapeutic relationship

As a nurse, it is important to acknowledge what you bring to your relationship with a person who has support needs around self-harming. This includes your assets, such as the skills and knowledge you have developed through education, training and experience (for example, the therapeutic skills covered in Chapters 20–25 of this textbook will be central to your work with people who self-harm). It is also important to be aware of the personal values and beliefs you hold which may shape your nursing practice. Research has found that nurses' attitudes towards self-harm are influenced by their **culture** and training, and their expectations around how a person in contact with mental health services should behave (James, 2015). The following are some examples we would like to share with you:

SEE ALSO CHAPTERS 20-25

Imran self-harms as a way of managing his feelings. His named nurse is Jamal and because they are both men and of the same faith, Imran was hopeful that he would have a rapport with Jamal that was lacking in his relationships with other staff members. However, Imran's self-harming behaviour challenged Jamal as it was contradictory to his religious beliefs – Jamal believes that it is a sin to harm or mark your body. This meant he found it difficult to support Imran. He told Imran he should stop self-harming as it caused him both physical and spiritual harm. As a consequence, Imran felt that Jamal didn't understand him and wasn't able to relate to him. This increased his sense of isolation and low self-worth and was stigmatising.

When supporting people who have challenges around self-harm, your practice must be guided by the values and responsibilities you hold as a nurse. Everyone has the right to hold strong personal beliefs, but, as a nurse, your role is to offer support which meets the needs of the person you are supporting. In many cases, this will mean accepting the person's need to self-harm. This is not always easy, but people have the right to makes choices about how they manage their own mental health, and more so, a right to be supported by professionals.

CRITICAL THINKING STOP POINT 39.1

Do you hold beliefs that self-harm is wrong or immoral? How might these beliefs affect the ways in which you support people who have challenges around self-harm? How can you ensure that your personal beliefs do not prevent you from meeting the needs of the person you are supporting?

Lawford works in a community mental health team and is Jennifer's care coordinator. Jennifer burns herself to remain present and distance herself from the trauma of upsetting memories. Jennifer feels voiceless and uncomfortable expressing how she feels and she suppresses her mental health challenges. Lawford hasn't explored different ways of supporting Jennifer to talk about her self-harm in a way that recognises these challenges. Because Lawford can't see that Jennifer is experiencing distress, he believes there is nothing wrong and she is just seeking attention. Lawford hasn't reflected on other explanations for her challenges around self-harm. This means that Jennifer isn't getting the support she needs and feels unable to seek support from Lawford.

Some people who self-harm can find it difficult to express how they are feeling, which can mean that they don't always seem in distress or in need of support. Self-harm also requires a response from you as a nurse, and so sometimes it might feel like someone is using self-harm to manipulate you. We know from research that the vast majority of people who self-harm will also be experiencing mental health challenges and holding such views will make it very difficult for you to support them. It might also have an impact on your own wellbeing – for example, nurses have described feeling upset, afraid, frustrated, powerless or angry when supporting people who self-harm (James et al., 2012). If you begin to feel that someone who self-harms is not deserving of support, then it is important that you try and find an alternative understanding for their behaviour. Understanding the individual's narrative around their self-harming challenges will help you to adopt a different view of their self-harm and will enable you to meet their needs. You can also draw on your knowledge of psychological theories and approaches (for example, attachment or behavioural theories).

After she self-harmed she said to me 'well you were busy, you couldn't talk to me this morning'. During my reflection I remembered reading about psychodynamic theory, and thought: 'this is about projection'. I think a transference and projection occurred, where perhaps somewhere in her past she had been met with hostility and told to go and deal with her feelings on her own.

Rebecca, mental health nurse

CRITICAL THINKING STOP POINT 39.2

Have you ever felt that people who self-harm are not really experiencing difficulties, or are undeserving of care? Why do you think this is? It might help to try and think about the individual's behaviour or challenges as being separate from the person themselves. Are there any alternative explanations you can draw on from the service user's narratives, psychological theory or therapeutic approaches that can help you develop a different understanding of their challenges?

Reflecting on the impact of the environment in which you are working

Sometimes the context or systems within which you are working can **affect** your nursing practice. This is a particular challenge for nurses working on inpatient wards. Often, ward policies will state that people should be prevented from self-harming, and to uphold these policies nurses may have to use observation, restraint or pro re nata medication. Whilst intended to keep people safe, these policies and practices can be detrimental to the **therapeutic relationship** and the overall wellbeing of the individual. In this context, it is particularly important to talk through these challenges with the person you are supporting to ensure that they feel heard and that you are enabling them to have as much choice and control over their support as possible.

Your practice might also be influenced by the people you work with; other nurses might have negative attitudes towards self-harm, and if you are working in a team where this is the dominant view, these beliefs can influence your own practice and the practice of others.

On my first placement the attitude from the other nurses was like, 'you don't tolerate this behaviour'. When a woman self-harmed the staff told me to ignore her and so I thought that was what I was supposed to do. But it didn't feel right and I spoke to my personal tutor about it. He said that I should talk to her because she probably needed support, especially because other nurses weren't responding to her. After speaking with her, I now understand some of the challenges she was experiencing, and this knowledge has helped me to develop my practice.

During reflection it is important to think about how these contextual factors might be influencing your practice or your view of self-harm. It might help to discuss these issues with your peers, or during supervision.

Joshua, mental health nursing student

WHAT'S THE EVIDENCE? 39.1

Very few high quality studies have investigated what works in supporting people who have challenges around self-harm, which means it is very difficult to make robust recommendations about the types of interventions or approaches that are most helpful. There is currently no evidence for the effectiveness of pharmacological interventions, but limited evidence that dialectical behavioural therapy (DBT) and problem-solving therapy can help to reduce self-harm, and improve outcomes such as depression and hopelessness (Hawton et al., 2015; NICE, 2011). A significant problem with research in this area is that researchers use different definitions of 'self-harm' and so it is difficult to compare results across studies. Another criticism is that these studies are not measuring the right outcomes; interventions are judged to be successful if they reduce rates of self-harm, however some people argue that there are other outcomes, such as mental wellbeing or quality of life, that are more important.

CRITICAL THINKING STOP POINT 39.3

What do you think are the most important 'outcomes' for people who self-harm? What is the difference you would like to make when you are supporting people who self-harm? How might this be measured in a study?

A NARRATIVE APPROACH TO WORKING ALONGSIDE PEOPLE WHO HAVE CHALLENGES AROUND SELF-HARM

In this section, we outline an approach to supporting people who self-harm which integrates narrative practices with **care planning**. Narrative practices focus on people as the experts in their own experiences, and recognise the many abilities, resources, values and commitments that will help them to manage the challenges in their lives. This is called a 'narrative' approach because it places an emphasis on the stories of people's lives and the difference that can be made by listening to and understanding their life experiences. We use the example of Veronica's relationship with Mandy to outline what this approach might look like.

The context

Personal context

Mandy is a primary school teacher and has a partner of four years. During her teenage years, Mandy experienced difficulties at school and was bullied. She told her mum but her mum was unsupportive. She said it was 'just one of these things that happens' and that she needed to get on with things and focus on her studies. Every time Mandy sought support and advice from her family, they minimised the impact that the bullying was having on her emotional wellbeing. Mandy began to feel unable to explore and express how she was feeling and believed the bullying was her fault. After a particularly traumatic incident, Mandy pulled her tie tight around her neck until it was difficult to breathe and found that this helped to stop the feelings. She used this as a way of managing her feelings about the bullying and about being unsupported for many years, but stopped when she met her partner, Jon, at university.

Mandy is now training to be a teacher, she has a very difficult class and her mentor is not supporting her. This has evoked feelings from her past and she has started self-ligaturing again (tying her headphones tight around her neck). In school, at lunchtime, she would self-harm in the toilets and this helped her to get through the day. One day, Jon comes home unexpectedly to find Mandy unconscious, but breathing, on their bed. He calls an ambulance. Mandy sees a psychiatric liaison nurse who recognises that she needs support and refers her to the community mental health team (CMHT). The CMHT believe she is trying to take her own life and pressure her to admit herself, voluntarily, to hospital to seek treatment.

Environmental context

Mandy is staying on a chaotic, busy ward with people who are acutely unwell. This causes her emotional wellbeing to deteriorate further and she increases her self-harming. The ward has an inconsistent way of supporting people who self-harm, but the policy states that people should be prevented from self-harming on the ward.

The mental health nurse

Veronica is Mandy's named nurse. During her training, Veronica had a placement on a ward where there was a lot of specialist knowledge about self-harm and the team used a **harm-minimisation** approach, which meant they supported people to self-harm in a safe way on the ward.

The conversation

Step 1: Starting the conversation

Veronica's first step in working with Mandy was to have a conversation with her that wasn't focused on her self-harm, but was about getting to know each other. They talked about shared interests and just spent some time listening to each other and being curious. Veronica made sure she set aside some time to do this without interruption, but Mandy didn't want to talk for long. Veronica respected Mandy's needs at that time and made sure Mandy knew that there would be other opportunities to pick up where they'd left off, and that she was available.

Step 2: Developing an understanding of the person's narrative

Veronica spent time asking Mandy about her life, paying special attention to what was most meaningful in her life story, for example influential relationships, turning points, important memories, events or decisions, and how these experiences related to each other.

A narrative is a personal account of an individual's life and it is important to consider how they have chosen to express this. This will help you to understand the person as a whole, including their wider social and cultural context, and will enable you both to reflect on the meaning of self-harm throughout the narrative.

Step 3: Developing an understanding of the person's support needs around their self-harm

Once Veronica felt that she had built a level of trust with Mandy, she began a conversation which helped her to understand the role of self-harm in her narrative, her support needs around self-harm, and how she could help her with these challenges.

This process could include the following questions:

- What is important to you and your community?
- What do you feel is going well in your life?
- What are your strengths? For example, abilities, knowledge, resources (such as important people and places).
- What would you like to change in your life?
- How can I support you to make these changes?
- What is important in the future? For example, hopes, dreams, aspirations.

As a nurse, it sometimes might feel like you need to tell people what to do about aspects of their lives (for example, that they should stop self-harming), and you might feel that you are responsible for changing their behaviour. However, your role is to support them to make the changes they want to make in their life. When someone honours you by sharing their narrative, it is important to listen without judgement and to give them space and allow them to own and lead the conversation. This approach will help you to develop an understanding of the person's experiences and self-harming behaviours, and develop a support plan that is truly person centered and based on their individual needs. The questions outlined above do not directly address self-harm, but they will elicit experiences that are related to these behaviours, and will help someone to share their narrative in a way that makes them feel stronger. This is because this approach is centered around the whole individual, and their assets as well as their support needs. As a nurse, you will play an important role in this process by using your knowledge and skills to support the person to reflect on their narrative journey, for example by using active listening skills such as questioning, summarising, clarifying and reflecting.

Step 4: Co-designing a plan to meet the support needs around self-harm

Veronica and Mandy used this narrative to put together a support plan (Table 39.1). This plan outlined how Veronica could support Mandy and how Mandy could use her assets to support herself. It recognised the strategies that Mandy had developed to manage her feelings as assets and not problems. For example, Mandy sees her self ligaturing as an asset because it enabled her to complete her teacher training course. Creating a support plan can involve:

- reflecting together on the person's narrative
- constructing an understanding of what self-harm means to that person
- exploring ideas and options together about what might help
- deciding on actions, drawing on the assets of the person and the nurse
- contingency planning (e.g. what to do if Veronica is not available or Mandy's mental health support needs increase)
- agreeing when, where and how to review the plan.

Step 5: Reviewing the support plan

Mandy and Veronica review their support plan every week. This means reflecting on the actions from both their perspectives (for example, after Veronica and Mandy's conversations with Jon, he told Mandy he felt much more confident and able to talk about her self-harm and support her) and together amending support needs and actions when necessary.

Table 39.1 Examples from Mandy's support plan

My support needs	I want to be able to talk to Jon about my self-harm.	I want to be able to manage my feelings when I am on the ward.
What I can do to meet these needs	I have asked Veronica for support with this. I have identified that Tuesday before ward round would be the best time to do this, in a local café.	Self-ligaturing helps me to manage my feelings and get through the day. I can ask Veronica for my headphones when I am feeling upset. If I self-harm I will speak with Veronica afterwards about how I am feeling.
What Veronica can do to support me	Veronica can help this process by using her skills and knowledge to offer Jon some support: I feel he avoids these conversations because he is anxious about making things worse.	Veronica can give me advice about how to self-harm in a safe way. If I self-harm she can make time to speak with me about it afterwards and can support me to understand the challenges I am experiencing, and identify how I can manage these challenges (e.g. explore what has worked for me in the past).

Step 6: Reflecting on endings and new beginnings

When your time supporting someone comes to an end, it is very important for you both to mark this occasion and reflect on what has been achieved during your time together.

For example, Veronica knows that Mandy is now able to manage her feelings, and that she has been able to support her to reach this point in her journey. Veronica has also gained new skills and knowledge and feels more confident in supporting others with similar challenges. Mandy feels less fearful about accessing services and is more able to talk about her way of managing her feelings.

Case studies 39.1 and 39.2 contain the narratives of two people who have experienced challenges around self-harm. Spend some time using the processes outlined above to reflect on these narratives and how you might be able to support these people.

CASE STUDY 39.1

Sharon's lived experience narrative account

I was in my mid thirties when I first told a GP I'd been self-harming. I'd actually been self-harming in various ways since the age of 13. The GP prescribed Effexor which just zombified me and I couldn't function at work so I stopped taking it after a few days. I saw the GP for other reasons but she never asked me about self-harming or even about the medication she'd prescribed.

I was sent to an occupational health doctor after I'd self-harmed at work in my early forties. The doctor told me I was self-harming as a form of attention seeking. He told my employers that I'd be fit to work after a week of sick leave but they sacked me. Apparently, self-harm made me a danger to others.

It took more incidents of self-harm and together with suicidal hysteria before another GP referred me to psychological services, aged 43. Eventually I had 18 months of psychodynamic psychotherapy which helped me to understand the origin of my self-harm (1970s domestic violence and ignored selective mutism) but it didn't give me any way of dealing with it. Often it left me feeling isolated, bereft, hopeless – the kind of feelings that often trigger self-harm for me.

One of the worst episodes for me was when I self-harmed in a GP's room and for some reason he put his hand on my hand. When I saw another GP in the same practice he told me that if I ever self-harmed again in the surgery he would bar me from the practice.

Aged 46 I finally had a diagnosis of BPD [borderline personality disorder] which led to me being able to access a DBT [dialectical behaviour therapy] course together with the type of input from a clinical psychologist that worked for me. I could phone in once a week, or they would phone me just to chat for 15 minutes about what I was doing and how I was coping. DBT is the only support I have had that has worked because it has enabled me to experiment with my own ideas and solutions and to share experiences in an empathetic supportive way.

This lived experience narrative demonstrates the role of other professionals and how this can shape a person's understanding of their self-harm.

Questions

Reflecting on the above narrative, what would you like to ask Sharon? What more would you want to know about her story to help you support her to manage her self-harm?

Some suggested solutions:

- Thinking about now, and when you were 13, is there a difference in how you understand your self-harm?
- Sharon, could you explain to me why this episode with the GP was so challenging for you? What could have been done differently?
- Can you tell me more about why you think DBT was so helpful?

CASE STUDY 39.2

David's lived experience narrative account

When I came to the UK I never imagined that I would have become unwell and end up being sectioned, and then it come to pass that I found myself in a place where the doors were locked and people were being abusive and talking in a language that I could not understand.

I felt worried and out of control of my body and mind. As a man that had grown and has some freedom, the fact that I could not express my inner feelings of anger and anxiety was hurting me at my core.

My anxiety become so bad that I need someone to talk to and the nurses on the ward were unable to speak Polish and I was trying to communicate but no one seemed to want to help and talk to me, not even touch me! I remember just feeling so alone and scared and thinking how was I going to get out of here if I couldn't communicate. The distress became something that was so unbearable that I could not take it anymore. I went to my room, and I don't know how or why, I cut my self with a plastic pen, but the feeling when I cut myself was that of freedom from the internal pain of my distress – it left my body for that moment and I felt so much better. For the first time I felt in control as they had taken my liberty away and then my access to

(Continued)

support by not giving access to interpreters, but they could not take my inner pain away. The blood and cutting made me feel alive and in control of my own body and mind. I felt liberated and free from the feeling of being nothing.

This lived experience extract is an account of how communication difficulties and also the inpatient environment can have an impact on self-harm.

Questions

How might you be able to support David? What would he need to be able to be heard?
    Some suggested solutions:

- protected engagement time with a translator to discuss his needs
- providing information and resources that are accessible to him.

SELF-HARM, SUICIDE AND SUICIDAL FEELINGS

The relationship between self-harm and suicidal feelings

For many people, self-harm helps them to continue living and we know from research that most people do not use methods that put their life at risk. However, there is a strong link between self-harm, suicidal feelings and suicide. Studies have found that people who self-harm are more likely to die by suicide than those who do not, and a history of self-harm is the strongest predictor of suicide, over and above other experiences such as depression, hopelessness and childhood abuse (Sakinofsky, 2000). This does not mean that everyone who self-harms is suicidal. Studies have found that between 45% and 58% of people who self-harm have thought about taking their own life, and around 3% of people who self-harm will die by suicide (Bebbington et al., 2010; Hawton et al., 2002). We are only just starting to understand the relationship between self-harm, suicidal feelings and suicide, but current evidence suggests that these are part of a complex spectrum of behaviours. Some people who self-harm will never feel suicidal, whilst others say that these feelings can fluctuate (so sometimes they feel suicidal when they self-harm, and at other times they don't). Sometimes, when people are feeling particularly distressed, an act of self-harm may escalate into something more dangerous which could put their life at risk. At other times, people will carry out a planned act of self-harm which they know might end their life. It is therefore important never to make any assumptions about whether or not a person who is self-harming is feeling suicidal. Instead, it is important to have ongoing conversations with them about how they are feeling.

Talking about suicidal feelings

During your conversations with someone who self-harms, they might mention that they have feelings that could be considered to be suicidal in nature. For example:

Joshua: 'I wish something bad would happen to me.'

Sabina: 'I just want to take all my medication and not wake up in the morning.'

Peter: 'When I'm at the bus stop and I see the bus coming, sometimes I think about jumping out in front of it.'

Ade: 'I feel like getting a rope and ending it all.'

Suicidal feelings and ideation can take many different forms and are very personal experiences, so it is important that you allow people to define these feelings for themselves. This involves looking beyond what they have said and considering what it means to them, what they are feeling, their understanding of the situation and what you could do to help. The following are some possible responses to some of the examples above.

Making assumptions about the meaning of what was said

Sabina felt safe enough to voice the above with her named nurse, Mia. Without talking to Sabina about this, Mia decided that Sabina was suicidal. She described this in her notes as 'active suicidal ideation' and it was discussed at ward round. As a result, Sabina had her leave suspended and was placed under observation. Sabina felt this was very intrusive and did not make sense as she did not have access to medication. For Sabina, this was a way of expressing how she was feeling inside (she felt that she had lost a lot of control since being on the ward), but it wasn't something she was planning to do.

In this example, Mia made an assumption about what Sabina was saying, and this had significant implications for Sabina, both in terms of her freedom and privacy (and consequently her wellbeing), and also her relationship with Mia, as she felt misunderstood.

Clarifying with the person the meaning of what was said

Ade said the above to his mum, who told his CPN, Martin. Martin called Ade and started to have a conversation with him:

Martin: 'I'm just calling to check in, I was wondering what you've been up to and what's been going on?'

Ade: 'I've not been feeling too well.'

Martin: 'What does "not feeling too well" mean'?

Ade: 'I'm just very low and I'm having bad images.'

Martin: 'Can you describe the images?'

Ade: 'I keep on thinking about buying a rope and hanging myself in the garden.'

Martin: 'OK, I'm not saying that you are going to do this, but I was just wondering if you could tell me on a scale of 1-10 how likely you think it is that you would?'

Ade: 'A seven.'

Martin: 'So how did you feel yesterday?'

Ade: 'About the same.'

Martin: 'Are you having these thoughts more often this week compared to last week? Is there anything you feel I could do to help you?'

Ade: 'No.'

Martin: 'I feel that I need to come and visit you as I have some concerns and I feel we need to have a bit more of a conversation about this and find a way of managing this together.'

Ade and Martin met and discussed how Ade was feeling, and agreed that Ade would attend a day hospital and that the home treatment team would visit at the weekend. Ade agreed to share his feelings with his support network (his mum and his friends). Ade said he would contact someone if these feelings increased.

This is an example of how you can have a conversation about suicidal feelings without making any assumptions about what the person is experiencing. It is important to have the conversation in a collaborative way (e.g. do not jump to conclusions, or make decisions about the actions you will take before speaking with the person). Your skills and knowledge are central to this process, and this is something that you will develop over time by having these conversations with people. As you develop new skills and gain confidence, it is also important to continue to have these conversations so that you do not overlook occasions when a person might be trying to tell you that they are suicidal.

'HARM-MINIMISATION' APPROACH

For a number of years now, some people with lived experience of self-harm have been calling for practitioners to adopt a 'harm-minimisation' approach, or 'supported self-harm'. This means 'accepting the need to self-harm as a valid method of survival until survival is possible by other means … and is about facing the reality of maximising safety in the event of self-harm' (Pembroke, 2009: 6). This approach is advocated by some people who find that being prevented from self-harming is unsupportive. **'Supported self-harm' practices** can include advising people on how to self-harm safely, how to clean their wounds, and supplying them with safer means to self-harm, such as clean blades. NICE guidance recommends 'tentative approaches to harm reduction for some people who self-harm' within the community (NICE, 2011: 259). However, research has found that nurses have mixed views of this approach, and some feel very strongly that it is wrong (James et al., 2017). There is currently very little research evidence for harm minimisation. There have been no studies exploring the experiences of people who are supported to self-harm and just one study has examined the impact of these practices on the incidence of self-harm. The study found that after a service had introduced supported self-harm practices, there was a significant decrease in the number of incidents during an admission (Birch et al., 2011). This research evidence has significant limitations as it only involved a small number of **service users** and no controls, however in our experience there is a lot of anecdotal evidence, from a wide range of people, including people with lived experience of self-harm, **carers** and practitioners, that harm minimisation is beneficial in the management of self-harm. For example, it is empowering, supports the development of trusting therapeutic relationships, is less stigmatising, and helps people who self-harm and professionals to see beyond the self-harming behaviour and focus on the assets of the individual (James et al., 2017).

CRITICAL THINKING STOP POINT 39.4

How do you feel about supported self-harm practices? Do you think they could be helpful? Why?

CHAPTER SUMMARY

This chapter has covered:

- The meaning of self-harm
- The importance of reflective practice and how you can develop this
- A narrative approach to supporting people who have challenges around self-harm
- The relationship between self-harm and suicidal feelings
- How to talk about suicidal thoughts and feelings with people who have challenges around self-harm.

BUILD YOUR BIBLIOGRAPHY

Books

- Babiker, G. & Arnold, L. (1997) *The language of injury: Comprehending self-mutilation*. Oxford: Blackwell. An excellent book about self-harm, including guidance for practitioners working in a range of different settings.
- Bassot, B. (2013) *The reflective journal*. London: Palgrave Macmillan. An introduction to critically reflective practice, including exercises and space where you can write your own reflections.
- Cutcliffe, J. & Stevenson, C. (2007) *Care of the suicidal person*. London: Churchill Livingstone. This book explains an evidence-based theory of how nurses can care for people who are feeling suicidal.

SAGE journal articles

Go to https://study.sagepub.com/essentialmentalhealth for further free online journal articles related to this chapter. If you are using the interactive ebook, simply click on the book icon in the margin to go straight to the resource.

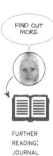

FIND OUT MORE

FURTHER READING: JOURNAL ARTICLES

- Edwards, S.D. & Hewitt, J. (2011) Can supervising self-harm be part of ethical nursing practice? *Nursing Ethics*, 18(1), 79-87. Covers key issues in the debate around supported self-harm practices from a nursing perspective.
- Hughes, N.D., Locock, L., Simkin, S., et al. (2015) Making sense of an unknown terrain: how parents understand self-harm in young people. *Qualitative Health Research*, 27(2), 215-225. An interesting study about how parents make sense of self-harm, including implications for practice.

Other journal articles

- Townsend, E. (2014) Self-harm in young people. *Evidence Based Mental Health*, 17(4), 97-99. A review of research evidence in this field and recommendations about how practitioners can support young people who self-harm.

Weblinks

Go to https://study.sagepub.com/essentialmentalhealth for further weblinks related to this chapter. If you are using the interactive ebook, simply click on the book icon in the margin to go straight to the resource.

FURTHER READING: WEBLINKS

- www.narrativetherapylibrary.com – includes free downloads and resources about narrative practices
- www.thesite.org/mental-health/self-harm – an online guide about self-harm, which includes video testimonies from people who have experienced challenges around self-harm
- www.thinklocalactpersonal.org.uk/personalised-care-and-support-planning-tool – a website to help with support planning.

Other resources

- Dace, A., Faulkner, A., Frost, M., et al. (1998) *The 'hurt yourself less' workbook*. Available at: http://studymore.org.uk/hylw.pdf. A resource to help people explore and understand their self-harm.

- National Institute for Health and Clinical Excellence (NICE) (2011) *Self-harm: longer-term management*. Clinical guideline CG133. London: NICE. Clinical recommendations about how to support people who self-harm.
- McPin Foundation (2015) *Wellbeing networks and asset mapping: Useful tools for recovery focused mental health practice*. Available at: http://mcpin.org/wp-content/uploads/Our-briefing-paper.pdf. A briefing paper outlining a person-centred, asset-mapping approach which you might find useful when developing a care plan with someone who self-harms.

ACE YOUR ASSESSMENT

ONLINE
QUIZZES &
ACTIVITY
ANSWERS

Revise what you have learned by visiting https://study.sagepub.com/essentialmentalhealth. If you are using the interactive ebook, simply click on the tick icon to go straight to the resource.

- Test yourself with multiple-choice and short-answer questions and flashcards.

REFERENCES

Bebbington, P.E., Minot, S., Cooper, C., et al. (2010) Suicidal ideation, self-harm and attempted suicide: results from the British psychiatric morbidity survey 2000. *European Psychiatry*, *25*(7), 427–431.

Birch, S., Cole, S., Hunt, K., et al. (2011) Self-harm and the positive risk taking approach. Can being able to think about the possibility of harm reduce the frequency of actual harm? *Journal of Mental Health*, 20(3), 293–303.

Briere, J. & Gil, E. (1998) Self-mutilation in clinical and general population samples: prevalence, correlates, and functions. *American Journal of Orthopsychiatry*, *68*(4), 609–620.

Glenn, C.R. & Klonsky, E.D. (2010) The role of seeing blood in non-suicidal self-injury. *Journal of Clinical Psychology*, *66*(4), 466–473.

Haines, J., Williams, C.L., Brain, K.L., et al. (1995) The psychophysiology of self-mutilation. *Journal of abnormal psychology*, 104(3), 471.

Haw, C., Hawton, K., Houston, K., et al. (2001) Psychiatric and personality disorders in deliberate self-harm patients. *The British Journal of Psychiatry*, *178*(1), 48–54.

Hawton, K., Rodham, K., Evans, E., et al. (2002) Deliberate self-harm in adolescents: self report survey in schools in England. BMJ, *325*(7374), 1207–1211.

Hawton, K.K., Townsend, E., Arensman, E., et al. (2015) Psychosocial and pharmacological treatments for deliberate self-harm. *Cochrane Database of Systematic Reviews*, *2*, CD001764.

Herpertz, S. (1995) Self-injurious behaviour: psychopathological and nosological characteristics in subtypes of self-injurers. *Acta Psychiatrica Scandinavica*, *91*(1), 57–68.

James, K. (2015) *The characteristics of inpatient self-harm and the perceptions of nursing staff*. PhD thesis, King's College London. Available at: https://kclpure.kcl.ac.uk/portal/en/theses/search.html (accessed 16/08/17).

James, K., Stewart, D. & Bowers, L. (2012) Self-harm and attempted suicide within inpatient psychiatric services: a review of the literature. *International Journal of Mental Health Nursing*, *21*(4), 301–309.

James, K., Samuels, T., Moran, P., et al. (2017) Harm reduction as a strategy for supporting people who self-harm on mental health wards: the views and experiences of practitioners. *Journal of Affective Disorders*, 214: 67–73.

Klonsky, E.D., Oltmanns, T.F. & Turkheimer, E. (2003) Deliberate self-harm in a nonclinical population: prevalence and psychological correlates. *American Journal of Psychiatry*, *160*(8), 1501–1508.

Moran, P., Coffey, C., Romaniuk, H., et al. (2012) The natural history of self-harm from adolescence to young adulthood: a population-based cohort study. *The Lancet*, *379*(9812), 236–243.

National Institute for Health and Clinical Excellence (2011) *Self-harm in over-8s: Long-term management*. Clinical guideline CG133. London: NICE.

Niedtfeld, I., Schulze, L., Kirsch, P., et al. (2010) Affect regulation and pain in borderline personality disorder: a possible link to the understanding of self-injury. *Biological psychiatry*, *68*(4), 383–391.

Pembroke, L.R. (2009) *Self-Harm: Perspectives From Personal Experience* Kindle edition. Chipmunkapublishing.com

Sakinofsky, I. (2000) Repetition of suicidal behaviour. In *The international handbook of suicide and attempted suicide*. Chichester: John Wiley & Sons. pp. 385–404.

Scoliers, G., Portzky, G., Madge, N., et al. (2009) Reasons for adolescent deliberate self-harm: a cry of pain and/or a cry for help? *Social Psychiatry and Psychiatric Epidemiology*, *44*(8), 601–607.

PALLIATIVE AND END-OF-LIFE CARE IN MENTAL HEALTH CARE

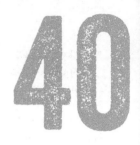

JAYNE BREEZE, CAROL COOPER, ANGELA KYDD, SUZANNE MONKS, JULIE SKILBECK, JAMES TURNER, ELEANOR WILSON

THIS CHAPTER COVERS

- Whether it is important to consider palliative and end-of-life care for people with mental health needs
- The terms that can be used when caring for people who may be in the last year of their life
- How to identify a service user who may be in the last year of their life
- The importance of identifying tools to aid communication and care planning, around palliative and end-of-life care needs
- What support is helpful for professional carers when caring for people in the last year of life.

> **"** When she comes [Nurse] she generally has a chat to me to see what I've been up to, make sure I'm active. They like to keep you active – still doing your crossword in the paper, and that sort of thing. Note the things I've done at church, because that's how you're social and you have to be talking quite a lot there. So she'll always do that first and then she can tell if I'm still the same or if I've got any worse ... It sounds just like chatter but it isn't really because it's important that she can tell whether I've got any better or worse. **"**
>
> **Service user (Wilson, 2013)**

> **"** With Huntington's you've got time to plan ... I've got a gentleman who is at end stage in a nursing home just now, and they're managing him fantastic with the GP. He's on full pain control. We've taken him off all the previous medication. I have regular contact with tissue viability [nurse] who goes in to just advise ... Other issues about palliative care are about what do people want near the end too. We do, as a team, try to gain that information from the user. It's a hard thing to actually broach when someone's still fairly healthy but, at some point they're not going to be able to communicate or there's going to be a question about capacity. **"**
>
> **Specialist nurse (Wilson, 2013)**

Visit **https://study.sagepub.com/essentialmentalhealth** to access a wealth of online resources for this chapter – watch out for the margin icons throughout the chapter. If you are using the Interactive ebook, simply click on the margin icon to go straight to the resource.

> I was working on a care of older people with Dementia ward and we were looking after a lady, diagnosed with Alzheimer's disease but still able to function quite well. She appeared to be deteriorating physically and the qualified nurses weren't sure how best to help. They had her transferred to a general ward but they quickly sent her back saying there was nothing they could do. A few days later she died and I was left thinking: could we have cared for her better?
>
> **Second-year mental health nursing student**

INTRODUCTION

In this chapter, we will focus on people with **dementia** and illustrate how the **palliative care** and the **recovery** approach are intertwined. Many nurses are uncertain about their role in **end-of-life** care and we intend to give you ideas on when, how and what you can contribute, both for **service users** who are inpatients and those who live in their own homes.

The concept of a recovery model in mental health has served to bring about positive changes in how people with mental illness and mental health **disorders** are viewed by both professionals and the public alike. The recovery model became popular in the 1990s (for example, Anthony, 1993) and gives a message of hope and optimism that individuals can live well with mental health problems. The model has its roots in spiritualty (Gomi et al., 2014), in that it enables people, with varying degrees of support, to find meaning, purpose and hope in their lives. It is not without its critics, with some authors such as Lukens and Solomon (2013) arguing that in giving vulnerable people choices at times when they are not ready to make such choices, this can result in poor treatment outcomes. In addition, a recovery model is not all embracing, as there are diseases that are progressive in their debilitating nature and that are life limiting. For people with dementia, a recovery model can serve to help people with these diseases, but given the fact that people die from dementia (or a related complication), it is important for mental health nurses to study the palliative care approach for those whose lives are limited. At first glance, palliative care and mental health care may seem to be poles apart, but when analysed more closely there are several links between these two areas. The recovery model and the palliative care approach can be seen as a logical continuum of care which complements the whole patient experience by helping an individual to live well with their disease and to die well with their disease.

WHY CONSIDER PALLIATIVE CARE AND END-OF-LIFE CARE FOR PEOPLE WITH MENTAL HEALTH PROBLEMS?

In the UK, the public health approach to end-of-life care has become increasingly prominent (Paul & Sallnow, 2012), with the recognition that the scope of palliative care service provision should be extended to those service users experiencing severe and enduring mental health problems. It is now widely acknowledged that service users with severe and enduring mental health problems are living longer and growing older (WHO, 2015), and there is evidence to suggest that service users with mental health problems are more likely to have comorbidities and complex health care needs towards the end of their life. As a mental health student and throughout your professional career, you are likely to care for many people approaching the end of their life (Watts & Davies, 2014). Before we go any further, we need to clarify what we mean by palliative and end-of-life care and recovery.

It is acknowledged that health and social care professionals and the general public find the terms used to describe end-of-life care confusing. The myriad of available terms can be interpreted differently in a variety of contexts, with the implication that it is difficult to work in partnership with service users in order to provide appropriate end-of-life care (Kydd, 2015). The common terms which are used are: palliative, end of life, terminal, advanced care planning and dying. In considering the relationship between recovery and palliative care and end-of-life care for people with mental health problems, we need to clearly define the terms we are using in this chapter.

What is palliative care?

Palliative care is an approach that improves the quality of life of patients and their families facing problems associated with life-threatening illness, through the prevention and relief of suffering by means of early identification and impeccable assessment and treatment of pain and other problems, physical, psychosocial and spiritual. Palliative care:

- provides relief from pain and other distressing symptoms
- affirms life and regards dying as a normal process
- intends neither to hasten nor postpone death
- integrates the psychological and spiritual aspects of patient care
- offers a support system to help patients live as actively as possible until death
- offers a support system to help the family cope during the patient's **illness** and in their own bereavement
- uses a team approach to address the needs of patients and their families
- enhances quality of life and may also positively influence the course of illness
- is applicable early in the course of illness, in conjunction with other therapies that are intended to prolong life, and includes those investigations needed to better understand and manage clinical complications.

Palliative care can be provided by a range of health and social care staff and may be done alongside treatment intended to reverse particular conditions (WHO, 2014).

What is end of life?

Patients are 'approaching the end of life' when they are likely to die within the next 12 months. This includes patients whose death is imminent (expected within a few hours or days) and those with: (a) advanced, progressive, incurable conditions; and (b) general frailty and coexisting conditions that mean they are expected to die within 12 months (Leadership Alliance for the Care of Dying People (LACDP), 2014a).

What are the last days/hours of life?

This time frame is more difficult to define as many people call it different things, such as the terminal phase, dying, the end stage. The latest evidence suggests that it is more useful to acknowledge this phase, where possible, as the last days or hours of life, which falls within the end of life (last 12 months of life) definition (see definition of end of life in LACDP, 2014b).

Everyone deserves the right to a good death with early recognition that a person may be approaching the end of their life, with honest and open communication between the service user and health and social care professionals. People are then provided with choice about the care they would like to receive and where they would like to receive that care. Current policies and guidance are readily available for health and social care staff to help guide care surrounding palliative and end-of-life care (see Table 40.1). The range of strategies reflects the fact that some people may be considered to have palliative care needs for a long period of time, or for non-curative conditions such as Huntington's disease, from diagnosis.

Table 40.1 Policies and guidance for palliative and end-of-life care

- National End of Life Care Strategy (DH 2008)
- Priorities of Care for the Dying Person (Leadership Alliance for the Care of Dying People 2014a)
- One Chance to Get it Right (Leadership Alliance for the Care of Dying People 2014b)
- National Dementia Strategy (DH 2009)
- NSF Neurological Long Term Conditions (DH 2005)
- Mental Capacity Act 2005
- NICE Supportive and Palliative Care (NICE 2004)

Key attributes from the policies include:

- treating service users and those identified as important to them with dignity and respect
- involving them both in decisions about treatment and care as much as they want to be
- identifying and actively exploring the needs of the dying person, and their families, and ensuring that they are explored, respected and met as far as possible; this includes recording preferences and wishes and creating an individual plan of care which is agreed, coordinated and delivered with compassion
- alleviating pain and other symptoms.

As the focus of this chapter is on dementia, let us now consider some facts relating to this range of conditions.

DEMENTIA FACTS

Dementia is a frequently used term which actually covers a wide range of different conditions that are connected by the fact that they all involve the death of brain cells. Brain cells cannot be replaced so, consequently, depending on which area of the brain is affected, a variety of challenges for individuals to surmount arise. The main types of dementia which you will encounter are Alzheimer's, Vascular, Lewy Body disease and rarer conditions such as Picks disease and Huntington's disease. Alzheimer's, Vascular and Lewy Body disease are more common in older people, while Picks and Huntington's disease are usually diagnosed at a much younger age.

According to the Alzheimer's Society (2015), it is estimated that there are currently 850,000 people with dementia (including Huntington's disease) living in the UK. Of this number, there are over 40,000 people with early-onset dementia (onset before the age of 65 years). This is expected to increase to over 1 million by 2025 and over 2 million by 2051. The National Dementia Strategy (DH, 2009) has highlighted the need for us to be aware that dementia is terminal and so the chasm between dementia and palliative care needs to be bridged (Dempsey et al., 2015). At least 100,000 people die each year with dementia, according to Lawrence et al. (2011). However, despite national policy which clearly promotes good end-of-life care for all, irrespective of diagnosis, evidence suggests that people with dementia and their families receive poor quality care at the end of life (Lawrence et al., 2011; Monroe & Hansford, 2010; Ryan et al., 2011). Some of the reasons put forward to explain this are that **carers** frequently do not realise that dementia is a terminal illness (Sleeman et al., 2014) and often attribute changes to deterioration in their dementia. Monroe & Hansford (2010) also argue that professionals too often fail to recognise the signs of impending death, so fail to address these needs appropriately. There can be issues of communication, decision making about nutrition and technologies of life support, and family care (Wilson et al., 2014), making long-term care planning difficult.

WHAT'S THE EVIDENCE? 40.1

Read the following article: Dempsey, L., Dowling, M., Larkin, P., et al. (2015) The unmet palliative care needs of those dying with dementia. *International Journal of Palliative Nursing, 21*(3), 126-133.
  Now consider the questions below:

- What do you think are the barriers to providing palliative and end-of-life care to service users with dementia?
- How could you get round some of these barriers in your workplace so that you can provide palliative and end-of-life care to service users with dementia?

RECOVERY AND END-OF-LIFE CARE

All professionals have a responsibility to provide a general level of palliative and end-of-life care. Palliative care comes under the umbrella term of supportive care (NICE, 2004). It embraces the 'holistic' approach to health care and focuses on quality of life, emphasising open communication, autonomy and choice. The WHO (2014) has adopted an explicitly public health **orientation** to palliative care, promoting a broad vision as relevant to all those with chronic illness and their families, whilst working collaboratively with other health and social care providers. Where people have complex conditions or symptoms, referrals can be made to specialist palliative care. This care is provided by trained health care professionals with specialist knowledge and skills.

The concept and application of recovery is now firmly ensconced in mental health care. The chief nursing officer, in her review of mental health nursing (DH, 2006: 4), asserted: 'Mental health nursing should incorporate the broad principles of the Recovery Approach into every aspect of their practice'. She goes on to point out that this includes palliative care.

Whilst the concept of recovery is a contested term, it is widely agreed that it is a way of living a satisfying, hopeful and contributing life, even with limitations caused by illness (as proposed by Anthony, 1993). Essentially, recovery is not dependent on diagnosis, prognosis or illness symptoms, and therefore is not precluded from end-of-life care.

The compatibility of the recovery approach with the palliative care model can be clearly seen when comparing the components of the process of recovery with some of the domains of the *Every Moment Counts* (EMC) document, produced for NHS England by National Voices in 2014 and incorporated into

'Actions for End-of-life Care' (NHS England, 2014). It has been suggested that there are four components to the process of recovery:

- finding and maintaining hope
- discovering (or re-discovering) a positive identity
- building a meaningful life
- taking responsibility and control. (Shepherd et al., 2010)

CASE STUDIES

We will now explore the relationship between recovery and end-of-life care in more detail. In particular, we will illustrate how you can use the four components of recovery, noted earlier, in your nursing care of people who have dementia and palliative care needs. We have drawn together a composite of service user experiences from the clinical setting to illustrate key issues relating to recovery and palliative and end-of-life care. These form two patient cases for the purpose of this chapter (Case studies 40.1 and 40.2); pseudonyms have been used to maintain confidentiality.

CASE STUDY 40.1

Sylvia, a 72-year-old widowed woman, was referred by her GP to the old adult community mental health team. She has a history of short-term memory loss and difficulties with the activities of daily living (driving, shopping, writing letters), which has been evident for the past six months. Her medical history showed no vascular risk factors. Her mother had a history of dementia and died in her 80s. Sylvia had worked as a teacher prior to retirement, was married for 42 years and had one child. She is a non-smoker and drinks 1-2 units of alcohol per week, and enjoys gardening, reading and walking. She scored 79/100 on Addenbrooke's Cognitive Examination (ACE-R) (Mioshi et al., 2006) and had a Mini-Mental State Examination (MMSE) score of 27/30 (Folstein et al., 1975). She has now been diagnosed with Alzheimer's disease.

Question

- Does Sylvia have any palliative care needs?

CASE STUDY 40.2

Michael is 56 years of age and has been diagnosed with Huntington's disease for 15 years. He is married to Jane, they have two children, one of whom still lives at home. Michael took early retirement from a government position due to his diagnosis. He has lived in a care home for the past three years. Michael is becoming increasingly unsteady on his feet and has recently fallen. He requires full assistance with washing and dressing. He has recently had a Percutaneous Endoscopic Gastrostomy (PEG) fitted as his swallowing and speech have now almost completely gone.

(Continued)

Question

- Does Michael have any palliative care needs?

As a student nurse when planning care, these are some of the issues that you would need to consider:

- How do you recognise when a service user is in the last year of life and/or dying?
- What informs the assessment, planning and delivery of their care?

Case studies 40.1 and 40.2 will feed into two sections highlighting areas that you might like to consider: (i) holistic and person-centred needs, including practical support; and (ii) advanced care planning, which also cover issues pertaining to capacity and autonomy. These two sections will also incorporate the relevant aspects of recovery, as previously discussed.

HOLISTIC AND PERSON-CENTRED NEEDS

Sylvia and Michael are clearly at different stages in their disease trajectory and therefore it is important to acknowledge and identify, where possible, the transition from living to actively dying with dementia. As Goodman et al. (2013) highlighted, it is important that we, as nurses, are able to consider the signs and symptoms that may help us identify that someone is approaching their end of life and therefore plan appropriate care with the person with dementia and their family.

Signs and symptoms indicating a person is reaching the last days of life

Signs include:

- **agitation**
- deterioration in levels of consciousness
- mottled skin
- noisy respiratory secretions
- progressive weight loss
- decreased urine output
- Cheyne–Stokes breathing (altered breathing patterns).

Symptoms include:

- increase in fatigue
- loss of appetite.

Functional observations include:

- changes in communication
- deteriorating mobility
- performance status (changes in the activities of daily living)
- social withdrawal. (Adapted from NICE, 2015)

As we can see from Sylvia's case study (40.1), she is an independent woman who is experiencing some problems autonomously in carrying out her activities of daily living. It will be important to reassure her that your role is to work alongside her and ensure that she remains independent for as long as possible (Sanderson & Bailey, 2014). One way to enhance this is through open and honest communication with Sylvia and her family about her future (Andrews et al., 2017).

Michael, in contrast (Case study 40.2), has multiple needs, for example he has fallen, he is unable to wash and dress, his swallow and speech have almost completely gone and he requires feeding through a PEG. These signs and symptoms indicate that Michael may be nearing the last months, weeks or even days of his life. However, he could also live for many years, so his wishes need to include how he wishes to live as well as how he would prefer to die.

Ryan et al. (2011) noted the significance of weight loss, motor disability and a decline in physical health and that they can be used as indicators that a person with dementia could be in the last year of life. Clearly, Michael and his family would need a full holistic assessment of his care requirements as he possibly enters the last year or last months of life, thus ensuring that his physical, emotional, spiritual and practical needs are met now and in the future. Knowledge of the principles of palliative care and symptom management, along with caregiving skills for people at the end of life, is essential. This would include, as Sampson et al. (2011) suggest, a focus on the most common problems experienced by people with dementia at the end of their lives, such as pain, pressure sores due to immobility and feeding problems – those that would benefit from good basic care. For example, in relation to pain it is important to undertake a comprehensive pain assessment, including signs that might indicate pain when a person cannot indicate this verbally. In Michael's case, the assessment of facial expressions, movements and changes in **personality** would be required (Lawrence et al., 2011). When symptoms become complex, referral to specialist care teams may be appropriate, however this should not overshadow attending to basic care needs such as eating, drinking and hygiene (Lawrence et al., 2011).

We would argue that this links nicely to one of the important aspects of recovery: hope.

Finding and maintaining hope

Hope is the gateway to recovery and involves believing in oneself and having some optimism for the future, which can be enhanced by having more agency and active control over one's life. This relates to the *Every Moment Counts* (EMC) domain of 'my physical, emotional, spiritual and practical needs are met', which involves receiving the information, care and support needed to feel 'at peace' with what will happen in the future. Hope-inspiring relationships are central to hope (Repper & Perkins, 2003) and this EMC domain suggests that nurses can help the person at the end of their life to feel safe, with as little fear as possible.

Now, if we look back at Sylvia and Michael, it is important that both they and their family have a chance to tell their carers about their life to date but also to discuss their future wants and wishes. As nurses, we must have knowledge of the person, and those significant to them, as well as of the disease process, in order to provide appropriate palliative and end-of-life care. In particular, Wilson (2013) identified that living while affected by Huntington's disease requires continued readjustment to maintain a balance between increasing disability, diminishing cognition and living well at home. The use of life story and family biographical approaches could provide opportunities to understand the person, looking beyond the diagnosis of dementia. McKeown et al. (2006) describe 'life story' as an opportunity to review and evaluate an individual's past life events. Here, it would involve working with Sylvia and Michael, and their families, to find out about their past and present lives, and recording that information in some way so that it could be used with Sylvia and Michael to guide the delivery of their person-centred care. As Thompson (2011) and Gibson and Carson (2010) point out, offering a critical review of life events enables the identification of present and future wishes. The 'This is me' programme (Alzheimer's Society & RCN, 2015) is one such tool that could be used to record Sylvia and Michael's past and present life in order to respect them as a whole in the context of living and dying.

Again, there seem to be clear links with our second important aspect of recovery: a new identity.

Re-discovering a positive identity

This is about finding a new identity, which incorporates illness, but retains a core, positive sense of self (Shepherd et al., 2010). This relates to the EMC domain 'we work for my goals and the quality of my life and death', which includes the aims 'I am respected as a whole person, not treated as an illness', 'my **care plan** records information about who I am: my life and past, what people **value** about me, my strengths and abilities, and my values' and 'people who care for and support me make a special effort to understand my life'.

Returning to our case studies, Sylvia may have the opportunity to meet new people in similar circumstances along with other forms of support to maintain her current lifestyle. For Michael, it will be important to maintain his current social relationships with his wife and children in spite of the current challenges posed by his increasing disability. He may be reassured that now he is receiving holistic care, this enables his family to re-establish their roles of child and wife rather than carer.

As Ryan et al. (2011) point out, palliative care for people with dementia should also include families and carers. The nurse needs to understand the stages of loss and bereavement, so that families and carers can receive appropriate and timely support to help them continue to care for their family member and also maintain their own personhood. Carers of people with dementia experience high levels of stress, strain and burden. Professionals should be aware of the differences between carers who have different relationships with the person with dementia, such as spouse or adult child, with different priorities and commitments (Davies et al., 2014). Relationships between the dying person and their significant others need to be forged and maintained in order to offer emotional support. This involves the sharing of information, spending time with and listening to them (Ryan et al., 2011).

This clearly parallels the third aspect of recovery: meaning in life.

Building a meaningful life

This involves making sense of the illness and finding a meaning in life despite the illness. Essentially, it means engaging in life. This relates to the same EMC domain as above. It is important to acknowledge the needs of the family/significant other as well as the person with dementia.

The second part of this involves continuing to achieve leisure- or work-related goals for as long as possible; maintaining social contacts; and living as actively and independently as possible at all stages of care and treatment.

ADVANCED CARE PLANNING

CASE STUDY: PALLIATIVE CARE TEAM

Looking back at our case studies, we believe that Sylvia should be approached to have her advanced care needs discussed and documented. For Michael, we would hope that this would have been undertaken at an earlier point in time. However, it is still not too late to ascertain his wishes, assuming that he still has capacity to do this.

Capacity and autonomy

There is now increasing evidence, particularly in relation to Huntington's disease, that changes in the brain take place long before the symptoms of dementia become evident (Harrington et al., 2012; Tribrizi, 2012). These prodromal symptoms not only produce subtle motor and psychiatric symptoms, but also cognitive changes. Changes continue throughout the disease trajectory, affecting cognition in a number of ways, including understanding and decision making. The Mental Capacity Act has been in force since 2005 to support people to make their own decisions.

There are five aspects to consider in relation to this. All adults are assumed to have the capacity to make their own decisions unless assessed otherwise. Second, any adult must be given all help available to make their own decisions before it is deemed that they lack capacity. Third, adults who make decisions that are seen as unwise cannot be deemed to be lacking capacity. Fourth, adults who are assessed as lacking capacity will be cared for using best interest decisions; and, fifth and finally, any of these decisions should be those that are least restrictive of their basic rights and freedom (Mental Capacity Act 2005).

There has been little to demonstrate what the effects of the Act have actually been for health and social care professionals working within this legislation. A study by Wilson et al. (2010) identified the need for a clearer understanding of the Mental Capacity Act, and particularly the terminology of the Act, in order for staff to hold discussions with patients and families for care planning. Similarly, social workers working with people with dementia were asked to reflect on the impact of the Mental Capacity Act on their casework and record keeping. Findings showed that the implementation of the Mental Capacity Act had significantly impacted the structure of decision making for the social workers, helping them to develop greater confidence in their assessment skills. Recognition of fluctuating capacity, involving people in their own decisions, and multi-disciplinary working were highlighted, as was the potential for social workers to take on roles as **advocates** and legal representatives (McDonald, 2010). Previous research with staff providing care to people with progressive long-term neurological conditions suggests capacity should be assessed according to the level of decision needed to be made (Wilson et al., 2010).

The Mental Capacity Act 2005 also provides for people who anticipate a loss of capacity at some future time, to draw up an 'advance decision' to refuse specified **medical treatment** in particular future circumstances (Wilson et al., 2010). An advance decision 'enables someone aged 18 and over, while still capable, to refuse specified medical treatment for a time in the future when they may lack the capacity to consent to or refuse that treatment' (Mental Capacity Act 2005). An advance decision will only come into effect when the individual has lost capacity to give or refuse consent to treatment (Halliday, 2009). **Advance care planning** has been highlighted as a beneficial strategy for people with dementia, as discussed by Dempsey (2013) and Sampson et al. (2011).

Advance care planning (ACP)

ACP is a discussion between an individual and their care provider to make clear a person's wishes and preferences. This will take place where there is an anticipated deterioration in a person's health, which may result in a loss of capacity and the ability to voice those wishes and preferences to others. With consent, the discussions should be documented, regularly reviewed and shared with key people involved in the person's care. Discussions could include: concerns raised by the individual, values and personal goals for care and the preference for certain types of treatment that may be beneficial in the future and the availability of these.

Advance care plans can include:

- Statement of wishes and preferences (such as the preferred priorities for care document): this is a term which embodies a range of written or verbally recorded oral expressions which can cover medical and non-medical elements. With consent, people can vocalise and have documented their wants, wishes and preferences in relation to future treatments or place of care, provide an explanation of their understanding of their current health condition and explain their beliefs and values which govern how they make decisions. These statements are not legally binding but should be used when decisions based on the best interests of the patient are made, in the event that they lose capacity to make those decisions or are not able to voice them.
- Lasting power of attorney: this is a legal form created by the Mental Capacity Act 2005. A person who has capacity may choose a person (an attorney) to make decisions on the person's behalf if they lose capacity. These can be financial decisions and/or health-related decisions.
- Advanced decisions to refuse treatment (ADRT): an ADRT is legally binding and relates to a refusal of specific medical treatment and can specify circumstances. The ADRT will come into effect when the person has lost capacity to give or refuse consent for treatment. It is essential to assess the validity and applicability of an advanced decision before it is used in clinical practice. (Department of Health, 2008)

Sampson et al. (2011) argue that ACP should be implemented in the earlier stages of dementia, whilst people are still able to make decisions and express their values and preferences clearly. However, it is not without challenges and, although it allows people to discuss and write down their wishes for future care (Thomas & Lobo, 2011), this is not commonplace for people with dementia (Dening et al., 2011). Difficulties with talking about dying equally make it difficult to plan for end-of-life care (Goodman et al., 2013). However, in the study by Goodman et al. (2013) it is clear that, if given the chance, people with dementia want to talk about how they should be cared for in the future. These conversations extend beyond the basics of physical needs and place of care (Moriaty et al., 2012). If these sometimes difficult conversations are left too late, then issues such as capacity to understand and consider information before communicating wishes can be compromised (Dempsey, 2013). Clearly, these decisions would need to be re-visited over time.

Place of care

Another aspect of taking control is thinking about where people want to be cared for and ultimately die, although it is important to recognise that this may change over time. Also, choices need to be achievable and feasible, for example many care homes and families are not equipped to deal with caring for people with dementia. This is a particular issue for those aged under 65. The hospice is seen as the gold standard when considering place of care, according to Sampson et al. (2011). However, hospitalisation is a frequent response to deterioration for people with dementia nearing the end of their lives (Sleeman et al., 2014). This may, in fact, increase confusion, worsen behavioural problems and lead to the development of pressure sores (Sleeman et al., 2014). What would be most important is that service users and their significant others have a choice in their place of care.

These issues are examples of the fourth component of recovery as identified earlier: control.

TAKING RESPONSIBILITY AND CONTROL

This involves feeling in control of illness and in control of life. It compares to the EMC domain – 'I have honest discussions and the chance to plan' – and involves professionals having timely and honest conversations with service users, no matter how difficult these might be for all concerned, in order that decisions about the best treatment, care and support can be made in partnership.

It can be argued therefore that the recovery approach and end-of-life care are underpinned by similar or shared values and can be implemented together. This would involve the mental health nurse seeing the person, and their life, before the illness; actively listening to what is important to the person and helping them to identify and prioritise their own goals for end-of-life care. Respect should be conveyed and a desire for true partnership working demonstrated. Regardless of the prognosis, we continue to show support for, and help with, achieving personal goals, i.e. maintaining hope.

As Dame Cicely Saunders, the founder of the modern hospice movement, said: 'You matter because you are you, and you matter to the end of your life' (NHS England, 2014: 4).

Nonetheless, it is also important to consider the professional carer's needs.

CRITICAL THINKING STOP POINT 40.1

Consider your own clinical supervision needs ... how often do you think you should receive support and how often does it actually happen? What might you do to manage this consistently?

CLINICAL SUPERVISION NEEDS

Working with service users with dementia at the end of life increases the complexity of care. Nurses need to support service users, their significant others and themselves, finding that although nursing is recognised as an occupation with stress, in both personal and professional areas, palliative care nursing is no more stressful than other specialities. In fact, Vachon (2000) noted that staff burnout is less than anticipated in palliative care settings, with staff experiencing less burnout than mental health professionals. However, mental health work is complex and demanding on many levels, and noticing the early signs of emotional exhaustion, fatigue and frustration can be the difference between feeling successful and positive compared to uncertainty. Because of this, it is important when we are working with service users with dementia at the end of life that we obtain clinical supervision within our work as it can provide an adequate intervention to manage emotional fatigue.

One student reflected on her experience of end-of-life care and supervision:

I did have supervision to discuss the emotions involved with working with the service user and their families. I also felt that my mentor was very supportive of helping me address any feelings I had towards the case, especially with it being such an emotive case and being my first year. We also discussed ways to remain professional but also display care and compassion whilst trying to not get too emotively involved. The support I had during that time was extremely valuable to me and really helped shape my nursing skills when I came across end-of-life care further into my nurse training.

Second-year nursing student

One of the first skills you have to develop is the 'listening to yourself' skill. If you find yourself feeling stressed and/or burned out, this should be a clear nudge towards taking up and managing your support and clinical supervision. In the authors' experience, supervision is a valuable reflective tool that not only helps with managing stress and complexity at work but also enables and supports learning and sets a 'bar' for a standard of work. Turner and Hill (2011a, 2011b; Hill & Turner, 2011) have reported on the development of clinical supervision within mental health services over a period of time and you might find their work useful if your service is struggling to implement or support practice.

Now that you have had a chance to read and reflect on this chapter, we will return to our original learning outcomes, identified in Critical thinking stop point 40.2, to see how you have developed.

CRITICAL THINKING STOP POINT 40.2

- Is palliative or end-of-life care important for those with mental health needs?
- What terms do you use when caring for people who may be in the last year of their life?
- How do you identify a service user who may be in the last year of their life?
- What tools to aid communication and care planning could you use with someone who may have palliative care needs?
- What support do you need when caring for people in the last year of life?

CRITICAL DEBATE 40.1

This chapter has explored the relationship between recovery and palliative and end-of-life care for people with dementia. It has identified that the process of recovery involves believing in oneself and having some optimism for the future, which can be enhanced by having more agency and active control over one's life. This is clearly challenging when a person with dementia is approaching the last year of life. For service users with a diagnosis of dementia, regardless of where they are in the illness trajectory, it is important to look beyond the diagnosis in order to understand the person. This can be achieved by accessing their life story in order to facilitate a person's wishes and wants for the present and the future in terms of end-of-life care. This can be challenging when a service user with dementia no longer has capacity. Now that you have worked through this chapter and considered the complex issues it raises, here are some questions to consider discussing with fellow students and colleagues:

1. How would you develop a relationship with a service user with dementia in order to ensure that their information, support and care needs are met?
2. What knowledge, skills and attitudes do you need to develop in order to work in partnership with the service user and other professionals to meet palliative and end-of-life care needs?

CHALLENGING CONCEPTS 40.1

Dementia is an umbrella term for diseases that cause brain cell death. Most dementias are progressive and degenerative and may result in death, but not all people with dementia die from this disease; they may die from other long-term conditions/disease. There are many different types of dementia, from dementias caused by injury (and these are not progressive) to dementias such as Huntington's disease where the symptoms of the disease can be very distressing and the progression rapid. Given the advances in dementia diagnostics, it is also the case that people with mild dementia can be diagnosed at a very early stage in their disease and these people may wish to get on with living their lives to the fullest extent they can – some remaining in employment, driving and caring for others. It may be that some people do not wish to consider advanced planning for their deaths – and such conversations should not be forced on them. As stated earlier, although dementia is progressive, some people will die from other, unrelated causes before their dementia becomes life-threatening. The key to recovery work and to palliative care/end-of-life care is finding out what is important to the individual.

CHAPTER SUMMARY

This chapter has covered:

- The clear links between palliative and end-of-life care and recovery. As a mental health nurse, this should offer some reassurance that you have some of the requisite knowledge and skills to work effectively with service users and their significant others when considering their needs at this time of life. Consequently, you can continue to provide holistic care for all service users throughout their life span
- Our case studies, Sylvia and Michael, who highlighted how to recognise a service user with palliative or end-of-life care needs. We also used these stories to discuss important care needs, including assessing, planning and delivering care at the end of life. An important aspect of this is that you remember to care for yourself as well as others. We argue that clinical supervision is an important part of this
- That in order to continue with improving palliative care for people with dementia, we are going to need more research, improvements in clinical care and education, as discussed by de Vries and Nowell (2011), to ensure we can meet these complex and challenging needs competently.

BUILD YOUR BIBLIOGRAPHY

Books

- Cooper, D. & Cooper, J. (2014) *Palliative care within mental health*. London: Radcliffe. This book has two chapters (11 and 12) devoted to the topic of dementia and palliative care as well as other topics that will be a useful starting point when learning about palliative care and dementia. It is written in a practical and easily accessible manner which makes it interesting and thought-provoking.
- Payne, S., Seymour, J. & Ingleton, C. (2008) *Palliative care nursing: Principles and evidence for practice*. Maidenhead: Open University Press. This book provides a comprehensive text for nurses working within palliative care.

- Repper, J. & Perkins, R. (2003) *Social inclusion and recovery*. London: Bailliere Tindall. This book focuses on ways in which direct care staff can assist people with mental health problems, reflecting on accounts of the nature and type of assistance which have been valuable, and the ways in which such help can best be offered. It addresses two key components of recovery: access to and inclusion in life opportunities, and acceptance.

SAGE journal articles

FURTHER READING: JOURNAL ARTICLES

Go to https://study.sagepub.com/essentialmentalhealth for further free online journal articles related to this chapter. If you are using the interactive ebook, simply click on the book icon in the margin to go straight to the resource.

- Ryan, T., Gardiner, C., Bellamy, G., et al. (2011) Barriers and facilitators to the receipt of palliative care for people with dementia: the views of medical and nursing staff. *Palliative Medicine*, *26*(7), 879–886.
- Wilson, E., Seymour, J.E. & Perkins, P. (2010) Working with the Mental Capacity Act: findings from palliative and specialist neurological care settings. *Palliative Medicine*, *24*(4), 396–402.

Other journal articles

- Sampson, E., Burns, A. & Richards, M. (2011) Improving end-of-life care for people with dementia. *The British Journal of Psychiatry*, *199*(5), 357–359.

Weblinks

FURTHER READING: WEBLINKS

Go to https://study.sagepub.com/essentialmentalhealth for further weblinks related to this chapter. If you are using the interactive ebook, simply click on the book icon in the margin to go straight to the resource.

- Curriculum for Dementia Education (HEDN, 2014): www.dementiauk.org/for-healthcare-professionals/free-resources/download-the-curriculum-for-dementia-education – this curriculum was created by senior academics who are also members of the UK dementia special interest group; core topic 9 outlines learning outcomes for student mental health nurses focusing on palliative care
- Implementing Recovery through Organisational Change (ImROC) programme: www.imroc.org – a website which supports local NHS and independent mental health service providers to become more 'recovery orientated'; it is a useful resource for accessing information on the principles of recovery and their application to practice
- National Council for Palliative Care (NCPC): www.ncpc.org.uk – the NCPC is the umbrella charity for all those involved in palliative, end-of-life and hospice care in England, Wales and Northern Ireland.

Briefing

- Moriarty, J., Rutter, D., Ross, P.D.S., et al. (2012) *SCIE research briefing 40: End-of-life care for people with dementia living in care homes*. London: Social Care Institute for Excellence. This briefing highlights many important aspects of end-of-life care that need to be considered.

Video link

VIDEO LINK 40: SOCIAL CARE TV

- Social Care TV: Dementia – End-of-life care: www.youtube.com/watch?v=3zKADdgcf14 –this interesting video showcases how palliative care can be delivered to individuals in a 24-hour care environment. Mrs Smart, a lady with advanced dementia, and her family are central to this explanation.

ACE YOUR ASSESSMENT

Revise what you have learned by visiting https://study.sagepub.com/essentialmentalhealth. If you are using the interactive ebook, simply click on the tick icon to go straight to the resource.

- Test yourself with multiple-choice and short-answer questions and flashcards.

ONLINE
QUIZZES &
ACTIVITY
ANSWERS

REFERENCES

Alzheimer's Society (2015) Home page. Available at: www.alzheimers.org.uk (accessed 23.11.17).

Alzheimer's Society & RCN (2015) *This is me*. London: Alzheimer's Society.

Andrews, S., McInerney, F., Toye, C., et al. (2017) Knowledge of dementia: do family members understand dementia as a terminal condition? *Dementia*, 16(5), 556–575.

Anthony, W.A. (1993) Recovery from mental illness: the guiding vision of the mental health service system in the 1990s. *Psychosocial Rehabilitation Journal*, 16, 11–23.

Davies, N., Maio, L., Rait, G., et al. (2014) Quality end-of-life care for dementia: what have family carers told us so far? A narrative synthesis. *Palliative Medicine*, 28(7), 919–930.

Dempsey, L. (2013) Advance care planning for people with dementia: benefits and challenges. *International Journal of Palliative Nursing*, 19(5), 227–234.

Dempsey, L., Dowling, M., Larkin, P., et al. (2015) The unmet palliative care needs of those dying with dementia. *International Journal of Palliative Nursing*, 21(3), 126–133.

Dening, K.H., Jones, L. & Sampson, E.L. (2011) Advance care planning for people with dementia: a review. *International Psychogeriatrics*, 23(10), 1535–1551.

Department of Health (2005) *National service framework (NSF) for longterm conditions*. London: DH. Available at: www.gov.uk/government/uploads/system/uploads/attachment_data/file/198114/National_Service_Framework_for_Long_Term_Conditions.pdf (accessed 16.08.17).

Department of Health (2006) *Chief nursing officer's review of mental health nursing*. London: The Stationery Office.

Department of Health (2008) *End-of-life care strategy*. London: The Stationery Office.

Department of Health (2009) *Living well with dementia: A national dementia strategy*. London: The Stationery Office.

De Vries, K. & Nowell, A. (2011) Dementia deaths in hospice: a retrospective case note audit. *International Journal of Palliative Nursing*, 17(12), 581–585.

Folstein, M.F., Folstein, S.E. & McHugh, P.R. (1975) 'Mini-mental state': a practical method for grading the cognitive state of patients for the clinician. *J Psychiatr Res*, 12(3), 189–198.

Gibson, F. & Carson, Y. (2010) Life story work in practice: aiming for enduring change. *Journal of Dementia Care*, 18, 20–22.

Gomi, S., Starnino, V. & Canda, E. (2014) Spiritual assessment in mental health recovery. *Community Mental Health Journal*, 50, 447–453.

Goodman, C., Amador, S., Elmore, N., et al. (2013) Preferences and priorities for ongoing and end-of-life care: a qualitative study of older people with dementia resident in care homes. *International Journal of Nursing Studies*, 50(12), 1639–1647.

Halliday, S. (2009) Advance decisions and the Mental Capacity Act. *British Journal of Nursing*, 18(11) 697–699.

Harrington, D., Smith, M., Zhang, Y., et al. & The PREDICT-HD Investigators of the Huntington Study Group (2012) Cognitive domains that predict time to diagnosis in prodromal Huntington disease. *Journal of Neurology, Neurosurgery & Psychiatry*, 83(6), 612–619.

Hill, A. and Turner, J. (2011) Implementing clinical supervision (part 3): an evaluation of a clinical supervisor's recovery-based resource and support package. *Mental Health Nursing (Online)*, *31*(5), 14–18.

Kydd, A. (2015) Palliative care: from oncology to all nursing arenas – good practice or scaring the patients? *Maturitas: The European Menopause Journal*, *81*(4), 446–448. Available at: www.maturitas. org/article/S0378-5122(15)00702-1/fulltext (accessed 16.08.17).

Lawrence, V., Samsi, K., Murray, J., et al. (2011) Dying well with dementia: qualitative examination of end-of-life care. *British Journal of Psychiatry*, *199*(5), 417–422.

Leadership Alliance for the Care of Dying People (LACDP) (2014a) *Priorities of care for the dying person*. London: NHS.

Leadership Alliance for the Care of Dying People (2014b) *One chance to get it right: Improving people's experience of care in the last few days and hours of life*. London: The Stationery Office.

Lukens, J.M. & Solomon, P. (2013) Thinking through recovery: resolving ethical challenges and promoting social work values in mental health services. *Journal of Social Work Values and Ethics*, *10*(1), 61–71.

McDonald, A. (2010) The impact of the 2005 Mental Capacity Act on social workers' decision-making and approaches to the assessment of risk. *British Journal of Social Work*, *40*(4), 1229–1246.

McKeown, J., Clark, A. & Repper, J. (2006) Life story work in health and social care: systematic literature review. *Journal of Advanced Nursing*, *55*(2), 237–247.

Mental Capacity Act 2005. Available at: www.legislation.gov.uk/ukpga/2005/9/contents (accessed 01.12.17).

Mioshi, E., Dawson, K. & Mitchell, J. (2006) The Addenbrooke's Cognitive Examination Revised (ACE-R): a brief cognitive test battery for dementia screening. *Int J Geriatr Psychiatry*, *21*, 1078–1085.

Monroe, B. & Hansford, P. (2010) Challenges in delivering palliative care in the community: a perspective from St Christopher's Hospice UK. *Progress in Palliative Care*, *18*(1), 9–13.

Moriarty, J., Rutter, D., Ross, P.D.S., et al. (2012) *SCIE research briefing 40: End-of-life care for people with dementia living in care homes*. London: Social Care Institute for Excellence.

National Institute for Clinical Excellence (2004) *Improving supportive and palliative care for adults with cancer*. Cancer Service Guideline (CSG4). London: NICE.

National Institute for Health and Care Excellence (2015) *Recognising when someone is in the last days of life*. London: NICE.

NHS England (2014) *Every moment counts: A new vision for coordinated care for people near the end of life*. London: NHS.

Paul, S. & Sallnow, L. (2012) Public health approaches to end-of-life care in the UK: an online survey of palliative care services. *BMJ Supportive and Palliative Care*, *3*, 196–199.

Repper, J. & Perkins, R. (2003) *Social inclusion and recovery*. London: Balliere Tindall.

Ryan, T., Gardiner, C., Bellamy, G., et al. (2011) Barriers and facilitators to the receipt of palliative care for people with dementia: the views of medical and nursing staff. *Palliative Medicine*, *26*(7), 879–886.

Sampson, E., Burns, A. & Richards, M. (2011) Improving end-of-life care for people with dementia. *The British Journal of Psychiatry*, *199*(5), 357–359.

Sanderson, H. & Bailey, G. (2014) *Personalisation and dementia: A guide for person-centred practice*. London: Jessica Kingsley.

Shepherd, G., Boardman, J. & Burns, M. (2010) *Implementing recovery: A methodology for organisation change*. London: Sainsbury Centre for Mental Health.

Sleeman, K.E., Ho, Y.K., Verne, J., et al. (2014) Reversal of English trend towards hospital death in dementia: a population-based study of place of death and associated individual and regional factors, 2001–2010. *BMC Neurology*, *14*, 59.

Thomas, K. & Lobo, B. (2011) *Advance care planning in end-of-life care*. Oxford: Oxford University Press.

Thompson, R. (2011) Using life story work to enhance care. *Nursing Older People*, *23*(8), 16–21.

Tribrizi, S. (2012) *Brain and body changes over time*. Presentation at Seeing beyond the gene: Second UK National Conference on Huntington's Disease, Stoke-on-Trent, UK.

Turner, J. and Hill, A. (2011a) Implementing clinical supervision (part 1): a review of the literature. *Mental Health Nursing (Online)*, *31*(3), 8–12.

Turner, J. and Hill, A. (2011b) Implementing clinical supervision (part 2): using proctor's model to structure the implementation of clinical supervision in a ward setting. *Mental Health Nursing (Online)*, *31*(4), 14–19.

Vachon, M. (2000). Burnout and symptoms of stress in staff working in palliative care. In H. Chochinov & W. Breitbart (eds) *Handbook of psychiatry in palliative medicine*. Oxford: Oxford University Press.

Watts, T.E. & Davies, R. (2014) Tensions and ambiguities: a qualitative study of final year adult field nursing students' experiences of caring for people affected by advanced dementia in Wales, UK. *Nurse Education Today*, *34*(8), 1149–1154.

Wilson, E. (2013) *A delicate equilibrium: living with Huntington's disease*. PhD thesis, University of Notthingham. Available at: eprints.nottingham.ac.uk/13487/2/A_delicate_equlibrium_Living_with_Revised.pdf (accessed 16/08/17).

Wilson, E., Pollock, K. & Aubeeiuck, A. (2014) Providing care services to people affected by Huntington's disease: an overview of the challenges. *British Journal of Neuroscience Nursing*, *10*(3), 139–143.

Wilson, E., Seymour, J.E. & Perkins, P. (2010) Working with the Mental Capacity Act: findings from palliative and specialist neurological care settings. *Palliative Medicine*, *24*(4), 396–402.

World Health Organization (2014) *Global atlas of palliative care at the end of life*. Geneva: World Health Organization. Available at www.who.int/cancer/publications/palliative-care-atlas/en (accessed 16.08.17).

World Health Organization (2015) *Mental health*. Geneva: WHO. Available at: www.who.int/topics/mental_health/en (accessed 16.08.17).

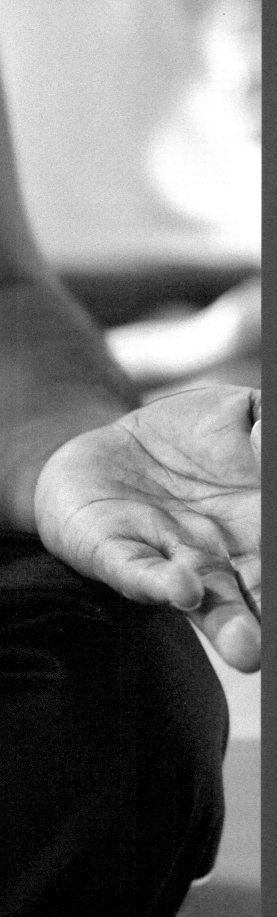

DEMOCRATIC LEADERSHIP FOR MENTAL HEALTH CARE

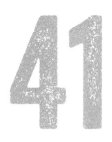

MICK McKEOWN, KAREN M. WRIGHT AND LYNDA CAREY

THIS CHAPTER COVERS

- The policy context for leadership
- An argument for democratic leadership and what is meant by this
- Ways in which informed leadership can improve practice
- The similarities between notions of democracy within therapy organisation and planning for services, and wider society
- The differences between 'leadership' and management
- The possibilities for more radical democratic transformations.

I have the privileged position of working for the mental health charity Rethink Mental Illness as the organiser and facilitator of a national network of involvement groups for people living in, working in and commissioning secure mental health services in England. Called the Recovery and Outcomes network, this initiative grew out of the increase in service user involvement in secure services that has taken place over the past 10 years. Held quarterly in nine regions throughout the country, Recovery and Outcomes Group meetings are a place where these three groups of people come together in an informal, non-hierarchical space. In a spirit of mutual respect, cooperation and a desire to effect positive change, the meetings are a place to share best practice, discuss difficulties and developments in mental health services and find solutions to common problems. More than this, the Groups facilitate development of a collective voice for people who otherwise might not be heard – a voice that increasingly influences the design, commissioning and delivery of services.

I first became involved with this work during my time spent in a secure mental health service myself – little did I know that this would lead to a position of leadership within this field. I was recognised as one of the Top 50 Health Service Journal Patient Leaders in 2015, a sign that the people with direct lived experience of health services are ideally placed to influence matters, not only as a result of their own experiences, but as with our network, by empowering the voices of others with similar experiences. Our network has been active for five years and during that time others have grown to become leaders themselves – initially by giving presentations

(Continued)

---

at meetings (usually the highlight of these events), and by co-facilitating discussions. Crucially, these peer leaders provide hope to others through much-needed peer support and showing that their own achievements and recovery journeys are a possibility for all. Seeming at times somewhat strange to be considered leaders, we now (as one person recently put it to me) 'sit at the top table' with organisations of influence and 'power' such as NHS England, the Department of Health and the Ministry of Justice. Increasingly we are considered the 'experts' in the room and recent national policy, such as the Five Year Forward View, has recognised this.

We live in exciting times, as services change and adapt to a new landscape in healthcare. I must say I have some ambivalence in being thought of as a leader – we should remember that change is made together so in that sense we are all 'leaders'. Nevertheless, as peer leaders and experts by our own experiences, we are truly beginning to drive that change.

Ian Callaghan former secure service user

The National Service User Awards are a celebration of the innovation, hard work and dedication of service users in secure services who through their projects have made a difference to their own lives and those of others. People in secure services are so often stigmatised by society as not being able to offer positive contributions, or forgotten behind high fences and walls. The awards are organised by and for service users to ensure that they receive the recognition they deserve. The planning process is characterised by positive values and participatory ideals so that in effect there is shared leadership.

Each year the awards have become bigger and more inclusive with participating service users taking on a greater responsibility for the event, with a diverse team leading the process. The event is now in its 6th year and it is my privilege to have been an event facilitator for this inspirational and humbling project. The role of the event facilitator is not to take ownership of the event but to guide and support the service users who are recruited onto the team to do this. The service users have the opportunity to apply for a number of different roles including team leader, deputy team leader, marketing, hospitality, admin, finance and entertainment leads. Many of the service users who apply for the roles are able to use skills that they have learnt whilst in hospital and also draw on previous work and community experiences.

Throughout the process there are many challenges and difficult decisions to be made whilst keeping within a set budget. This tests the team's problem solving skills and their resilience to the limit but also supports them to gain valuable skills and enhance their recovery. Part of the event facilitator role is to ensure that the team are provided with supervision and support both individually and as a peer group to explore challenges and work together for a solution. As well as working with the team within Cygnet Hospitals we also work with service users in high secure services to ensure no-one is excluded. This in itself poses challenges but the team have been creative in ensuring that they are able to communicate with their peers and ensure representation in meetings and at the event. The most rewarding part of the whole process is seeing the team grow in terms of their friendship and support of each other. It is also seeing the team grow in confidence from sitting quietly in a corner at a meeting to speaking in front of 200 delegates at the event itself.

Louise Bannister, ward manager

INTRODUCTION

Scholars of leadership in the nursing context have remarked that we have never been in more need of effective leadership at the same time as so much effort has been wasted in presenting such weak formulations of what good leadership actually might be (Grossman & Valiga, 2016). This chapter will consider nurse leadership through the lens of democracy. In doing so, the nurse leader is seen as a person who role-models an inclusive style of compassionate leadership in keeping with democratic principles. Unfortunately, many nurses experience distinctly undemocratic management of their work, resulting in diminished job satisfaction and low morale. Compounding this, there has been a relative lack of attention to how power is distributed within prevailing managerial systems and hierarchies (Cleary et al., 2011). More democratic leadership directly addresses any imbalances of power, evening these out for fairer inclusion of diverse viewpoints and arguably better results.

It is our view that transformational and democratic leaders act as change champions, improving the quality of care, challenging constraining **cultures** and ritualistic practices. Such leadership is empowering of colleagues – supporting their actions with a sound evidence base and developing a positive learning climate. Moreover, if we consider more fully realised democratisation processes, then the very idea of individual leadership and leaders becomes less of an issue within horizontal, collectivised democracies. Such possibilities include opportunities to bring together empowered staff and **service user** voices into forms of conjoint democratic organisation and decision making. These would be highly congruent with current proposals for **co-production**, but would actually extend the logic of co-production towards creating fully democratised working practices and organisational management. Conjoint leadership for change, transacted by service users and staff together, also portends openings for service users to be acknowledged as leaders in their own right or to share responsibilities within distributed models of leadership.

Whilst once naysayers might have accused us of being 'idealistic', we have arguably reached a point where democratised leadership is a necessity. Various system failings and subsequent policy pronouncements have bolstered the case for more democracy and distributed or transformative leadership (Berwick, 2013; Clwyd & Hart, 2013; Francis, 2013). Not all of this activity is completely radical, rather there is a spectrum of proposals and opportunities that affords openings for a democratic impulse to a greater or lesser degree. We will discuss some of these that are most relevant to mental health, beginning with more mainstream offerings, before turning to certain radical, perhaps utopian ideas.

We contend that all options are worth pursuing, and even the less radical of these can create the time and space for critical shifts in relationships that would move us on towards greater democracy. At stake may be a recalibration of power between care staff and service users and the potential to reimagine professional roles and identity (Fisher, 2016). Amidst more fully realised democratic practices, our professionalism may lay more authentic claims to a sense of who we are that embraces compassionate, cooperative, empathic and supportive selfhood.

DEVELOPING LEADERSHIP: THE POLICY

The King's Fund (2017) proposes that people should be informed and supported sufficiently to be able to make their own decisions about how their care is managed. The intention is for mental health nurses to be proactive, fully engaged, demonstrate personal commitment and act on situations rather than be acted on. In turn, this facilitates the inclusion of service user perspectives which are central to problem solving, innovation, creativity and time-management activities, which can be embedded within future practice.

The King's Fund (2017) calls for the 'developing and strengthening of leadership at all levels' and, at the same time, admits that leadership vacancies are hard to fill due to the pressure to do more with less, within a context of increasing regulation. To help us to lead improvements to care, the NHS's National Improvement and Leadership Development Board (2016: 18) has published a framework centred on the creation of five conditions common to high-performing health and care systems.

These five conditions are:

(i) Leaders equipped to develop high quality local health and care systems in partnership: leaders of organisations in local health and care systems are able to collaborate with partners, including patient leaders across organisational, professional and geographical boundaries in trusting relationships to achieve the same clear, shared system goals for their communities.

(ii) Compassionate, inclusive and effective leaders at all levels: compassionate leadership means paying close attention to all staff; really understanding the situations they face; responding empathically; and taking thoughtful and appropriate action to help.

(iii) Knowledge of improvement methods and how to use them at all levels: individuals and teams at every level know established improvement methods and are using them in partnership with patients, communities and citizens to improve their work processes and systems.

(iv) Support systems for learning at local, regional and national levels: there is sufficient training, coaching and organisation development capacity to meet development needs and enable and support learning and improvement.

(v) Enabling, supportive and aligned regulation and oversight: at the same time, central organisations help local systems find the support and resources they need. The constituent parts of the oversight system behave consistently and 'speak with one voice'.

The words 'inclusive' and 'compassionate' are repeatedly used to describe care, treatment and leadership. We contend that both inclusivity and compassion can be achieved through *democracy*.

DEVELOPING LEADERSHIP: THE PRACTICE

There has been much recent attention to how more democratised models of leadership can underpin practice change and innovation. Democratised practices must be grounded in shared **values** that enable constructive, respectful dialogue (Fulford & Woodbridge, 2004). Such interaction supports people to establish co-supportive relationships, which work to even out power imbalances and seek to achieve respect, regardless of difference. Fulford (1998), now at the Centre for Values Led Practice, pointed out that a values-driven dialogue need not be aimed at easy consensus building. Indeed, the idea of a constructive and creative 'dissensus' might be equally appealing, especially if there is a concern with a plurality of care and treatment alternatives.

Effective principles and practices in this regard are highlighted by Helen Bevan and Steve Fairman (2014) in the UK Government White Paper: *The new era of thinking and practice in change transformation: A call to action for leaders of health and care*. These authors describe a distributed model of leadership and the basis of innovation and change as essentially relational: 'change is increasingly about commitment to a common cause, built on a foundation of relationships' (2014: 8).

This relationship-forming process builds **social capital**, facilitating the development of meaningful communities of practice, which in turn support practice change and consciousness raising. To achieve all of this, participatory forms of democratic leadership are essential. These work to decentralise decision making and render it inclusive of all service users and colleagues. Associated with this can be a notion of leading 'the edge' of organisations: with key actors cooperating to identify radical thinking for transformative change, ideally ensuring faster innovations, negotiation of barriers to change and better service outcomes.

There are a plethora of textbooks and research papers that list the qualities and tasks of a good nurse leader, some of which you will also encounter within this chapter. McCloughen et al. (2009) suggest that a good leader should possess the following qualities:

- altruism
- a genuine interest in developing others
- the ability to provide unconditional support and honest feedback
- the ability to promote independence and capacity to deal with challenging situations
- good professional boundaries
- trustworthiness.

It is easier to trust the judgement of managers or leaders if you trust them as a person; they make you feel safe and you believe that they don't just want to get the job done, they also want you to be the best you can be. Hence, the parallels with the **therapeutic relationship** are quite clear. They can be seen in Horvath and Greenberg's (1989) Working Alliance Inventory (WAI), which assesses the three essential components of the working alliance:

1. Agreement between service user and therapist on the goals of the therapy
2. The person's agreement with the therapist that the tasks of the therapy will address the problems the individual brings to treatment
3. The quality of the interpersonal bond between the individual and the therapist. (Hatcher & Gillaspy, 2006: 12)

These three tenets, a shared goal, agreement about the collective task and the bond between the leader and the team, are similarly fundamental to democratic leadership. Furthermore, The Kim Alliance Scale (Kim et al., 2001) identifies four dimensions which frame the effectiveness of the alliance: **collaboration**, communication, integration and empowerment.

In summary, we suggest that the core skills of a good, transformational and democratic leader are:

- the ability to influence and inspire others, within a shared vision
- the motivation to achieve collectively, where success is shared and people are valued
- the insight and imagination to transform practice, enable the workforce and empower service users to see the possibilities
- to understand the impact of change on the individual, the service and the system.

DEVELOPING COLLECTIVE LEADERSHIP

Traditional models of management deal with how organisational goals are achieved and focus on processes and procedures, wrapped up with an imperative to exert control and disciplinary power. Leadership is perhaps more concerned with innovation and change, built on relationships and mutual interests (Jennings et al., 2007). In the traditional, usually top-down management model, leadership will typically be embodied in inspirational managers who persuade employees to get behind new initiatives and assist in their implementation. More progressive approaches to both management and leadership reject simple distinctions between superiors and subordinates and value the collective and relational contribution of all in strategic thinking and day-to-day working practices (Van Vactor, 2012). Moreover, evidence shows that relational rather than task-orientated leadership styles produce greater job satisfaction for nurses (Cummings et al., 2010). These more enlightened approaches have informed

CASE STUDY:
HOME
TREATMENT
TEAM

the development of courses delivered by the NHS Leadership Academy, but there are still tensions in the extent to which these are valued over more directive approaches (Storey & Holti, 2013).

Collective leadership has been referred to by the NHS Improvement and Leadership Development Board (2016) as 'leadership of all, by all and for all', inferring that all staff have the opportunity to get involved and to change practice. The Board describes this as being 'empowered', and this is evident in the following:

- everyone understands and embodies the vision and values
- everyone has clear objectives and data on performance
- there is an open, supportive and compassionate approach to people management and how all staff interact with each other day to day
- there is a high level of staff engagement
- learning and quality improvement are embedded
- good team and inter-team working are standard.

There are different forms of collective leadership that share common features. These have been variously titled: distributed leadership (Martin et al., 2015), servant leadership (Jackson, 2008a) and transformational leadership (Hutchinson & Jackson, 2013). There is a strong emphasis on cooperation and shared decision making that are essentially collectivised and concerned with flattening power differentials. Cooperative working and decision making have been remarked on as being implicitly satisfying, in contrast to the more alienating hierarchical processes of organising work (Sennett, 2012).

Coincidentally, these are similar principles to the aforementioned empowering principles of therapeutic alliances. Hence, establishing an alliance with a team, as well as with service users and their families, can create not only the catalyst for **recovery**, but also precipitate change in an organisation. The term *empowerment* is a particularly interesting concept here, since it is cognisant of the potential for service users to take control and responsibility for their recovery, whilst still inferring the worker's role in revealing this potential and initiating the recovery (Clark & Nayar, 2012).

Co-production and democratised professions

Co-production has been vaunted as the ideal way of organising contemporary public services and reshaping them to be fit for the 21st century (Alford, 2009; Cahn, 2000; Durose & Richardson, 2016; Dzur, 2008; Fisher, 2016). The idea of co-produced mental health care is highly compatible with the forms of democratised leadership we favour. As such, co-produced services offer a platform for actually re-imagining how professional care workers might practice and develop critical thought about their very identity. A co-produced professional encounter begins with a healthy scepticism about simplistic notions of empowerment. Proper attention must be paid to power imbalances between staff and service users, every effort made to minimise such discrepancies in power. One route to ensure that power is more evenly distributed across services is to democratise the relations between professionals, and between them and service users. Arguably, authentic co-production is more likely in a context of relationship-centred care and alternatives to singular biological psychiatry (Fisher, 2016).

Through the history of therapeutic interventions, certain therapeutic approaches have been designed to be more democratic, most obviously therapeutic communities including versions of these enacted by Ronnie Laing and others such as Kingsley Hall (Crossley, 1998). Hannah Proctor (2016), in an article broadly sympathetic but also critical of the work of Peter Sedgwick (2015/1982), highlights the left-politics-inspired Red Therapy, developed as self-help by radical workers as a form of collective support. This was an example of a critical reaction to the perceived individualising and pathologising focus of most mainstream psycho-therapies. Such a shift in emphasis is important, as it is also reflected in other examples of more innovative working practices, such as **Open Dialogue**, where the focus is on transparent communication with people and their family networks (Seikkula & Olson, 2003).

In a more general sense, the impulse to democratise care and even out power amongst the people involved can be seen as in tune with a particular politics of change. This is the notion of 'prefiguration', whereby participants in a group or system attempt to shape the sort of relationships they would like to see in a future, ideal, state in the course of trying to achieve this. Such ideas have, for a long time, been associated with various progressive theological and political trains of thought, notably the anarchism of philosophers and revolutionaries such as Kropotkin and Serge, or Marxist-tinged Latin American liberation theology, such as that exemplified in the work of Paolo Freire.

Freire (1971), in particular, has been influential amongst critically minded nurses, mainly for his contribution to models of participatory learning and research. Kropotkin (1908) is often credited as being a founder of the discipline of human geography, concerned with the social relations of place and space: a field with much to offer those of us caught up in change practices in mental health care (Curtis, 2010; Parr, 2008; Philo, 2005). Prefiguration is also emphasised powerfully by the human geographer Simon Springer (2012, 2016), with a focus on challenging the inequities of **neo-liberalism**. Victor Serge (1963/2012), the anarchist who joined the Bolshevik revolution, inspired Sedgwick to develop his ideas for prefiguring new approaches to mental health care, particularly noting the Geel model, and wishing for more constructive political alliances between service users/**survivors** and workers.

Sadly, Sedgwick did not live to see the more contemporary prefigurative developments or indeed the growth in service user movements, but his book *Psychopolitics* was reissued in 2015 because of its continued relevance (Cresswell, 2016; Spandler et al., 2015). For Sedgwick, the task of transforming psychiatry has always been a relational task, and in this sense it is commensurate with the task of transforming society as a whole. If this is seen as utopian, that is because it is; and in this regard, all prefigurative politics is about trying to achieve small-scale, situated utopias that could show how larger-scale change could work. In his comprehensive study of UK mental health **social movements**, Crossley (1999, 2006) explicitly refers to the sort of examples we have already mentioned as 'mini working utopias'. For progressive thinkers such as Springer (2016), notions of utopia, literally places that exist 'nowhere', ought to be dealt with sceptically at the very least, lest they are thought of with pessimism as unachievable. Similar observations have been made about ideal versions of co-production (Stone & Teifouri, 2017).

Working democratic utopias

Any new model of working or service organisation must survive within prevailing social and political conditions. The current neo-liberal policy has placed mental health services and wider health and welfare systems under extreme pressures that, for many, precipitate a degree of pessimism that meaningful democratisation can be delivered. Bauman (2000), for example, sees failings within services as symptomatic of a state of liquid modernity, under which continuity of care, insecurity of employment, and the quality of caring relationships, interact with, and are perhaps fatally undermined by, inadequate funding and privatisation. In publically funded services, so-called systems of 'new public management' serve neo-liberal interests, whilst rhetorically also presenting a case for involvement and empowerment practices (Clarke, 2007; Dahl & Soss, 2014). Whilst the threats posed by such developments are very real, collectively facing up to them may actually assist in advancing us towards greater democracy in health care services (Randall & McKeown, 2014).

Commentators such as Clarke (2007) highlight how pessimism in the face of powerful neo-liberal forces may be somewhat misplaced. Rather than resign ourselves to the assumed omnipotence and omnipresence of neo-liberalism, we ought to consider seeking out the places and spaces where neo-liberalism is not always looking. Clarke argues that large public service bureaucracies are full of interstitial places where more radical ideas can be enacted and even thrive; where the power of neo-liberalism is less obviously exerted. If Clarke is correct, then rhetorically supported policy initiatives such as co-production could become a vehicle for pursuing the more thorough and radical forms of democratisation that might be transformative of service organisations.

Workplace democracy is one possible route towards the emancipation of service users and staff, may be a necessary foundation for innovation and change, and is congruent with the most progressive models of distributed leadership (McKeown & Carey, 2015; McKeown et al., 2014). Most organisations, at least at the level of rhetoric, value employee voice, yet models of partnership working with trade unions are often weak and other forms of staff engagement can be similarly lacking. A lack of formal engagement with staff concerns has been implicated in service failings such as at Mid Staffs Hospital and in many whistleblowing examples (Jackson, 2008b). Service user involvement can also be less well provided for than policy directives or celebratory services suggest (Hodge, 2009). In the absence of true power sharing, these opportunities for self-expression and involvement can be illusory or enmeshed with wider tendencies towards social control (Cooke & Kothari, 2002).

We could envisage democracies for organising mental health care hospitals, wards or community teams that bring together staff and service users and the public to shape the way care is enacted and how professional work is organised. This would be truly co-production. Such democracy would need to be collectively built on effective solidarity and political alliances, appreciative of diverse service user and survivor criticisms of established services and the challenging political economy within which they are organised. A big part of the workforce being open to democratic change may have to be a commitment to engage in healing past and current hurts and grievances within the system. To this end, calls have been made for some sort of truth and reconciliation process as a foundation for the progressive alliances necessary to take us forward in solidarity (McKeown, 2016; Slade, 2009; Spandler & McKeown, 2017; Wallcraft & Shulkes, 2012).

CRITICAL DEBATE 41.1

- How feasible do you think the idea of a workplace democracy might be in mental health settings?
- What might the enabling or impeding factors be?
- How best might barriers be surmounted?

CONCLUSION

It is difficult to offer an exemplar of fully realised, co-produced democratic leadership. In many respects, the literal meaning of utopia prevails, and such mental health democracies do not exist at present. It may, however, be left to the power of our imagination to envisage all of the potential and possibilities for fully democratised mental health care and the extent to which this might more completely address the ideals of reconciliation and recovery, or lead to a plurality of alternative services.

CHAPTER SUMMARY

This chapter has covered:

- Approaches to leadership in health care settings
- The difference between leadership and management

- The desirability of democratic models of leadership and congruence with therapeutic ideals
- A suggestion that fully-fledged workplace democracy represents a solution to a history of service failures.

BUILD YOUR BIBLIOGRAPHY

Books

- Gopee, N. & Galloway, J. (2017) *Leadership and management in healthcare*. London: SAGE.
- Sennett, R. (2012) *Together: The rituals, pleasures and politics of cooperation*. London: Allen Lane.
- Yeoman, R. (2014) *Meaningful work and workplace democracy: A philosophy of work and a politics of meaningfulness*. London: Palgrave Macmillan.

SAGE journal articles

Go to https://study.sagepub.com/essentialmentalhealth for further free online journal articles related to this chapter. If you are using the interactive ebook, simply click on the book icon in the margin to go straight to the resource.

FURTHER READING: JOURNAL ARTICLES

- Checkland, K. (2014) Leadership in the NHS: does the emperor have any clothes? *Journal of Health Services Research & Policy*, 19(4), 253–256.
- Nicol, E. & Sang, B. (2011) A co-productive health leadership model to support the liberation of the NHS. *Journal of the Royal Society of Medicine*, 104(2), 64–68.
- Stanton, A. (1989) Citizens of workplace democracies. *Critical Social Policy*, 9(26), 56–65.

Weblinks

Go to https://study.sagepub.com/essentialmentalhealth for further weblinks related to this chapter. If you are using the interactive ebook, simply click on the book icon in the margin to go straight to the resource.

FURTHER READING: WEBLINKS

- Change Management Institute introduces an NHS White Paper on leading organisational change: http://webarchive.nationalarchives.gov.uk/20160506182942/http://theedge.nhsiq.nhs.uk/white-paper-the-new-era-of-thinking-and-practice-in-change-and-transformation-a-call-to-action-for-leaders-of-health-and-care
- Mary O'Hagan, the notable antipodean survivor activist, lets her imagination run free to envisage an alternative future in this short film: www.youtube.com/watch?v=Tle1trJhs2g
- NHS Leadership Academy: www.leadershipacademy.nhs.uk
- Russell Razzaque who is in the vanguard of introducing Open Dialogue to the UK makes a link to this social experiment in democracy in war torn Kurdistan – The Revolution Starts in Rojava: www.youtube.com/watch?v=JNWQfQkUCtM&feature=youtu.be&app=desktop

CHECK YOUR ANSWERS

ACE YOUR ASSESSMENT

Revise what you have learned by visiting https://study.sagepub.com/essentialmentalhealth. If you are using the interactive ebook, simply click on the tick icon to go straight to the resource.

- Test yourself with multiple-choice and short-answer questions and flashcards.

ONLINE QUIZZES & ACTIVITY ANSWERS

REFERENCES

Alford, J. (2009) *Engaging public sector clients: From service delivery to co-production*. Basingstoke: Palgrave Macmillan.

Bauman, Z. (2000) *Liquid modernity*. Cambridge: Polity Press.

Berwick, D. (2013) *A promise to learn: a commitment to act – improving the safety of patients in England*. London: Department of Health.

Bevan, H. & Fairman, S. (2014) *The new era of thinking and practice in change transformation: A call to action for leaders of health and care*. An NHS Improving Quality (NHSIQ) White Paper. Available at: theedge.nhsiq.nhs.uk/wp-content/uploads/2016/02/nhsiq_white_paper.pdf (accessed 16/08/17).

Cahn, E.S. (2000) *No more throw-away people: The co-production imperative*, 2nd edition. Washington, DC: Essential Books.

Clark, M. & Nayar, S. (2012) Recovery from eating disorders: a role for occupational therapy. *New Zealand Journal of Occupational Therapy*, *59*(1), 13.

Clarke, J. (2007) Citizen-consumers and public service reform: at the limits of neo-liberalism? *Policy Futures in Education*, *5*, 239–248.

Cleary, M., Horsfall, J., Deacon, M., et al. (2011) Leadership and mental health nursing. *Issues in Mental Health Nursing*, *32*, 632–639.

Clwyd, A. & Hart, P. (2013) *A review of the NHS hospitals complaints system: Putting patients back in the picture*. London: Department of Health.

Cooke, B. & Kothari, U. (2002) *Participation: The new tyranny?* London: Zed Books.

Cresswell, M. (2016) Marxism and psychiatry: rethinking mental health politics for the twenty-first century. *Social Theory & Health*, *14*, 510–523.

Crossley, N. (1998) R.D. Laing and the British anti-psychiatry movement: a socio-historical analysis. *Social Science & Medicine*, *47*(7), 877–889.

Crossley, N. (1999) Working utopias and social movements: an investigation using case study materials from radical mental health movements in Britain. *Sociology*, *33*(4), 809–830.

Crossley, N. (2006) *Contesting psychiatry: Social movements in mental health*. Abingdon: Routledge.

Cummings, G., MacGregor T., Davey, M., et al. (2010) Leadership styles and outcome patterns for the nursing workforce and work environment: a systematic review. *Int J Nurs Stud*, *47*(3), 363–385.

Curtis, S. (2010) *Space, place and mental health*. Aldershot: Ashgate.

Dahl, A. & Soss, J. (2014) Neoliberalism for the common good? Public value governance and the downsizing of democracy. *Public Administration Review*, *74*(4), 496–504.

Durose, C. & Richardson, L. (2016) *Designing public policy for co-production: Theory, practice and change*. Bristol: Policy Press.

Dzur, A.W. (2008) *Democratic professionalism: Citizen participation and the reconstruction of professional ethics, identity, and practice*. Pennsylvania, PA: Pennsylvania State University Press.

Fisher, P. (2016) Co-production: what is it and where do we begin? *Journal of Psychiatric and Mental Health Nursing*, *23*(6–7), 345–346.

Francis, R. (2013) *Report of the Mid Staffordshire NHS Foundation Trust public inquiry*. London: TSO.

Freire, P. (1971) *Pedagogy of the oppressed*. Harmondsworth: Penguin.

Fulford, K.W.M. (1998) Dissent and dissensus: the limits of consensus formation in psychiatry. In H.A.M.J. ten Have & H.-M. Sass (eds) *Consensus formation in health care ethics*. Dordrecht: Kluwer. pp. 175–192.

Fulford, K.W.M. & Woodbridge, K. (2004) *Whose values? A workbook for values-based practice in mental health care*. London: Sainsbury Centre for Mental Health.

Grossman, S. & Valiga, T.M. (2016) *The new leadership challenge: Creating the future of nursing*, 5th edition. Philadelphia, PA: F.A. Davis.

Hatcher, R.L. and Gillaspy, J.A (2006) Development and validation of a revised short version of the Working Alliance Inventory. *Psychotherapy Research*, *16*(1), 12–25.

Hodge, S. (2009) User involvement in the construction of a mental health charter: an exercise in communicative rationality? *Health Expectations*, *12*(3), 251–261.

Horvath, A. O. & Greenberg, L.S. (1989) Development and validation of the Working Alliance Inventory. *Journal of counseling psychology*, 36(2), 223–233.

Hutchinson, M. & Jackson, D. (2013) Transformational leadership in nursing: towards a more critical interpretation. *Nursing Inquiry*, *20*(1), 11–22.

Jackson, D. (2008a) Servant leadership in nursing: a framework for developing sustainable research capacity in nursing. *Collegian, 15*, 27–33.

Jackson, D. (2008b) Editorial: what becomes of the whistleblowers? *Journal of Clinical Nursing, 17*, 1261–1262.

Jennings, B., Scalzi, C., Rodgers III, J., et al. (2007) Differentiating nursing leadership and management competencies. *Nursing Outlook, 55*, 169–175.

Kim, S.C., Boren, D. & Solem, S.L. (2001) The Kim Alliance Scale: development and preliminary testing. *Clinical Nursing Research*, *10*(3), 314–331.

King's Fund, The (2017) *Priorities for the NHS and social care in 2017*. Available at: www.kingsfund.org. uk/publications/priorities-nhs-social-care-2017 (accessed 16.08.17).

Kropotkin, P. (1908) *Mutual aid*. London: Heinemann.

Martin, G., Beech, N., MacIntosh, R., et al. (2015) Potential challenges facing distributed leadership in health care: evidence from the UK National Health Service. *Sociology of Health & Illness*, *37*(1), 14–29.

McCloughen, A., O'Brien, L. and Jackson, D., (2009) Esteemed connection: creating a mentoring relationship for nurse leadership. *Nursing Inquiry*, *16*(4), 326–336.

McKeown, M. (2016) Can we put the hurt behind us? *Asylum: the magazine for democratic psychiatry*, *23*(4), 8–9.

McKeown, M. & Carey, L. (2015) Editorial: democratic leadership – a charming solution for nursing's legitimacy crisis. *Journal of Clinical Nursing*, *24*(3–4), 315–317.

McKeown, M., Cresswell, M. & Spandler, H. (2014) Deeply engaged relationships: alliances between mental health workers and psychiatric survivors in the UK. In B. Burstow, B.A. LeFrançois and S.L. Diamond (eds) *Psychiatry disrupted: Theorizing resistance and crafting the (r)evolution*. Montreal, QC: McGill/Queen's University Press.

National Improvement and Leadership Development Board (2016) *Developing people – improving care: A national framework for action on improvement and leadership development in NHS-funded services.* Updated 2017. Available at: https://improvement.nhs.uk/resources/developing-people-improving-care (accessed 16/08/17).

Parr, H. (2008) *Mental health and social space: Towards inclusionary geographies?* Oxford: Blackwell.

Philo, C. (2005) The geography of mental health: an established field? *Current Opinion on Psychiatry*, *18*, 585–591.

Proctor, H. (2016) Lost minds: Sedgwick, Laing and the politics of mental illness. *Radical Philosophy*, *197*, 36–48.

Randall, D. & McKeown, M. (2014) Failure to care: nursing in a state of liquid modernity? *Journal of Clinical Nursing, 23*, 766–767.

Sedgwick, P. (2015/1982) *Psychopolitics*. London: Unkant.

Seikkula, J. & Olson, M.E. (2003) The open dialogue approach to acute psychosis: its poetics and micropolitics. *Family Process*, *42*(3), 403–418.

Sennett, R. (2012) *Together: The rituals, pleasures and politics of cooperation*. London: Allen Lane.

Serge, V. (1963/2012) *Memoirs of a revolutionary, 1901–41*. New York: New York Review of Books.

Slade, M. (2009) *Personal recovery and mental illness*. Cambridge: Cambridge University Press.

Spandler, H. & McKeown, M. (2017) Exploring the case for truth and reconciliation in mental health services. *Mental Health Review Journal*, *22*(2), 83–94.

Spandler, H., Dellar, R. & Kemp, A. (2015) Foreword. In P. Sedgwick, *Psychopolitics*. London: Unkant Books.

Springer, S. (2012) Anarchism! What geography still ought to be. *Antipode*, *44*, 1605–1624.

Springer, S. (2016) Fuck neoliberalism. *ACME: An International Journal for Critical Geographies*, *15*(2), 285–292.

Stone, B. & Teifouri, S. (2017) *The impossibility of co-production*. ESRC seminar: Re-imagining professionalism in mental health – towards co-production. York University, 3 March. Available at: https://coproductionblog.wordpress.com/tag/seminar-5 (accessed 16/08/17).

Storey, J. & Holti, R. (2013) *Towards a new model of leadership for the NHS*. Available at: www.leadership academy.nhs.uk/wp-content/uploads/2013/05/towards-a-new-model-of-leadership-2013.pdf (accessed 16.08.17).

VanVactor, J. (2012) Collaborative leadership model in the management of health care. *Journal of Business Research*, *65*, 555–561.

Wallcraft, J. & Shulkes, D. (2012) Can psychiatry apologise for crimes against humanity? *Open Mind*, Jan.–Feb., 12–13.

CLINICAL SUPERVISION IN MENTAL HEALTH CARE

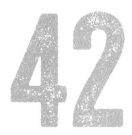

42

NATALIE MILES AND KAREN M. WRIGHT

THIS CHAPTER COVERS

- What clinical supervision is
- What the NMC has to say about clinical supervision
- Models and approaches to supervision
- Looking after your service users … looking after you!
- What is expected of you and your supervisor
- Contracts and records for supervision.

INTRODUCTION

This chapter presents clinical supervision (CS) as an essential part of professional practice for contemporary mental health nurses. There are tens of thousands of books and journal articles published on this subject already, so we have concentrated on the core issues that establish clinical supervision as a mechanism to help you to develop safe, competent, reflective and evidence-based practice. We'll also look at two nurses' experiences of supervision and a **service user's** perspective.

NOTES ON VOICES

In this chapter, two mental health nurses, Gemma and Fleur, were interviewed and part of those narratives are provided to share their experiences of clinical supervision. Both provide examples of what they believe is good about supervision – for example, being listened to, having time out to share their thoughts with somebody who doesn't judge them, and the safety of knowing that their disclosures will be dealt with respectfully, sensitively and professionally.

In many ways, their description of clinical supervision resonates with our understanding of a **therapeutic relationship** since they both **value** the trustworthiness and safety of the relationship formed with the supervisor and both see this as pivotal to their engagement with the process. Fiona's thoughts about supervision are included in the chapter and provide an insightful account of the observed pressure that nursing staff encounter every day as part of their jobs.

BACKGROUND: 'WHAT IS IT'?

Supervision is a core national standard and one of the ten essential capabilities of a mental health practitioner (DH, 2004: 29); it is also regarded as an *essential ingredient* in modern mental health care (DH, 2008) in developing and maintaining complex relationships in modern mental health services. It is a regulatory and professional requirement (CQC, 2013) and, according to Sloan (2006), a central and valuable intervention in mental health nursing practice. The NMC issued a clinical supervision advice sheet (NMC, 2006) but it is not, however, mentioned specifically in the Nursing and Midwifery Council's (NMC) Code (2015a). Despite this, we argue that, fundamentally, CS aims to assist the nurse to achieve the essence of the Code, which is to:

- prioritise people
- practise effectively
- preserve safety
- promote professionalism and trust.

━━━━━━ 'WHAT'S THE EVIDENCE'? 42.1 ━━━━━━

A number of health and social care failures have contributed to the debate on the need for clinical supervision, which is cited as the 'single most important contributor to training effectiveness' (Gonsalvez & Milne, 2010: 233). Despite its apparent importance (Felton et al., 2012), clinical supervision is often 'thrown in' at the end of investigations, reports and audits that seek to provide recommendations for better practice. Ashburner et al. (2004) highlight its importance in creating safe practice and, although produced some years ago, *The Clothier Report* (DH, 1994), which concentrated attention on the issue of safe and accountable practice in nursing in the wake of the Beverley Allitt case, is still referred to as a significant report on nursing misconduct. Subsequently, two distinct types of supervision became the subject of much debate, namely performance development review supervision and facilitative clinical supervision (DH, 1993).

CS AND THE CODE: WHY IS IT IMPORTANT FOR NURSES?

The Nursing and Midwifery Council (NMC, 2016) advice sheet guides the implementation of clinical supervision as an important aspect of clinical governance to support nurses to achieve high quality standards of care, but a recent statement by the NMC chief executive and registrar included the following: 'There is no doubt that access to good clinical supervision is essential for all health care professionals. However, it is for employers, not regulators, to take responsibility for this important function.' (Smith, 2016).

FIND OUT MORE

NMC ADVICE SHEETS (2016)

Hence, it is clear that, irrespective of directives, regulations and national guidance, we, as nurses, need to be clear that we have a professional and personal duty to provide informed and ethical care. Clinical supervision is one way of working towards this.

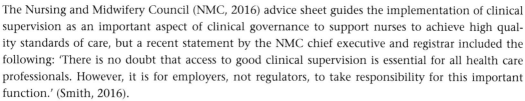

CRITICAL THINKING STOP POINT 42.1

As nurses, we have a duty to provide safe, supportive care. Do you think that we also have a duty to engage in clinical supervision?

THE FUNCTION AND DEFINITION OF CLINICAL SUPERVISION: WHAT DOES IT DO?

In many ways, it is easier to describe what CS does for the nurse, i.e. its function, rather than to define it, since it is defined by its utility and interpreted, and understood by professionals in different ways depending on their practice and theoretical foundation. There are several functions of supervision, such as skill development, process, focus and case management. Patricia Benner's (1984) concept of the 'novice to expert' is exemplified within CS, which aims to develop nurses' confidence and expertise by reflection on their practice. The overall purpose of supervision is to assist supervisees to work as effectively as possible at any stage of their career.

Proctor (1986) identifies three functions of clinical supervision:

- a normative function, which ensures safe and effective practice by the supervisee and the protection of clients/patients
- a formative function, which relates to education process and development
- a restorative function, which seeks to help the supervisee manage any negative effects or concerns in relation to their practice/work.

Brunero and Stein-Parbury (2008) refer to these when concluding that clinical supervision provides **peer support** and stress relief for nurses (restorative function) as well as a means of promoting professional accountability (normative function) and skill and knowledge development (formative function).

There have been a number of international reviews which consider the outcomes of, and the evidence to support the use of clinical supervision (Watkins, 2011; White & Winstanley, 2011, 2014). It is purported that effective clinical supervision has a causal effect on lowering the stress levels of individual supervisees when carefully measured by research instructions with established psychometric properties. There are growing indications that clinical supervision may also have positive effects on the improvement of clinical care, and improved outcomes for mental health service users may also be detected (Bambling et al., 2006; Bradshaw et al., 2007; White & Winstanley, 2010).

CLINICAL SUPERVISION FOR NURSES

A popular definition of supervision by Bernard and Goodyear (2004: 88) is:

> an intervention provided by a more senior member of a profession to a more junior member or members of that same profession. The relationship is evaluative, extends over time and has the simultaneous purposes of enhancing the professional functioning of the more junior person(s), monitoring the quality of professional services offered to the clients, she/he or they see, and serving as a gatekeeper for those who are to enter the particular profession.

Milne (2007), however, critiques Bernard and Goodyear's (2004) definition of supervision, suggesting that it is not always replicable, that there is a lack of specification about supervision interventions and that it is a 'sorely neglected topic' (Milne, 2009: vii). Worse still, nurses are aware of their responsibility to take supervision and hence feel that they are neglectful themselves. It is important to remember that CS is the responsibility of the organisation (Butterworth et al., 2008), not just the nurse.

Crucially, CS aims to facilitate the tasks, roles and functions of nursing as well as assisting the nurse to 'unpick' some of the complexities of their work in a way that isn't accessible 'on the floor', but is enabled by the confidential CS relationship. Indeed, the self-disclosure that occurs within the CS relationship has been compared by Banks et al. (2013) to a 'confessional' act.

It is important that CS is not confused with managerial supervision. Faugier and Butterworth (1994) argued that clinical supervision should be considered a necessary part of the clinical governance agenda for safer nursing practice in Britain and should focus on issues of competency and professionalism. If clinical supervision is to increase confidence and competence in the nurse, then Falender and Shafranske (2007: 233) are right to define supervision as *competency-based*, as it is:

> an approach that explicitly identifies the knowledge, skills and values that are assembled to form a clinical competency and develops learning strategies and education procedures to meet criterion-referenced competence standards in keeping with evidence-based practices and requirements of the local clinical setting.

Managerial supervision, on the other hand, is usually where a nurse reports to and is accountable to their line manager. It tends to relate to issues of caseload, workload, competence in relation to the expectations of the nurse's role and service focus. Line management supervision often sets priorities and objectives; it can identify personal training/development needs; and it serves more the process of monitoring the quality of the nurse's practice (CQC, 2013).

There are also other models of supervision such as peer supervision.

Peer supervision

Peer supervision can be an opportunity for mutual learning in an atmosphere of safety and trust (Proctor & Inskipp, 2001) whereby two or more peers can supervise and learn from each other.

Kirk (2010) makes the point that in peer supervision, if facilitated well:

> a good supervisor can help you identify blind spots in your understanding, possibly those associated with unhelpful beliefs of your own; and help you to become aware of gaps in skills and knowledge ... providing you with support and reassurance if you are dealing with distressing and difficult material. (Kirk, 2010: 293)

Hawkins and Shohet (2000) discuss the notion that peer group supervision can provide learning and also be supportive and normative in the sense that one may discuss challenges and dilemmas in practice as well as identify with others' experiences. In today's climate of additional pressures on mental health professionals in relation to targets, outcomes, waiting lists and limitations on resources in the form of shortage of time, money and expertise, group supervision could be a positive choice rather than a compromise.

CRITICAL THINKING STOP POINT 42.2

Think about whether you would prefer one-to-one supervision or peer group supervision, and what the benefits are of each.

MODELS OR APPROACHES TO SUPERVISION: HOW DO I DO IT?

There is no hard and fast rule about how to conduct or engage in CS (Hawkins & Shohet, 2000) and there are many different models or approaches to clinical supervision developed from different psychotherapy-based supervision models that are also suitable for and transferable to mental health practitioners. They (Hawkins & Shohet, 2000) propose seven 'modes' or tasks within supervision :

- the content of therapy
- the strategies and interventions used in therapy
- the therapeutic relationship
- the therapist's process that includes countertransference and parallel processes
- the supervisor's own processes (including reaction to the supervisee)
- the supervisor–client relationship
- the wider context that the supervisee professionally functions within, such as the organisation where they practise and their relationships with colleagues.

These seven modes are not necessarily in each supervision session and depend on the developmental stage of the supervisee, but each of the modes is fundamental within a quality, collaborative relationship between supervisor and supervisee. However, as a rule of thumb, we suggest that CS sessions adopt a structure similar to that shown in Figure 42.1.

In order that clinical supervision may be successfully implemented and sustained, White and Winstanley (2010) suggest that a number of environmental conditions should be met; mainly that clinical supervision should be universally considered as part of the core of contemporary professional mental health nursing practice; and that there is positive support for clinical supervision at management level as part of organisational **culture**. The following list is derived by Scaife (2001: 7), as suggested for supervisees:

- considering how to share your current understanding of your strengths and points for development with the supervisor
- taking a position of openness to learning, which includes communicating your thoughts and feelings in supervision
- noticing what you find threatening in supervision
- noticing how you typically show defensiveness
- identifying your own ideas about boundaries in supervision and working out how to let your supervisor know if they begin to stray beyond them
- being prepared for and having the skills to negotiate disengagement
- identifying your expectations about the focus of supervision
- being clear about the roles that you expect of your supervisor
- working out how to stay in control of feedback that might be given by your supervisor
- working out how to show your supervisor your fears and anxieties without undue apprehension in anticipation of negative evaluation
- letting your supervisor know what is proving helpful and unhelpful to your learning and development
- acknowledging errors with a view to learning from them.

The figure below is our representation of the flow of activity in CS.

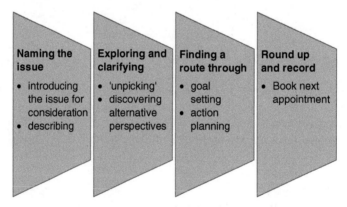

Figure 42.1 Supervision (see Chapter 42 of this text) – hour-long sessions model

Here's what *Fleur*, a mental health nurse, says about her experience of supervision and what works best for her:

> I've had good supervision and I've had bad. No two supervisors are the same and their approaches vary widely.
>
> The worst supervision is where you come away feeling judged, or feel that the session has met the supervisor's agenda not mine. There have been occasions when it is clear that the supervisor effectively hijacks the session and I am sat there busting to talk about what is

> bothering me and I've just not been able to express myself at all … the session has met their needs and not mine.
>
> The best supervision is when I can sit down with someone I can trust and I can just spill my guts. I can just throw all my toys out of the pram and I can let off steam. Supervisors really need to appreciate that sometimes the work is overwhelming and that those 60 minutes are a safe place to let it all out. I don't just mean a whinge-fest, I mean an out-pouring, where I can get it all out on the table and then we can pick through it together.
>
> A good supervisor picks through it with me, helps me to reflect, to organise it, to get some perspective and then work up an action plan with me. It's like I put all the toys back in the boxes and I end up with a sense of organisation and purpose. But this can only happen if you trust the supervisor. So, today, for example, I did feel quite troubled when we sat down, but she listened whilst I got it all out of my system and then she helped me to tease out three main issues for an action plan.
>
> It's all about reflection. I put it on the table, we look at it together, we sort it out, pick through it and look at it again, reflectively. I really enjoyed it actually.
>
> **Fleur, mental health nurse**

There are clearly established frameworks for reflection (one being the *critical incident technique*, described in Chapter 2) which is considered to be fundamental to caring and compassionate nursing (Benner, 1984). In Benner's text, *From Novice to Expert*, she describes the skills required to reflect on practice in order to develop expert practice and increase self-awareness (Benner, 1984). Benner, like Schön (Schön, 1984), considered that nurses often act intuitively; consequently, she demanded that nurses looked at what they did, reflected on why they did it, the impact or response of their actions and how they could do things differently (better).

Such reflection and disclosure depend on a trusting relationship very similar to the therapeutic relationship that exists between a nurse and their patient. So, in the same way that 'therapeutic relationships seem to be more about a way of being rather than doing' (Wright , 2015: 436), we need to accept that, for Fleur, being accepted, never judged and being given the space to reflect in order to move forward, have got to be fundamental to the process. The greatest challenge may be to find the time to reflect, hence supervision can provide the space for both reflection and consideration of practice, with another.

LOOKING AFTER YOUR SERVICE USERS; LOOKING AFTER YOU

There are many functions, definitions and models of supervision, however, ultimately, the main purpose of supervision is to ensure that care is evidence-based and safe. In modern mental health care, which increasingly requires evidence-based practice, it is fundamental to consider the practitioner's cognitive and emotional wellbeing and functioning as well as that of service users. Indeed, Maplethorpe et al. (2014) suggest that service-user-facilitated CS is one option.

Burnout has regularly been cited as a factor for nurses working in tiring and demanding **environments**, but Edwards et al. (2006) have suggested that effective CS lowers levels of burnout in mental heath nurses. *Fiona*, a mental health service user, voices her concerns about the impact of working as a mental health nurse and offers suggestions for how clinical supervision could be a supportive mechanism to prevent 'burnout':

I think, from my perspective, clinical supervision really is essential because of the things that nurses are facing nowadays. They are unable to spend a lot of time with patients and they are ill-informed when it comes to special populations of patients, for example, those with Borderline Personality Disorder and those who self-harm. They can't just be nurses, as there are a lot of social problems that are difficult to manage as well. So, with the lack of available supervision I think that nurses feel quite scared, they feel out of control and not equipped, and they have no one to talk to about it.

Staff are hesitant to share for fear of blame and looking like they're not up to the job. They have a lack of management support and they daren't admit that they aren't coping well, for fear of recriminations; so they won't want to inform people they know. It's hard to admit that sometimes things are difficult to deal with; that some patients are difficult to deal with and sometimes other staff are difficult to deal with too.

I think that it's a really good idea to have a supervisor that's not their manager and is not from that ward/service. They need someone who won't judge them and will give them time away from the ward to think and consider the decisions they are making. What they see can have an effect and they have no chance to talk about it, so go home feeling emotional … and what do they do with those emotions? I think that some nurses just go home via the off-licence! And that's contributing to burnout that is not good for staff nor for patients. Emotional and physical wellbeing is affected and there is a lot of sickness and reliance on agency staff. Staff could try to prepare for difficult situations in supervision to enable them to cope better and not feel that they are fire-fighting the whole time. This would be good if they knew that somebody was being admitted that self-harmed (for example) so that they could prepare themselves for how to be, rather than being 'reactive'.

In my opinion, in an ideal world staff would have 24 hour access to someone on the phone to talk about what has happened to them during their shift and access to someone face to face as soon as they need it.

Fiona Edgar, service user

CRITICAL THINKING STOP POINT 42.3

Fiona has suggested that staff could try to prepare for difficult situations to enable them to be more resilient. Can you think of an example of when this might have been helpful and how you would prepare for a clinical supervision session to do this?

We 'use ourselves' so much in our practice that it is inevitable that we will be personally affected by our interactions. Travelbee (1971) believed that the nurse's 'use of self' was a basic principle of nursing as the human-to-human relationship is the means through which the purpose of nursing is fulfilled. Travelbee (1971: 19) explains this as occurring within a conscious process which she refers to as the therapeutic use of self, and defines this as: 'When a nurse uses self therapeutically she consciously makes use of her **personality** and knowledge in order to effect a change in the ill person. This change is considered therapeutic when it alleviates the individual's stress.'

Unfortunately, not all nurses are self-aware, but a trusting clinical supervisory relationship can be one way of creating introspection, insight and self-awareness. According to Freshwater, the goal of any therapeutic alliance is to 'facilitate the emergence of the authentic self' and the 'therapeutic use of self' which are integral to nursing, amongst other caring **professions** (Freshwater, 2002: 4). Therefore, a care worker who has poor self-awareness and does not recognise the impact that their presence and manner may have on the patient is unlikely to develop a therapeutic relationship which is professional.

CRITICAL THINKING STOP POINT 42.4

How might you be able to develop self-awareness through clinical supervision?

IMPORTANCE OF THE SUPERVISORY RELATIONSHIP

An important key to good supervision for mental health practitioners is to have a positive, respectful and trusting working relationship to facilitate the practitioners to be open and transparent about their practice. Milne (2009: 152) discusses, in relation to supervision, that 'it takes two' and Crook Lyon & Potkar (2010) consider *disclosure* to be pivotal:

> Disclosure about clients, practice, self and the supervisory relationship is considered essential for the supervisee to gain maximum benefit from the supervision process and that failure to disclose is closely linked with the perceived quality of the supervision. (Crook Lyon & Potkar, 2010: 24)

There can often be various interpersonal, interprofessional dynamics, issues and responsibilities in mental health practice that can be complex and require the benefit of supervision to identify, discuss and promote effective working relationships. For *Gemma*, the relationship with the supervisor was the most significant part of the process:

Clinical supervision is really important to me because it gives me the opportunity to meet with someone regularly, to discuss ongoing issues, and to reflect on my practice.

I've been really lucky because my ward brings in an independent clinical supervisor with specialist knowledge in eating disorders who understands my field. It's really good just to get off the shop-floor and off-load sometimes. I sometimes feel like I'm going stir crazy so seeing her and talking things through helps massively as she can direct me. It's reassuring to hear them say that it's normal to feel like that. Sometimes you think that you're the only one that's ever felt like that as people don't always admit how the patients make you feel. She doesn't

(Continued)

tolerate whinging though, so I soon have to get my thoughts back to how to make things better rather than wallowing in how difficult things are! So it makes it possible for me to be honest and confront the impact that the work has on me.

It's nice to establish a relationship with the person too; it's empowering and good to hear that you're doing things well. Seeing the same person every month and developing a mutual understanding means that I don't need to go over stuff again and again, we have a foundation and trusting relationship. She remembers things right back to when I started and will remind me how far I have come. I know that she will never breach my confidence and that makes it possible to talk frankly and openly. I would never be offended if she expressed concern about me or my practice as I know that she is helping me to be better, not criticising me. It's helpful to have a different pair of ears and eyes on each scenario that I take to supervision.

Seema, mental health nurse

THE EXPECTATIONS OF THE SUPERVISOR

The CQC (2013: 6) comments that 'importantly clinical supervision has been linked to good clinical governance by helping to support quality improvement, managing risk and by increasing accountability'.

Likewise, the CQC (2013: 9) recommends that supervisors should:

- adopt a supportive and facilitative approach to help supervisees identify issues
- ensure that a supervision contract is in place to ensure both are aware of roles, responsibilities and boundaries
- keep a record and appropriately share information where there are serious concerns about conduct, competence or health of a practitioner
- keep up to date with their own professional development and also have access to their own supervision.

THE EXPECTATIONS OF THE SUPERVISEE

CASE STUDY:
STUDENT
NURSE
TO STAFF
NURSE

It is not unusual for nurses to raise issues that cause them **anxiety** and that are hence often closely related to risk. The CQC (2013: 9) recommends that supervisees should:

- prepare for supervision sessions, which include identifying issues from practice for discussion with their supervisor
- take responsibility for effective use of time and for actions taken as a result of supervision.

CONTRACTS AND RECORDS

There are many reasons to adopt both a contract and a record of supervision sessions, not least because of our professional requirements for revalidation (NMC, 2015b), but also because of what Grant refers to as the 'accountability culture' (Grant & Townend, 2007: 613). Ideally, a supervision contract identifying the role, responsibilities and boundaries of the supervision relationship should be agreed and signed and kept by both supervisor and supervisee.

CRITICAL DEBATE 42.1

Engagement with CS

The most frequently cited reason for not engaging with clinical supervision is lack of time/an inability to leave the ward. Some would argue that if clinical supervision is undertaken, then the nurse will work better and more effectively. Others suggest that clinical supervision is mainly used when they are having problems and, thus, things have already gone wrong and it's too late.

Discuss: Clinical supervision should be a proactive, not reactive, activity.

CHALLENGING CONCEPTS 42.1

Burnout and clinical supervision

Burnout has regularly been cited as a factor for nurses who work in tiring and demanding environments. Although clinical supervision is cited as one way of creating resilience in nurses as they are supported, guided and developed through this process, others suggest that when a nurse reaches the point of burnout, they are too exhausted to find the motivation to change.

Is it the clinical supervisor's role to inspire and motivate? What should they do if they feel that a nurse is not functioning to the point that service users are not receiving adequate care?

CONCLUSION

Many professional issues can be challenging or, at worst, overwhelming, but being able to discuss, reflect on and, if required, seek further reading, training or support can only help enhance and sustain professional practice to be rooted in evolving evidenced-based practice.

Clinical supervision should aim to provide a safe working professional relationship for mental health nurses to actively engage in and reflect on their clinical practice, and to be able to discuss difficult situations, problems, concerns and professional issues that may occur with their clients and colleagues, or at times even personal issues that may impact on or **affect** their working practice, such as their own mental/emotional wellbeing that at times may feel overwhelming. Clinical supervision is one vehicle to enhance practice or make changes to ultimately benefit the wider context of their work by reducing stress, limiting emotional exhaustion and preventing burnout.

In our current world of increased requirements for evidenced-based practice in mental health, we have a desire to know what works and what makes a positive difference. As mental health nurses, we know that the area we practise in is increasingly challenging and, has no absolutes in relation to human interpersonal work with our clients or, at times, our colleagues. Hence, clinical supervision should be an integral part of mental health professionals' working life and be both rooted in staff support and a part of management and ongoing professional development for each individual within each team.

--- **CHAPTER SUMMARY** ---

This chapter has covered:

- What clinical supervision is
- The professional duty of the nurse with regard to clinical supervision
- A range of perspectives about clinical supervision
- How to use CS to look after your service users and yourself
- The expectations of you and your supervisor within clinical supervision.

--- **BUILD YOUR BIBLIOGRAPHY** ---

Books/book chapters

- Caroll, M. & Holloway, E. (eds) (1999) *Counselling supervision in context.* London: SAGE.
- Power, S. (1999) *Nursing supervision: A guide for clinical practice.* London: SAGE.
- Pryjmachuk, S. (2011) *Mental health nursing: An evidence based introduction.* London: SAGE.
- Roberts, M. & Walker, S. (eds) (2015) *Critical thinking and reflection for mental health nursing students.* London: SAGE.
- Walker, S. (2014) *Engagement and therapeutic communication in mental health nursing.* London: SAGE.

SAGE journal articles

FURTHER
READING:
JOURNAL
ARTICLES

Go to https://study.sagepub.com/essentialmentalhealth for further free online journal articles related to this chapter. If you are using the interactive ebook, simply click on the book icon in the margin to go straight to the resource.

- Berggren, I. & Severinsson, E. (2000) The influence of clinical supervision on nurses' moral decision making. *Nursing Ethics,* 7(2), 124-133.
- Davey, B., Desousa, C., Robinson, S., et al. (2006) The policy-practice divide: who has clinical supervision in nursing? *Journal of Research in Nursing,* 11(3), 237-248.
- Ellis, M.V., Berger, L., Hanus, A.E., et al. (2013) Inadequate and harmful clinical supervision: testing a revised framework and assessing occurrence. *The Counseling Psychologist,* 42(4), 434-472.

Weblinks

FURTHER
READING:
WEBLINKS

Go to https://study.sagepub.com/essentialmentalhealth for further weblinks related to this chapter. If you are using the interactive ebook, simply click on the book icon in the margin to go straight to the resource.

- Flying Start NHS: www.flyingstart.scot.nhs.uk/learning-programmes/safe-practice/clinical-supervision – an online learning resource for clinical supervision

- The Royal College of Nursing, which provides authoritative resources on clinical supervision: www.rcn.org.uk/get-help/rcn-advice/clinical-supervision
- Nursing & Midwifery Council: http://revalidation.nmc.org.uk – the NMC's website provides a step-by-step approach to revalidation; clinical supervision and reflectivity can count towards this process and are supported by the NMC as learning activities

ACE YOUR ASSESSMENT

Revise what you have learned by visiting https://study.sagepub.com/essentialmentalhealth. If you are using the interactive ebook, simply click on the tick icon to go straight to the resource.

ONLINE
QUIZZES &
ACTIVITY
ANSWERS

- Test yourself with multiple-choice and short-answer questions and flashcards.

REFERENCES

Ashburner, C., Meyer, J., Cotte, A., et al. (2004) Seeing things differently: evaluating psychodynamically informed group clinical supervision for general hospital nurses. *NT Research, 9,* 38–48.

Bambling, M., King, R., Raue, P., et al. (2006) Clinical supervision: its influence on client-rated working alliance and client symptom reduction in the brief treatment of major depression. *Psychotherapy Research, 16*(3), 317–331.

Banks, D., Clifton, A.V., Purdy, M.J., et al. (2013) Mental health nursing and the problematic of supervision as a confessional act. *Journal of psychiatric and mental health nursing,* 20(7), 595–600.

Benner, P. (1984) *From novice to expert: Excellence and power in the clinical nursing process.* Menlo Park, CA: Addison-Wiley.

Bernard, J.M. & Goodyear, R.K. (2004) *Fundamentals of clinical supervision,* 3rd edition. London: Pearson.

Bradshaw, T., Butterworth, A. & Mairs, H. (2007) Does structured clinical supervision during psychosocial intervention education enhance outcome for mental health nurses and the service users they work with? *J Psychiatr Ment Health Nurs,* 14(1), 4–12.

Brunero, S. & Stein-Parbury, J. (2008) The effectiveness of clinical supervision in nursing: an evidence based literature review. *Australian Journal of Advanced Nursing,* 25(3), 86–94.

Butterworth, T., Bell, L., Jackson, C. & Pajnkihar, M. (2008) Wicked spell or magic bullet? A review of the clinical supervision literature. *Nurse Education Today, 28,* 264–272.

Care Quality Commission (CQC) (2013) *Supporting information guidance: Supporting effective clinical supervision.* Available at: www.cqc.org.uk/sites/default/files/documents/20130625_800734_v1_00_supporting_information-effective_clinical_supervision_for_publication.pdf (accessed 16.06.2016).

Crook Lyon, R.E. & Potkar, K.A. (2010) The supervisory relationship. In N. Ladany & J.E. Bradley (eds) *Counsellor supervision,* 4th edition. Abingdon: Routledge. pp. 15–52.

Department of Health (1993) *A vision for the future.* London: DH.

Department of Health (1994) *The Allitt Inquiry: Independent inquiry relating to deaths and injuries on the children's ward at Grantham and Kesteven General Hospital during the period February to April 1991* (Clothier Report). London: HMSO.

Department of Health (2004) *The ten essential shared capabilities.* London: DH. p. 29.

Department of Health (2008) *Improving access to psychological therapies (IAPT) commissioning toolkit.* London: DH.

Edwards, D., Burnard, P., Hannigan, B., et al. (2006) Clinical supervision and burnout: the influence of clinical supervision for community mental health nurses. *Journal of Clinical Nursing*, 15(8), 1007–1015.

Falender, C.A. & Shafranske, E.P. (2007) Competence in competency-based supervision practice: construct and application. *Professional Psychology: Research and Practice*, 38, 232–240.

Faugier, J. & Butterworth, T. (1994) *Clinical supervision: A position paper.* Manchester: University of Manchester.

Felton, A., Sheppard, F. & Stacey, G. (2012) Exposing the tensions of implementing supervision in pre-registration nurse education. *Nurse Education in Practice*, 12, 36–40.

Freshwater, D. (2002) Therapeutic nursing. In D. Freshwater (ed.) *Therapeutic use of self in nursing.* London: Sage.

Gonsalvez, C.J. & Milne, D.L. (2010) Clinical supervisor training in Australia: a review of current problems and possible solutions. *Australian Psychologist*, 45, 233–242.

Grant, A. & Townend, M. (2007) Some emerging implications for clinical supervision in British mental health nursing. *Journal of Psychiatric & Mental Health Nursing*, 14(6), 609–614.

Hawkins, P. & Shohet, R. (2000) *Supervision in the helping professions: An individual group and organisational approach*, 2nd edition. New York: Open University Press.

Kirk, J. (2010) Going it alone: working in private practice. In M. Mueller, H. Kennerley, F. McManus & D. Westbrook (eds) *Oxford guide to surviving as a CBT therapist.* Oxford: Oxford University Press. pp. 275–299.

Maplethorpe, F., Dixon, J. & Rush, B. (2014) Participation in clinical supervision (PACS): an evaluation of student nurse clinical supervision facilitated by mental health service users. *Nurse Education in Practice*, 14(2), 183–187.

Milne, D.L. (2007) An empirical definition of clinical supervision. *British Journal of Clinical Psychology*, 46, 437–447.

Milne, D.L. (2009) *Evidence-based clinical supervision: Principles and practice.* Oxford: Blackwell.

Nursing and Midwifery Council (2006) *Clinical supervision: A–Z advice sheet.* London: NMC. Available at: www.supervisionandcoaching.com/pdf/page2/CS%20Advice%20Nursing%20Midwifery%20Council%20(UK)(2006).pdf (accessed 15.06.16).

Nursing and Midwifery Council (2015a) *NMC code.* London: NMC. Available at: www.nmc.org.uk/standards/code (accessed 16.06.16).

Nursing and Midwifery Council (2015b) *How to revalidate with the NMC.* London: NMC. Available at: www.nmc.org.uk/globalassets/sitedocuments/revalidation/how-to-revalidate-booklet.pdf (accessed 16.06.16).

Nursing and Midwifery Council (NMC) (2016) *NMC Responds to Midwifery Supervision Report.* Available at: www.nmc.org.uk/press-releases/nmc-responds-to-midwifery-supervision-report (accessed 04.12.17).

Proctor, B. (1986) Supervision: a co-operative exercise in accountability. In M. Marken and M. Payne (eds) *Enabling and ensuring.* Leicester: National Youth Bureau and Council for Education and Training in Youth and Community Work. pp. 21–23.

Proctor, B. & Inskipp, F. (2001) Group supervision. In J. Scaife (ed.) *Supervision in the mental health professions: A practitioner's guide.* Hove: Brunner-Routledge.

Scaife, J. (2001) *Supervision in the mental health professions: A practitioner's guide.* Hove: Brunner-Routledge.

Schön, D.. (1984) *The Reflective Practitioner.* London: Temple Smith.

Sloan,G.(2006) *Clinical Supervision in Mental Health Nursing.* Chichester: Whurr.

Travelbee, J. (1971) *Interpersonal aspects of nursing*, 2nd edition. Philadelphia: F.A. Davies.

Watkins, C.E., Jr. (2011) Does psychotherapy supervision contribute to patient outcomes? Considering 30 years of research. *The Clinical Supervisor*, 30(2), 1–22.

White, E. & Winstanley, J. (2010) A randomised controlled trial of clinical supervision: selected findings from a novel Australian attempt to establish the evidence base for causal relationships with quality of care and patient outcomes, as an informed contribution to mental health nursing practice development. *Journal of Research in Nursing*, *15*(2), 151–167.

White, E. & Winstanley, J. (2011) Clinical supervision for mental health professionals: the evidence base. *Social Work and Social Sciences Review*, *14*(3), 77–94.

White, E. & Winstanley, J. (2014) Clinical supervision and the helping professions: an interpretation of history. *The Clinical Supervisor*, *33*(1), 3–25.

Wright, K.M. (2015) Maternalism: a healthy alliance for recovery and transition in eating disorder services. *Journal of psychiatric and mental health nursing*, *22*(6), 431–439.

COMMISSIONING FOR MENTAL HEALTH SERVICES

43

GED McCANN, MICK BURNS AND IAN CALLAGHAN

THIS CHAPTER COVERS

- A brief outline of the process of commissioning, its background, and how it relates to the nurse in everyday practice
- Service user and practitioner voices in the commissioning process – the importance of establishing a tri-partite relationship between service users, clinicians and commissioners in delivering on the commissioning process
- Multiple systems – engaging with and harnessing the multiple stakeholders involved across the health, social care and criminal justice systems, to improve patient pathways and outcomes
- Using the evidence – developing and utilising clinical information and published guidance and the importance of improving and analysing provider data in the commissioning process.

> I have worked in the NHS for over seven years and have a genuine passion for mental health nursing. Whilst I have enjoyed working as a frontline member of staff, I also felt the need to learn about the role of a nurse within a Clinical Commissioning Group. Through my participation in an eight-week placement, I had sought to understand what commissioning really means at the frontline, and to understand how the '6Cs' (NHS England, 2013) is embedded into the commissioning framework. The placement gave me the opportunity to meet with commissioners and partner organisations across a number of local CCGs, in fact a key message I took from my mentor, the Chief Nurse at Erewash CCG, was the importance of how working together can really help to achieve more with less energy. The evidence for this can be clearly seen in the new models of integration in health and social care – the Vanguard sites (NHS England, 2014).
>
> The role of a nurse within this setting can be empowering and I found the whole experience really useful, allowing me a better understanding of the holy trinity of efficiency, clarity, and accountability. Participating in quality assurance groups and contract meetings, which oversee and monitor provider CQUIN's (DH, 2008), I was able to
>
> *(Continued)*

Visit **https://study.sagepub.com/essentialmentalhealth** to access a wealth of online resources for this chapter - watch out for the margin icons throughout the chapter. If you are using the interactive ebook, simply click on the margin icon to go straight to the resource.

understand how the basic principles of 'health economics and quality' impact on care delivery at the frontline. I can see how a basic understanding of commissioning will allow frontline nurses to fully participate in planning, implementing and evaluating programmes which may have a great impact on the health of the community.

With the rapid development of CCGs across the country it is increasingly difficult to ignore the role of the nurse within the commissioning arena. I have gained a better awareness of my own practice and its implications on commissioning and patient care, which has increased my level of motivation and enthusiasm to want to make a real difference at the frontline. I have also developed a greater insight into how my own efforts can contribute to the efforts and the performance of others, with whom I work. With all of the difficulties the NHS faces I have come to realise that 'cooperation' is the bedrock of commissioning because this will recognise and allow human endeavour to flourish within nursing practice.

Femi Ogundipe, mental health nurse

Around 5 years ago, during my stay in a secure hospital, I was at a meeting for service users, staff and commissioners looking at ways of improving secure services, and as I went to talk to one of the commissioners, someone said to me 'you can't talk to her, she's a commissioner!' I paid no attention of course, and did indeed go up to speak to her, but this illustrates the disconnect that had existed for a long time between many commissioners and service users. Somehow, paradoxically, commissioners were seen as distant from the actual experience of service users, which was probably also felt by many of the staff working hard to deliver the services that were being commissioned. Fortunately, times have changed and many service users have gone on to work with commissioners and others at NHS England to bring about significant improvements to the mental health system and, in particular, the way secure mental health services are commissioned and delivered.

I'd been fortunate to have experience of the important role that commissioners can play in the care that people receive while in hospital as my case manager usually attended my CPA meetings and took a keen interest in my progress. I didn't ever get to speak to her directly however, the attitude expressed at that earlier meeting still prevailed at that time, but things have changed considerably since then. It was such a breath of fresh air when I finally became involved in the project that was to have such an impact on the delivery of secure mental health services and the experience of service users, which we called My Shared Pathway (Ayub et al., 2013). Without the foresight and encouragement of commissioners, this undoubtedly wouldn't have had the impact it has had – there has been such an improvement in the collaborative nature of the commissioning and delivery of secure care and the continued input and drive from commissioning teams and the importance placed on working with service users has been central to this. Services are now much more recovery focused, outcomes are clearer, and the relationship between commissioning and service user experience is stronger than ever.

Tom, service user

INTRODUCTION

What is commissioning?

Commissioning is simply the process used in a local context to decide how we spend available funds to improve health (Sobanja, 2009). In its widest sense, commissioning is about understanding health care delivery for populations as well as individuals, and designing systems to ensure that the best health outcomes are achieved for the resources available. As a mental health nurse, this process may seem a little peripheral or even irrelevant to planning care for individuals on a day-to-day basis. However, this chapter will aim to challenge that view, and argue that an understanding of commissioning will transform the way nurses view all aspects of care delivery, as well as ignite a passion for innovation. The concept of commissioning will be explored as well as how **service users** and practitioners can harness the commissioning process to achieve tangible benefits. For commissioning is about engaging with individuals, like the individuals in the stories above demonstrate, in a pragmatic, hands-on way. It means changing the behaviours of individuals and organisations to achieve real health outcomes, and it means developing close relationships, setting boundaries and taking risks.

In fact, commissioning is a simple cyclical process that in many ways mirrors the stages nurses utilise in planning care. Just as nurses assess, plan, implement and evaluate care for individuals, commissioners are responsible for assessing the health needs of individuals or a population, planning health care services to meet those needs, procuring or contracting those services to meet the need and then evaluating how well this has been done. The cycle then starts again.

The initial phase of the commissioning process is therefore understanding need and this can be done in a number of ways. Clearly, as a nurse, the more you can engage with an individual and develop a trusting relationship, the more effective the **care plan** will be. This is because the needs of the individual become clearer the more you know them, and the more they are willing to engage with you. Similarly, the commissioning process begins by engaging with individuals and communities to understand what health outcomes need addressing, whilst at the same time brokering a partnership relationship in meeting those needs. In mental health services, this means working closely with clinical colleagues and service users to develop a detailed knowledge of services in a given locality, or setting, and to understand the issues they face in providing care. On a population basis, it also means working with colleagues in public health to understand the needs of a given population and what these might look like over time, and perhaps what works in other populations based on the evidence.

Commissioners will also use a combination of methods and public health approaches, drawing on epidemiological studies, population-based health research and local mental health statistical information. More importantly, commissioners will need to engage with frontline clinicians and service users to understand how care operates within a given service, and how it might be improved, and that will mean talking directly to staff and patients, to build up a detailed picture. Just as a nurse will use **assessment tools** to understand an individual, a wealth of data exists relating to populations that commissioners can draw upon. Minimum data sets and qualitative information collated by hospitals and community services can be collated across a particular geography in order to understand and prioritise need, upon which future services can be planned. Drawing together clinicians that deliver a whole-care pathway is an effective means of understanding how care can be directed to achieve the best outcomes. Similarly, organising a workshop of all clinicians working in a particular service setting across a geographical area can identify gaps in services for a local population.

As an example, in order to develop a 3–5 year strategy for women's secure mental health services across Yorkshire and the Humber, a number of workshops were organised to draw together clinicians, commissioners and service users to discuss how services could be improved. These meetings allowed for **collaboration** across multiple hospital sites, at varying levels of secure care, to identify how the current pathway for service users could be developed in order to reduce lengths of stay, and the quality of care. Topics for discussion focused on defining admission criteria; care planning outcomes; the configuration and location of services; caring for people closer to home; innovation; and specialist clinical programmes. The result was an agreed strategy for the Yorkshire and Humber population, the development of a secure service in Wakefield, and York, and an innovative therapeutic locked service also in York as part of an integrated pathway for women.

LEADERSHIP AND RELATIONSHIPS

Whatever method is used, to understand need it is important to build up relationships with clinicians and service users in order for them to engage in any planned changes, and this requires leadership. Commissioners need to provide leadership within the health care system they are working with; sometimes this is a local system such as an inpatient service within a hospital trust, sometimes a regional system such as all medium secure services across a geographical area. In certain circumstances, it is necessary to work across a national system, depending on the population that is being served, for instance attempting to establish health care systems within the prison population in England (James, 2016). In whatever setting commissioning takes place, the relationship with clinicians and service users will be instrumental in effecting change, and this requires a certain level of clinical credibility, an ability to build trust and a vision of how things could change – the same qualities expected of all nurses who wish to see the best health outcomes. This relationship, however, is complex in that it is collaborative, not hierarchical, and dependent on a number of mutually agreed outcomes, some of which may require significant negotiation. The relationship is further complicated because it is usually transactional, in that it is driven through a contractual agreement, underpinned by a legal framework. In essence, the commissioner needs to be able to develop and communicate a strategic vision for a community or a pathway of services that providers want to subscribe to, underpinned by minimum standards, and again these skills resonate with the core nurse competencies.

PLANNING

Once we understand what health outcomes need to be addressed, a range of services can then be planned and procured. This can involve the reorganisation or refocusing of an established network of services, or it may require commissioners to go out to tender for new services and innovation. Commissioners are therefore required to manage complex processes and projects to ensure that contracts are awarded in a way that avoids legal challenge, whilst ensuring that service provision meets strategic objectives. It is not unusual for commissioners to plan in five- or even ten-year cycles in order to have the time to understand, and redesign, services to meet current and future needs.

Once services have been contracted to provide a service, the contract then needs to be monitored. This process again requires significant collaboration with clinicians, managers, service users and other commissioners to establish mechanisms by which the quality of services and the experience of those receiving the services can be measured. Commissioners are essentially responsible for managing this approach and holding providers of services to account on behalf of the public.

THE DEVELOPMENT OF COMMISSIONING

The background to how commissioning has developed across the UK has not been straightforward, and only recently has the process been articulated and described (DH, 2007). Its development has hinged on a number of political initiatives designed to manage NHS resources effectively, within the context of a number of societal pressures, behaviours and expectations. In 1991, John Major's Conservative government introduced legislation to promote competition between health care providers (HM Government, 1989), and this was achieved by separating NHS organisations into 'purchaser/provider' roles. District health authorities, established in 1982 to run local hospitals on behalf of the Department of Health, became purchasers of care and were mandated to buy health services from local hospitals on behalf of their local communities. This initiative ran alongside a GP fundholding scheme that saw groups of GPs collaborating to buy some episodes of elective care on behalf of their patients. The intention was for the new internal market to **drive** down price and improve the quality of services through economic market mechanisms.

In opposition, the Labour Party campaigned against marketisation of the NHS, arguing that the 'internal market' had caused fragmentation. However, on gaining power in 1997 the New Labour administration published an equally radical manifesto of reforms that rejected the old 'command and control' and 'internal market' models (HM Government, 1997) and laid the ground for the introduction of further market reforms in 2002 (National Health Service Reform and Health Care **Professions** Act 2002). By 2002, the 'purchasers' of 1991 had evolved into 'commissioners' – commissioners who would help patients navigate a complex web of choice about which provider (including private providers) to use for a range of elective procedures. This new system was given additional leverage by the withdrawal of block contracts (annual blocks of money to provide a service but with little incentive to change practice), which were then replaced by a complex 'payment by results' system which rewarded providers for seeing and treating more patients, thus driving down waiting times in the process. These reforms allowed greater sophistication within existing contracts, and began to place more emphasis on patients being customers, whilst at the same time introducing a greater expectation of better **value** for the funding.

The controversial Health and Social Care Act 2012, introduced by the Conservative/Liberal Democrat coalition government, laid the ground to open up the NHS to competition from 'any willing' (qualified) provider. The much feared explosion in private competition didn't materialise, and, against a backdrop of public concern with NHS hospitals prompted by the Mid Staffordshire Trust inquiry (Francis, 2013), and a change in health secretary, much of the focus in the NHS during the latter part of the coalition term and the subsequent Conservative majority government was on strengthening the role of the regulator in the NHS (HSJ, 2015) and encouraging providers to work collaboratively rather than competitively (NHS England, 2014). All of these recent changes to health legislation have enabled the opportunity for greater patient say over the services they receive, whilst commissioners have assumed a greater role in improving quality across patient pathways.

Within this changing political landscape, the discipline of commissioning has struggled to establish itself as being credible in the NHS since its introduction as 'purchasing' in 1991 (Britnell et al., 2008; Davies, 2007). Various theories have been put forward to explain this failure to thrive: a lack of clarity around what commissioning is and does (Britnell et al., 2008); the NHS tendency to reorganise itself at frequent intervals, denying the discipline the chance to mature (Davies, 2007); and a lack of evidence about what skills and competencies commissioners require (Woodin & Wade, 2007).

Despite this, the high level policy framework, driven by changing demographics, has inexorably moved the health care system towards a model that reinforces the need for the health economy to be underpinned by robust commissioning (EFILWC, 2003). The phenomena of 'triple ageing' across the European Union (Coomans, 1999), an increase in the expectations of users of health care services and technological advances in medicine and medical devices, mean that there is significant potential for the costs of health and social care to spiral out of control (EFILWC, 2003). A strong commissioning framework is therefore seen as vital in moving the UK health system away from a reactive provider-driven system towards a more proactive, preventative and economically viable approach (Britnell et al., 2008; NHS Institute for Innovation and Improvement, 2008).

The introduction of the World Class Commissioning assurance framework (DH, 2007) was a deliberately ambitious attempt by the Department of Health to push commissioning to a new level (Britnell et al., 2008). This was a recognition that commissioning in the NHS had failed to reach its potential and that power within the NHS still sat within large provider organisations. The competency framework proposed under World Class Commissioning was therefore an attempt to raise ambitions for commissioning in a way that has not been achieved in any of the modern health economies internationally. The ambition was to shift the balance of power away from provider organisations back to local communities, ensuring that health provision was based on population need and not provider interest (DH, 2007). This policy may well be resurrected under the current regime with the Tory Secretary of State for Health, Jeremy Hunt, proposing 'Ofsted' style ratings for clinical commissioning groups (CCGs) covering a range of clinical areas (cancer, **dementia**, learning disabilities, mental health and maternity) (HSJ, 2015).

CRITICAL THINKING STOP POINT 43.1

The chronology, as outlined above in terms of the development of commissioning and the purchaser-provider split across the NHS, would suggest that some order of logic and intellectual thinking has gone into the process. In reality, the NHS is prone to the whims and political leanings of successive governments as they grapple with its complexities on a four- to five-year rota. Many would argue (e.g. Walshe, 2015) that the problems that the NHS continues to attempt to resolve are not best served by frequent reorganisations, or by changes in the direction of policy that are brought about by speed dating with a succession of health secretaries that change about every two years. Many policy and structural changes take many years to embed before they begin to produce any results, and this requires stability and sustainable planning. Yet more reform is planned. Devolution of NHS budgets to local governments such as Manchester is one of the current government's flagship policies (McKenna & Dunn, 2015), yet significant policy issues remain unresolved. Other changes, such as the development of sustainable transformation plans by each health and social care group in England, and the development of new care models at pilot sites in England (NHS England, 2014), will seek to transform local commissioning arrangements. Many of these changes seek to deliver a number of commendable policy objectives, but are often generated and implemented without the close involvement of practitioners, commissioners or service users.

- In selecting one local initiative or policy objective, consider the following:

    i. What level of practitioner, service user or commissioner involvement has taken place?
    ii. How does the initiative fit with other planned changes across the wider context of health and social care policy objectives?

- Consider how commissioning processes might continue to change in the current rapidly changing landscape of health service provision.

WHAT'S THE EVIDENCE? 43.1

The World Class Commissioning initiative (Sobanja, 2009) provided a very detailed commissioning framework that not only allowed the process to be articulated, but also identified the core competencies required of commissioners. The 11 competencies required as a commissioner and identified to achieve world class commissioning are as follows. Commissioners:

- are recognised as the local leader of the NHS
- work collaboratively with community partners to commission services that optimise health gains and reductions in health inequalities
- proactively seek and build continuous and meaningful engagement with the public and patients, to shape services and improve health
- lead continuous and meaningful engagement with clinicians to inform strategy, and drive quality, service design and resource utilisation
- manage knowledge and undertake robust and regular needs assessments that establish a full understanding of current and future local health needs and requirements
- prioritise investment according to local needs, service requirements and the values of the NHS
- effectively stimulate the market to meet demand and secure required clinical and health and wellbeing outcomes
- promote and specify continuous improvements in quality and outcomes through clinical and provider innovation and configuration
- secure procurement skills that ensure robust and viable contracts
- effectively manage systems and work in partnership with providers to ensure contract compliance and continuous improvement in quality and outcomes
- make sound financial investments to ensure sustainable development and value for money.

SERVICE USER AND PRACTITIONER VOICES IN THE COMMISSIONING PROCESS

CASE STUDY:
MENTAL
HEALTH
SERVICES

So far, we have argued strongly for the need to involve clinicians when commissioning services as they have a wealth of information in relation to need, service provision, and in terms of being a strong partner in designing and delivering services. We have also described how they can be engaged in the commissioning process. Equally, service users have a powerful voice when it comes to describing what services are actually like to experience, what their needs are and what outcomes they would like to achieve. Moreover, they are crucial at every step of the process and provide a perspective that clinicians and service managers cannot. As active participants in the commissioning process, their involvement has demonstrated key improvements in the quality of services, as well as numerous personal benefits through the act of involvement itself (McKeown et al., 2014). For commissioning to be really effective, there needs to be a balance between the three perspectives of service user, clinician and commissioner, in order to ensure that health benefits are maximised with the available resources. Fundamentally, it is involvement in the decision-making processes aligned to clinical practice and policy that is the key to successful service design and real outcomes for service users, which is reflected in current NHS policy. How service users can be engaged at each step of the process is much more difficult to achieve however, although examples of good practice are available. Here, one service user, Ian Callaghan, involved closely with commissioning in the past few years, gives his views:

I was diagnosed with bipolar disorder in 1987 at the age of 23 in my final year at medical school. Periods of severe depression interrupted my career at which I was otherwise very successful and the 1990s saw several admissions to hospital on an informal basis. I'd tried a whole range of medications and talking therapies seemed not to work. Things spiralled out of control in the mid 2000s and after a catastrophic crisis, I was admitted to a secure unit in 2007. While in the secure unit, I received some good as well as some not such good care. At times, there was a lack of clear direction or meaningful involvement in care planning and less collaboration in my care than I would have liked. For some of us, it wasn't clear what we had to do to move on and out of secure care. I became committed to trying to improve things – for myself and for others. Involvement in governance structures proved very frustrating: if it wasn't financial problems it was procedural rules; change was so difficult to effect. There was often a will on the part of management, but there often wasn't a way.

It was 2010 and the grounds for change across the country on the part of people in secure care, was increasing. Some enlightened commissioners in Yorkshire & the Humber, including the other two authors of this chapter, and Rosie Ayub (Ayub et al., 2013), were encouraging regional service user involvement groups that were having a great effect on the way many services were delivered. There was appetite for change elsewhere and a national meeting of service user representatives, staff, managers and commissioners was held in York. It was the first time people had come together in this way and the atmosphere was electric – there was incredible enthusiasm and commitment to improving an inadequate system. We wanted to be involved and to be the drivers for change. After all, secure services were there to support us to get well, learn how to keep ourselves and others safe and return to living in the community.

People were saying how they felt they were staying in inpatient secure care for too long. Some people actually said they didn't know why they were there in the first place. Many people felt staff knew about their clinical history but didn't know them as people, with experiences and skills that were more important to them than their mental health history. People felt that they had been locked up and the key thrown away. They described experiencing increasingly complex layers of stigma, with a forensic history trumping even the widespread prejudice towards people with severe mental illness. And many reported negative attitudes amongst their caregivers: people reported being told that they deserved to be locked up for what they'd done.

So there was a great desire for change to the system. Development groups were set up with representatives from across the country looking at the whole secure care pathway and, in particular, the areas where the process could be improved. Care planning, CPA (care programme approach) meetings, greater collaboration in risk assessment and safety planning, more meaningful activities, access to education and occupation, contact with family and friends and improving relationships were all areas that were identified as in need of improvement. We wanted the whole of our care to be more recovery focused and we wanted clearer, more explicit outcomes to work towards. Working with commissioners, both locally and nationally, was key to achieving the changes we were trying to make – without their support it is unlikely that progress would have been made.

Out of this, a recovery-focused programme called 'My Shared Pathway' was born, with materials to support people to think about and develop clearer care plans in the areas service users said were important to them: Reaching a Shared Understanding; Me and My Recovery;

(Continued)

My Health; My Safety and Risks; and My Relationships. Some suggested outcomes and their measures were drawn up in 'My Outcome, Plans and Progress' and for staff, managers and commissioners, they developed a clearer 'Pathway Process'. With the help of two Commissioning for Quality and Innovation (CQUIN) quality incentive targets, developed by and driven by service users and commissioners, My Shared Pathway was implemented in secure units across the country. For some, there was little change in already great practice, but for others it posed a real challenge. However, some people felt that giving service users more control and responsibility would increase risk. Some staff found the new goal-focused 'coaching style' difficult as it challenged the way they lived their own lives. Some just couldn't adapt at all. The drive placed on these changes by commissioning teams and the benefits to the way our care was commissioned and delivered became central to the implementation of My Shared Pathway – fortunately a momentum was generated and there was no going back.

To support the implementation of My Shared Pathway, a network of nine regional Recovery and Outcomes Groups was set up, bringing together service users, staff, managers and commissioners in the same geographical area. Designed to facilitate the sharing of best practice, difficulties and developments, the groups also gave service users a greater voice and confidence. They were able to meet service users from neighbouring units, speak face-to-face with commissioners and feed their views into national work, encouraged greatly following the formation of NHS England in 2013. Something very magical happened when people were taken out of a clinical environment and brought together in an informal setting with lunch and time to mingle. We often overheard conversations between service users and commissioners that ended with the commissioners saying 'that's something I can fix as soon as I get back to the office'.

Following years of hard work, service users in secure care now have much more control over and responsibility for their care and pathway. Perhaps most importantly, there is an increased sense of hope and optimism for many people. And thanks to the Recovery and Outcomes Groups, people now have a stronger voice locally with their own commissioners and nationally with NHS England and have provided crucial input into the development of the Five Year Forward View for Mental Health (the Mental Health Taskforce). Such collaboration between service users and commissioners is a clear win-win situation – a better experience for people in care, with a clearer, more optimal pathway and better long-term outcomes. Let's hope the situation continues to improve, and there are still definitely areas of improvement that need to be addressed, such as better crisis care and greater support for people to avoid secure care in the first place. Here I have described the collaboration between service users and commissioners in NHS England directly commissioned services – such close involvement is often not the case when it comes to Clinical Commissioning Groups. However, things have changed so much since I was first in the secure hospital in 2007. I'm sure things will continue to improve in the years ahead. Following confirmation of funding from NHS England, my role in coordinating the Recovery and Outcomes Groups nationally has been secured and I am now employed by the national charity Rethink Mental Illness as the Recovery and Outcomes Manager.

Ian Callahan, former secure service user

1. The scenario above demonstrates how service users can be involved in the commissioning process, something that is often overlooked. Consider why this is important and what benefits might be achieved in involving service users in commissioning.
2. Consider how *you* might be able to influence commissioning decisions by introducing service users into the process.

MULTIPLE SYSTEMS

Consider:

- the competing demands between providers, clinicians, patients and commissioners
- the impact of the CQC, **safeguarding**, monitoring, the government, the public, local authorities, criminal justice agencies
- priorities of national versus regional versus local commissioning
- financial restraints, cost-efficiencies, rationing, changing demographics.

Commissioners in mental health services are required to occupy a difficult boundary position between systems (the purchaser/provider system, between NHS and independent/third-sector organisations, between providers of and regulators of services), between organisations and even between clinicians and the service users in their care. This complex dynamic means those commissioners have a very difficult role to manage, acting both within and outside the various systems and often acting as a repository for the anxieties in the various systems (Cardona, 1999; Menzies Lyth, 1988). It is therefore important for commissioners to be aware of the potential for these tensions to interfere with delivery of the primary task in hand and to attend to these tensions through supervision and through the careful management of relationships in the system. This requirement again resonates with mental health nursing and perhaps explains why so many nurses make effective commissioners. Some of these tensions include the following:

- The needs of individuals versus the needs of a population are a fundamental cause of tension. Clearly, resources are finite and need to be rationed in meeting multiple needs. In a cash-limited NHS, how do commissioners decide what resources to invest in cancer care compared to mental health?
- When trying to understand need, there is a difference between what individuals need and what they want, and this is further confused by expectations based on perceptions of what the NHS can deliver. Multiple demands on the NHS need to be understood in terms of what needs should be addressed, in order to have the greatest impact on health, and these decisions are not always popular.
- The involvement of service users in the decision-making process also creates a tension in terms of managing the expectations of individuals and the priorities of the NHS. Listening to patients cannot be tokenistic, however this has the potential to lead to bias in allocating resources.
- Stimulation of the market and the generation of private providers in order to lead to competition and cost-effective services mean that profits are made in the provision of essential care. This creates tension in meeting the core values and principles underpinning the NHS.
- Commissioning organisations create barriers and tensions in commissioning priorities between local clinical commissioning groups and national specialist commissioning groups, and these tensions are further complicated through the introduction of provider commissioning, and individual patient budgets. How these varying priorities at the different commissioning levels are managed is a key concern.

Over and above these tensions are the competing demands of other organisations, including the Care Quality Commission, local authorities, the Ministry of Justice, the national probation service and prison system. These key players, who have such an impact on the delivery of health care, mean that commissioners are required to understand how they operate and actively seek to coordinate their competing needs with those of the NHS.

It is these systemic tensions which highlight how important it is for commissioners to lead and manage the system in a collaborative psychologically informed manner, and to forge effective relationships with these agencies in order to achieve cost-effective services. To assist in this process and manage system pressures across the care pathway for patients, the introduction of case managers has had a significant effect.

Case Management as a discipline was introduced into commissioning in 2000; this followed the devolution of the commissioning of high secure services from a national to a regional level and was aimed at the accelerated discharge of service users from high **secure hospitals** following the Tilt review of security (Tilt et al., 2000). **Mental health case management** is essentially a process which allows a mental health specialist (usually a nurse but not exclusively) to oversee pathways of care with a view to ensuring prompt and appropriate access to and discharge from services and an optimum length of stay within those services. They also fulfil a fundamental role in the monitoring of the quality of care within services, on behalf of commissioners, and in ensuring that the individual needs of patients are addressed effectively. There is also evidence to suggest that mental health case management, as part of a well-organised commissioning infrastructure, can have a positive impact on length of stay within hospital services as well as helping to establish a positive **culture** and good experience for service users within those services (McKeown et al., 2014).

WHAT'S THE EVIDENCE? 43.2

- Information and data development and analysis
- Real outcomes, proxy outcomes in mental health, recovery-focused outcomes.

As discussed earlier in the chapter, commissioning is sometimes seen as a transactional process. Providers are given money to provide services for a population under the auspices of a contract. The contract 'currency' has generally been 'output' based, meaning that providers are paid for how many contacts they have with a service user or how many 'bed days' have been occupied by a particular service user, rather than being 'outcome' based, i.e. looking at how service users progress in a service. In some areas, this system has created perverse incentives for providers to extend the time that service users spend in hospital or remain under the care of a clinical team in the community, as discharging service users from a service often means that income attached to those service users is lost to a service.

In recent years, there has been an increased focus on commissioning for outcomes within services and attempts to redefine the 'currency' by which services are paid from output to outcome based. This has seen a change in the range and type of data that commissioners request from providers through the contract. Traditional output-based contracts require services to report activity to commissioners (numbers of contacts or occupied bed days), so that these can be reconciled with invoices against a given service line. This activity data is useful for commissioners in helping them plan for future service delivery – knowing how many service users with a particular demographic and clinical profile from a given district are in a particular hospital, and how long on average they stay there, can be helpful in identifying how many beds of a particular type might be needed in a given locality over a period of time. However, this type of data is not very helpful for commissioners when they are trying to make judgements about the quality of care in a given service. In making informed judgements about the quality of a service, commissioners also require providers to submit data that aims to capture the quality of an **environment** and the quality and nature of the experience of service users within that environment.

Capturing data that accurately describes how service users experience services, and agreeing what outcomes are important for services to help service users achieve is a complex process. Identifying suitable 'metrics' to measure these outcomes is even more complex and requires commissioners to facilitate a process that captures the views of clinicians within services, of other professional groups within provider organisations and, of course, of service users.

The NHS Standard Contract was first introduced into the NHS in 2010–11. Prior to this date, contractual relationships between commissioners and providers were managed through a series of locally negotiated 'service level agreements'. For the first time, this gave all providers and commissioners a standard, legally binding template within which to agree what, and more importantly how, services should be provided. The Standard Contract also introduced an incentive scheme for providers. The Commissioning for Quality and Innovation Scheme – known by the acronym CQUIN – introduced as part of the 2010–11 contract, allowed providers to access extra funds for developing innovations in services that improved quality and/or improved service user experience. This process allowed commissioners, service users and providers to work together to develop a series of proposals that began to change the shape of services. Over subsequent years, these initiatives assimilated into routine service provision and allowed a series of quality measures to be developed that better allowed commissioners and providers to judge the quality of provision available within a provider.

Within the Yorkshire and Humber NHS England hub, the concept of improving the quality of services by directly involving service users, and then embedding these changes into contracts, was grasped enthusiastically. The CQUIN initiative paved the way for a number of service user-developed initiatives to find their way into the Standard Mental Health Contract in secure mental health services, as it provided a focus for the existing 'involvement network' of service users, staff and commissioners of secure services in Yorkshire and the Humber. The network had an informal structure and involved skilled facilitation by two 'involvement leads' employed in the NHSE commissioning team, using a number of 'action methods' workshops. A series of priorities for services were agreed in an open and democratic fashion, and through this process a series of recovery-focused 'contract products' were developed for inclusion in the Standard Mental Health Contract. These included standards around **advance directives**: positive dining experience within services which emphasised the importance of interacting during mealtimes; the quality of therapeutic activities within services; and, significantly, agreement on a number of CPA meeting standards. A number of these initiatives, and the importance of this involvement network, are highlighted in the literature (McKeown et al., 2014) and helped to dramatically impact on the culture and quality of service delivery in this field. The initiatives established within Yorkshire and the Humber later led to the development of the national '**Recovery** and Outcomes' network, which again led to further consolidation of the voice of the service user in the national strategic framework for delivery of secure mental health services. These initiatives have demonstrated the importance of the tri-partite relationship of service user, practitioner and commissioner in working together toward a common endeavour, and how this can be translated into contracts and care delivery.

The development of networks of service users and the linking in of these networks into the commissioning cycle has allowed the development of a helpful dialogue about what 'outcomes' are important to service users and how these might best be measured. Unsurprisingly, this has seen a focus on the quality of relationships in services, the importance of networks and relationships beyond mental health services and, most importantly, the importance of happiness and hope in recovery for service users, rather than the absence of symptoms or reduction of 'risk' as measured by psychometric tools.

The 2016–17 Standard Mental Health Contract will, for the first time, include the requirement that services administer a patient reported outcome measure (PROM) and initiate a service development in response to this measurement. The PROM was developed by service users working in partnership with commissioners and service providers and will be used as part of a national initiative to redefine the currency in secure mental health services in the coming years.

In this section, we have seen how important data is to the work of commissioners. Activity data, which is quantitative in nature, allows commissioners to understand how much of a given type of service is needed in a given area, and quality data allows commissioners to make judgements about the quality of service, gathering evidence from successive CQUIN schemes and assimilating this into the range of provision services are expected to deliver. This qualitative endeavour has allowed commissioners to develop a more detailed understanding of what service users feel is important in services and has furnished them with the necessary evidence to ensure that these elements are included in the portfolio of things that services are expected to deliver.

As an aspiring nurse, this chapter is aimed at introducing the concept and practice of commissioning early on in your professional practice, in the hope that the wider perspective of understanding need on a population basis, and planning services across a wider geography, will help to place your individual practice within a wider context. More importantly, we hope to impart a level of understanding that can actually influence practice in terms of ensuring service users are involved at all stages of the therapeutic and service delivery process. For this is the key to transforming the way services are delivered. We have to find ways to engage and involve service users, not only in the development of individual care plans, but also in the way services are planned, developed and evaluated. Without the involvement of service users in these key aspects of care delivery, the NHS will continue to steer away from its founding principles and will inevitably flounder in the reality of insufficient resources. The tri-partite relationship between service users, commissioners and practitioners, in true collaboration with each other, is the only way to ensure that the resources available are maximised for the benefit of individuals, and the population as a whole.

CRITICAL DEBATE 43.1

Mental health services are traditionally measured in terms of the quality of the environment and the interventions provided to service users. Measures might include the availability of specific treatments or interventions, the evidence base associated with the intervention, or the range of facilities or activities available to service users. Despite policy imperatives to focus on 'payment by results', these have had little impact on mental health services.

Service users expect more tangible outcomes such as a secure place to live, meaningful things to do, paid employment and supportive relationships.

It is argued that if services were able to articulate and focus on outcomes rather than interventions, and services were measured on the outcomes they achieved with service users, then real progress on effectiveness and an evidence base would be made.

Consider the questions below:

(a) How can the care planning process be re-orientated to focus on service user outcomes rather than planned interventions, and how can these be measured?
(b) How can the commissioning of services be developed to support these approaches?

CHALLENGING CONCEPTS 43.1

Integrating commissioning to create seamless pathways for service users remains a significant goal which is yet to be realised. Pathways become blocked or slow down for a number of reasons, often because there are gaps in services or insufficient resources at one point along the pathway. For example, a service user who is currently in a secure mental health hospital may no longer require secure care, but cannot move on because of a lack of supported accommodation in the community. This block in the pathway can be further exacerbated because these services are commissioned by another commissioner, in a separate organisation, with different priorities.

A number of initiatives are being tested to improve mental health pathways. These include the formation of shared commissioning budgets across commissioning organisations such as CCGs and local authorities to better align the range of services required. This allows funding to flow with the service user, as in personalised budgets, so that services can be commissioned by the service user as and when required. Alternatively, it may place the responsibility of commissioning into the hands of a provider organisation that can then resource and provide the whole pathway based on the needs of service users (NHS England, 2014).

Each of these methods creates its own perverse incentives and unwanted dynamics. Pooled budgets have a greater range of priorities and policy imperatives to deal with, whilst personalised budgets are difficult to manage across a large population. New Care Models (NHS England, 2014) are based on the concept that providers will be more efficient in delivering pathways if they are responsible for their own commissioning budget. This concept has not yet been evaluated.

CHAPTER SUMMARY

This chapter has covered:

- What commissioning is and its four steps which are very similar to the nursing process
- The importance of the tri-partite relationship between service users, commissioners and practitioners in the process of commissioning
- The wider political context and the multiple organisational tensions within the health and social care landscape.

BUILD YOUR BIBLIOGRAPHY

Books

- Heginbotham, C. (2012) *Values-based commissioning of health and social care*. Cambridge: Cambridge University Press.
- Glasby, J. and Tew, J. (2015) *Mental health policy and practice*. London: Palgrave Macmillan.
- Beresford, P. (2016) *All our welfare: Towards participatory social policy*. Bristol: Policy Press.

SAGE journal articles

Go to https://study.sagepub.com/essentialmentalhealth for further free online journal articles related to this chapter. If you are using the interactive ebook, simply click on the book icon in the margin to go straight to the resource.

- Glover-Thomas, N. (2014) The Health and Social Care Act 2012: The emergence of equal treatment for mental health care or another false dawn? *Medical law international, 13*(4), 279–297.
- Lewis, L., 2014. User involvement in mental health services: a case of power over discourse. *Sociological Research Online, 19*(1), 1–15.
- Watson, N. (2013). Clinical Commissioning – what is all the fuss about? *InnovAiT, 6*(6), 379–385.

Weblinks

Go to https://study.sagepub.com/essentialmentalhealth for further weblinks related to this chapter. If you are using the interactive ebook, simply click on the book icon in the margin to go straight to the resource.

- Commissioning for Better Outcomes: www.local.gov.uk/sites/default/files/documents/commissioning-better-outc-bbc.pdf – gives a very good account of 'what good looks like' for a wide range of services, with an emphasis on person-centred commissioning
- Health Policy Insight (HPI): www.healthpolicyinsight.com
- Joint Commissioning Panel for Mental Health (JCPMH): www.jcpmh.info/wp-content/uploads/jcpmh-commissioningframework.pdf; www.jcpmh.info/wp-content/uploads/jcpmh-publicmentalhealth-guide.pdf – the JCPMH has published a framework for local authority and NHS commissioners of mental health and wellbeing services, and useful information about the commissioning of mental health services
- My Shared Pathway: www.recoveryandoutcomes.org/my-shared-pathway/my-shared-pathway.html – this includes a video about recovery and My Shared Pathway at: https://vimeo.com/100461311
- NHS England: www.england.nhs.uk/commissioning/spec-services/key-docs

GREAT FOR REVISION!

ACE YOUR ASSESSMENT

Revise what you have learned by visiting https://study.sagepub.com/essentialmentalhealth. If you are using the interactive ebook, simply click on the tick icon to go straight to the resource.

- Test yourself with multiple-choice and short-answer questions and flashcards.

REFERENCES

Ayub, R., Callaghan, I., Haque, Q., et al. (2013) Increasing patient involvement in care pathways. *Health Service Journal*, 3 June.

Britnell, M., Farrar, M., Richardson, T., et al. (2008) Commission impossible? Is world class commissioning achievable in the NHS? Debate hosted by Civitas, Grand Committee Room, House of Commons, London, 16 July.

Cardona, F. (1999) 'The team as a sponge': how the nature of the task affects the behaviour and mental life of a team. In V. Vince & R. French (eds) *Group relations, management and organisation*. Oxford: Oxford University Press.

Coomans, G. (1999) *Europe's changing demography: Constraints and bottlenecks*. Demographic and social trends issue paper. IPTS Futures Report Series No. 08.

Davies, P. (2007) Your shout: interview with Mark Britnell. *In View*, 15, 3.

Department of Health (DH) (2007) *World class commissioning vision*. London: HMSO.

Department of Health (DH) (2008) *Using the Commissioning for Quality and Innovation (CQUIN) payment framework*. Available at: http://webarchive.nationalarchives.gov.uk/20130105012233/ http:/www.dh.gov.uk/prod_consum_dh/groups/dh_digitalassets/@dh/@en/documents/digitalasset/ dh_091435.pdf (accessed 22.09.17).

European Foundation for the Improvement of Living and Working Conditions (EFILWC) (2003) *Sector futures: The future of health and social services in Europe*. Dublin: EMCC.

Francis, R. (2013) *Report of the Mid Staffordshire NHS Foundation Trust public inquiry*. London: The Stationery Office.

HM Government (1989) *Working for patients*. White Paper. London: HMSO.

HM Government (1997) *The new NHS: Modern, dependable*. White Paper. London: HMSO.

HSJ (2015) Health secretary announces Ofsted style ratings for CCGs, 9 November. Available at: www. hsj.co.uk/home/video-health-secretary-announces-ofsted-style-ratings-for-ccgs/5091754.article (accessed 17.08.17).

James, E. (2016) Inside the special prison unit where rehabilitation rules the roost. *The Guardian*, 24 May.

McKenna, H. & Dunn, P. (2015) *Devolution: what it means for health and social care*. London: The Kings Fund

McKeown, M., Jones, F., Wright, K., et al. (2014) It's the talk: a study of involvement initiatives in secure mental health settings. *Health Expectations, 19*(3), 570–579.

Menzies Lyth, I. (1988) The functioning of social systems as a defence against anxiety. In *Containing anxiety in institutions: Selected essays, vol 1*. London: Free Association Books.

National Health Service Reform and Health Care Professions Act 2002. Available at www.legislation. gov.uk/ukpga/2002/17/contents (accessed 22.9.17).

NHS England (2013) *Transforming participation in health and care: 'The NHS belongs to us all'*. Patients and Information Directorate, NHS England Publications Gateway Reference No. 00381. Available at: www.cityandhackneyccg.nhs.uk/Downloads/Get%20involved/trans-part-hc-guid1.pdf (accessed 17.08.17).

NHS England (2014) *Five year forward view*. Available at: www.england.nhs.uk/wp-content/ uploads/2014/10/5yfv-web.pdf (accessed 17.08.17).

NHS Institute for Innovation and Improvement (2008) *Commissioning to make a bigger difference: A guide for NHS and social care commissioners on promoting service innovation*. London: HMSO.

Sobanja, M. (2009) *What is world class commissioning?* Available at: www.bandolier.org.uk/painres/ download/whatis/what_is_wc_comm.pdf (accessed 17.08.17).

Tilt, R., Perry, B., Martin, C., et al. (2000) *Report of the review of security at the high secure hospitals*. London: Department of Health.

Walshe, K. (2015) Re-organising the NHS: never again? University of Manchester policy blog. Available at: http://blog.policy.manchester.ac.uk/featured/2015/04/reorganising-the-nhs-never-again (accessed 17.08.17).

Woodin, J. & Wade, E. (2007) *Towards world class commissioning competency*. A report produced for West Midlands Strategic Health Authority by the Health Services Management Centre, University of Birmingham.

TRANSFERABLE SKILLS AND TRANSITION: BECOMING A MENTAL HEALTH NURSE AND BEYOND

KEVIN MOORE AND MARIE O'NEILL

THIS CHAPTER COVERS

- Key aspects of making the transition from student to staff nurse
- Personal development and preceptorship
- The importance of developing confidence, competence and a true sense of professional practice and integrity, whilst adapting to transition
- Developing emotional resilience.

> I have had no choice but to adapt to the daily routine within the clinical area to enable me to survive the day, and for me, it was a complete and utter culture shock.
>
> **Caine, a newly qualified mental health nurse working in a medium secure unit**

> If I could give a first year staff nurse any advice it would be to listen carefully, observe a lot and don't talk too much. I think for me the core thing for any mental health nurse is to see past my disability, please see me for whom and what I am.
>
> **Denise, service user**

Visit **https://study.sagepub.com/essentialmentalhealth** to access a wealth of online resources for this chapter – watch out for the margin icons throughout the chapter. If you are using the interactive ebook, simply click on the margin icon to go straight to the resource.

INTRODUCTION

Role transition has been extensively reported within the literature and much of this has been as a con-sequential result of radical changes to the delivery of nurse education within the UK and Ireland over the past two decades. The need to ensure that nurses are competent and fit to practise as a registered nurse has resulted in an analysis of this transition, specifically that transition from being a student to being a registered nurse. Much of this literature specifically reports on adult nursing experiences, but some authors have taken a broader view and include mental health and learning disability students within their studies. The concept of this transition has been linked to a sustainable mental health nursing workforce (Cleary & Happell, 2005), the importance of mental health clinical experiences and appropriate preparedness (Happell, 2008) for the 'expectations' and the 'unexpected' (Mooney, 2006). Higgins et al. (2010) conducted a systematic review of such experiences within the UK and reported that transition remains a stressful experience for newly qualified nurses, and Hayman-White et al. (2016) also reported that there are additional and specific problems unique to the mental health nurse graduate commencing a career within a mental health setting that could impact significantly on their level of confidence and competence.

This chapter will explore in further detail some of these core issues related to and reported on within this transition for the mental health nurse and will be specifically related to mental health prac-tice. Hoffart et al. (2011) have reported the transition as a continued reality shock which they believe can have a demonstrable effect on patient safety, quality of care and nurse retention.

It is envisaged also that working though this chapter will equip the mental health nurse to transition much more easily and to develop personally and professionally as a result.

> I am constantly anxious in my nursing role and do not think that this will ever change, due to the responsibility and accountability involved. It is a very demanding role and I come home each evening mentally exhausted from gaining new knowledge and experiences.
>
> **Karen, newly qualified mental health nurse working in a nursing home**

KEY ASPECTS OF MAKING THE TRANSITION FROM STUDENT TO STAFF NURSE

The voices of the two practitioners, Caine and Karen, resonate clearly with some of the earlier pub-lished literature within transitions (Kramer, 1974; Holland, 1999; Gerrish, 2000), and yet more current authors have also articulated and recognised that such a transition from student nurse to staff nurse can be an extremely stressful experience (Deasy et al., 2011; Kumaran & Carney, 2014; Hayman-White et al., 2016) and one in which the new practitioner requires personal support, environmental support and effective preceptorship to enable them to gain the confidence and competency levels commensu-rate with becoming a registered nurse. Personal and professional development at this time must take due cognisance of the myriad of factors that may impinge on such development if the practitioner feels in a state of shock or fearful all the time. The interconnected nature of linking their undergradu-ate theoretical preparation to that of the existing clinical **environment** must become an important element in the development of their role and growing expertise in a nurturing environment, which will enhance their confidence and competence aligned to advancing skills with **reflective practice**.

Transition period and models

It is clear from reviewing the literature that the initial transition period can therefore be a time of significant change for the newly qualified nurse, and role stress and adaptability to the change process are common problems experienced. Indeed, the assertions made by the practitioner Karen clearly identify ambiguity with her role and what has been referred to within the literature as role overload (Bowles & Candela, 2005).

Meleis et al. (2000) have pointed out that transition is a central concept of nursing and extensively examined transitions within nursing using an integrative approach to theory development, suggesting that it is a period of time during which change takes place within the individual and the environment. Meleis et al. (2000) proposed that a theory of transitions consists of types and patterns of transitions, properties of transition experiences, facilitating and inhibiting conditions, process and outcome indicators and nursing therapeutics, and advocated that transition experiences need to be further explored within the nursing literature. Kumaran & Carney (2014) also suggested that Meleis et al.'s (2000) theories had several implications for role transition from student nurse to staff nurse and offered strategies that promote and support role transition. They explored these broad concepts within their study and identified two emergent themes: (1) *initial feelings and experiences and inherent highs and lows of qualification* and, (2) *standing on their own two feet*. Within this chapter, some aspects of the practitioners' narrative is clearly identifiable within these two themes. Kumaran & Carney (2014) concluded that independent responsibility is the biggest step in the transition process, as well as the need for support and time to adjust to new roles and responsibilities, and suggested that supportive staff and good team working were identified as the most important factors in easing the transition process.

PERSONAL DEVELOPMENT AND PRECEPTORSHIP

Personal development

CASE STUDY:
KNOWING
ONE'S SELF

Continuing professional development (CPD) encompasses experiences, activities and practices that contribute to the development of a nurse as a health care professional. CPD is, thus, a lifelong process of both structured and informal learning.

It is essential for each nurse to engage in CPD, following registration, in order to acquire new knowledge, skills and competence to practise effectively in an ever-changing health care environment. Continuing professional and personal development are essential in order to 'revalidate' (NMC, 2016) and enhance professional standards and to provide quality, competent and safe patient care.

Examples of activities that might contribute to a nurse's professional development include formal education programmes, reflective practice, journal clubs, case conferences, clinical supervision, preceptorship, mentorship, workshops, distance learning, blended learning, e-learning, sourcing information and self-directed learning.

It is important, therefore, for newly qualified registrants to successfully prepare themselves for their first nursing role. In order to enter or remain on the register, the nurse must:

- maintain/achieve appropriate standards of proficiency
- ensure they are of good health and good character
- adhere to principles of good practice set out in the rules, standards guidance and information.

In addition, all nurses and midwives are currently required to renew their registration every three years. Revalidation will strengthen the renewal process by introducing new requirements that focus on:

- up-to-date practice and professional development
- reflection on the professional standards of practice and behaviour as set out in the Code (NMC, 2015)
- engagement in professional discussions with other registered nurses or midwives.

We have clearly identified that the beginning of a newly qualified practitioner's career can be a challenging and stressful time. Initial experiences can influence how they progress in their career. To ensure the best possible start for newly qualified nurses, a quality preceptorship programme is essential and this is well supported and documented within the literature (Higgins et al., 2010; Kumaran & Carney, 2014). It is important when undertaking your first nursing position that gaining a preceptorship opportunity is discussed with your future employer.

Preceptorship

In the UK, preceptorship is the process of supporting newly qualified nurses over the transition period from student to registered nurse (RN). The NMC strongly recommends that all 'new registrants' have a period of preceptorship on commencing employment: this applies to those newly admitted to the NMC register who have completed a pre-registration programme in the UK for the first time, or have subsequently entered a new part of the register. New registrants also include those newly admitted to the register from other European Economic Area States and other nation states (NMC, 2006) Moreover, preceptorship is defined as 'a period of structured transition for the newly registered practitioner during which he or she will be supported by a preceptor to develop their confidence as an autonomous professional, refine skills, **values** and behaviours and to continue on their journey of lifelong learning' (DH, 2010:11).

From the time of registration, you as a practitioner are autonomous and accountable. Preceptorship should, consequently, be considered as a transition phase when continuing your professional development, building confidence and further developing competence to practise. Therefore, it is highly recommended that all new registrants have a period of preceptorship in which support and guidance are provided.

The NMC believe that the 'new registrant' who is receiving preceptorship has a responsibility to:

- practise in accordance with the Code
- identify and meet with their preceptor as soon as is possible after they have taken up post
- identify specific learning needs and develop an action plan for addressing these needs
- ensure that they understand the standard, competencies or objectives set by their employer that they are required to meet
- reflect on their practice and experience
- seek feedback on their performance from their preceptor and those with whom they work.

A positive preceptorship experience plays an essential role in supporting registrants as they integrate into their new role and team. This is the time when they need an individualised period of structured support under the supervision of an experienced clinician. The benefits of positive preceptorship should enable, encourage and assist registered practitioners to consider their future career pathway and create an appropriate foundation for this in their personal development plan (Willis, 2015).

The transition from student nurse to staff nurse was a journey that was filled with fear of the unknown for Steve who has been a qualified mental health nurse for over a year now. Steve outlines the importance of being supported in clinical practice and talks honestly about his experience of preceptorship:

> On receiving my first post I was told by the company owner that I would receive 6 months preceptorship, this had given me confidence that I would have the support of fellow nursing professionals to help guide me and support me. This didn't happen and I felt let down and disappointed. I left this post just after 6 weeks. I received an interview for a second post as staff nurse and was offered the job. The manager assured me that I would have a mentor appointed, and would have guidance and support throughout the whole 6 months. This was duly provided and with the support of my mentor and the guidance and knowledge I received whilst doing my degree, I feel that my confidence has grown from day to day. I have made mistakes, but have learned and reflected upon these. I feel that anyone who is graduating from student to staff nurse must have a preceptorship programme in place as it helps to build confidence in practice. This has made me a better nurse in my decision-making processes to enhance the best outcomes for the patients in my care.
>
> **Steve, mental health nurse**

The transition from student to newly qualified nurse can certainly be a daunting one, with high expectations placed on oneself to know everything and be familiar with all experiences added to the pressure of succeeding within the nursing role. Supporting new registrants to maximise their potential as autonomous and accountable practitioners is an important part of this. Brenda, a staff nurse who has been qualified for three years and who is working in an **acute** admissions ward, reflects:

> I feel what impacted on my own transition from being a student were the staff in the teams that I was joining, supportive, patient staff willing to guide, mentor and value me within their team made me grow in confidence and establish the type of nurse I am today.
>
> **Brenda, mental health nurse**

CRITICAL THINKING STOP POINT 44.1

Read Karen's experience of becoming a new registrant below and consider the following statements:

- Making the transition from student nurse to staff nurse can be a stressful experience.
- For some newly qualified nurses, being thrown in at the *deep end* can help them to develop their analytical skills and boost confidence.
- Ensuring a smooth transition should be a concern for nurse managers.

> My first post as a staff nurse is in a nursing home for older people living with dementia. The first shock was the amount of residents within the care home with only two staff nurses allocated in the morning and one in the evening. The carers carried out the 'hands on' work with the residents and did so in a manner I was not happy about. All aspects of care were carried out at an extremely fast pace – taking short cuts which compromised care and was task orientated rather than the person-centred care I was hoping to be part of. There was no time to talk to and get to know residents. I was not receiving the support I needed as a newly qualified nurse. Staff morale was extremely low and I was not getting the preceptorship I needed. I felt out of my depth and inadequate.
>
> **Karen, mental health nurse**

The environment where newly qualified nurses first work is crucial to a smooth transition process. Mooney (2007) stated that the majority of newly qualified nurses experience a lack of support whilst in the clinical environment. Karen has identified an obvious lack of support in her role and has experienced role ambiguity and overload, as identified by Bowles and Candela (2005). The development of confidence and professional competence as a newly qualified nurse in a supportive environment with teamwork have all been identified as important precursors to change and transitions. Read below how Karen addressed in a professional manner the lack of support with her manager:

> I spoke with the home manager to put forward my concerns. She explained to me that unfortunately it was not a good time to start as a newly qualified nurse in that particular unit due to staff shortages, although she was unaware of the poor practice being carried out and was genuinely quite shocked. The manager was very sympathetic and understood my need to work in an environment which supported me as a new registrant. I was moved to a general unit and I am now undertaking my preceptorship programme with plans to move to an EMI unit once my preceptorship programme is successfully completed. I am gaining knowledge with physical illnesses which will enhance my skills for further practice.
>
> Care is carried out as it should be and to a very high standard and staff genuinely care for the residents' wellbeing. My current role will give me the experience and confidence in future roles. I never imagined having to report poor practice within my first couple of weeks as a staff nurse. However, the fact that doing so has put in place important things to change and address the issues identified gives me some sense of personal and professional satisfaction that I acted in accordance with the NMC Code of Conduct.
>
> **Kathryn, mental health nurse**

CRITICAL THINKING STOP POINT 44.2

- Consider the duty of care and a legal liability Kathryn has with regard to the care of her patients, including the delegation of duties to health care assistants.
- How did Kathryn enhance clinical standards and her professional competence whilst improving the level of patient safety and care standards?
- What aspects of the interactions between Kathryn and her line manager make this a positive outcome, and for whom?
- What do you believe were the antagonists for change that perhaps motivated Karen to act in this situation?

THE IMPORTANCE OF DEVELOPING CONFIDENCE, COMPETENCE AND A TRUE SENSE OF PROFESSIONAL PRACTICE AND INTEGRITY, WHILST ADAPTING TO TRANSITION

Confidence, competency and true professional practice

The period of transition from student to newly qualified nurse has been seen and described as a 'reality shock' for many newly qualified nurses who find themselves in work situations for which they often feel inadequately prepared. This transition period is a time when nurses need to consolidate their knowledge and skills, and adjust and adapt in a meaningful and reflective manner to the inherent challenges of their new role. The potential benefits of minimising a 'reality shock' associated with this transition could be a reduction in perceived stress and **anxiety** levels for the new staff nurse, accompanied by enhanced job satisfaction levels and improved retention rates or longevity of employment status for the new graduates.

The experience of transition for the new graduate entering professional practice is distinguished by Duchscher (2008) as the process of making a significant adjustment to changing personal and professional roles at the start of one's nursing career. Although not explicit, the period of time during which the initial transition to professional practice in nursing is generally thought to occur encompasses the first 12 months as a graduate and then as a registered nurse. Therefore, the newly qualified nurse needs to consider the challenges they may face during this transitional period. It is essential that the newly qualified nurse communicates effectively with their manager/employer to ensure their learning needs are being met and to ease the transition process. This is important and necessary to uphold personal and professional **ethics** and values, taking into account the values of the organisation and respecting the **culture**, beliefs and abilities of all individuals concerned.

Read Caine's experience of becoming a new registrant below and consider the points identified within Critical thinking stop point 44.3:

I am beginning to understand the accountability and responsibility that the role entails. Like any new job in healthcare I spent the first few weeks getting to know my colleagues and more importantly trying to get to know my patients and gaining an understanding of their histories. I have found the transition extremely difficult from the very first day. I now appreciate the role and the extreme pressure our team work under each and every day. I understand the accountability

(Continued)

and responsibility of the nurse within this team. I have seen, first hand, and been involved in split-second decision making, often in hostile environments. I have completed complex risk assessments and care planning. However, I feel that I still have a lot of development to do before I will be confident to be in charge of the ward, and feel like the preceptorship programme my employer offers will help me do this.

Caine, mental health nurse

CRITICAL THINKING STOP POINT 44.3

As an autonomous and accountable professional, you need to make informed and reasonable decisions about your practice to ensure that you are safe and competent to practice within the NMC standards:

* From your reading to date, can you suggest how the clinical environment might be enhanced to facilitate a new registrant's learning and adaptation?
* Consider the ongoing actions that the practitioner Caine might take to develop his knowledge, skills and experiences as a new registrant?

As a registered nurse, it is important to remember that the environment within which you work and the nature of the changing and evolving role are clearly reflected within the NMC Code (2015). As a registrant, you must always adhere to the four themes: prioritise people, practise effectively, preserve safety, and promote professionalism and trust.

Thus far within the chapter, it is clear from the voices of the practitioners that practising in accordance with the Code will require a commitment to continuing professional development. You should also consider getting advice and support from education providers, your employers, professional bodies, other professional colleagues and, of course, **service users**, as this will enable you to make sure that you uphold these four themes and are competent to practise in accordance with the Code at all times.

Adaptability

The voice of the practitioner, Caine, demonstrates that his adaptability within the clinical environment is crucial to his transition as a staff nurse, and suggests that such adaptability remains challenging and complex. Moreover, the added complexity herein for this practitioner is the nature of his clinical environment, which is a medium secure unit, and the evidence would appear to support the view that the clinical environment can add to the reality shock for the nurse in transition. Further, a review of the literature suggests that there remains a need to ensure that the clinical environment is supportive and collegiate for nurses within the transition from student to staff nurse, and those environments that are, appear to enable practitioners to 'stand on their own two feet' much more quickly, as also evidenced and supported by the voice of Karen (Kumaran & Carney, 2014). The resultant challenge to adapt to changes in the level of responsibility, level of accountability, level of autonomy, becoming the prescribing practitioner for all aspects of nursing care, completing and documenting the mental health assessment, fitting into the **multi-disciplinary** team as an effective team player, administering prescribed medications and dealing with potential mental health emergencies, can all be an overwhelming experience for the new staff nurse.

Moreover, Kumaran & Carney (2014) have postulated various themes and assert that the ability to stand on 'one's own two feet' is linked to the importance of familiarity with the new work situation and the development of competence necessary to assume full responsibility. This suggests that such familiarity, both with the work and the environment, and the practitioner's adaptation to these resultant changes can have a positive impact during the transition period. The concomitant need for effective support mechanisms must therefore be in place, both within team structures and the respective clinical environments.

One of the main difficulties I had was, on my very first day, the health care assistants coming to me for direction and to make decisions about patient care, when in fact I felt that they were more informed to make these decisions than I was, as they knew the patients and I didn't.

Caine, mental health nurse

It is clear that practitioners' fear or trepidation in responding to the changes faced are very real and require the practitioner to respond in a positive and proactive manner to limit the stressors within the environment and to embrace the concept of autonomy and accountability in accordance with the NMC guidelines. However, this is a significant challenge that the practitioner must embrace and the individual level of preparedness is critical. It has also been argued that some pre-registration graduate programmes are not preparing students well enough to enable them to embrace these challenges (Hayman-White et al., 2016), in that there is insufficient attention paid to theoretical and clinical mental health content, which, it is argued, impacts significantly on confidence and competency levels for the new graduate.

Adaptation within a nursing context has been underpinned by some explicit assumptions within the literature (Roy, 1989; Roy & Andrews, 1991), in that adaptation is linked to responding positively to environmental changes and that the person's adaptation is a function of the stimuli that one is exposed to, and one's own adaptation levels and self-reflection and choice help to create human and environmental integration. Hayman-White et al. (2016) support the view that to maximise and sustain the development of the mental health workforce, there is a need for further research to identify those aspects that are most useful in providing supportive learning environments and to extrapolate further on those that negatively impact on the experiences of new graduates.

It was within my first month as a staff nurse working in an acute psychiatric admissions unit that I encountered some very serious challenges to my sense of professionalism and seriously considered leaving mental health nursing for good because of these feelings. No one seemed to be as concerned about the situation as I was and this saddened me, yet terrified me also. My 22-year-old male school friend was an inpatient in our admission unit, and had been an inpatient

(Continued)

for about two weeks and he had just returned the day previously from day leave, and for all intents and purposes it had apparently gone well for him. I remember feeling good that he appeared to be improving and on the road to recovery. He had presented as a first admission with some classical signs and symptoms of depression, and thoughts that his life was not worth living, all of which appeared to be triggered by his recent break down of a long-term relationship and his growing dependence on alcohol. I can remember vividly speaking with him whilst he had his afternoon tea and I distinctly remember that I picked up on no evidence or concerns that his mental health was deteriorating. There were clearly no cues to suggest that he, at this point, had a plan to take his own life. He was fully conversant with me and appeared to be improving quite well. Imagine my extreme horror when just a few hours later he was missing and later found in the woods and had taken steps to end his own life. I was devastated, shocked, dismayed and felt that I had failed him? I felt that I had perhaps missed essential cues due to my inexperience? I could not, for a long time, shift the belief that it was my inexperience that had resulted in this catastrophic sequence of events.

Lynn, mental health nurse

CRITICAL THINKING STOP POINT 44.4

- How may your own level of self-esteem and self-efficacy be linked to your own resources and personal levels of strength to meet competing clinical demands within the transitional process?
- How may your own personal motivational processes, expectations and/or personal belief systems prepare you for the realities of clinical practice and in coping with stressful situations or mental health emergencies?
- How may our practitioners, Caine, Kathryn and Lynn, have dealt with their feelings about autonomous decision making and taken definitive steps to help to promote positive outcomes and environmental and personal adaptation?
- Which specific themes within the NMC Code should these practitioners take due cognisance of within their course of action?

The NMC Revalidation (2016) implemented new changes to PREP (Professional Requirements for Education and Practice) requirements for all nurses as part of revalidation to renew their registration every three years. Within this process, the registrant must have obtained five pieces of practice-related feedback in the three-year period since the last registration, or in the case of a new registrant in transition, since they joined the register. Moreover, each registrant must have prepared five written reflective accounts in the three-year period since registration was last renewed, or since joining the register, and have provided a template to record these reflections, as outlined in NMC online.

The NMC (2016) suggests that each reflective account must be recorded on the approved form and must refer to:

- an instance of your CPD, and/or
- a piece of practice-related feedback you have received, and/or
- an event or experience in your own professional practice

and how they relate to the Code.

Reflective Account:
What was the nature of the CPD activity and/or practice-related feedback and/or event or experience in your practice?
What did you learn from the CPD activity and/or feedback and/or event or experience in your practice?
How did you change or improve your practice as a result?
How is this relevant to the Code? Select one or more themes: Prioritise people – Practise effectively – Preserve safety – Promote professionalism and trust

Figure 44.1 NMC Template for written reflective accounts

I am a married woman aged 56 and I have six sons and three daughters now and I married my husband in 1980 when I was 20. I would say that I have suffered from depression most of my life, possibly since I was 15, when I also began to deliberately self-harm. I was brought up by my grandparents as my mother was not married and she left us to go to England. I think that I had a happy childhood from what I can remember. I had my own first child at 16, and then a second son at 18, neither of them to my current husband. I was supposed to marry my boyfriend at this time also, but alas this fell through when he met someone else and decided to tell me this, three weeks after moving into my own flat with two young sons. I reinvested my life into the father of my first son at this time, but again this was a disaster as he had an affair with my cousin at the time. I started cutting myself again at this time as I was lost again. I remember that at an early age my uncle used to give me lifts home if I had sometimes missed the bus home to my grandfather's. As I think back now I realise that I was a victim of sexual abuse at my uncle's hands from the age of 11 and all of this is now to the forefront of my mind and is perhaps the reason I am the way I am today and feeling always so sad, so lost, hurt and confused. These actions have resulted in a complex court case so that I can begin to feel like a survivor and not so much the victim, and I also wish this was all behind me and wasn't taking so much time. At times I am unable to get out of bed, and I just want to cry and be alone. I have found Nexus to be the most helpful, my lifeline, as they are genuinely interested in me as a person and will listen to what I have got to say and do not judge me, I feel. So often the CMHT nurses change and I am not sure that they truly understand how I am feeling. As I write this short piece I realise I have lots of issues going on in my life at this time and this is only a small insight into my life.

Rosie, service user

CRITICAL THINKING STOP POINT 44.5

- What would guide and inform you in the development of a therapeutic relationship with Rosie at this difficult time in her life, whilst you are within the transition from student to staff nurse?
- How would you as a practitioner be available and present for Rosie at this time and demonstrate genuine concern for her, whilst also managing and knowing your level of professional involvement, taking due cognisance of your strengths and limitations?

- In what way can you as a nurse practitioner know what is desirable for Rosie at this time and what do you think should guide your possible course of action, cognisant of the ethical principles of autonomy, beneficence and non-maleficence?
- What specific themes within the Code do you feel are directly relevant here as you approach the mental health assessment with Rosie?

The work of a mental health nurse has been acknowledged as emotionally demanding. As seen in the complexity of Rosie's situation, mental health nurses work with patients and their families during emotionally challenging times. In addition, nurses find themselves working in increasingly busy and stressful environments. It is important therefore for the nurse to develop resilient strategies to allow them to adapt more positively to the increased stressors of their work. Participating actively in reflection must be seen as a core requisite skill for the nurse at all times, particularly during the transition period. Development of such skills will also enable the nurse to develop emotional resilience.

DEVELOPING EMOTIONAL RESILIENCE

Although organisations have a duty of care to protect the wellbeing of their employees, it is widely recognised that employees need to enhance their personal resilience to survive and prosper. It is asserted that emotional resilience may be an essential quality for helping professionals, as it can help them adapt positively to stressful working conditions, manage emotional demands, foster effective **coping** strategies, improve wellbeing and enhance professional growth (McDonald et al., 2012; Stephens, 2013).

The concept of emotional resilience embraces the knowledge, personal qualities and skills required for a sustained and successful career in nursing (McDonald et al., 2012). According to Chen (2010), resilient nurses are reflective, optimistic and socially competent; they also possess good problem-solving skills and have a sense of purpose. Moreover, social confidence, assertiveness and well-developed communication and conflict-resolution skills are essential qualities in helping professionals; they have also been associated with emotional resilience in this working context (McDonald et al., 2012; Pines et al., 2012).

Knowledge of the ways in which emotional resilience can be fostered is likely to help nurses to prosper in their career and make a positive contribution to the lives of their patients and clients. The need to develop evidence-based interventions to enhance resilience among professionals has been widely emphasised (McAllister & McKinnon, 2008). Moreover, the government strategy for mental health (DH, 2011) highlights the importance of individuals and employers recognising and building resilience. The Francis Report (2013) emphasises the importance of organisations creating a compassionate culture. Resilient cultures will start with compassionate leaders who build resilience individually and organisationally (Dutton et al., 2014). Furthermore, resilience is influenced by the interaction between individual and environmental factors (McCann et al., 2013).

Jackson et al. (2007: 6) proposed specific self-development strategies that can help build personal resilience to workplace adversity, particularly adversity grounded in interpersonal problems:

- Building positive nurturing professional relationships and networks: it is generally agreed that social support is one of the most important mechanisms by which helping-professionals can build their resilience. It is especially important to develop networks with people outside the immediate work area. Professional networks should include relationships that are nurturing in nature.

- Maintaining positivity: understand that you do have a choice about your attitude. Resilient people are able to see the positive aspects and potential benefits of a situation, rather than being continually negative or cynical.
- Developing emotional insight: understanding one's own emotional needs gives you insight into how to cope with stress. Moreover, developing insight into negative and positive emotions could be a beginning step in strengthening personal resilience.
- Achieving life balance and spirituality: it is important to participate in a range of healthy activities outside one's professional life. These activities should ideally include those that are physically, emotionally and spiritually nurturing. In this way, it is possible to retain some balance in life, even when occupied in a very demanding career such as nursing.
- Becoming more reflective: reflection is a way of developing insight and understanding into experiences, and of developing knowledge that can be used in subsequent situations. In reflection, concrete experience is used as a catalyst for thinking and learning.

Developing emotional resilience for practice is a key skill that will enhance wellbeing, job satisfaction and retention in the helping **professions**. Ahern (2006) reported that characteristics found in resilient nurses include hope, self-efficacy, effective coping, which in turn promote wellbeing and positive outcomes in vulnerable populations. Therefore, it is important that the newly qualified nurse actively seeks out the support they require to safeguard their own wellbeing, and develop the confidence to **advocate** for working environments and services to optimise the wellbeing of patients in their care.

OUR TOP TEN TIPS FOR TRANSITION FROM STUDENT TO STAFF NURSE

The following top ten tips are not intended to be a definitive list, nor is it our intent to suggest that one is more of a priority than the other. Rather, the intent herein is to give you our interpretation of the top ten things that might enable you to cope and manage better your transition from student to staff nurse based on our own experiences in mental health nursing and education, and most importantly from talking to service users. We believe that with experience will come more confidence, with confidence comes increasing levels of competence, and this is aligned to both professional and personal growth and development. We assert that it is a privilege to work in a holistic and person-centred way with the person with mental ill health and that the positivity and nature of the care environment within which nursing care is delivered are central to both the person's **recovery** and your transition from student to staff nurse.

Top Ten Tips for Transition from Student to Staff Nurse

1. Always have a sense of excitement and humour with a deep passion for mental health nursing and be knowledgeable, giving of one's self in a meaningful manner, with sincerity, demonstrating genuine interest in the person's growth and recovery.
2. Listen attentively at all times, reflect in and on your actions, ensuring that you communicate effectively with the person always.
3. Listen attentively at all times, and trust your gut instincts and the development of your own 'ways of knowing'.

---

4. Note that transparency in your interactions and dealings are fundamental to the maintenance of the therapeutic relationship with your client, so be authentic, be credible, be a nurse and an educator with compassion and heart.

5. Remember that participating in practical day-to-day experiences will be helpful as you develop, but never be afraid to say 'I don't know something' as pretending to know is contrary to No. 1 above; and it is not the 'not knowing something' that is the real problem – it's the not doing something about it to effect positive professional change that can become the problem.

6. Be generous in giving your time, care and commitment to the person and remember that continuous engagement with the person is central to truly knowing that person and responding with effective interpersonal skills.

7. Take note that involvement of the person in their own decision making in a collaborative and collegiate way is crucial to their own sense of hope and recovery and to your sense of effective engagement.

8. Develop a sense of personhood that demonstrates respect for the person's diversity, culture, norms, values and beliefs.

9. Manage yourself well and project manage other aspects around you that are central to your personal and role development within the team.

10. Take due cognisance of the NMC guidelines and the Code at all times within your professional practice, and deliver care that ensures that no act or omission on your behalf could result in any harm to the person.

CONCLUSION

We have identified within this chapter that making the transition from student to qualified nurse can be a stressful experience for some, and assert that if this process is managed appropriately through personal reflection in and on one's practice, combined with preceptorship support from clinical colleagues, the transition may not be as stressful or problematic. Working as a newly qualified nurse with a degree of preparedness and some realistic expectations with a sense for dealing with and managing the unexpected will be core personal characteristics. The environment where a newly qualified nurse first works is crucial for a smooth transition and it is imperative that the new registrant gets the support and guidance required to become a competent and confident practitioner, from their fellow colleagues within the multi-disciplinary team. Adaptation within the change process to both the work and the environment can have a positive impact on the transition process. We have identified, from our own experiences and reflections, what we feel are the top ten tips to help ease this transition, as identified above, and we assert that these are interconnected in a meaningful manner with an understanding of the personal and professional self within the **therapeutic relationship**.

CHAPTER SUMMARY

This chapter has covered:

- Acknowledging the possible 'reality shock' of becoming a registered nurse
- Making the transition from student to staff nurse
- Some possible suggestions for personal development and preceptorship to enable the transition

- The importance of developing confidence, competence and a true sense of professional practice and integrity, whilst adapting to the transition
- Some commentary on how emotional resilience can be developed to enable and facilitate the transition from student to staff nurse.

BUILD YOUR BIBLIOGRAPHY

Books

- Elcock, K., and Sharples, K., (2011). *Preceptorship for Newly Qualified Nurses*. Exeter: Learning Matters.
- Mutsatsa, S. (2015) *Physical Healthcare and Promotion in Mental Health Nursing*. London. SAGE.
- Roberts, M. (2015) *Critical Thinking and Reflection for Mental Health Nursing Students*. London. SAGE.
- Trenoweth, S. (2017) *Promoting Recovery in Mental Health Nursing*. London. SAGE Publications.
- Walker, S. (2014) *Engagement and Therapeutic Communication in Mental Health Nursing*. London. SAGE.

FIND OUT MORE

FURTHER READING: JOURNAL ARTICLES

SAGE journal articles

Go to https://study.sagepub.com/essentialmentalhealth for further free online journal articles related to this chapter. If you are using the interactive ebook, simply click on the book icon in the margin to go straight to the resource.

- Delaney, K.R., Hamera, E. & Drew, B.L., (2010) National survey of psychiatric mental health advanced practice nursing: The adequacy of educational preparation: Voices of our graduates. *Journal of the American Psychiatric Nurses Association*, 15(6), 383-392.
- Shu-Yueh, C. & Hui-Chen, H., (2014). Nurses' reflections on good nurse traits: Implications for improving care quality. *Nursing Ethics*, 22(7), 790-802.
- Thrysoe, L., Hounsgaard, L. & Bonderup Dohn, N. (2011). Expectations of becoming a nurse and experiences on being a nurse. *Nordic Journal of Nursing Research*, 31(3), 15-19.

FURTHER READING: WEBLINKS

Weblinks

Go to https://study.sagepub.com/essentialmentalhealth for further weblinks related to this chapter. If you are using the interactive ebook, simply click on the book icon in the margin to go straight to the resource.

- Revalidation: What all nurses need to know about Revalidation and the Nursing and Midwifery Council. http://revalidation.nmc.org.uk/
- Newly Qualified Nurses and Transitions: Evidence-based information for newly qualified nurses on interventions to improve transition from student to newly qualified nurse from the Royal College of Nursing and the National Institute for Health and Care Excellence. www.evidence.nhs.uk/search?q=newly+qualified+nurses
- Preceptorship for newly qualified staff, NHS Employers: www.nhsemployers.org/your-workforce/plan/education-and-training/preceptorships-for-newly-qualified-staff

ACE YOUR ASSESSMENT

Revise what you have learned by visiting https://study.sagepub.com/essentialmentalhealth. If you are using the interactive ebook, simply click on the tick icon to go straight to the resource.

ONLINE
QUIZZES &
ACTIVITY
ANSWERS

- Test yourself with multiple-choice and short-answer questions and flashcards.

REFERENCES

Ahern, N.R. (2006) Adolescent resilience: an evolutionary concept analysis. *Journal of Pediatric Nursing, 21*, 175–185.

Bowles, C. & Candela, L. (2005) First job experiences of recent RN graduates: improving the work environment. *Journal of Nursing Administration, 35*, 130–137.

Chen, J-Y. (2010) Problem-based learning: developing resilience in nursing students. *Kaohsiung Journal of Medical Sciences*. 27, 230–3. [DOI:10.1016/j.kjms.2010.11.005]

Cleary, M. & Happell, B. (2005) Promoting a sustainable mental health nursing workforce: an evaluation of a transition mental health nursing programme. *International Journal of Mental Health Nursing, 14*, 109–116.

Deasy, C., Doody, O. & Tuohy, D. (2011) An exploratory study of role transition from student nurse (general, mental health and intellectual disability) in Ireland. *Nurse Education in Practice, 11*, 109–113.

Department of Health (2010) *Preceptorship framework for newly registered nurses, midwives and allied health professionals*. London: DH.

Department of Health (2011) *No health without mental health: A cross government mental health outcomes strategy for people of all ages*. Available at: www.gov.uk/government/uploads/system/uploads/attachment_data/file/213761/dh_124058.pdf (accessed 01.11.16).

Duchscher, J.B. (2008) A process of becoming: the stages of new nursing graduate professional role transition. *The Journal of Continuing Education in Nursing, 39*(10), 441–450.

Dutton, J.E., Workman, K.M. & Hardin, A.E. (2014) Compassion at work. *Annual Review of Organisational Psychology and Organisational Behaviour, 1*, 277–304.

Francis, R. (2013) *Report of the Mid Staffordshire Foundation Trust public inquiry*. London: The Stationery Office.

Gerrish, K. (2000) Still fumbling along? A comparative study of the newly qualified nurse's perception of the transition from student to qualified nurse. *Journal of Advanced Nursing, 32*, 473–480.

Happell, B. (2008) The importance of clinical experience for mental health nursing – Part 1: undergraduate nursing students' attitudes, preparedness and satisfaction. *International Journal of Mental Health Nursing, 17*(5), 326–332.

Hayman-White, K., Happell, B., Charleston, R., et al. (2016) Transition to mental health nursing through specialist graduate nurse programs in mental health: a review of the literature. *Issues in Mental Health Nursing, 28*, 185–200.

Higgins, G., Spencer, R.L. & Kane, R. (2010) A systematic review of the experiences and perceptions of the newly qualified nurse in the United Kingdom. *Nurse Education Today, 30*, 499–508.

Hoffart, N., Waddell, A. & Young, M.B. (2011) A model of new nurse transition. *Journal of Professional Nursing, 27*(6), 334–343.

Holland, K. (1999) A journey to becoming: the student nurse in transition. *Journal of Advanced Nursing, 29*(1), 229–236.

Jackson, D., Firtko, A. and Edenborough, M. (2007) Personal resilience as a strategy for surviving and thriving in the face of workplace adversity: a literature review. *Journal of Advanced Nursing, 60*(1), 1–9.

Kramer, M. (1974) *Reality shock: Why nurses leave nursing.* St Louis, MO: C.V. Mosby.

Kumaran, S. & Carney, M. (2014) Role transition from student nurse to staff nurse: facilitating the transition period. *Nurse Education in Practice, 14,* 605–611.

McAllister, M. & McKinnon, J. (2008) The importance of teaching and learning resilience in the health disciplines: a critical review of the literature. *Nurse Education Today, 29,* 371–379.

McCann, C.M., Beddoe, E., McCormick, K., et al. (2013) Resilience in the health professions: a review of recent literature. *International Journal of Wellbeing, 3,* 60–81.

McDonald, G., Jackson, D., Wilkes, J., et al. (2012) A work-based educational intervention to support the development of personal resilience in nurses and midwives. *Nurse Education Today, 32,* 378–384.

Meleis, A., Sawyer, L.M., Eo, I.M., et al. (2000) Experiencing transitions: an emerging middle-range theory. *Advances in Nursing Science, 23*(1), 12–28.

Mooney, M. (2007) Facing registration: the expectations and the unexpected. *Nurse Education Today, 27,* 840–847.

Nursing and Midwifery Council (2006) *Preceptorship guidelines.* NMC Circular 21/2006, 4 October. Available at: www.nmc.org.uk/.../circulars/2006circulars/nmc-circular-21_2006.pdf (accessed 17.08.17).

Nursing and Midwifery Council (2015) *The code for nurses and midwives.* Available at: www.nmc.org.uk/standards/code (accessed 11.16).

Nursing and Midwifery Council (2016) *Revalidation.* http://revalidation.nmc.org.uk/welcome-to-revalidation (accessed 11.16).

NMC online. http://revalidation.nmc.org.uk/what-you-need-to-do/written-reflective-accounts

Pines, E.W., Rauschhuber, M.L., Norgan, G.H., et al. (2012) Stress resiliency, psychological empowerment and conflict management styles among 23 baccalaureate nursing students. *Journal of Advanced Nursing, 68*(7), 1482–1493.

Roy, C. (1989) *Roy's adaptation model.* Available at: http://currentnursing.com/nursing_theory/Roy_adaptation_model.html (accessed 11.16).

Roy, C. & Andrews, A.A. (1991) *The Roy Adaptation Model: The definitive statement.* Norwalk, CT: Appleton and Lange.

Stephens, T. (2013) Nursing student resilience: a concept clarification. *Nursing Forum, 48*(2), 125–133.

Willis, P. (2015) *Raising the bar. Shape of caring: A review of the future education and training of registered nurses and care assistants.* London: Health Education England in partnership with the Nursing and Midwifery Council.

COMPASSIONATE MENTAL HEALTH CARE IN TIMES OF UNCERTAINTY

45

KAREN M. WRIGHT, MICK McKEOWN AND MIKE THOMAS

THIS CHAPTER COVERS

- Compassionate care for service users and mental health nurses
- Shifting terminology away from hollow policy rhetoric such that compassion is properly valued and resituated at the centre of improved systems of care
- Suggestions of some means by which mental health nurses can protect themselves and service users from the vicissitudes of operating environments that squeeze out compassion, and creatively envisage the alternatives
- The value of compassionate mental health nurses, occasionally interjecting our own voices and recollections into the text.

Visit **https://study.sagepub.com/essentialmentalhealth** to access a wealth of online resources for this chapter - watch out for the margin icons throughout the chapter. If you are using the interactive ebook, simply click on the margin icon to go straight to the resource.

INTRODUCTION

A notion of compassion is central to latterday debates over the **value** of mental health nursing. On the one hand, an assertion that mental health nurses ought to be compassionate and caring would seem to be axiomatic, reflected in the NHS Mandate (DH, 2017: 9):

> Everyone deserves care that is safe, compassionate and effective, at all times and regardless of their condition.

On the other hand, however, it would seem foolhardy to take this for granted as mental health services and the nurses within them are alleged to lack compassion with reference to the findings of inquiries into neglect and abuse. Furthermore, commentators, not least from the **service user** and **survivor** movement, but also including critically minded nurses, are highly disparaging of the offer from a narrowly defined biological psychiatry, apparently more defined by **compulsion** and **coercion** than compassion and care (Burstow et al., 2014; LeFrançois et al., 2013; Sidley, 2015). Overlain on this, the economic restrictions of austerity exacerbate and exaggerate **restrictive practices**, further deepening moral objections to psychiatry and the psy-professions. In these circumstances, mental health nurses can struggle to maintain compassionate practice, and the emphasis on compassion in framing a positive professional identity can appear to be more about public relations' imaginaries than real experiences (Cleary, 2004).

We believe that mental health nurses are, on the whole, compassionate individuals who can be supported and relied on to provide compassionate care. Indeed, it would be odd if hordes of uncompassionate people were lining up to do this work with the intention of neglecting and abusing service users. Similarly, if mental health nurses adhere to a positive, compassionate and caring self-image, but find themselves working in conflict-ridden, coercive situations, then we argue that this is unsettling and damaging for them as well as for service users. Hence, we return to the emphasis we have placed in this text on criticality and critical self-reflection and suggest that one way out of this compassion crisis is for mental health nurses, collectively and individually, to think critically about their role and prevailing social factors, to contemplate critically informed solutions and to act accordingly.

MENTAL HEALTH NURSING AND CARING

In an era of nursing where it is rare not to find Jane Cumming's 6Cs in a student nurse's essay (Cummings & Bennett, 2012), Karen recalls her student nurse interview in 1981, at which she proudly announced that 'I want to be a nurse because I *care about people*'. More than 35 years later, this is still the foundation for mental health nursing and nurses are the vehicle by which care is delivered. In a collective effort to 'prioritise people':

> You [nurses] put the interests of people using or needing nursing or midwifery services first. You make their care and safety your main concern and make sure that their dignity is preserved and their needs are recognised, assessed and responded to. You make sure that those receiving care are treated with respect, that their rights are upheld and that any discriminatory attitudes and behaviours towards those receiving care are challenged. (NMC, 2015: 48)

Travelbee (1971) believed that the nurse should 'know thyself' and, hence, that the nurse's 'use of self' was a basic principle of nursing, as the human-to human relationship should be the means through which the purpose of nursing is fulfilled. Travelbee (1971: 19) explains this as occurring within a conscious process which she refers to as the 'therapeutic use of self':

When a nurse uses self therapeutically she consciously makes use of her personality and knowledge in order to effect a change in the ill person. This change is considered therapeutic when it alleviates the individual's stress.

Contemporary concerns about compassion and anxieties over its absence are not necessarily new. Travelbee asserted that nursing needed a 'humanistic revolution' and a return to compassion, which she believed was lacking but could be restored though interpersonal relationships that involved empathy and sympathy. Mental health nursing's attachment to humanist, relational ideals has continued to the present day, with evidence for the therapeutic value of such engagement (McAndrew et al., 2014). According to Freshwater, the goal of any therapeutic alliance is to 'facilitate the emergence of the authentic self' and the 'therapeutic use of self' which are integral to nursing, amongst other caring **professions** (Freshwater, 2002: 4). A **therapeutic relationship** can only be established if we are trusted (Peplau, 1952), and trust cannot be taken for granted. For Kate Granger (2014), who started the #hellomynameis campaign, if compassionate care is the goal then it cannot be achieved without first making some sort of human connection, and it is on this basis that trust is established and deepened. In the main, trust is considered from an individual perspective; that is, the individual needs to trust us as we deploy ourselves and our skill set to meet their needs. However, we argue that nurses are not only 'vehicles' for the delivery of care, but neither are they *catalysts* for change since a catalyst creates change and reaction but is not changed itself. Mental health nurses have their own agency and are personally affected by their interactions with service users and colleagues.

Compassionate caring in contemporary health care can take its toll. To be an effective nurse, we need compassion, skill, knowledge and resilience in equal measure, or, as described in the preface: we need to present with *humility, humanity and honesty*. Notions of trauma-informed care (Sweeney et al., 2016) alert us to the damaging effects of psychiatric systems for service users, but harm can be complexly shared with the workforce, nurses included, who may also at times make use of services. We have to recognise that working in services can also be detrimental for staff who might experience forms of actual or vicarious trauma. This may be due to having to cope with the consequences of poor funding, being subject to authoritarian management, or worrying over the welfare of service users or the threat of violence. Consequently, workplace stress is common for the mental health care workforce who are recorded as having high rates of sickness/absence and mental health problems (Health and Safety Executive, 2016; Rössler, 2012).

If we 'prioritise people', then we prioritise *their* needs, and in order to do this we need to understand what these are and what people's preferences are. Throughout this text, many authors have referred to how we put the service user first, individualise their needs and provide a plethora of helpful and insightful advice that creates a toolkit for mental health nursing practice. We are reminded that we need to *listen* but also acknowledge that compassionate communication requires a level of self-awareness and understanding about how we are perceived by others as well as how we view them. All too often, service users are seen as different to 'us', thus constructing a sense of 'otherness' with regard to those in our care (MacCallum, 2002).

Additionally, whilst we refer constantly to 'person-centred care', we must remember that we are interpersonal beings who exploit our 'humanness' in our work as nurses. In the provision of care and **collaboration** within the care team, we are reminded that communicative relationships are fundamental to care coordination, and nursing care relies on partnerships with **carers**, health and social care agencies and mental health services. It can sometimes take a very tenacious care coordinator to pull these together as, effectively, supportive systems aren't always readily available. Thus, compassionate care is not merely about people – we need the right systems, the right **environment** and the right organisations to function compassionately.

WHEN CARING IS NOT ENOUGH

Simply caring is not enough: the context in which care is practised is a crucial determinant of outcome, and evidence for what works best in terms of help and support is equally important. Despite some misgivings regarding dogmatic commitments to a **culture** of 'evidence-based' nursing (which may actually serve to consolidate biomedical approaches) (Holmes et al., 2006), dismissing scientifically informed approaches is an untenable position. It is worth noting, however, that substantially large proportions of practice are not supported by evidence but this need not mean that they are ineffective, rather relevant research just has not yet been undertaken (Rousseau & Gunia, 2016). Human beings are the vehicle for therapy, which is interpersonal in nature, bringing to bear communication skills in ways that can exemplify both an art and science of nursing (Norman & Ryrie, 2013).

Notwithstanding this, critical commentators have disputed both the art and science of nursing (Hopton, 1997). The softer relational skills which arguably make up the art do not exclusively belong to nursing, and together with the wider critique of psy-science, the science of nursing is problematised in terms of its provenance and utility claims (Barker, 2003; Clarke, 1999). Many typical nursing interventions were originally derived from the behavioural experiments of Ivan Pavlov (1849–1936) and Burrhus Skinner (1904–90), raising moral concerns over their applicability to human relations. The **advocates** for cognitive behavioural therapy emphasise a scientific foundation, suggesting the therapeutic relationship is necessary but not sufficient to bring about change (Beck, 1976). Conversely, studies of the efficacy of a range of psychotherapy interventions suggest that common factors such as alliance and empathy are influential, regardless of the specific therapy modality (Wampold, 2015).

ALLOWING COMPASSION INTO A CHALLENGING SYSTEM

Despite professional and policy rhetoric committing nurses to compassionate care, actually making this happen consistently in practice has been challenging, not least because of implicit constraining factors within the mental health system. Karen Wright reflects on her 'early years' as a post-registered student nurse on the RMN course, back in the 1980s, when she trusted the words of her mentors and felt bemused by the lack of evidence for 'writing off' those in their care to the treadmill of psychiatry:

> I can vividly remember a staff nurse on my first mental health ward as a post-registration RMN student, I'll call her 'Alison'. We had just left the room of a young mum (I'll call her 'Sally') and her baby. Alison had known Sally for some years, she had been on that ward a few times. As we walked away Alison said, 'there you go … another schizophrenic baby'. At the time, I wasn't sure what to say, I didn't want to look ignorant, but it was 1986 and I was a cardio-thoracic nurse with a very limited knowledge of psychiatry. The term *schizophrenic baby* made me cringe, I didn't think that schizophrenia was hereditary, but I didn't know enough to argue about the theory and I felt too junior to argue about the language. I also wasn't sure if Alison meant that Sally's baby was now 'in the system'.
>
> **Karen Wright, mental health nurse**

The asylums were contemplating closure, many people had been incarcerated within their walls and had effectively been damaged by the system. Goffman (1961) famously referred to 'asylums' as 'total institutions' that were closed and sat apart from the rest of society. He observed that the inmates were institutionalised by the rigid routine and enforced isolation from the rest of society in rather the same way as prisons and concentration camps. At the time, these practices were rationalised in terms of individual and public safety, in much the same way as contemporary forms of compulsion and coercion are legitimated (Slemon et al., 2017).

In 1928, John A. Shedd published a collection of sayings titled *Salt from my Attic*, and the following popular aphorism was included: *A ship in harbour is safe, but that is not what ships are built for.*

This reminds us not be afraid to take a positive risk, to be adventurous, to try something new. It also reminds us to plot our route, plan our journey, gather our supplies, and set sail. Just as ships are not designed to sit in port but are built to cross the horizon, into places we cannot immediately see, this is as true for people; for mental health nurses and those in our care. It would be comforting to believe that the totalising systems that Goffman observed are no longer around, but it is clear that closed and coercive environments still exist within mental health services and negatively impact on therapeutic relationships and continue to disable people (Sheehan & Burns, 2011; Sidley, 2015). Recognising this can be part of the motivation to move away from coercive practice and create a solid foundation on which to provide therapeutic, relational care supported by enabling environments that ideally reduce oppression and violence in mental health services (Bowers, 2014; Duxbury, 2015; Johnson & Haigh, 2011).

For critics of the system, the legitimately acceptable limits of compulsion are yet to be adequately defined, and current practices are beset with risk aversion and some dubious risk management practices (Coffey et al., 2016; Sidley, 2015). However, we accept that the use of legislation (e.g. the Mental Health Act in England and Wales) remains, sadly, a necessity for some who pose a risk to self or others. Indeed, almost ironically, there is anecdotal evidence that lack of bed provision and community resources is a factor in increasing levels of compulsion, as a device for ensuring care is provided rather than necessarily risk mitigation. In this sense, in austere economic times concerns may shift from matters of abuse of compulsory powers to the prospect of neglect (Spandler, 2016).

Mick reflects that role dilemmas regarding compulsion are never clear-cut and are both personally and professionally difficult:

In my time as a mental health nurse perhaps the most awful situations I have had to deal with have been after a person has taken their own life. A very good friend of mine killed himself not long after I qualified as a mental health nurse. Meeting with his family before the funeral was an excoriating experience that will always stay with me. I have similarly witnessed the devastating impact upon families and care teams when persons under the care of services have taken their own life. As much as we may consider and value individual autonomy, and as much as I am personally critical of shortcomings in mental health services, it is events such as these that cause me to believe that some powers of compulsion are necessary.

Mick McKeown, mental health nurse

The fact that personal vulnerabilities or risk may necessitate a degree of compulsion is not the same as accepting industrial levels of compulsion and coercion or acquiescing in services becoming a stop-gap for societal failures in justice and welfare. Better alternatives must include improving services so that people in need would actually want to be there rather than have to be compelled into admission. Service users need to feel safe in order to access care and in order to trust those who deliver the care, and this must be a foundational basis for the provision of compassionate services. Clearly, we have a duty to report any concern over the vulnerability of any individual if we believe they are at risk. NHS England (2015) reminds us of our responsibility to have effective arrangements in place to safeguard children and adults at risk of abuse or neglect. Mental health care systems, moreover, represent a complex mix of service user, institutional and worker interests, with the potential for both cooperative or conflictual relationships. Arguably, all interests can be served at one and the same time as ensuring compassionate care, but this requires meaningful attention to systems and will not just happen of its own accord.

SUPPORTING COMPASSIONATE CARE

So, how do we provide compassionate care within mental health care services and overcome various constraints, including addressing the impact of the system on both service users and workers? The **safeguarding** of people's rights and promoting increased choice and control over their lives is an important place to start, but we go one step further and emphasise the need to safeguard both the person, the family (carers) and the workforce (McKeown & Foley, 2015). Services appoint 'safeguarding leads' and establish processes, policies and protocols for managing rapid referrals and the protection of those in our care. We must also remind ourselves that these same guidelines stipulate that we must have safe recruitment practices, effective training, effective supervision arrangements, arrangements for engaging and working in partnership with other agencies, and that we should develop an organisational culture that makes staff aware of their personal responsibility to report concerns and to ensure that poor practice is identified and tackled. It is clear that the fundamental principles of safeguarding align very closely with the duty of care and professional responsibilities of the nurse, and which are highlighted within this text. In this regard, we have to protect service users and we also have to protect nurse colleagues.

Compassionate care requires *kindness*, respect and collaboration with co-workers, service users and carers. Cleary and Horsfall (2016) discuss this further in relation to the relevance of kindness for those working in mental health services and the effect that that has on service users, causing them to feel 'cared for'. Similarly, nurses are acutely aware of their *duty of care* to others, a professional duty which relates to underpinning moral values including kindness and compassion, but not, however, obliging us to be kind to ourselves. We must recognise that compassion cannot simply exist at an individual, interpersonal level but that it must also be supported at a collective or organisational level (Hungerford et al., 2016). Long all-day shifts, for example, take their toll on staff and impact on caring; it's quite a challenge to maintain patience and kindness for the duration (Shaw & Wright, 2013). Clearly, such organisational matters require collective and organisational solutions. Ethical organisational leadership is required, grounded in an **ethics** of compassion that recognises the fact that many workers such as nurses often provide an amount of discretionary labour, over and above what they are contracted for (Thomas & Rowland, 2014). Similarly, relationally organised trade unions can provide an important check on unenlightened employers, providing valuable protection for workers, but also opening up opportunities for progressive political alliances with service user interests (Saundry & McKeown, 2013).

COMPASSIONATE LEADERSHIP

What does compassionate leadership actually mean in a mental health context? As has already been pointed out, it seems odd that practitioners of nursing have to be told via central government that they should be more compassionate and caring. Are the inquiries into neglect and abuse capturing poor leadership as well as poor practices? Work by Upenieks (2003) showed clearly that if a clinical leader of nurses wishes to attract and retain staff, they have to demonstrate credibility (being knowledgeable and skilful regarding the practice of nursing), be visible, responsive and hold a passion for the profession – in other words, be an authentic leader.

The child psychotherapist Winnicott (1988) discussed the skill of understanding the world view of the other as essential to developing empathy, but many forget that he also stated that it was not one-way traffic. The leader interested in mental health and wellbeing has to apply their own developed skills of listening and understanding and also open themselves up so that others can understand their world view. Empathy requires both parties to engage with each other's perceptions. It is a risk many leaders are not prepared to take.

Applying kindness and compassion is personal risk taking; for example, some people view it as a sign of not being a strong enough leader, of lacking the objectivity (read lack of compassion) to implement change. Yet, paradoxically, being kind takes more effort, resilience and courage in leadership than implementing a hierarchical instructive model. That is because compassion involves relational issues, which encompass caring and nurturing others, whilst balancing pragmatism and decision making.

Irving Yalom (1980) talks at great length about the psychotherapeutic relationship and there is much to learn from his approach which can be applied to compassionate leadership. The humanistic principles of genuineness, trust, authenticity and empathy support practice, but he also emphasises four elements of compassion which direct the therapeutic journey. Yalom cannot conceive of an individual who is genuinely applying the craft of relational management doing so without thinking about how they nurture people, care for them, provide hope for the future and actively seek to know more about the individuals they lead.

Martha Nussbaum (1997) argues that relational empathetic skills can be learned, and one way of exercising and developing empathy is through the reading of literature that explores human dilemmas and the internal dynamics of the protagonists. We take her work in a slightly different direction in defining literature as story-telling. The compassionate leader can apply relational skills by focusing on the stories people reveal, about their work, practice, backgrounds, fears and hopes. It means actively listening and using wisely the modern currency of time.

Compassionate leadership is much harder to apply than mere management. In mental health, there is every opportunity to practise core skills to a higher level of expertise within a compassionate leadership approach. The skills of courage, resilience, tolerance and reflection act as the bedrock for improving teamwork, quality and compassion which benefit the individual and the organisation.

Within my own university, we are applying concepts of Trust, Teamwork, Common Sense, Attention to Detail and Compassion as signposts to support the university strategy. Bringing different constituents together has meant a degree of pragmatism to reach a consensus regarding definitions and applications. Interestingly, some colleagues have felt that applying kindness could be perceived as soft management and it has taken time and much discussion to gain their understanding that compassionate leadership is more difficult but also more rewarding as an approach to strategic improvement. Compassionate leadership challenged their own perceptions of how good their abilities were to manage relationships and come out of 'role' to reveal more authentic leadership qualities – again, another risk to self which some leaders were not prepared to take.

People can't pretend to be kind; it is both a virtue and an act. Compassionate leadership defines the **personality** of the leader and inauthenticity is quickly discovered by colleagues. Just as trust is an integral part of mental health nursing, it should also be an integral part of compassionate leadership.

Good use of clinical supervision is one way to support nurses to be compassionate leaders and practitioners, whilst protecting them from the stress and burnout that are becoming pervasive in mental health services (Breen & Sweeney, 2013). Unfortunately, in times of service pressures, commitments to provide clinical supervision can tend to '*go out of the window*'. Hence, many UK mental health staff report having no access to regular structured supervision and models of team supervision may represent a solution (Tuck, 2017) Interestingly, there is evidence that mindfully building self-compassion can be a protective and resilience-enhancing personal strategy for staff attempting to cope with stress and work pressures, and may have a subsequent positive impact on service users (Devenish-Meares, 2015; Sinclair et al., 2017).

We can all be a bit 'ratty' or short-tempered when we've not had enough sleep, and this can be a vicious circle; we don't sleep because of the stress of work and, consequently, not getting a restful night's sleep **affects** our concentration and performance, impacting on relationships and making us more anxious about making mistakes. There is no doubt that sleeplessness has a negative impact on our health, but research also reveals that this compromises mindfulness and reduces self-compassion (Kemper et al., 2015). So, in a nutshell, being kind to ourselves can help us to be kind to others. Whilst this statement might appear superficially banal, there is no doubt that we have less capacity to *care* when we are tired and preoccupied.

Nursing is a role that demands emotional labour, a term coined to describe the way in which two contrasting occupational groups – flight attendants and debt collectors – managed their emotions in their daily work, by Arlie Hochschild, an American sociologist. Workers in such service industries can be required to present a smiling, emotionally engaged presence, even when they feel the burden of dealing with challenging individuals and situations. The intimacy of interpersonal relationships prominent in the work of mental health nurses is implicitly stressful, and this emotional labour can be compounded by an insensitive managerialism and routinisation of nursing work that undermine inclinations to practise more person-centred models of care (James, 1992). When researching the therapeutic relationship, Wright and Schroeder (2016) discovered, however, that patience and kindness can only be maintained for so long, and workers can find themselves alienated in the relationship. Furthermore, finding oneself in conflictual relations can unsettle nursing identities, especially if nurses prefer to see themselves as caring and kind rather than authoritarian (McKeown & Spandler, 2006).

Perhaps unlike other occupations, nurses value the extent to which communication engages their emotions and interacts with the emotional state of service users in the context of caring; expressing support and compassion demands no less (Riley & Weiss, 2016). For such reasons, historical calls for nursing professionalisation have emphasised a need to depart from archetypal professions and ensure a professional identity that properly values a caring ethos, avoids distancing from service users and prioritises relational skills over technologies (Davies, 1995). Such alternative constructs of professionalism reflect feminist ideals and concerns with the importance of gender in understanding nursing practice. Similarly, Karen's (Wright, 2015) work speaks of a *maternalistic* approach, referring to the protective and nurturing role of both the nurse and the mother; remembering always that a good mother enables their child to reach a position of self-reliance and independence. Maternalism has a flexible appreciation of professional boundaries and is quite different to paternalism which is dependency inducing and disempowering. This resonates with Yalom's (2010: 26) exhortation:

Let your patients matter to you, let them enter your mind, influence you – and not conceal this from them.

CONCLUSION

Arguably, never before has there been such recognition that there really is *No Health Without Mental Health*, precipitating calls for a fairer redistribution of funding such that mental health gets a more just share, and where mental health nursing is concomitantly seen to have parity of esteem with adult nursing. Not all practitioners will recognise our critique of mental health care services, especially, perhaps, those who work in well-organised and resourced environments with teams fully committed to progressive ideals of good practice. For such staff, and others who are convinced of the value of psychiatry, the more radical strands of criticism can seem misplaced or even hurtful. Similarly, not all service users are radical critics of bio-psychiatry and, thankfully, many are helped by and satisfied with current services. Even in such circumstances, we argue that mental health nurses still require a critical disposition, for the following reasons:

- Examples of progressive practice are sparsely spread through the system, so a nursing career may infrequently or never encounter them.
- Compulsion and coercion, or their implicit threat, are ever present, however tempered. Thus, the disempowerment of service users is endemic, however well-meaning the staff who work in services.
- Nursing remains subordinate to and less powerful than other positions within professional hierarchies, necessitating ongoing challenges to power imbalances.
- Particularly when working under resource pressures, nurses can become habitiuated to lowering standards of care or even neglect and abuse (Roberts & Ion, 2015)

Our appeal for compassionate mental health nursing is twofold. First, nurses can utilise their therapeutic and relational skills to soften and humanise mental health care services as they are at present. This would hopefully ensure that many more service users have positive experiences of care. Second, mental health nurses can be part of a movement for transforming services, including participation in the critical debate regarding the legitimate limits of compulsion and coercion. Together with service users and carers, we can thus be part of a collective re-imagining of how mental health care is organised. Ideally, this would represent a radical turn away from a singular bio-psychiatric model and would more fully embrace the potential for nurses to practise authentic, compassionate, relational care.

Rachelle is a young woman who was in a specialist eating **disorder** unit at the time of speaking. We have chosen her story to close our book and hopefully reinforce our commitment to both the value of compassionate mental health nursing and the imperative to maintain a critical reflexive disposition to care:

My thoughts about myself and my body had spiralled into negativity that pervaded my very existence, I didn't eat, and eventually anorexia took control. My thoughts got too much, I acted on them, lost weight. My mum and dad noticed. I hid it as best I could, I didn't want people to know, ironically, because they cared, and I was protective of them, but in the process of doing so deteriorated rapidly. In the end, I told them everything. It was the worst time of my life. I thought that I was a bad daughter, but I couldn't stop myself. My dad told me that he thought that I was going to drop dead. In my head, I thought 'I wish I would' as I wanted the pain to go away, but didn't want my family to suffer any more. I didn't really want to die but I felt that my body was giving up on me, every bit of me hurt. In the end it was a relief to tell them, to get help and to embark on my recovery.

Rachelle, service user

Rachelle was acutely aware of her frailty and fragility and desperately needed kindness and gentleness. She talked of the things that matter to her the most:

- It helps a lot when the nurses are positive, when they are happy and joking and laughing with us.
- It's good when the nurses talk to me about how I'm feeling; they let me get it all out.
- They always know what to say.
- They are really caring, and know when I just need a hug.
- It really helps when I can feel the compassion of the nurses when they comfort me.

Conversely, Rachelle recognised that for some nurses it was clearly 'just a job'. These nurses appeared not to be approachable, functioning in a very distant, task-orientated way. Rachelle knew that the nurses that offered her comfort really cared. We can wax lyrical about the research that underpins our practice, and should never trivialise the importance of the evidence behind our work but, if care is to be delivered compassionately with humility, humanity and honesty, we must listen to Rachelle, and others, who offer us salient and insightful observations on the practice of mental health nursing. We have much to learn, especially from people like Rachelle and the other service user contributors to this text who speak to us from the vital perspective of lived experience of health care. This book has brought together the lived experience of service users, practitioners and academics to present a rounded, informed and inclusive perspective on the essentials of mental health nursing. We sincerely hope it is of use to nurses wishing to develop confident, knowledgeable, skilled and, above all, compassionate and caring nursing careers.

REFERENCES

Barker, P. (2003) The Tidal Model: psychiatric colonization, recovery and the paradigm shift in mental health care. *International Journal of Mental Health Nursing*, 12(2), 96–102.

Beck, A.T. (1976) *Cognitive therapy and the emotional disorders*. New York: International Universities Press.

Bowers, L. (2014) Safewards: a new model of conflict and containment on psychiatric wards. *Journal of Psychiatric and Mental Health Nursing*, 21(6), 499–508.

Breen, M. & Sweeney, J. (2013) Burnout: the experiences of nurses who work in inner city areas: Maria Breen and John Sweeney describe the factors that influence practitioners' ability to cope with job stress. *Mental Health Practice*, 17(2), 12–20.

Burstow, B., LeFrançois, B. & Diamond, S.L. (eds) (2014) *Psychiatry disrupted: Theorizing resistance and crafting the revolution*. Montreal, QC: McGill/Queen's University Press.

Clarke, L. (1999) Nursing in search of a science: the rise and rise of the new nurse brutalism. *Mental Health Care*, 2, 270–272.

Cleary, M. (2004) The realities of mental health nursing in acute inpatient environments. *International Journal of Mental Health Nursing*, 13(1), 53–60.

Cleary, M. & Horsfall, J. (2016) Kindness and its relevance to everyday life: some considerations for mental health nurses. *Issues in Mental Health Nursing*, 37(3), 206–208.

Coffey, M., Cohen, R., Faulkner, A., et al. (2016) Ordinary risks and accepted fictions: how contrasting and competing priorities work in risk assessment and mental health care planning. *Health Expectations*, 20(3), 471–483.

Cummings, J. & Bennett, V. (2012) *Compassion in practice: Nursing, midwifery and care staff – our vision and strategy*. London: NHS Commissioning Board.

Davies, C. (1995) *Gender and the professional predicament in nursing*. London: McGraw-Hill Education.

Department of Health (DH) (2017) *The government's mandate to NHS England for 2017–18*. Available at: www.gov.uk/government/uploads/system/uploads/attachment_data/file/601188/NHS_Mandate_2017-18_A.pdf (accessed 30.04.17).

Devenish-Meares, P. (2015) Call to compassionate self-care: introducing self-compassion into the workplace treatment process. *Journal of Spirituality in Mental Health, 17*(1), 75–87.

Duxbury, J.A. (2015) The Eileen Skellern Lecture 2014: physical restraint – in defence of the indefensible? *Journal of Psychiatric and Mental Health Nursing, 22*(2), 92–101.

Freshwater, D. (2002) Therapeutic nursing. In D. Freshwater (ed.) *Therapeutic use of self in nursing*. London: Sage.

Goffman, E. (1961) *Asylums: Essays on the social situation of mental patients and other inmates*. Harmondsworth: Penguin.

Granger, K. (2014) *Hello my name is*. Available at: hellomynameis.org.uk (accessed 29.04.17).

Health and Safety Executive (2016) *Work related stress, anxiety and depression statistics in Great Britain 2016*. London: HSE. Available at: www.hse.gov.uk/statistics/causdis/stress/stress.pdf (accessed 29.04.17).

Holmes, D., Perron, A. & O'Byrne, P. (2006) Evidence, virulence, and the disappearance of nursing knowledge: a critique of the evidence-based dogma. *Worldviews on Evidence-Based Nursing, 3*(3), 95–102.

Hopton, J. (1997) Towards a critical theory of mental health nursing. *Journal of Advanced Nursing, 25*(3), 492–500.

Hungerford, C., Sayers, J. & Cleary, M. (2016) Facilitating goodwill in workplace relationships: the benefits and challenges. *Issues in Mental Health Nursing, 37*(7), 530–532.

James, N. (1992) Care = organisation + physical labour + emotional labour. *Sociology of Health and Illness, 14*, 488–509.

Johnson, R. & Haigh, R. (2011) Social psychiatry and social policy for the 21st century: new concepts for new needs – the 'Enabling Environments' initiative. *Mental Health and Social Inclusion, 15*(1), 17–23.

Kemper, K.J., Mo, X. & Khayat, R. (2015) Are mindfulness and self-compassion associated with sleep and resilience in health professionals? *Journal of Alternative & Complementary Medicine, 21*(8), 496–503.

LeFrançois, B., Menzies, R. & Reaume, G. (eds) (2013) *Mad matters: A critical reader in Canadian mad studies*. Toronto, Ontario: Canadian Scholars' Press. pp. 122–129.

MacCallum, E.J. (2002) Othering and psychiatric nursing. *Journal of Psychiatric and Mental Health Nursing, 9*(1), 87–94.

McAndrew, S., Chambers, M., Nolan, F., et al. (2014) Measuring the evidence: reviewing the literature of the measurement of therapeutic engagement in acute mental health inpatient wards. *International Journal of Mental Health Nursing, 23*, 212–220.

McKeown, M. & Foley, P. (2015) Reducing physical restraint: an employment relations perspective. *Journal of Mental Health Nursing, 35*(1), 12–15.

McKeown, M. & Spandler, H. (2006) *Alienation and redemption: The potential for alliances with mental health service users*. Published conference proceedings. Alternative Futures & Popular Protest, 11th International Social Movements Conference, 19–21 April, Manchester Metropolitan University.

NHS England (2015) *Safeguarding vulnerable people in the NHS: Accountability and assurance framework safeguarding*. Available at: www.england.nhs.uk/.../safeguarding-accountability-assurance-framework.pdf (accessed 29.04.17).

Norman, I. & Ryrie, I. (2013) *The art and science of mental health nursing: Principles and practice*, 3rd edition. Maidenhead: Open University Press.

Nursing & Midwifery Council (2015) *NMC code*. London: NMC. Available at: www.nmc.org.uk/standards/code (accessed 10.08.17).

Nussbaum, M.C. (1997) *Cultivating humanity: A classic defence of reform in liberal education*. Cambridge, MA: Harvard University Press.

Peplau, H.E. (1952) *Interpersonal relations in nursing*. New York: G.P. Putman's Sons.

Riley, R. & Weiss, M.C. (2016) A qualitative thematic review: emotional labour in healthcare settings. *Journal of Advanced Nursing, 72*(1), 6–17.

Roberts, M. & Ion, R. (2015) Thinking critically about the occurrence of widespread participation in poor nursing care. *Journal of Advanced Nursing, 71*(4), 768–776.

Rössler, W. (2012) Stress, burnout, and job dissatisfaction in mental health workers. *European Archives of Psychiatry and Clinical Neuroscience, 262*(2), 65–69.

Rousseau, D.M. & Gunia, B.C. (2016) Evidence-based practice: the psychology of EBP implementation. *Annual Review of Psychology, 67*, 667–692.

Saundry, R. & McKeown, M. (2013) Relational union organising in a healthcare setting: a qualitative study. *Industrial Relations Journal, 44*, 533–547.

Shaw, T. & Wright, K. (2013) The impact of caring. *Asylum, 20*(2), 20–22.

Shedd, J.A. (1928) *Salt from my attic*. Portland, ME: The Mosher Press.

Sheehan, K.A. & Burns, T. (2011) Perceived coercion and the therapeutic relationship: a neglected association? *Psychiatric Services, 62*, 471–476.

Sidley, G.L. (2015) *Tales from the madhouse: An insider critique of psychiatric services*. Wyastone Leys: PCCS Books.

Sinclair, S., Kondejewski, J., Raffin-Bouchal, S., et al. (2017) Can self-compassion promote healthcare provider well-being and compassionate care to others? Results of a systematic review. *Applied Psychology: Health and Well-Being, 9*(2), 168–206.

Slemon, A., Jenkins, E. & Bungay, V. (2017) Safety in psychiatric inpatient care: the impact of risk management culture on mental health nursing practice. *Nursing Inquiry, 24*(4), e12199.

Spandler, H. (2016) From psychiatric abuse to psychiatric neglect? *Asylum Magazine, 23*(2), 7–8.

Sweeney, A., Clement, S., Filson, B. et al. (2016) Trauma-informed mental healthcare in the UK: what is it and how can we further its development? *Mental Health Review Journal, 21*(3), 74–92.

Thomas, M. & Rowland, C. (2014) Leadership, pragmatism and grace: a review. *Journal of Business Ethics, 123*(1), 99–111.

Travelbee, J. (1971) *Interpersonal aspects of nursing*, 2nd edition. Philadelphia: F.A. Davies.

Tuck, J.A. (2017) A new approach to team clinical supervision on an acute admissions unit. *Mental Health Practice, 20*(5), 24–27.

Upenieks, V.V. (2003) What constitutes effective leadership? Perceptions of magnetic and non-magnetic nurse leaders. *Journal of Nursing Administration, 33*(9), 456–467.

Wampold, B.E. (2015) How important are the common factors in psychotherapy? An update. *World Psychiatry, 14*(3), 270–277.

Winnicott, D.W. (1988) *Human nature*. London: Free Association Books.

Wright, K.M. (2015) Maternalism: a healthy alliance for recovery and transition in eating disorder services. *Journal of Psychiatric Mental Health Nursing, 22*(6), 431–439.

Wright, K.M. & Schroeder, D. (2016) Turning the tables: the vulnerability of nurses treating anorexia nervosa patients. *Cambridge Quarterly, 25*(2), 219–227.

Yalom, I.D. (1980) *Existential psychotherapy.* New York: Basic Books.

Yalom, I.D. (2010) *The gift of therapy.* London: Piatkus.

APPENDIX

MENTAL HEALTH LEGISLATION IN THE UK
KEVIN MOORE AND MARIE O'NEILL

Most nations internationally have a legal framework for the safeguarding of persons with mental illness or issues related to vulnerability or to lack of mental capacity. These will have much in common with each other, not least, defining the legal requirements for compulsory admission for assessment and treatment. Within the United Kingdom there are three discrete jurisdictions, England and Wales, Scotland and Northern Ireland, and thus three pieces of different legislation exists.

ENGLAND AND WALES

In England and Wales two specific pieces of legislation govern how people with mental health conditions received care and treatment and these were The Mental Health Act 1983 and the Mental Capacity Act 2005. The Mental Health Act 2007 was introduced on the 19th July 2007 to amend these two pieces of earlier legislation. The Mental Health Act 2007 is divided into three discrete parts. *Part 1* details the Amendments to the Mental Health Act of 1983, and contains eight distinct chapters therein. *Part 2* relates to Amendments to other Acts, whilst *Part 3* relates to General information.

SCOTLAND

The Mental Health (Care and Treatment) (Scotland) 2003 legislation was passed by Parliament on 20th March 2003and was the primary legislation for this jurisdiction until the introduction of the Mental Health (Scotland) Act on the 4th August 2015. *Part 1* details the provision about the operation of the Mental Health (Care and Treatment) (Scotland) Act 2003. *Part 2* relates to the amendments to the Criminal Procedure (Scotland) Act 1995 in relation to the treatment of mentally disordered offenders. It amends timescales for assessment and treatment orders and provides for variations of certain orders. *Part 3* of the Act creates a new notification scheme for victims of some mentally disordered offenders. This will allow certain information to be provided to victims of offenders subject to certain orders and to allow victims to make representations in certain circumstances in connection with the release of the patient from detention. The timescale for full implementation of the Act has been outlined within the legislation but individuals are advised to consult with their legal representatives during the transitional phases.

NORTHERN IRELAND

Mental Health Legislation in Northern Ireland (NI) is governed by the Mental Health Order (NI) 1986. The revised GAIN Mental Health (NI) Order Guidelines, to accompany the Order, were issued in 2011 some 25 years later to take account of changes in the Order and its interpretation of developments in legislation, practice and services as far as was possible. The 1986 Order and the 2011 GAIN Guidelines will eventually be replaced by a significantly revised and robust piece of new legislation called The Mental Capacity Act (NI) 2016.

The Mental Health (Northern Ireland) Order 1986

The Mental Health (Northern Ireland) Order came into effect on the 26th March 1986 and has remained as the core aspect for mental health legislation in NI since this date. The Mental Health Order (NI) 1986 has a total of 11 discrete Parts to the Order. *Part 1* relates to an Introduction and herein contains a definition of mental disorder. *Part 2* relates to Compulsory Admission to Hospital and Guardianship and this Part covers significantly the powers related to Detention and outlines the Nurses Holding Powers therein and renewals for Compulsory Detention. *Part 3* relates to Patients Concerned in Criminal Proceedings or under Sentence. *Part 4* relates to Consent to Treatment. *Part 5* relates to The Mental Health Review Tribunal for NI. *Part 6* relates to The Mental Health Commission for NI. *Part 7* relates to the Registration of Private Hospitals and *Part 8* relates to the Management of Property and the Affairs of Patients. *Part 9* relates to miscellaneous functions of Department and Boards. *Part 10* relates to Offences and *Part 11* relates to Miscellaneous and Supplementary.

The GAIN Mental Health (NI) Order 1986 Guidelines 2011

According to Professor Robin Davidson Chairman of the GAIN Operational Committee the GAIN Mental Health (NI) Order 1986 Guideline offered a practical, accessible, available e-learning package for all the agencies involved in mental health care, who had significant powers to intervene in people's lives. The GAIN Guidelines 2011 developed due to the absence in recent guidance that reflected changes that had occurred over the past 25 years. The Guideline took account of developments in legislation, practice and service as far as possible and was accompanied and supported by a list of resources that were made available for download at: www.gain-ni.org It is fair to say that the Guideline provided significant clarity for the application of the Order, particularly Parts 2, 3, 4, 5 & 6 and introduced pathways for consideration for Compulsory Admission for Assessment and Treatment under the Order. Moreover the Guideline provided a clearer pathway for the introduction and planning for the new Mental Capacity Act (NI) 2016 and the e-learning packages and modules of learning that accompanied the Guideline 2011 were an important instrument that enabled practitioners to address the needs for an important vulnerable group in society taking due cognisance of their human rights.

The Mental Capacity Act (Northern Ireland) 2016

The Mental Capacity Act (NI) 2016 is the state's first independent legislation that provides details of the safeguards that are now in place to protect the care, treatment and personal welfare for those persons who lack capacity. It covers the legalities surrounding a lack of mental capacity that was enacted in May 2016, and is now available for public access on the UK Government website and ensures that NI legislation is now in line with the rest of the United Kingdom. The full timescale for full implementation of the Act is not yet clear and individuals are advised to consult with their legal representatives during the transitional phases. This is the first time that **mental health** and **mental capacity** have been combined in the one piece of legislation and it ensures that those individuals who have a lack of capacity due to their mental health issues are clearly protected.

Divided into 15 parts, with multiple chapters and sub-chapters therein the Act starts by clearly defining key terms such as 'lacking capacity' and 'best interests decision making', making this the first time that NI has explicitly defined mental capacity through legislation. It also defines the High Court's role in making decisions on a person's behalf, including their ability to appoint deputies to act on someone's behalf. *Part 1*of the Act outlines The Principles, whilst *Part 2* details Lack of Capacity: Protection from Liability and Safeguards. *Part 3* relates to the Nominated Person and *Part 4* details Independent Mental Capacity Advocates. *Part 5* details the Lasting Powers of Attorney, whilst *Part 6* relates to High Court Powers: Decisions and Deputies. *Part 7* details Public Guardian and Court Visitors and *Part 8* relates to Research. *Part 9* details Powers of Police to Remove Person to Place of Safety. *Part 10* relates to Criminal Justice and *Part 11* details Transfer between Jurisdictions. *Part 12* relates to Children and *Part 13* Offences. *Part 14* details Miscellaneous and *Part 15* Supplementary.

REFERENCES

Guideline and Audit Implementation Network (GAIN) (2011). *Guidelines on the Use of the Mental Health (Northern Ireland) Order 1986.* Available at: https://rqia.org.uk/RQIA/files/4e/4ee9f634-be47-4398-afc9-906a20ff3198.pdf (accessed 29.05.17).

Mental Health (Care and Treatment) (Scotland) (2003). Available at: www.legislation.gov.uk/asp/2003/13/contents (accessed 29.05.17).

Mental Health (Scotland) Act 2015. Available at: www.legislation.gov.uk/asp/2015/9/contents/enacted (accessed 29.05.17).

The Mental Capacity Act (Northern Ireland) 2016. Available at: www.legislation.gov.uk/nia/2016/18/pdfs/nia_20160018_en.pdf (last accessed 29.05.17).

The Mental Health (Northern Ireland) Order 1986. Available at: www.legislation.gov.uk/nisi/1986/595/pdfs/uksi_19860595_en.pdf (accessed 29.05.17).

The Mental Health Act 2007 Available at: www.legislation.gov.uk/ukpga/2007/12/contents (accessed 29.05.17).

GLOSSARY OF TERMS

Caveat: Mental health care is notable for a degree of contention regarding many commonly used terms or concepts. This glossary is not necessarily intended as an endorsement of any particular term. The mental health workforce and service users arguably need to have knowledge of the range of terminology without necessarily agreeing with all of it.

Absolute poverty: Occurs when there is severe deprivation of basic human needs, including food, safe drinking water, sanitation facilities, health, shelter, education and information. Whilst is is often expressed as an income measure it depends not only on income but also on access to services.

Acute: Acute, in medicine, refers to an intense illness or affliction of abrupt onset.

Addiction: An organism's psychological or physical dependence on a drug, characterised by tolerance and withdrawal.

Adherence: The extent to which a patient's behaviour (in terms of taking medication, following a diet, modifying habits or attending clinics) coincides with medical or health advice.

Adjustment disorder: A pathological psychological reaction to trauma, loss or severe stress. Usually these last under six months, but may be prolonged if the stressor, e.g. pain or scarring, is enduring.

Advance care planning (ACP): A process of discussion between an individual and their care providers in order to make clear a person's wishes, and will usually take place in the context of an anticipated deterioration in the individual's condition in the future, with attendant loss of capacity to make decisions and/or ability to communicate wishes to others.

Advance directive: A document used to register advance instructions about future treatment in the event of an incapacitating psychiatric crisis. It is intended to support patients' self-determination at a time when they are vulnerable to loss of autonomy, to help them ensure their preferences are known and to minimise unwanted treatments.

Advanced decisions to refuse treatment (ADRT): An ADRT is legally binding and relates to a refusal of specific medical treatment and can specify circumstances. The ADRT will come into effect when the person has lost capacity to give or refuse consent for treatment. It is essential to assess the validity and applicability of an advanced decision before it is used in clinical practice (http://endof lifecareambitions.org.uk/wp-content-uploads/2016/09/Advance-Decisions.pdf).

Advocate: An advocate may act to assist a service user to represent themselves well and ensure that their opinions are heard. Advocates also provide help and information about rights under mental health legislation, including the rights of the nearest relative, when making complaints in relation to health and social care services.

Affect: A person's affect is their immediate emotional state which the person can recognise subjectively and which can also be recognised objectively by others. A person's mood is their predominant current affect. Common examples of affect are sadness, fear, joy and anger. The normal range of expressed affect varies considerably between different cultures and even within the same culture. Types of affect include: euthymic, irritable, constricted, blunted, flat, inappropriate and labile.

Affective disorders: Disorders of mood. Examples would include major depressive disorder, depressive disorder, adjustment disorder with depressed mood, and bipolar disorder.

Age-associated memory impairment (AAMI): The mild disturbance in memory function that occurs normally with ageing; a benign senescent forgetfulness. Such lapses in memory are lately humorously referred to as representing 'a senior moment'.

Aggression: Feelings of anger or antipathy that may lead to constructive or destructive actions but that usually has long-term negative consequences; whilst violence is the harmful use of force or strength. A violent person is generally understood to refer to someone who attacks another.

Agitation: (psychomotor agitation) Excessive motor activity that accompanies and is associated with a feeling of inner tension. The activity is usually non-productive and repetitious and consists of such behaviour as pacing, fidgeting, wringing of the hands, pulling of clothes and an inability to sit still.

Alienation: The estrangement felt in a setting one views as foreign, unpredictable or unacceptable. For example, in depersonalisation phenomena, feelings of unreality or strangeness produce a sense of alienation from one's self or environment. In the workplace, alienation occurs for workers who lack control over how their work is organised, or the products of their efforts. Not being able to support or help others when one wants to represents a particular form of alienation from sense of self or being.

Ambivalence: The coexistence of contradictory emotions, attitudes, ideas or desires with respect to a particular person, object or situation. Ordinarily, the ambivalence is not fully conscious and suggests psychopathology only when present in an extreme form.

Amnesia: Loss of memory. Types: anterograde is loss of memory of events that occur after the onset of the etiological condition or agent; retrograde is loss of memory of events that occurred before the onset of the etiological condition or agent.

Anorexia nervosa: Anorexia nervosa is an eating disorder characterised by excess control – a morbid fear of obesity leads the sufferer to try and limit or reduce their weight by excessive dieting, exercising, vomiting, purging and use of diuretics. Sufferers are typically more than 15% below the average weight for their height/sex/age. Usually, they have amenorrhoea (if female) or low libido (if male); 1–2% of female teenagers are anorexic.

Anti-psychiatry: Either a movement or loose collection of different critics of psychiatry. Notable in the late 1960s and 1970s and associated with the ideas of Foucault, Szasz, Laing and Goffman. A new variant can be seen in the writing and activism of people like Bonnie Burstow who speaks of dismantling psychiatry in a process of attrition.

Antipsychotic: The word antipsychotic is applied to a group of drugs commonly, but not exclusively, used to treat psychosis.

Anxiety: The apprehensive anticipation of future danger or misfortune accompanied by a feeling of dysphoria or somatic symptoms of tension. The focus of anticipated danger may be internal or external. Anxiety is often distinguished from fear in that fear is a more appropriate word to use when there exists threat or danger in the real world. It has been claimed that we live in an age of anxiety.

Apathy: Lack of feeling, emotion, interest or concern.

Appropriate adult: A person who is independent of the police and who is responsible for ensuring a mentally disordered person is treated fairly, if they are in police custody.

Appropriate treatment: References to 'appropriate medical treatment' or 'appropriate treatment', in relation to a person suffering from mental disorder, are references to medical treatment which is appropriate in his or her case and takes into account the nature and degree of the mental disorder and all other circumstances of his or her case.

Approved clinician: Some decisions under the Mental Health Act (2007, England & Wales) can only be taken by approved clinicians. An approved clinician is a mental health professional who has been approved, for the purposes of the Mental Health Act, by the Secretary of State (England) or by Welsh ministers (Wales). Approved clinicians may be doctors or non-medically qualified mental health professionals such as psychologists, nurses, occupational therapists and social workers. A **Responsible Clinician** is the Approved Clinician who has been given overall responsibility for a patient's care.

Approved mental health practitioner (AMHP): Approved mental health practitioners may be social workers, nurses, occupational therapists or psychologists who have been approved by a local social services authority to carry out certain functions under the Mental Health Act (2007, England & Wales). The Mental Health Act 1983 gives them the power to make an application for admission to hospital under a section of the Act where necessary and proper. Before doing so, the AMHP must interview the patient and satisfy him- or herself that detention in hospital is, in all the circumstances, the most appropriate way of providing the care and medical treatment the patient needs.

Assessment process: An ongoing process aimed at understanding and exploring a service user's experiences and the impact on their health and functioning.

Assessment tools: Means of gathering information about a service user/client's physiological, psychological, sociological and spiritual status, and helping inform the identification of current and ongoing needs.

Auditory hallucination: A hallucination involving the perception of sound, most commonly of voices. Some clinicians and investigators would not include those experiences perceived as coming from inside the head and would instead limit the concept of true auditory hallucinations to those sounds whose source is perceived as being external.

Biophilia: The idea that humans have an instinctual need to affiliate with nature.

Bisexual: A person who is sexually and/or romantically attracted to women and men. You may see this shortened to 'bi'.

Blunted affect: An affect type that represents significant reduction in the intensity of emotional expression.

Body image: One's sense of the self and one's body.

Bulimia nervosa: Described by Russell in 1979, bulimia nervosa is an eating disorder characterised by lack of control. Abnormal eating behaviour, including dieting, vomiting, purging and particularly bingeing, may be associated with normal weight or obesity.

Care plan: Care plans are a record of a service user's current needs and risk factors. It should also include the responses to those needs, how to meet those needs, by whom, and desired outcome. They are a way of communicating this information to everybody involved. They also record who is to be involved, when the overall plan is to be reviewed and whether unmet needs have been identified.

Carer: A relative or close friend who assumes an unpaid and unanticipated responsibility for another, the client, who has mental health problems.

Carer attributions: The process of inferring the causes of actions or behaviours, particularly in relation to their friend/relative's mental health.

Carer burden: The stressors encountered by carers that are either directly or indirectly related to mental health problems.

Carer psychoeducation: Professionals provide information on the development and maintenance of mental health problems and ways in which they could be alleviated or made worse. Cognitive therapy approaches are often included.

Carer support: Groups where carers receive information and mutual assurance from other carers.

Catharsis: The healthful (therapeutic) release of ideas through 'talking out' conscious material, accompanied by an appropriate emotional reaction. Also, the release into awareness of repressed ('forgotten') material from the unconscious.

Cis/cisgender: A cis person is someone who does identify with the gender that they were assigned at birth, i.e. a person who is not trans.

Citizenship: Citizenship involves playing an active part in society. In the main, it refers to being a member of a state or a nation. It encompasses the process of being a member of society and how we make society work, together. Active citizenship can help make society fairer and more inclusive. It supports a democracy in which people participate and belong.

Clarifying assessment: An ongoing process of expounding on the information gathered during broad-based assessment using specific symptoms or need-based assessment tools.

Classification: In psychiatry, the set of illnesses, diseases, disorders or syndromes defined in terms of symptoms. The two main classificatory systems are the Diagnostic and Statistical Manual (in the USA) and the World Health Organization's International Classification of Diseases (in the rest of the world). These are revised in new editions every few years. For example, DSM-5 was published in 2013. The study of classification or, more formally, taxonomy is sometimes called, even more formally, 'nosology'. These frameworks have attracted concerted criticism.

Coercion: Unlike other areas of health care – with the exception of some communicable diseases – mental health care allows for the detention and treatment of adults who have committed no crimes, against their will. The need for coercion is usually balanced against the conflicting need to respect patient autonomy. The precise justification for coercion remains conceptually and morally challenging.

Cognition: Cognition is another word for 'thought'.

Cognitive behaviour therapy (CBT): Cognitive behaviour therapy is a talking treatment designed to alter unwanted patterns of thought and behaviour; it addresses personal beliefs which may result in negative emotional responses, concentrating on understanding behaviour rather than the actual cause of a problem.

Collaboration: An active and ongoing partnership, often between people from diverse backgrounds, who work together to solve problems or provide services.

Commissioning: The process used, in a local context, to decide how to spend available funds to improve health.

Community treatment order (CTO): CTOs were introduced into the Mental Health Act in November 2008. In the NMC Code, it is called a supervised community treatment; in the Act, those subject to CTOs are called community patients. A CTO allows a detained service user to leave hospital and be treated safely in the *community* rather than in hospital.

Comorbidity: With respect to diagnostic practices, the simultaneous appearance of two or more illnesses, such as the co-occurrence of schizophrenia and substance abuse or of alcohol dependence and depression. The association may reflect a causal relationship between one disorder and another or an underlying vulnerability to both disorders. Also, the appearance of the illnesses may be unrelated to any common aetiology or vulnerability. One of the criticisms of DSM-5 is that more or less everything is potentially comorbid with everything else.

Compensation: A defence mechanism, operating unconsciously, by which one attempts to make up for real or fancied deficiencies. Also a conscious process in which one strives to make up for real or imagined defects of physique, performance skills or psychological attributes. The two types frequently merge.

Compulsion: Repetitive ritualistic behaviour such as hand washing or ordering or a mental act such as praying or repeating words silently that aims to prevent or reduce distress or prevent some dreaded event or situation. The person feels driven to perform such actions in response to an obsession or according to rules that must be applied rigidly, even though the behaviours are recognised to be excessive or unreasonable. For instance, for a person obsessed by the idea that they are dirty, repeated ritual hand washing may serve to reduce anxiety.

Compulsion: the legally legitimated forced entry to mental health services.

Concrete thinking: Thinking characterised by immediate experience, rather than abstractions. It may occur as a primary, developmental defect, or it may develop secondary to organic brain disease or schizophrenia.

Confabulation: Changing, loosely held and false memories created to fill in organically derived amnesia. Fabrication of stories in response to questions about situations or events that are not recalled.

Coping: The process of responding to a perceived threat through an appraisal of the situation and of a person's resources.

Coping mechanism: A way of adjusting to environmental stress without altering one's goals or purposes; may be conscious and/or unconscious.

Co-production: A process which is jointly developed using both expert by profession and expert by experience perspectives. In this process, each perspective holds equal value and the unique skills and experiences are valued as a means to develop a rounded perspective.

Culture: The cumulative deposit of knowledge, spatial relations, experience, beliefs, values, attitudes, notions of time, meanings, hierarchies, religion, roles, concepts of the universe, and material objects and possessions acquired by a group of people in the course of generations through individual and group relations. It can also describe a particular way of thinking, working or behaving that exists in a place or organisation.

Delusion: An irrational belief which is out of keeping with the person's cultural context, intelligence and social background and which is held with unshakeable conviction.

Delusional perception: A normal perception which has become highly invested with significance and which has become incorporated into a delusional system, e.g. 'when I saw the traffic lights turn red I knew then that the spies were after me'.

Dementia: A global deterioration in cognitive abilities and which usually runs a deteriorating course.

Denial: A defence mechanism where certain information is not accessed by the conscious mind. Denial is related to repression, a similar defence mechanism, but denial is more pronounced or intense. Denial involves some impairment of reality. Denial would be operating (*as an example*) if a cardiac patient who has been warned about the potential fatal outcome of engaging in heavy work, decides to start building a wall of heavy stones.

Depersonalisation: An experience where the self is felt to be unreal, detached from reality or different in some way (e.g. feeling like one is in a dream). Depersonalisation can be triggered by tiredness, dissociative episodes or partial epileptic seizures.

Depression: An affective state characterised by a profound and persistent sadness.

Deprivation of liberty safeguards: The Mental Capacity Act (England & Wales) allows restraint and restrictions to be used, but only if they are in a person's best interests. Extra safeguards are needed if the restrictions and restraint used will deprive a person of their *liberty*.

Disorientation: Confusion about the time of day, date or season (time), where one is (place), or who one is (person).

Dose-response relationship: Also known as an exposure-response relationship, it is the idea that repeated or prolonged exposure causes increased change. For example, increased exposure to urban environments is associated with an increased risk of mental health difficulties.

Drive: A basic urge or motivation; a term used to avoid confusion with the more purely biological concept of instinct.

Dyslexia: Inability or difficulty in reading, including word-blindness and a tendency to reverse letters and words in reading and writing.

Dystonia: Disordered tonicity of the muscles.

Early warning signs: Subtle signs of change that indicate that a person may need to take action to avoid a worsening of their mental health. Again, these are unique to each individual and might include: becoming forgetful, sleeping too much or too little, not leaving the house, being confrontational.

Elevated mood: An exaggerated feeling of wellbeing, or euphoria or elation. A person with elevated mood may describe feeling 'high', 'ecstatic', 'on top of the world' or 'up in the clouds'.

End of life: Patients are 'approaching the end of life' when they are likely to die within the next 12 months. This includes patients whose death is imminent (expected within a few hours or days) and those with: (a) advanced, progressive, incurable conditions; or (b) general frailty and coexisting conditions that mean they are expected to die within 12 months (LACDP, 2014).

Environment: The combination of external physical conditions that affect and influence the growth, development and survival of an organism.

Epidemiology: The study and analysis of the patterns, causes and effects of health and disease conditions in defined populations. It is the cornerstone of public health, and shapes policy decisions and evidence-based practice by identifying risk factors for disease and targets for preventive health care.

Ethics: At its simplest, *ethics* is a system of moral principles. They affect how people make decisions and lead their lives. *Ethics* is concerned with what is good for individuals and society and is also described as moral philosophy.

Ethnicity: Identification with a group that shares a distinctive culture, common language, ancestral or national background, allegiance, association, language or religion.

Euthymia: A person's normal mood state.

Euthymic: Mood in the 'normal' range, which implies the absence of depressed or elevated mood.

Expressed emotion: A measure of the emotional temperature within a family. Family environments are assessed on three domains; critical comments; hostility; emotional over-involvement, with those family environments that reach a threshold being rated as high in expressed emotion. High expressed emotion is associated with high levels of psychosocial stress and relapse.

Family therapy: An intervention where the family group is the focus. The therapy is concentrated on the interpersonal processes rather than on individual problems within the family.

Fantasy: An imagined sequence of events or mental images (e.g. daydreams) that serves to express unconscious conflicts, to gratify unconscious wishes, or to prepare for anticipated future events.

First-rank symptoms: Schneider classified the most characteristic symptoms of schizophrenia as first-rank features of schizophrenia. These included third-person auditory hallucinations, thought echo, thought interference (insertion, withdrawal and broadcasting), delusional perception and passivity. Such approaches to diagnosis have been heavily criticised by commentators favouring continua frameworks.

Flashback: A recurrence of a memory, feeling or perceptual experience from the past.

Flat affect: An affect type that indicates the absence of signs of affective expression.

Flourishing: A state of high psychological wellbeing.

Gay man: A man who is sexually and/or romantically attracted to other men.

Grandiose delusion: A delusion of inflated worth, power, knowledge, identity, or special relationship to a deity or famous person.

Grandiosity: An inflated appraisal of one's worth, power, knowledge, importance or identity. When extreme, grandiosity may be of delusional proportions.

Green space: A space situated within an urban area that is predominantly made up of grass, vegetation and trees, and is considered to have both aesthetic and recreational value.

Gustatory hallucination: A hallucination involving the perception of taste (usually unpleasant).

Hallucination: A sensory perception that has the compelling sense of reality of a true perception but that occurs without external stimulation of the relevant sensory organ. Hallucinations should be distinguished from illusions, in which an actual external stimulus is misperceived or misinterpreted. The person may or may not have insight into the fact that he or she is having a hallucination. One person with auditory hallucinations may recognise that he or she is having a false sensory experience, whereas another may be convinced that the source of the sensory experience has an independent physical reality. The term hallucination is not ordinarily applied to the false perceptions that occur during dreaming, while falling asleep (hypnagogic) or when awakening (hypnopompic). Transient hallucinatory experiences may occur in people without a mental disorder.

Harm minimisation: Policies, programmes or interventions that aim to reduce the health-related harms of a behaviour.

Hedonism: Pleasure-seeking behaviour; may be contrasted with anhedonia.

Hypomania: An affective disorder characterised by elation, over-activity and insomnia.

Ideas of reference: Incorrect interpretations of casual incidents and external events as having direct reference to oneself. May reach sufficient intensity to constitute delusions.

Illness, disease, disorder, syndrome: In general use, these words all mean the same and refer to particular conditions. However, some philosophers and psychiatrists, such as Boorse, use 'illness' to pick out the subjective aspect of feeling unwell, and 'disease' to refer to the underlying cause.

Independent Mental Health Advocate (IMHA): A mental health advocate granted specific roles and responsibilities under the Mental Health Act (2007, England & Wales). They support qualifying service users to understand what they are entitled to in terms of rights and safeguards. They help people exercise their rights by actively involving them in decision-making processes.

Inequality: Typically measured in terms of the difference between the 20% richest and the 20% poorest in a country.

Insight: In psychotic mental disorders and organic brain syndromes, a patient's insight into whether or not they are ill and therefore requiring treatment may be affected. In depression, a person may lack insight into their best qualities and in mania a person may overestimate their wealth and abilities. The notion of insight is often challenged as meaning little more than the extent to which a person agrees with a psychiatric frame; similarly linked to compliance with treatment.

Interprofessional collaboration: A type of interprofessional work which involves different health and social care professions who regularly come together to solve problems or provide services.

Interprofessional coordination: A type of work, similar to interprofessional collaboration (see above), as it involves different health and social care professions. It differs as it is a 'looser' form of working arrangement, whereby interprofessional communication and discussion may be less frequent in nature.

Interprofessional education: This occurs when members (or students) of two or more health and/or social care professions engage in learning with, from and about each other to improve collaboration and the delivery of care.

Interprofessional teamwork: A type of work which involves different health and/or social care professions who share a team identity and work closely together in an integrated and interdependent manner to solve problems and deliver services.

Intersexed person: An intersexed person (previously used term = hermaphrodite) is someone who has physical characteristics that differ from the typical male or female arrangements. Most likely to be intermediate between the sexes, having some male and some female characteristics, or to have underdeveloped sex characteristics. Around 1 in 2000 people are identified as intersexed at birth. May have chromosomal or hormonal differences – if an intersexed person is identified at birth, doctors usually test chromosomes and hormones to help them advise parents which gender to bring their baby up as. The notion of intersex complicates the legal insistence on a two-option (male/female) model. The system does not allow for sex or gender expressions other than male or female, although, for many people, their sex is not so clear-cut.

Labile affect: An affect type that indicates abnormal sudden rapid shifts in affect.

Languishing: A state of low psychological wellbeing.

Lesbian: A woman who is sexually and/or romantically attracted to other women.

Locus of control: The extent to which individuals feel in control of their lives and outcomes, where an external locus of control refers to the belief that control is coming from an external force.

Long-term memory: The final phase of memory in which information storage may last from hours to a lifetime.

Lunacy: The term *'lunatic'* derives from the Latin word *lunaticus*, which originally referred mainly to epilepsy and madness, as diseases thought to be caused by the moon. This language used to be enshrined in mental health legislation.

Maastricht Approach: Also known as the *hearing voices approach*, it was first developed in Maastricht, in the Netherlands, by psychiatrist Marius Romme and researcher and science journalist Sandra Escher. It is based on three central tenets, that the phenomena of hearing voices is: (1) more prevalent in the general population than is generally understood by the mental health community; (2) a personal reaction to life stresses, whose meaning or purpose can be deciphered; and (3) best considered a dissociative experience and not a psychotic symptom.

Mad Pride: A social movement committed to celebrating madness and challenging stigma, borrowing tactics from the Queer movement. Mad Pride activists resist negative dispositions to diverse experiences and subjective states; this also involves resistance to psychiatric interference in people's lives.

Mad Studies: A new discipline and movement that emerged out of Canadian activism and scholarship with the breakout text, *Mad Matters: A Critical Reader in Canadian Mad Studies* (LeFrançois et al., 2013).

Magical thinking: The erroneous belief that one's thoughts, words or actions will cause or prevent a specific outcome in some way that defies commonly understood laws of cause and effect. Magical thinking may be a part of normal child development.

Medical treatment: Any reference in the Mental Health Act to medical treatment in relation to mental disorder refers to medical treatment which has the purpose of alleviating, or preventing a worsening of, the disorder or one or more of its symptoms or manifestations. It includes nursing, psychological intervention and specialist mental health habilitation (learning skills), rehabilitation (relearning skills) and care.

Mental disorder: 'Any disorder or disability of mind', as defined in section 1 of the Mental Health Act (1983/2007 England & Wales) as mental illness, arrested or incomplete development of mind, psychopathic disorder or any other disorder or disability of mind. This wide definition includes all forms of mental illness, learning disability, brain injury and personality disorder.

Mental Health Act Commission: A special health authority in England and Wales authorised to keep under review all aspects of the care of formal patients; now subsumed under the Care Quality Commission. It can investigate complaints, appoint panels to give a second opinion on consent to treatment (including treatment given to community patients under supervised community treatment (SCT) and certain informal child patients), and draw up codes of practice for mental health workers. The Commission produces informative annual reports.

Mental health case management: Essentially a process which allows a mental health specialist (usually a nurse but not exclusively) to oversee pathways of care with a view to ensuring prompt and appropriate access to and discharge from services, and an optimum length of stay within those services.

Mental health law: In the UK, the devolved nations, Scotland and Northern Ireland have separate legislation from England and Wales. The latter nations rely on the Mental Health Act (MHA) 1983 – an Act of Parliament covering the care and treatment of people with mental health problems, amended in 2007. Scotland has the Mental Health Care & Treatment Act 2003; and Northern Ireland the Mental Health Order 1986.

Mood: A pervasive and sustained emotion that colours the perception of the world. Common examples of mood include depression, elation, anger and anxiety. In contrast to affect, which refers to more fluctuating changes in emotional 'weather', mood refers to a more pervasive and sustained emotional 'climate'. Types of mood include dysphoric, elevated, euthymic, expansive and irritable.

Multi-disciplinary team: A group of health care workers who are members of different disciplines (professions, e.g. psychiatrists, social workers), each providing specific services to the patient.

Narrative approach: A respectful, non-blaming approach, which centres on people as the experts in their own lives. It views problems as separate from people and assumes people have many skills, competencies, beliefs, values, commitments and abilities that will assist them to change their relationship with the problems in their lives.

Needs assessment: A systematic process for determining and addressing gaps between a current situation and a desired situation.

Negative symptoms: Most commonly refers to a group of symptoms characteristic of schizophrenia diagnosis that include loss of fluency and spontaneity of verbal expression, impaired ability to focus or sustain attention on a particular task, difficulty in initiating or following through on tasks, impaired ability to experience pleasure, to form emotional attachment to others, and blunted affect.

Neo-liberalism: The dominant global political and economic system. Typified by unbridled faith in free markets, concentration of wealth with a minority, and privatisation of public services.

Non-binary: A person who identifies outside the gender binary, i.e. a person who identifies as neither a man nor a woman. Genderqueer, androgyne and gender fluid are non-binary gender identity terms you might hear used.

Obsession: An unpleasant or nonsensical thought which intrudes into a person's mind, despite a degree of resistance by the person who recognises the thought as pointless or senseless, but nevertheless a product of their own mind. Obsessions may be accompanied by compulsive behaviours which serve to reduce the associated anxiety.

Olfactory hallucination: A hallucination involving the perception of odour, such as of burning rubber or decaying fish.

Open Dialogue: An intervention approach developed in Finland characterised by democratic meetings involving the service user, carers and the extended social network.

Orientation: Awareness of one's self in relation to time, place and person.

Palliative care: An approach that improves the quality of life of patients and their families facing problems associated with life-threatening illness, through the prevention and relief of suffering by means of early identification and impeccable assessment and treatment of pain and other problems, physical, psychosocial and spiritual.

Panic attack: A discrete period of sudden onset of intense apprehension, fearfulness or terror, often associated with feelings of impending doom. During these attacks, there are symptoms such as shortness of breath or smothering sensations; palpitations, pounding heart or accelerated heart rate; chest pain or discomfort; choking; and fear of going crazy or losing control. Panic attacks may be unexpected (uncued), in which the onset of the attack is not associated with a situational trigger and instead occurs 'out of the blue'; situationally bound, in which the panic attack almost invariably occurs immediately on exposure to, or in anticipation of, a situational trigger ('cue'); or situationally predisposed, in which the panic attack is more likely to occur on exposure to a situational trigger but is not invariably associated with it.

Pansexual: A person who has the capability of attraction to others, regardless of their gender identity or biological sex. A pansexual could be sexually and/or romantically attracted to someone who is male, female, transgender, intersex or genderqueer.

Paranoid ideation: Ideation of less than delusional proportions, involving suspiciousness or the belief that one is being harassed, persecuted or unfairly treated.

Peer support: Offering and receiving help, based on shared understanding, respect and mutual empowerment between people in similar situations (ImROC, 2013). In mental health services, peer support is often formalised into paid or volunteer roles. In these contexts, the peer support worker is somebody who has relevant lived experience and is explicit in the use of this to support other people in their recovery.

Persecutory delusion: A delusion in which the central theme is that one (or someone to whom one is close) is being attacked, harassed, cheated, persecuted or conspired against.

Personality: Enduring patterns of perceiving, relating to and thinking about the environment and oneself. Personality traits are prominent aspects of personality that are exhibited in a wide range of important social and personal contexts. Only when personality traits are inflexible and maladaptive and cause either significant functional impairment or subjective distress are they deemed to constitute a personality disorder.

Phobia: A persistent, irrational fear of a specific object, activity or situation (the phobic stimulus) that results in a compelling desire to avoid it. This often leads either to avoidance of the phobic stimulus or to enduring it with dread.

Place of safety: A locally agreed place to where the police may remove someone, usually a police station or a hospital.

Primary mental health: The World Health Organization describes primary mental health services as providing first contact, accessible, continued, comprehensive and coordinated care (WHO, 2016).

Profession: An occupational group which in general provides services to others, such as nurses or social workers. It can be used as a term of self-ascription to avoid the need to apply regulatory criteria which differ between groups.

Psychosis: The word psychosis is used to describe a range of experiences that can include unusual or distressing perceptions, e.g. hallucinations and delusions, which may be accompanied by a reduced ability to cope with usual day-to-day activities and routine. There is ongoing controversy whether so-called psychotic symptoms exist on a continuum with normal experiences rather than indicate distinct mental disorders.

Psychotropic medication: Medication that affects thought processes or feeling states.

Race: A group of people united, classified together or identified as distinct from other groups owing to supposed physical and/or genetic traits or on the basis of common history, nationality or geographic distribution. Most biologists agree that there is no genetic basis for distinguishing between races.

Rating scale: Focuses the service user/client on relevant areas and assigns a value to each area/symptom.

Recovery: In mental health care, this does not mean simply getting better or returning to a prior state of health. Rather, it means being able to live a flourishing life expressive of one's own values, whether or not symptoms of illness persist. Recovery is a deeply personal, unique process of changing one's attitudes, values, feelings, goals, skills and roles. It is a way of living a satisfying, hopeful and contributing life, even with the limitations caused by illness. Recovery involves the development of new meaning and purpose in one's life as one grows beyond the catastrophic effects of mental illness (Anthony, 1993).

Recovery college: An educational paradigm to deliver comprehensive, peer-led education and training programmes. The identity shift from service user to student is seen to be an empowering means of supporting recovery and organisational change.

Reflective practice: Paying critical attention to the theory, values, emotions and beliefs which inform your actions so as to engage in a process of continuous learning.

Refusers: Individuals who could use mental health services but refuse to do so unless coerced.

Relative poverty: Takes into account societal context and recognises the strong relationship between low income and social exclusion. Relative poverty is calculated using household income adjusted for family size. Household income is then compared to the country's median and those with an income at 60% or more below the mean are judged to be in relative poverty.

Restrictive practices: Deliberate acts on the part of other person(s) that restrict an individual's movement, liberty and/or freedom to act independently.

Safeguarding: Protecting people's health, wellbeing and human rights, and enabling them to live free from harm, abuse and neglect.

Schizophrenia: A psychotic illness, not a 'split personality', as some would believe.

Secure hospital: Provides accommodation, treatment and support for people with severe mental health problems who pose a risk to the public. Secure services work predominantly with people who have been imprisoned or admitted directly to hospital following a criminal offence.

Selective serotonin reuptake inhibitor (SSRI): A group of antidepressant drugs used to treat depression. They are also used to treat other conditions such as bulimia, panic disorder and obsessive-compulsive disorder.

Self-harm: Any act of self-poisoning or self-injury carried out by an individual, irrespective of motivation.

Service user: A person receiving the services of a health authority or voluntary or independent organisation. In this book, the term usually refers to someone who is using mental health services. Some people prefer the terms 'client', 'patient' or 'consumer'. The terminology has been taken up within various participation and involvement practices, hence the term *service user involvement.*

Sick role: An identity adopted by an individual as a 'patient' that specifies a set of expected behaviours, usually dependent.

Social capital: Social networks and norms that benefit individual members of groups. Progressive models of social capital are concerned with processes that facilitate social cohesion, trust and cooperation for the common good.

Social determinants: The conditions in which people are born, grow, live, work and age. These circumstances are shaped by the distribution of money, power and resources at global, national and local levels.

Social movement: An organised grouping of people who seek social change. So-called new social movements, these include service user and survivor movements who campaign for the transformation of or even abolition of psychiatric services.

Spectrum disorder: Here, symptoms and characteristics can present themselves in a wide variety of combinations, from mild to severe.

Stigma: An attribute or characteristic that marks a person out as different from others, and that extensively discredits their identity. Anti-stigma campaigns have made some progress in challenging negative attitudes. Critics have in turn challenged the typical anti-stigma claim that 'mental illness is an illness like any other' as equally stigmatising.

Supported self-harm practice: This can include advising people on how to self-harm safely, how to clean their wounds, and supplying them with safer means to self-harm, such as clean blades.

Survivor: Radical patients and service users (including service refusers) reject labels that link them to service use and prefer to refer to themselves as survivors of mental health systems, which they often see as detrimental.

Symptom assessment: A valid and reliable tool that assesses common symptoms that are associated with a given diagnosis, or provides a more in-depth understanding of a particular symptom.

Tardive dyskinesia: A serious potential side-effect of antipsychotic medication which includes involuntary movements of the face, mouth, tongue, upper or lower limbs. Can occur on withdrawal from antipsychotic drugs and may be irreversible.

Theory of mind: The ability to infer another individual's emotional and mental state.

Therapeutic relationship: The relationship between a mental health professional and a service user. It is the means by which the professional hopes to engage with, and effect change in, a service user. (Also called the helping alliance, the therapeutic alliance and the working alliance.)

Thorn programme: A UK training programme aimed at developing community psychiatric nurses' skills in psychosocial interventions for people with severe mental health problems and their carers. It has evolved into various incarnations, such as COPE (Collaboration for Psychosocial Education).

Thought blocking: The unpleasant experience of having one's train of thought curtailed absolutely, often more a sign than a symptom.

Thought broadcasting: The experience that one's thoughts are being transmitted from one's mind and broadcast to everyone.

Thought disorder: A disorder of the form of thought, where associations between ideas are lost or loosened; often only recognised because of unintelligible speech.

Trade-off: Evolutionary theorists argue that an increase in any trait will inevitably come at an evolutionary cost.

Trans: A trans person is someone who does not identify with the gender that they were assigned at birth. Trans (sometimes written trans) is an umbrella term to describe a wide range of identities. Some trans people suffer from gender dysphoria, a sense of intense discomfort caused by the mismatch between their physical sex and their gender identity. This may cause them to seek out medical interventions such as hormone therapy or surgery.

Transgender: Usually, this refers to a trans person who socially and/or medically transitions from one binary gender to another. You may also hear the term transsexual used, which implies a greater focus on medical transition which some consider to be pathologising.

Transitioning: The process of changing the way one's gender is lived publicly. Transitioning may involve changes in clothing and grooming, a name change, change of gender on identity documents, hormonal treatment and surgery.

Triggers: External events or circumstances likely to set off a chain reaction of behaviours, thoughts or feelings. These are unique to each individual and might include: significant dates or anniversaries, feeling rejected, loss, a change of environment or the prospect of change.

Unrecovery: A wry contribution from critically minded service users who object to the co-option and over-valorisation of the language of recovery within services and the proliferation of assessments such as Recovery Star. Unrecovery denotes a political standpoint that highlights the challenges of recovery under a neo-liberal economic system. See *The Unrecovery Star* by Recovery in the Bin (2015).

Urban penalty effect: A robust set of epidemiological statistics that demonstrate poorer health in urban areas.

Urbanicity effect: The increased risk of mental health difficulties in urban areas.

Value: Having a dimension of goodness or badness. Characterising something in value-laden terms expresses a positive or negative attitude to it, whether or not it also describes it in a further descriptive way. Thus, saying that an act is 'good' tells us that the speaker approves of it but very little else about the nature of the act. For example, calling something 'theft' implies some sort of taking and also a negative attitude to it (contrast: 'liberate'). Ethical values are a subset of values.

Values-based practice: An important counterpart to evidence-based practice. It is based on the argument that clinical and ethical dilemmas arise because of the conflicting values of the people involved. Values-based practice suggests that, traditionally, the values of the person using services is often not considered or is ignored, and that by exploring it, mental health practice will become more patient-centred.

Wellness plan: A framework whereby an individual documents their patterns of wellbeing with the aim of using this to regulate and reflect on them. This is commonly written using an established format, but may take other creative forms.

REFERENCES

American Psychiatric Association (APA) (2013) *Diagnostic and statistical manual of mental disorders (DSM–V)*, 5th edition. Arlington, VA: APA.

Anthony, W.A. (1993) Recovery from mental illness: the guiding vision of the mental health service system in the 1990s. *Psychosocial Rehabilitation Journal, 12*, 55–81.

ImROC (2013) www.imroc.org.

Leadership Alliance for the Care of Dying People (LACDP) (2014) *Priorities of care for the dying person.* London: NHS.

LeFrançois, B., Menzies, R. & Reaume, G. (eds) (2013) *Mad matters: A critical reader in Canadian mad studies.* Toronto: Canadian Scholars Press

Recovery in the Bin (2015) *The unrecovery star.* Available at: https://recoveryinthebin.org/unrecovery-star-2 (accessed 17.08.17).

Repper, J., Aldridge, B., Gilfoyle, S., et al. (2013) *Peer support workers: Theory and practice.* Londo: IMROC.

Russell, G. F. M. (1979) Bulimia nervosa: an ominous variant of anorexia nervosa. *Psychological Medicine*, 9, 429–448.

World Health Organization (1992) *International classification of disease (ICD)*, 10th edition. Geneva: WHO.

World Health Organization (2016) Main terminology. Available at: www.euro.who.int/en/health-topics/Health-systems/primary-health-care/main-terminology (accessed 13.07.16).

INDEX